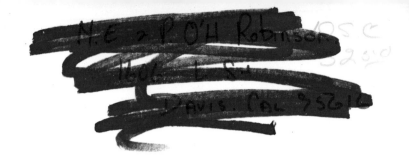

D1558428

STEPHEN J. ETTINGER, D.V.M.

STAFF CARDIOLOGIST; ASSISTANT HEAD OF MEDICINE;
THE ANIMAL MEDICAL CENTER, NEW YORK, N. Y.

PETER F. SUTER, Dr. med. vet., Privatdozent

ASSOCIATE PROFESSOR, UNIVERSITY OF CALIFORNIA, DAVIS,
SCHOOL OF VETERINARY MEDICINE; FORMERLY, STAFF
RADIOLOGIST, THE ANIMAL MEDICAL CENTER, NEW YORK, N. Y.

CANINE
CARDIOLOGY

W. B. SAUNDERS COMPANY - PHILADELPHIA - LONDON - TORONTO
1970

W. B. Saunders Company: West Washington Square
                          Philadelphia, Pa.   19105

                          12 Dyott Street
                          London, WC1A 1DB

                          1835 Yonge Street
                          Toronto 7, Ontario

Canine Cardiology   SBN 0-7216-3437-0

Print No.:   9   8   7   6   5   4   3   2   1

TO OUR WIVES
SANDRA and EVELYN

PREFACE

In presenting courses and seminars at The Animal Medical Center and elsewhere, it became apparent to us that a convenient source and reference book was needed in canine cardiology. Although a great deal of basic scientific and clinical information relating to canine cardiology has been accumulated in the veterinary and human medical literature, there is no veterinary textbook which fully meets the needs of modern veterinary cardiology.

The aims of this textbook are to meet the needs of practicing veterinarians and students and to stimulate their interest in cardiology. Therefore, the emphasis throughout has been placed on practical methods of diagnosis and treatment of heart disease. Information relating to etiology and physiologic and detailed pathologic findings for specific conditions is provided where it seems necessary to enhance the understanding of a disease, the rationale for therapy, or the prognosis. Sophisticated diagnostic techniques such as vectorcardiography, cardiac catheterization, and angiocardiography are included so that the potentials of such methods can be appreciated.

The design of the book is based on the assumption that an understanding of the basic concepts applied in making a cardiovascular diagnosis (Chapters 1 through 6) and a thorough clinical knowledge of cardiovascular therapeutic agents (Chapters 7 through 10) are essential to the diagnosis and treatment of cardiac disease (Chapters 11 through 19). Throughout the text, except as otherwise stated, electrocardiograms were recorded at a paper speed of 50 mm. per sec. and standard amplitude of 10 mm. = 1 mv. Similarly, phonocardiograms and cardiac catheterization tracings were recorded at a paper speed of 100 mm. per sec. and an interval between time lines of 0.1 sec. Vectorcardiograms were consistently recorded with the teardrops equal to 0.002 sec., their direction being from the broad to the narrow end.

It is our hope that we have succeeded in presenting the complex field of cardiology in a comprehensive and clinically relevant manner for students and practitioners alike. In presenting data in this book it was impossible to provide an exhaustive presentation of every disease relating to cardiology. We trust that the specialist will excuse us for resorting to oversimplification, especially in the discussions of complex arrhythmias and in the diagnosis of both acquired and congenital heart diseases.

This book makes pretention neither to originality nor to completeness. Notice of omissions or errors will be greatly appreciated. The findings of many who have accumulated data over the years have been referred to frequently. To this data we have added the results of our own investigations and experience. We are sincerely indebted to the pioneers in the field of veterinary cardiology. We would particularly like to acknowledge the work of Drs. James Buchanan, David Detweiler, Robert Hamlin, Nils Lannek, Donald Patterson, Robert Pensinger, C. Roger Smith, Robert Tashjian, Charles Wallace, and the late Erwin Gratzl. As is readily apparent in the reference lists, we have frequently referred to the work of many other investigators, to whom we are also appreciative. In addition, we have cited and excerpted generously from human cardiology texts and journals, especially when descriptions of experimental canine studies have proved directly applicable.

We express our gratitude to Drs. Edward Baker, Gerard Rubin, and Joe Morgan for reviewing the manuscript and for criticism and advice. We must also express our sincere appreciation to Drs. Philip Ettinger and Lawrence Gould, physicians who have given freely of their time in helping to review the manuscript.

The authors wish to acknowledge the assistance of Dr. Robert J. Tashjian, Director of The Animal Medical Center. Dr. Tashjian has also been Project Director of Program-Project Grant HE-06936-05 from which the start, facilities, and programs in comparative cardiovascular disease were initiated at The Animal Medical Center. The Animal Medical Center later established the Heartworm 75 Project Grant which further supplemented these studies. These funds thus established the cardiopulmonary laboratories and the basis of much of the data that was made available for this textbook. We wish to express our gratitude to these sources from which pioneering studies in canine angiocardiography and this textbook have been made possible. Dr. Ettinger's postdoctoral training fellowship (1-F2-31, 587-01 to -02) from the National Institutes of Health is similarly acknowledged. We have frequently called upon our colleagues at The Animal Medical Center for their critical comments while writing this book. To these doctors, past and present, we offer our grateful appreciation.

The preparation of the manuscript has been a difficult and at times a tedious job. Specific recognition is due our willing editorial secretary, Mrs. Mary B. Brown, for the frequent suggestions and many hours spent in preparing the manuscript. Also, we wish to thank Mrs. Nancy Böhning for her secretarial assistance and Mrs. Virginia Lundeen for providing many of the drawings in the text. We acknowledge, too, the genuinely fine work of the W. B. Saunders Company, especially Mr. John Dyson, Veterinary Editor, and Mr. George Laurie, Production Manager.

STEPHEN J. ETTINGER, D.V.M.
PETER F. SUTER, DR. MED. VET.

CONTENTS

SECTION I   RECOGNITION OF CARDIAC DISEASE

Chapter 1
CLINICAL EXAMINATION 3

Chapter 2
HEART SOUNDS AND PHONOCARDIOGRAPHY 12

Chapter 3
RADIOGRAPHIC EXAMINATION.. 40

Chapter 4
ELECTROCARDIOGRAPHY.. 102

Chapter 5
CARDIAC CATHETERIZATION AND ANGIOCARDIOGRAPHY 170

Chapter 6
THE RECOGNITION OF CARDIAC DISEASE AND CONGESTIVE
HEART FAILURE.. 214

**SECTION II   PHARMACOLOGIC AND OTHER THERAPY IN
CARDIAC DISEASE**

Chapter 7
DIGITALIS AND THE CARDIAC GLYCOSIDES... 225

Chapter 8
ANTIARRHYTHMIC THERAPY... 239

Chapter 9
DIURETICS 249

Chapter 10
LOW SODIUM DIETS AND OTHER DRUGS AND METHODS INDICATED IN
CARDIAC THERAPY 257

SECTION III ARRHYTHMIAS: DISTURBANCES OF THE CARDIAC RATE AND RHYTHM

Chapter 11
ARRHYTHMIAS: DISTURBANCES OF THE CARDIAC RATE AND RHYTHM 271

SECTION IV ACQUIRED AND CONGENITAL HEART DISEASE

Chapter 12
THE INCIDENCE OF HEART DISEASE IN DOGS 313

Chapter 13
ACQUIRED VALVULAR AND ENDOCARDIAL HEART DISEASE 321

Chapter 14
ACQUIRED DISEASES OF THE MYOCARDIUM 383

Chapter 15
DISEASES OF THE PERICARDIUM 403

Chapter 16
COR PULMONALE 421

Chapter 17
MISCELLANEOUS CONDITIONS AFFECTING THE CARDIOVASCULAR
SYSTEM 456

Chapter 18
CONGENITAL HEART DISEASES 477

Chapter 19
SURGICAL CORRECTION OF PATENT DUCTUS ARTERIOSUS AND
VASCULAR RING ANOMALIES (By Dr. W. D. DeHoff) 579

INDEX 603

SECTION I

RECOGNITION OF CARDIAC DISEASE

CHAPTER 1   CLINICAL EXAMINATION

CHAPTER 2   HEART SOUNDS AND PHONOCARDIOGRAPHY

CHAPTER 3   RADIOGRAPHIC EXAMINATION

CHAPTER 4   ELECTROCARDIOGRAPHY

CHAPTER 5   CARDIAC CATHETERIZATION AND
            ANGIOCARDIOGRAPHY

CHAPTER 6   THE RECOGNITION OF CARDIAC DISEASE
            AND CONGESTIVE HEART FAILURE

CHAPTER

1

CLINICAL EXAMINATION

A review of the history and an examination of the patient constitute the basis of a complete medical examination. Emphasis in this chapter is focused on the cardiac symptomatology recognized during an examination.

EXAMINATION RECORDS

A thorough written record of the cardiac examination is essential for following patient progress. Since recording the results of an examination is time consuming, we have developed forms that may be filled out quickly and clearly (Figs. 1-1 and 1-2). These forms require simple symbols or check marks, rather than a detailed written description. Comprehensive records of the physical and special cardiac examinations (e.g., electrocardiogram and radiographs) are thus made easier to review.

ANAMNESIS

After the owner has described the condition for which his pet is being presented, the veterinarian should begin a thorough search of the medical history for information related to the pet's present illness. Brief inquiry about disease or causes of death in related animals might yield pertinent information.

Develop the chronologic history of the present illness after the past medical history, including medical and surgical procedures and vaccination history, has been obtained. All previous diagnoses, as well as the specific drug therapy (i.e.,

THE ANIMAL MEDICAL CENTER
CARDIOVASCULAR CLINIC EXAMINATION REPORT

CASE NO. ______ DATE ______

Owner______ Ward______

Breed______ Age______ Sex M M_C F F_S Weight______ Name______

History

1. Out of State/Country 2. Last Immunization - Dist.______ Rabies______
3. Related Diseases in Family or Pets______
4. Previous Surgery______
5. Previous Illness______ X Ray Taken ☐ Yes ☐ No
6. Present History (signs, tests, and medications)______ Blood Taken ☐ Yes ☐ No
7. Suspected Diagnosis______
8. Doctor Requesting Examination______

DO NOT WRITE BELOW THIS LINE

CARDIAC EXAMINATION

Physical Examination:

1. General Attitude........ ☐ Alert ☐ Depressed ☐ Lethargic ☐ Prostrate
2. General Condition........ ☐ Normal ☐ Thin ☐ Emaciated ☐ Obese
3. Hydration........ ☐ Normal ☐ Mod. Dehydrated ☐ Very Dehydrated
4. Mucous Membranes........ ☐ Normal ☐ Pale ☐ Injected ☐ Jaundiced
5. Head and Neck........ ☐ Normal ☐ Abnormal______
6. Uro-genital system........ ☐ Normal ☐ Abnormal______
7. Gastro-intestinal........ ☐ Normal ☐ Abnormal______
8. CNS........ ☐ Normal ☐ Abnormal______
9. Musculo-Skeletal........ ☐ Normal ☐ Abnormal______
10. Respiratory System........ ☐ Normal ☐ Abnormal______

Palpation:

Cardiac Region:

☐ Normal ☐ Abnormal Chest

Maximum Impulse - Location and force

Other

Abdomen:

Abnormalities______

Pulse:

Venous. ☐ Jugular pulse ☐ Venous engorgement ☐ Other______

Arterial. ☐ Rapid ☐ Slow; ☐ Strong ☐ Weak ☐ Thready; ☐ Early ☐ Late;
☐ Sinus arrhythmia ☐ Arrhythmia; ☐ Other______

left

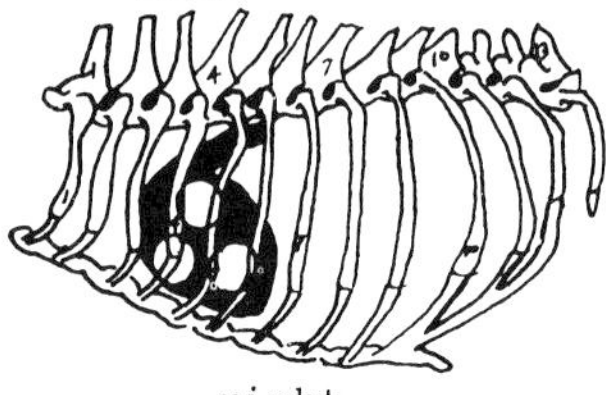

DESCRIBE

Hi. Freq. I I I I

Low Freq. ∿∿

Mixed Freq. XXX

Intensity 6 4 2

S1 S2 S1

Description Other Heart Sounds

Description of Lung Sounds

right

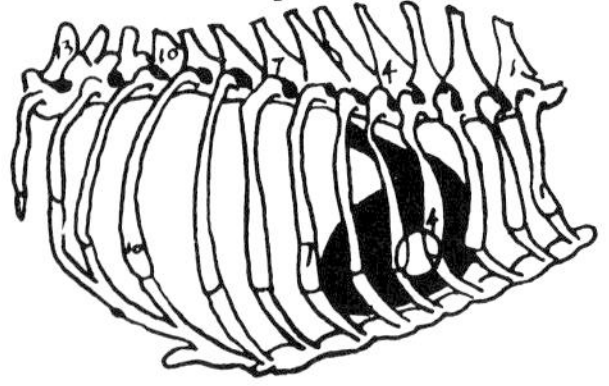

Examining Doctor's Signature______

CV COPY

FIGURE 1-1 Cardiovascular examination sheet. The results of the history and physical examination may be permanently recorded with a minimum number of words, as well as with check marks and lines. Changes in the patient's condition over a period of time are noted easily and concisely.

CARDIOVASCULAR EXAMINATION SHEET

CASE NO.   DATE

NAME_____

ELECTROCARDIOGRAM:

    Heart Rate_____Rhythm_____
    P_____; P-R_____; QRS_____; Q-T_____; ST-T_____
    Axis_____
    Other

VECTORCARDIOGRAM:

    Frontal Projection

    Horizontal (transverse) Projection

    Sagittal Projection

ELECTROCARDIOGRAPHIC DIAGNOSIS: N. Y. Heart Code

                                                 _____

                                                   _____

PHONOCARDIOGRAM: Description (sounds, murmurs, area, etc.)

ROENTGENOGRAPHY:

                                              N. Y. Heart Code

                                                 _____

OTHER EXAM SYNOPSIS:

DIAGNOSIS (Complete only applicable categories):   N. Y. Heart Code
    1. No Heart Disease; unexplained manifestation.
    2. Etiologic Cardiac Diagnosis   _____

    3. Anatomic Cardiac Diagnosis (congenital or acquired)   _____

    4. Physiological Cardiac Diagnosis

RECOMMENDATIONS:

ICDA Code:_____

                          Examining Doctor's Signature _____
C V CLINIC

FIGURE 1-2   The results of specialized cardiovascular examinations are indicated on a second record form.

noticeable increase in the angulation of the rib cage and must work hard to force air in and out of the lungs (Jackson, 1969).

Other conditions that may be observed prior to the physical examination include peripheral or jugular venous engorgement, abdominal distention, peripheral edema, and discoloration of the tongue or mucous membranes.

Color of mucous membranes. Cyanosis, or insufficient oxygenation of the blood, results in a bluish tinge of the mucous membranes and tongue. Cyanosis is rarely present in cardiac conditions except in certain heart diseases when unoxygenated blood is shunted from the right to left side of the heart (congenital conditions); when pulmonary edema or other advanced lung pathology interferes with the normal aeration of blood passing through the lungs; or when advanced heart disease results in a diminished cardiac output, thereby causing peripheral pooling of blood with stasis and peripheral cyanosis. The appearance of the mucous membranes in advanced atrioventricular valvular insufficiency is usually muddy or dirty reddish. In polycythemia, whether spontaneous or secondary to dehydration (hemoconcentration), the tongue and mucous membranes have a dark-blackish color. Jaundice is an unusual finding in heart disease, although it may occur if chronic passive congestion of the liver is prolonged and severe. Anemia from any cause, producing pallor of the mucous membranes, does not aggravate cardiac disease unless it is chronic. If severe, it may be accompanied by cardiac signs such as a systolic murmur, thready pulse, and tachycardia.

Jugular pulse. A jugular pulse due to retrograde transmission of pressure from the heart, as well as generalized engorgement of the peripheral veins, is caused by elevated venous pressure and suggests right heart failure. Pericardial effusion, cardiac tamponade, and obstruction of the venae cavae may produce similar findings. A jugular pulse should be differentiated from pounding of the carotid artery in nervous animals. Intermittent, bounding jugular venous pulsations (cannon 'a' waves) occur when disturbances of the cardiac rhythm cause the right atrium to contract on a closed atrioventricular valve, thus forcing the blood to move retrograde into the jugular veins.

Edema. Subcutaneous peripheral edema in the dog rarely occurs without ascites unless it is of local origin. Cool tissue may suggest a local noninfectious disturbance. When the edema is bilateral there may be a central circulatory disturbance, whereas unilateral edema usually results from a regional or peripheral lesion.

PHYSICAL EXAMINATION

The rectal temperature should always be taken, regardless of the apparent urgency of the condition. Temperatures below 99° F., except when associated with whelping, reflect shock or a moribund condition. The temperature may be moderately elevated in the nervous dog, but this may also suggest an infectious process. Temperature elevations greater than 105° F. in a dog presented with tachypnea and tachycardia of sudden onset may indicate heat prostration. Marked fluctuations in environmental heat and humidity may adversely affect chronic heart disease due to impairment of the normal heat-dissipating mechanisms (Pittman and Cohen, 1964).

Although the heart rate may be a diagnostic indicator, one study (Hamlin et al., 1967) has shown that all dogs had heart rates within limits established for normal dogs except those that were agitated, in pain, or in atrial fibrillation. During spontaneous sleep the mean heart rate in healthy, untrained dogs was 62 beats/min. (minimum, 38/min.; maximum, 90/min.). On the examination table the mean rate was 130 beats/min. (minimum, 86/min.; maximum, 185/min.). The heart rate of dogs with heart disease other than congestive heart failure and atrial fibrillation was within one standard deviation (± 25) of the mean for normal dogs. Dogs with painful conditions such as pancreatitis, fractures, or anal sac infections had heart rates greater than one standard deviation from the mean.

The head and neck should be examined for abnormalities of anatomic structures and for pallor, injection, or icterus of the mucous membranes. Dental abscess and decay, enlargement of lymph nodes, and the ease with which tracheal palpation elicits a cough are observed.

Palpation of the thorax and abdomen is best accomplished from the rear of the relaxed, standing dog by gently palpating caudally from the thorax. The thorax is examined first for evidence of trauma, deformities, and healed fractures. The point of maximal intensity (P.M.I.) is normally palpated near the cardiac apex at the left sternal border from the fourth to sixth intercostal spaces. Displacement of the cardiac apex suggests a thoracic or abdominal mass or cardiac enlargement. Extensive movement of the left thoracic wall, referred to as a left ventricular heave, also suggests cardiac enlargement. Palpable vibrations (thrills) synchronous with the heart beat may be present over the precordium if a loud heart murmur is present. In younger dogs, the presence of a thrill over a portion of the thorax suggests a congenital defect. Moving caudally, the abdomen is examined for ascites, splenic and hepatic enlargement, pulsations, and abnormal masses.

In the normal dog, the liver borders are palpated within the costochondral arch near the sternal borders. The liver should not extend significantly beyond the rib cage and is usually not palpable in the obese dog. The spleen is usually palpable only in very relaxed dogs. Enlargement of the liver or spleen may be detected by gentle palpation of the region caudal to the ventral costochondral arch. Splenic enlargement is often less diffuse than hepatic enlargement and is recognized by digital ballottement. In association with chronic passive congestion of the abdominal organs, the borders of the liver and spleen may be palpably rounded rather than sharp as they are in the normal patient. The liver may infrequently pulsate in coordination with the heart beat, reflecting right atrial pressure being transmitted retrograde by the posterior vena cava. Enlargement of other abdominal organs independent of hepatic and splenic engorgement is not likely to be related to cardiac diseases.

Ascites or abdominal fluid collection is recognized by a pendulous abdomen. Palpation of the abdominal organs may not be possible, although ballottement of a mass may be accomplished. Paracentesis of a small amount of fluid for chemical, microscopic, and cytologic analysis should be performed. Ascitic fluid is usually straw-colored (or blood-tinged) and has a specific gravity under 1.018 (Gillmore, 1962), although it may be greater than 1.018 in the presence of an infection or large quantities of blood cells. Microscopic examination usually demonstrates some neutrophils and mononuclear cells. In contrast to the ascites of congestive heart failure, fluids grossly appearing red with a specific gravity greater than 1.030 indicate that hemorrhage into the abdominal cavity has occurred. Microscopic examination of this fluid would demonstrate erythrocytes and white cell elements in about the same ratio as found on a peripheral blood smear. Abdominal tumors often are responsible for fluid collection. Analysis of fluid may differ according to the origin of the tumor. However, the specific gravity of the fluid usually exceeds 1.018 and cellular elements are abundantly present when examined microscopically. To categorize the etiology of the malignant growth, cytology is especially useful. Abdominal infections (bacterial, nonbacterial, or mycotic) are characteristically exudates, the specific gravity usually being greater than 1.020 (Gillmore, 1962). Red and white cells are abundantly present in the fluid. When stained and examined microscopically, bacteria or fungal organisms are recognized and culture may further define their identity.

Palpation of the femoral arteries for rate, rhythm, and fullness of pulse is an important diagnostic procedure. The normal pulse is rhythmic, and the artery is felt to distend rapidly and then relax slowly with each cardiac contraction. The character of the pulse is at times directly related to specific cardiac defects. When shock or cardiovascular collapse develops, on palpation the pulse is weak and small. A jerky pulse, also referred to as a "B-B shot" or "waterhammer" pulse, describes the typical pulse palpated in association with a patent ductus arteriosus. This pulse has a rapid upstroke and downstroke as compared to the normal pulse. A similar but less accentuated pulse is palpated in most advanced cases of mitral insufficiency, aortic insufficiency (Gould, Ettinger, and Lyon, 1968), and ventricular septal defects. The pulse of congenital aortic stenosis is small and late-rising in comparison with the normal pulse. In addition to the pulse variations described, irregularities of the pulse suggest the presence of congestive heart failure (pulsus alternans) or cardiac arrhythmias. Proceeding distally, the limbs are examined for subcutaneous edema, noting the character and extent of the edematous area as well as the degree of involvement (limited, unilateral, or general).

The rate and rhythm of the heart should be correlated with that of the femoral pulse. A sign of serious heart disease is a pulse deficit. When the cardiac contraction occurs so close to the preceding beat that ventricular diastolic filling is impaired, the resultant contraction is ineffectual and not felt in the peripheral arteries. Thus when the heart is auscultated simultaneously with palpation of the pulse, it is recognized that the number of cardiac contractions auscultated is greater than the number of arterial pulses palpated. A pulse deficit is most often associated with atrial fibrillation and premature cardiac contractions. Tachycardia (heart rate greater than 160 to 180) or bradycardia (heart rate less than 70) may also be confirmed.

When percussion of the thorax reveals excessive dullness or variations from the normal sounds, cardiomegaly, pericardial effusion, or thoracic fluid or masses should be suspected. A more tympanic sound would likewise suggest pneumothorax or emphysema. The value of percussion in examination of the thorax has not been recognized by the authors, although it is used successfully by some.

Auscultation of the heart sounds is the most important part of the cardiovascular examination. Irregularity of the heart sounds necessitates a more intensive study (see Chapter 2). Muffled, soft, or tinny sounds suggest obesity, pericardial or pleural effusion, or diaphragmatic herniation. Loud sounds are associated with chronic mitral valvular fibrosis, tachycardia, anemia, fever, or excitement and are often heard in thin-chested, young dogs. A diagnosis of the severity of heart disease based on the intensity of the heart sounds or murmur alone is often unreliable. Instead, all portions of the cardiac examination must be considered and weighed before making such a conclusion.

Auscultation of the normal thorax reveals soft inspiratory and expiratory sighing sounds. The presence of coarse, crackling bronchial tones with inspiratory or expiratory wheezing, an inspiratory effort, or expiratory grunting suggests pulmonary disease. The presence of moist râles or fluid sounds within the pulmonary tree occurs in association with congestive cardiac disease as well as pulmonary diseases such as pneumonia. Pulmonary abnormalities may be primary, but they frequently accompany cardiac disease. The absence of respiratory sounds suggests the abnormal presence of fluid or masses in the thorax obstructing the normal transmission of lung sounds.

Ophthalmologic examination, often a successful method of visualizing vascular abnormalities in man, has been generally unrewarding in helping to confirm a diagnosis of cardiac disease in the dog (Vainisi and Ettinger, 1968). Systemic venous distention is observed in the eye grounds only in dogs with advanced, clearly recognizable congestive heart failure.

Clinical pathology cannot be covered in detail in this chapter. Individual changes will be discussed with each specific disease. It is essential, however, that the thorough cardiac examination include a hematocrit and urinalysis. In endemic areas a microfilarial count is also a necessity. It would in no way be excessive for the routine examination to include at least a complete blood count (CBC), blood urea nitrogen (BUN), blood glucose, serum glutamic pyruvic transaminase (SGPT), and serum sodium and serum potassium levels.

References

Ettinger, S.: Isoproterenol Treatment of Atrioventricular Block in the Dog. J. A. V. M. A., 154 (1969):398.
Gillmore, C.: Characteristics of Abnormal Chest Fluids. Small Anim. Clin., 2 (1962):334.
Gould, L., Ettinger, S. J., and Lyon, A. F.: Intensity of the first heart sound and arterial pulse in mitral insufficiency. Dis. Chest, 53 (1968):545.
Hamlin, R. L., Olsen, I., Smith, C. R., and Boggs, S.: Clinical Relevancy of Heart Rate in the Dog. J. A. V. M. A., 151 (1967):60.
Jackson, W. F.: Physical Examination of the Heartworm Patient. J. A. V. M. A., 154 (1969): 377.
Otto, G. F.: Geographical Distribution, Vectors, and Life Cycle of *Dirofilaria immitis*. J. A. V. M. A., 154 (1969):370.
Pittman, J. G., and Cohen, P.: The Pathogenesis of Cardiac Cachexia. New England J. Med., 271 (1964):403 and 453.
Thrasher, J. R., and Clanton, J. R.: Epizootiologic Observations of Canine Filariasis in Georgia. J. A. V. M. A., 152 (1968):1517.
Vainisi, S., and Ettinger, S.: Unpublished observations. 1968.

CHAPTER

2

HEART SOUNDS AND PHONOCARDIOGRAPHY

AUSCULTATION OF THE HEART

The stethoscope is one of the most useful diagnostic aids in clinical medicine, and the importance of auscultation as part of the cardiac examination cannot be overemphasized.

Although stethoscopes vary in quality and sound transmission, no single product can be considered superior. The best stethoscope is the one which fits the ear canals comfortably. When used frequently, abnormal sounds are easily recognized and differentiated. A stethoscope recommended for daily use consists of both a bell and a diaphragm. When the bell is placed gently on the thorax, it transmits low-frequency sounds; when the diaphragm is placed firmly on the thorax, it transmits a wider band of frequencies including the higher frequencies. Diaphragms vary from pediatric to larger adult sizes. The large diaphragm transmits sounds from a wider area, so that extraneous noises may be present when hairy dogs are examined. The length of tubing should be as short as possible since the intensity of the transmitted sound is diminished with length. Imperfections in the tubing, valves, or chest piece, or wax lodged in the ear tips may interfere with normal sound conduction. The ear tips should be parallel with the external auditory canal of the listener's ear.

Figure 2-1 indicates the range of frequencies within which heart sounds and murmurs occur in contrast to normal human speech frequencies (Butterworth et al., 1960). Within the frequency range that heart sounds and murmurs are heard, there is a limit to the normal human threshold of audibility. Figure 2-1 demonstrates that a sound at 32 cycles per second (c.p.s.) requires 100 times the intensity to make it as audible as a sound being transmitted with a frequency of 256 c.p.s. Therefore, it should be recognized that the human ear does not hear all

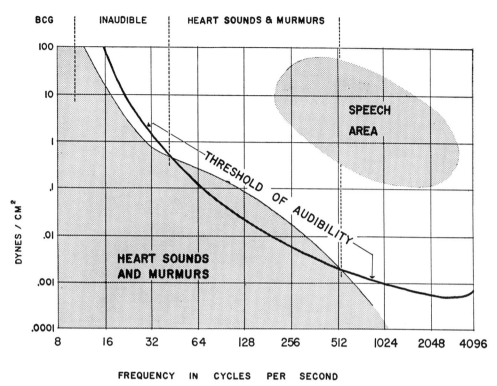

FIGURE 2-1 Common frequency ranges of heart sounds and murmurs. Because of the intrinsic limitations of the human ear, only a small segment of the total vibratory energy of murmurs is audible. (From Butterworth, J. S. et al.: Cardiac Auscultation, Grune & Stratton, 1960, p. 25. Used by permission.)

sounds of equal intensity with equal ease, and, in addition, the threshold of audibility may differ from person to person depending upon individual hearing ability.

A permanent written recording of the heart sounds is a phonocardiogram (PCG). The electrocardiogram (ECG) is usually recorded simultaneously with the heart sounds for timing. Arterial pressures, respiration, or both may also be concurrently recorded if instrumentation is available. Heart sound recordings serve several purposes. A sound or murmur recognized on auscultation is more clearly displayed on a photographic copy. This is helpful if various sounds cannot be differentiated with the stethoscope. Phonocardiograms are also excellent for teaching and have comparative value when recorded prior to and following treatment. Most phonocardiographic units can record a wide range of sounds (50 to 500 c.p.s.) as well as sounds within bands of the most important heart sound frequencies (low frequency, 50 to 100 c.p.s.; mid frequency, 100 to 200 c.p.s.; and high frequency, 200 to 500 c.p.s.). Logarithmic channels that record the audible components of heart sounds but place emphasis on the higher frequency components are especially useful if very high frequency sounds or murmurs need accentuation. In all phonocardiographic illustrations in the book the channels are marked low, medium, high, wide, or logarithmic and correspond to the frequencies just noted. Whenever possible, tracings were taken with the patient standing.

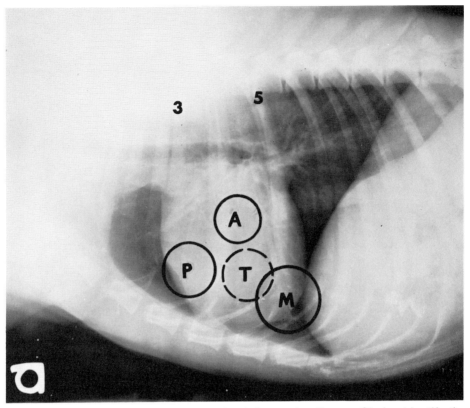

FIGURE 2-2 Left lateral radiograph of the canine thorax. Circles identify the valve areas. M = Mitral valve area; P = pulmonic valve area; A = aortic valve area; T = tricuspid valve area. Because the tricuspid valve area is located on the right side of the thorax, it is indicated by a broken circle.

Failure to use a systematic procedure for auscultation of the valve areas may prevent sounds that are more audible over one area than another from being heard. The sounds produced by the *mitral valve* are best heard at the mitral valve area, which is at the lower third of the thorax above the left sternal border from the fifth to sixth intercostal spaces. These sounds are the loudest heart sounds heard in most normal dogs, and the area of the mitral valve is usually identical with the palpable point of maximal intensity (PMI). By advancing the stethoscope cranially along the left sternal border to the third to fourth intercostal spaces, the region of the *pulmonic valve* is auscultated. The *aortic valve* region is dorsal and slightly caudal to the pulmonic valve area in the middle third of the left thorax in the fourth intercostal space. Sounds transmitted from the *tricuspid valve* are best heard from the third to fifth intercostal spaces at the junction of the lower and middle thirds of the right thorax (Fig. 2-2).

HEART SOUNDS

Some heart sounds are known to originate directly from valve movements, and others are due to vibrations in the adjacent blood column initiated by the

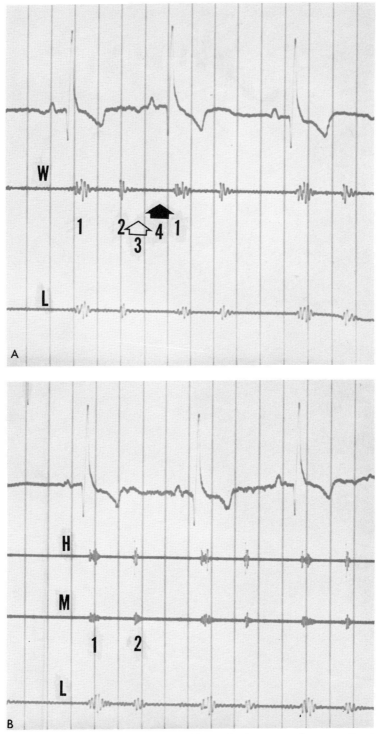

FIGURE 2-3 *A,* Simultaneous recording of electrocardiogram (lead II) and phonocardiogram of a normal dog. The first (1) and second (2) heart sounds are seen. The arrows indicate the timing of the third (3) and fourth (4) heart sounds; however, they were not detected in this recording. W = Wide-frequency band (50 to 500 c.p.s.); L = low-frequency band (50 to 100 c.p.s.).

B, Simultaneous recording of electrocardiogram (lead II) and phonocardiogram of a normal dog at high- (200 to 500 c.p.s.), middle- (100 to 200 c.p.s.), and low-frequency (50 to 100 c.p.s.) bands. Note the first (1) and second (2) heart sounds.

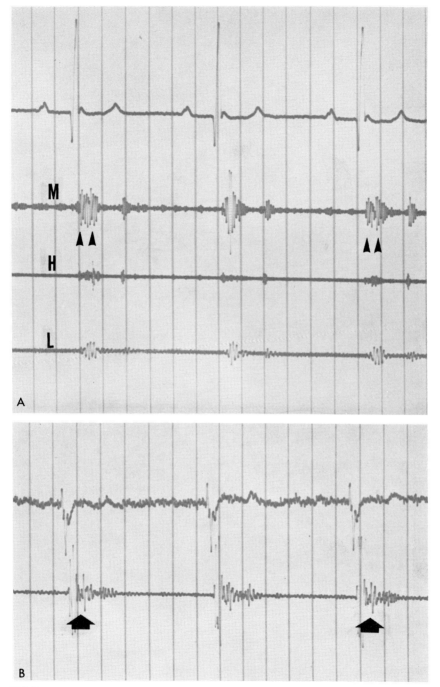

FIGURE 2-4 *A,* Splitting of the components of the first heart sound on the middle-frequency band phonocardiogram is shown by arrows. Respiratory variations cause splitting of the first heart sound in the first and third complexes, whereas summation of the components is seen in the second complex. Recording is from a normal 6-year-old Saluki.

B, Splitting (arrows) of the first heart sound due to asynchronous activation of the ventricles in a dog with right bundle branch block. Wide-band phonocardiogram from the pulmonic valve position was recorded simultaneously with the electrocardiogram (lead II).

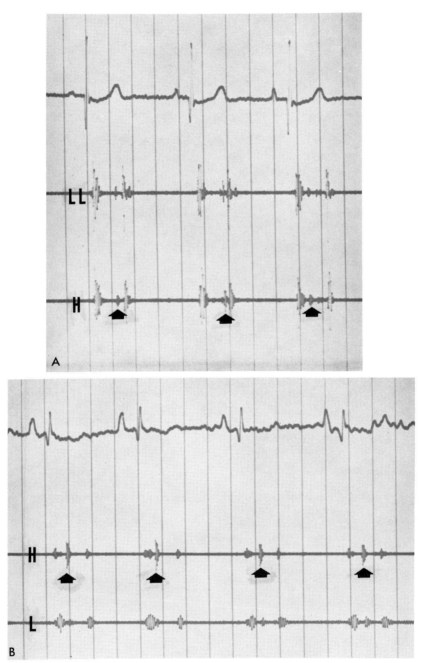

FIGURE 2-5 *A*, High-frequency systolic clicks (arrows) occurring at varying points during systole in an otherwise normal dog. High-frequency (H) and logarithmic (LL) phonocardiograms were recorded simultaneously with the lead II electrocardiogram.

B, High- (H) and low-frequency band (L) phonocardiograms demonstrate the presence of a mid-systolic click. Note the greater intensity of the sound when only the high-frequency vibrations were recorded. This dog had chronic lung disease, as demonstrated by P waves of abnormal amplitude.

sounds is not clear and in man is often attributed to extracardiac causes. The systolic clicks may be single or multiple (Fig. 2-5) and can be misinterpreted as a systolic murmur or split heart sound on auscultation. In the dog, this sound has often been related to early mitral valvular insufficiency, although it is also reported to be transient in normal dogs (Detweiler and Patterson, 1965).

THE SECOND HEART SOUND

The onset of the second heart sound (S_2) occurs near the end of the T wave on the electrocardiogram (Fig. 2-3). This sound, composed first of the aortic (A_2) and then of the pulmonic (P_2) components, is produced by closure of the aortic and pulmonic valves and by the subsequent vibrations produced in the blood columns (Butterworth et al., 1960). The second heart sound is a short (0.06 sec.) (Detweiler, 1961) and high-pitched sound usually best auscultated over the aortic and pulmonic valve regions. The aortic component is loud and sharp. Respiratory splitting of the second heart sound is normal in some dogs and is best recognized over the pulmonic valve. When it occurs, the pulmonic component occurs slightly later in the cardiac cycle and is further from the aortic component during inspiration. During expiration the two components approximate each other, and there is no splitting. Inspiration increases the negative intrathoracic pressures, drawing an increased amount of blood into the right ventricle; this requires a longer period for right ventricular ejection, which momentarily delays closure of the pulmonic valve. Normal respiratory splitting of the second heart sound is recognized less frequently in dogs than in man because of the shorter separation between A_2 and P_2 and because the increase in heart rate accompanying a normal sinus arrhythmia nullifies the diastolic filling that occurs during inspiration (Patterson and Detweiler, 1963). Pathologic splitting (doubling or reduplication) of the second heart sound occurs when a cardiac disease delays the pulmonic component of the second heart sound so that two audible components of S_2 are consistently heard (Fig. 2-6) (Patterson and Detweiler, 1963). This occurs in dogs with pulmonary hypertension (as in heartworm disease), and with congenital heart diseases such as atrial septal defects, anomalous pulmonary venous drainage, and pulmonic stenosis. It may also be associated with right bundle branch block (Fig. 2-6) and with ventricular ectopic beats (Detweiler and Patterson, 1967). The pulmonic component is accentuated and best heard when disease produces pulmonary hypertension.

Paradoxical splitting of the second heart sound. When closure of the aortic valve is delayed, as in left bundle branch block, aortic stenosis, and patent ductus arteriosus, the aortic component may follow the pulmonic component of the second heart sound. In one dog with congenital aortic stenosis, the pulmonic component was reported to occur 0.05 to 0.07 sec. before the aortic component (Carmichael et al., 1968). Whereas the pulmonic component normally diverges from the aortic component with inspiration, with paradoxical splitting the sounds approximate each other during inspiration because of increased filling and delayed right ventricular ejection (Detweiler and Patterson, 1967). In one case of left bundle branch block, paradoxical splitting of the second heart sound was recorded with the aortic component following the pulmonic component from 0.03 to 0.04 sec. (Patterson and Detweiler, 1963).

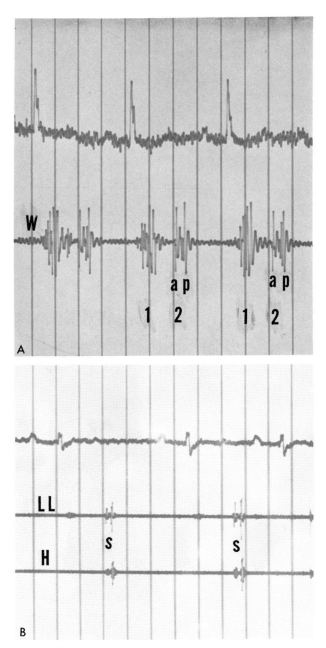

FIGURE 2-6 *A,* Splitting of the aortic (a) and pulmonic (p) components of the second heart sound (2) (0.05-sec. separation) in a dog with moderately advanced heartworm disease. The cause of this splitting was thought to be pulmonary hypertension.

B, Asynchronous activation of the ventricles resulted in splitting (S) of the second heart sound in a dog with right bundle branch block. Lead II electrocardiogram and logarithmic (LL) and high-frequency (H) phonocardiograms recorded simultaneously demonstrate that the split sound is clearest in the high-frequency band. The first sound is predominantly a low-frequency vibration and is therefore not well seen in this recording.

THE THIRD HEART SOUND

The third heart sound (S_3), a low frequency sound, is heard best with the bell of the strethoscope at the cardiac apex along the left sternal border. The sound may be verbally characterized as "lub-dub-thud." On the phonocardiogram it is a low-pitched sound seen 0.10 to 0.15 sec. after the second heart sound (Fig. 2-3). The distensibility of the ventricle when blood flows rapidly into it from the corresponding atrium determines the intensity of the third heart sound. Loud third heart sounds are considered pathologic in the dog (see Gallop Rhythms).

THE FOURTH HEART SOUND

The fourth heart sound (S_4) is produced by atrial systole. It is always inaudible in normal dogs but may occasionally be demonstrated on the normal phonocardiogram (Detweiler, 1961). Vibrations initiated by forceful ejection of the atrial blood column into an already distended ventricle produce this low-pitched, low-frequency heart sound (Fig. 2-3). Audible fourth heart sounds are pathologic in the dog (see Gallop Rhythms).

GALLOP RHYTHMS

A gallop is a sequence of three sounds consisting of the first and second heart sounds and an extra sound, which is an intensified third or fourth heart sound, or both. Gallop rhythms usually indicate advanced myocardial disease or heart failure (Detweiler and Patterson, 1965), and the prognosis is poor. The following types of gallop rhythms are heard in the dog.

PROTODIASTOLIC GALLOP.   This sound is present during the period of rapid ventricular filling and thus represents an accentuation of the third heart sound. This is the most common gallop rhythm in dogs. Pathologic third heart sounds are heard in association with diastolic overloading of the ventricle, as occurs in mitral and tricuspid insufficiency. In dogs with mitral insufficiency, an accentuated third heart sound may be mistaken for the second heart sound if a loud pansystolic murmur extends through the second heart sound (Fig. 2-7).

PRESYSTOLIC GALLOP.   This sound, heard just before the first heart sound, represents accentuation of the fourth heart sound (Fig. 2-8). In man, the fourth heart sound is present in cardiac conditions associated with left ventricular hypertrophy as long as sinus rhythm is preserved. It has also been recognized in acute mitral insufficiency associated with ruptured chordae tendineae (Getzen and Diamond, 1968). The fourth heart sound is not infrequently heard in the dog with mitral valvular insufficiency. It may indicate that the disease has progressed from the compensated stage to early congestive heart failure.

SUMMATION GALLOPS.   When the third and fourth heart sounds merge at rapid heart rates, the single accentuated gallop is called a summation gallop. The summation gallop is caused by the same conditions that produce individual protodiastolic or presystolic gallops (Fig. 2-9).

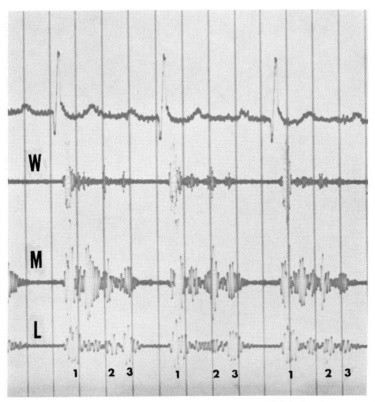

FIGURE 2-7 Accentuation of the third heart sound (3) is best seen on the low- (L) and mid-frequency (M) bands of the phonocardiogram. Accentuation of this heart sound produces a gallop rhythm and usually indicates heart failure. It is common in advanced mitral valvular disease. The systolic murmur of mitral insufficiency is also present in this recording.

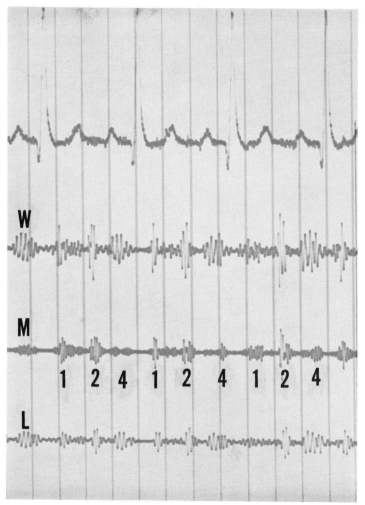

FIGURE 2-8 Accentuation of the fourth heart sound may occur when the left atrium enlarges. The increased intensity of the fourth heart sound (4) is evident in this dog which had advanced mitral valvular regurgitation. The fourth heart sound is identified as a series of low-frequency vibrations beginning after the onset of the P wave on the electrocardiogram and terminating before the onset of the QRS complex. Both left atrial dilatation and left ventricular hypertrophy are indicated on the electrocardiogram.

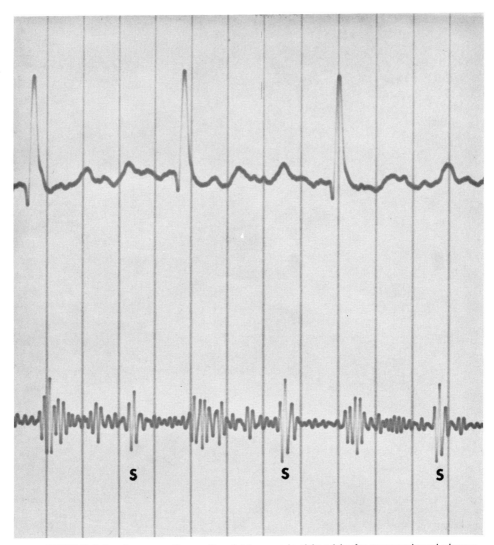

FIGURE 2-9 A summation gallop (s) is seen in this wide-frequency band phono-cardiogram. This abnormal sound signifying heart failure occurs when the abnormal third and fourth heart sounds are summated. It is most often present when the heart rate is rapid (180 beats/min. in this recording). It is not unusual for the gallop sound to be the loudest heart sound, as it is in this recording. Therefore, erroneous inter-pretations of the heart sounds may result if the gallop is not identified properly.

VARIATIONS IN INTENSITY AND RHYTHM
OF HEART SOUNDS

Heart sounds are loudest in young dogs, in dogs with thin thoracic walls, and in dogs with tachycardia, hyperthyroidism, anemia, or fever. The intensity of the heart sounds is diminished in obese dogs, in dogs with emphysema, pleural or pericardial effusions or thoracic masses, or diaphragmatic hernias, and in states when contractility of the heart is diminished and cardiac output is lowered. Diminished intensity of the first heart sound, associated with first degree heart block in man, has not been consistently observed in dogs with this condition.

The most common reason for variability in cardiac rate is related to respiratory sinus arrhythmia. This arrhythmia occurs normally in most dogs. During inspiration, vagal tone decreases (partially in response to the Bainbridge reflex) and the heart rate increases. Then the rate slows as vagal tone increases during expiration. This waxing and waning of the heart rate produces a rhythmic arrhythmia which diminishes during anesthesia.

Variations in the degree of ventricular filling in pathologic states in turn produce heart sounds of varying intensity as unequal quantities of blood are expelled with successive contractions. Such variations occur when cardiac arrhythmias such as atrial fibrillation, supraventricular and ventricular premature contractions, heart block, and ventricular tachycardia alter the normal rhythm and ventricular filling time of the heart.

Atrial fibrillation is characterized by a rapid, irregular heart rate. The intensity of the first heart sound varies continuously. The second heart sound may be absent if the contraction was of magnitude inadequate to open the semilunar valves. If a valvular murmur was present prior to the onset of atrial fibrillation, it may be of variable intensity, especially if the ventricular rate is rapid (Fig. 2-10).

When premature ectopic contractions interrupt the normal cardiac rhythm, the ectopic beat occurs early in the rhythm and is followed by a pause. Atrial, junctional, and ventricular premature beats are auscultated as early heart sounds of low intensity (Fig. 2-11). The pause following atrial and junctional ectopic beats is usually shorter than that following a ventricular premature contraction. Since differentiation of these premature beats requires considerable practice the presence of early beats suggests the need for an electrocardiographic tracing. In some ventricular ectopic beats, right ventricular activation may be delayed and splitting of the second heart sound produced. This split is accentuated by inspiration (Patterson and Detweiler, 1963).

Paroxysmal atrial or ventricular tachycardias are characterized by bursts of rapid, regular beats which usually cease abruptly. Any murmurs present are often inaudible during this paroxysmal tachycardia.

Heart block, usually confirmed electrocardiographically, is first recognized during auscultation at the cardiac apex. The first heart sound may be of diminished intensity with first degree heart block, because the prolonged P-R interval (prolonged atrioventricular conduction) permits the mitral and tricuspid valve leaflets to return passively to a coapted state before ventricular contraction begins. In second degree heart block atrioventricular conduction is periodically blocked, which is recognized by a pause in the slow ventricular rhythm. The fourth heart sound, a low-pitched atrial sound, may be auscultated during the pause. Variations in the intensity of the first heart sound occur when atrioventricular conduction is

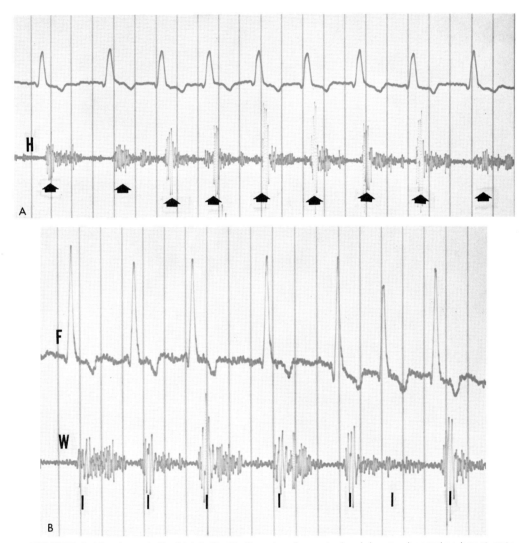

FIGURE 2-10 *A* and *B,* Atrial fibrillation is characterized by an irregular heart rate (variable R-R intervals), inconstant intensity of the first sound due to incomplete ventricular filling (arrow in *A*; [1] in *B*), and variation in the intensity of the murmur, all of which can be identified in these recordings.

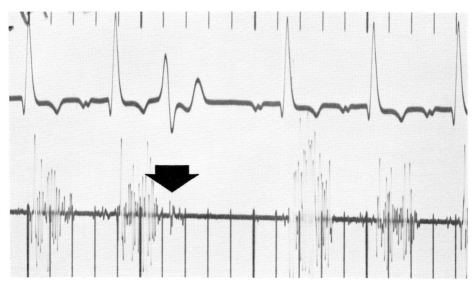

FIGURE 2-11   Premature contractions do not permit the ventricles to fill completely during diastole. The resultant contraction may then be ineffectual, and the intensities of both the first heart sound and the murmur are diminished (arrow). The second heart sound is often absent, since the ventricular contraction fails to generate enough pressure to open the valves initially. The negative P waves in the lead II electrocardiogram reflect an aberrant atrial rhythm produced by digitalis intoxication.

inconsistent. In complete heart block, two independent rhythms exist: the slow, but loud and forceful, first and second heart sounds produced by the ventricular contractions, and the more rapid, low-pitched atrial sounds (Ettinger, 1969) (Fig. 2-12).

CARDIAC MURMURS

Murmurs are sounds that occur when hemodynamic or physical changes within the cardiovascular system produce turbulence. Turbulence is created when the size of the vessel changes or when the velocity of the blood flow increases. Blood viscosity and blood density variations can also be responsible for turbulence within the cardiovascular system. When the Reynolds' number rises over a given level, streamline or laminar flow becomes turbulent and murmurs occur (Reynolds, 1970).

$$\text{Reynolds' number} = \frac{(\text{Radius}) (\text{Velocity}) (\text{Density})}{\text{Viscosity}}$$

Heart murmurs are classified as innocent, functional, or pathological. To describe a murmur or abnormal heart sound accurately, its timing, intensity, and pitch (frequency) over each of the four valve regions should be noted. *Timing* refers to the period of the cardiac cycle during which the murmur occurs. It may occur during early, mid, or late systole or diastole. When it lasts throughout

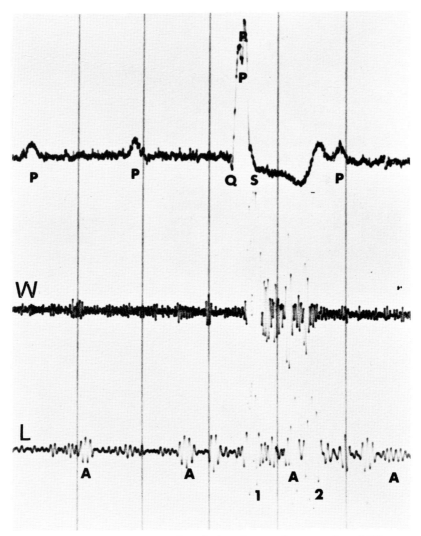

FIGURE 2-12 Low-frequency fourth heart sounds occurring 0.08 sec. after the onset of atrial depolarization (best seen on the low-frequency band). The first (1) and second (2) heart sounds are produced by ventricular depolarization and occur at a rate independent of the atrial sounds (A).

systole or diastole it is called a pansystolic or holosystolic murmur (or pandiastolic, holodiastolic). Murmurs are graded by intensity from I to V (Detweiler and Patterson, 1965), or from I to VI as follows:

I to V System (Detweiler and Patterson, 1965)
Grade I — ". . . softest audible murmur."
Grade II — ". . . faint murmur heard after a few sounds auscultation."
Grade III — ". . . heard immediately when auscultation begins and is audible over a fairly large area."
Grade IV — ". . . loudest murmur . . . audible when the chest piece is just removed from the thoracic wall."
Grade V — ". . . remain audible when the stethoscope chest piece is just removed from the thoracic wall."

I to VI System

Soft
- I/VI — a nearly imperceptible murmur.
- II/VI — a very soft murmur.

Medium
- III/VI — a murmur of low intensity.
- IV/VI — a murmur of moderate intensity which does not produce a precordial thrill.

Loud
- V/VI — a loud murmur heard with the stethoscope barely touching the thorax.
- VI/VI — the loudest murmur, heard when the stethoscope is held just away from the thorax.

A precordial thrill is always present with a grade V/VI or VI/VI murmur. The pitch indicates whether the sound is of low frequency, mixed frequency, or high frequency. The quality of the murmur may be further described as harsh or regurgitant and ejection or blowing. Whereas different grading systems exist, it should be noted that more important than the system chosen is the strict adherence to the same grading system from case to case.

Systolic murmurs begin with or after the first heart sound and end with or before the second heart sound, whereas diastolic murmurs begin with or after the first component of the second heart sound and end prior to the first heart sound.

MITRAL INSUFFICIENCY

The mixed frequency murmur of mitral insufficiency (MI) begins immediately after the first heart sound. It occurs initially early in systole, and as the valvular insufficiency increases it progresses to a harsh, holosystolic (pansystolic) murmur of constant intensity (Fig. 2-13). The murmur is best heard over the left caudal sternal border, but it radiates dorsally and to the right as it increases in intensity. The sound may be high-pitched or muscial (whooping) in quality at times, and its pitch often varies from examination to examination. The intensity of the murmur may range from grade I/VI to grade VI/VI, but when the intensity is above grade III/VI its severity need not indicate the severity of the valvular disease. In advanced mitral insufficiency (grade V/VI to VI/VI), a thrill palpable over the entire precordium is usually accentuated over the left caudal sternal border.

When mitral insufficiency is present the first heart sound is of increased intensity (Gould, Ettinger, and Lyon, 1968). When the murmur is loud and holosystolic, the second heart sound may not be clearly audible. The pulmonic component of the second heart sound can be accentuated due to pulmonary hypertension.

When valvular insufficiency produces heart failure, an excessive volume of blood remains in the left ventricle during diastole. The rapid flow of atrial blood into the incompletely emptied ventricle then produces an accentuated third heart sound and a protodiastolic gallop is heard. A gallop sound suggests cardiac failure (Detweiler and Patterson, 1967). When therapeutic measures improve the hemodynamic status of the ventricle, the intensity of the third heart sound diminishes (Fig. 2-14).

MITRAL STENOSIS

An early diastolic rumbling sound is associated with this extremely uncommon condition in the dog. Thus murmur was heard in a dog at the left fifth

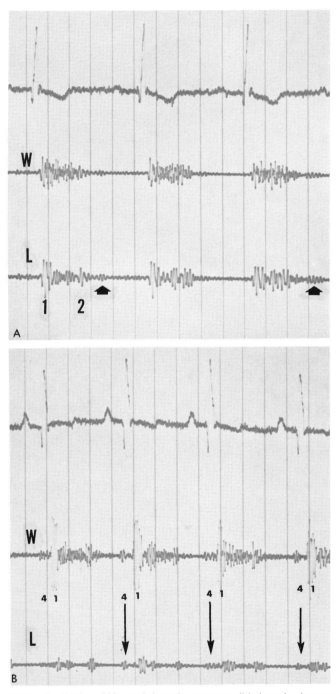

FIGURE 2-13 *A,* Wide- (W) and low-frequency (L) band phonocardiograms demonstrate the holosystolic murmur of equal intensity throughout that characteristically occurs with mitral and tricuspid valvular insufficiency. Notice that the second heart sound (2) is nearly obliterated by the murmur. The arrow indicates the low-frequency, low-amplitude third heart sound that could not be heard on auscultation.

B, The holosystolic murmur of mitral insufficiency is seen on the wide-frequency band phonocardiogram (W). The first heart sound (1) is characteristically loud in mitral insufficiency, and a fourth heart sound (4) of low intensity occurs prior to the onset of ventricular systole.

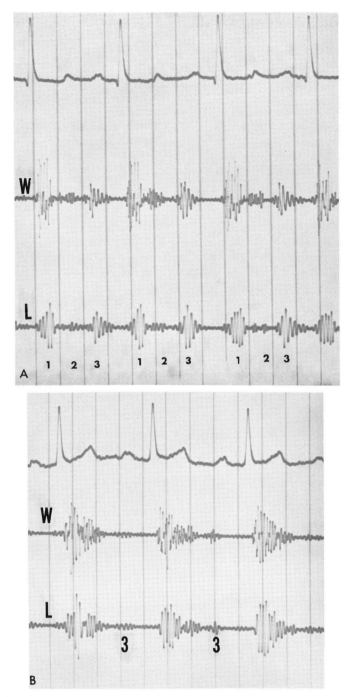

FIGURE 2-14 *A,* A diastolic gallop (3) and a holosystolic murmur associated with mitral valvular insufficiency were recorded prior to therapy in a dog in congestive heart failure. Part of the loud third heart sound may be summation with a fourth heart sound.

B, Following digitalization and cage rest, the heart failure was relieved, and the intensity of the gallop sound (3) was markedly diminished.

intercostal space at the costochrondral junction Tashjian and McCoy, 1960).
Patterson and Detweiler (1963) mention this unusual condition but give no
additional information, other than the absence of an opening snap during systole.

AORTIC INSUFFICIENCY AND PULMONIC INSUFFICIENCY

A retrograde flow of blood resulting from incompetency of the aortic or
pulmonary semilunar valves during early diastole results in a high-pitched, blowing, decrescendo murmur beginning immediately after the aortic or pulmonic
component of second heart sound. Aortic insufficiency (AI) (Fig. 2-15) is associated with bacterial endocarditis of the aortic valve leaflets or with congenital
aortic stenosis with some degree of aortic valve incompetence. If mitral insufficiency is also present, the systolic murmur is loud and extends through the
second heart sound, preventing the perception of the less intense murmur of
aortic insufficiency.

Isolated pulmonic insufficiency (PI) is occasionally described in association
with heartworm disease (Detweiler and Patterson, 1967).

AORTIC STENOSIS

Aortic stenosis (AS) is a congenital heart defect in the dog, characterized by
a loud, harsh, systolic murmur heard over the left dorsal cranial intercostal spaces
(Fig. 2-16). Because the dilated aortic arch courses craniad and rightward, there
can be transmission to the cranial right thorax (Detweiler and Patterson, 1965).
If the murmur is sufficiently intense, it is accompanied by a precordial thrill.
The murmur begins after the first heart sound and increases in intensity until mid
or late systole, when its intensity begins to decrease. Because of this crescendo-
decrescendo pattern the murmur is described as "diamond-shaped." The greater
the degree of stenosis, the later in systole is the peak intensity of the sound. An
aortic ejection sound was heard in one dog with subvalvular aortic stenosis and
may have been related to poststenotic aortic dilatation (Carmichael et al., 1968),
or opening of the aortic valve. The murmur is transmitted to the thoracic inlet
and/or the carotid arteries owing to arterial transmission of the sound. Aortic
stenosis is usually associated with some aortic insufficiency.

PULMONIC STENOSIS

A high frequency systolic ejection murmur is heard over the pulmonic valve
in this congenital heart disease (Fig. 2-17). The intensity of the murmur usually
varies with the degree of stenosis. A nearly imperceptible, high-pitched sound
may be heard, as may a crescendo-decrescendo (diamond-shaped) holosystolic
murmur with maximum intensity in mid systole in less advanced cases of pulmonic stenosis (PS). Loud murmurs are usually accompanied by palpable precordial thrills, often restricted to the cranial thoracic region on the left side. Over
the remainder of the thorax the murmur is less intense, and in some cases a
murmur is heard only over the pulmonic valve. As the pressure gradient between
the right ventricle and pulmonary artery widens, the murmur becomes louder and
peaks later in systole. Splitting of the second heart sound is noted on the phonocardiogram but is usually not heard because of the murmur produced (Patterson
and Detweiler, 1963).

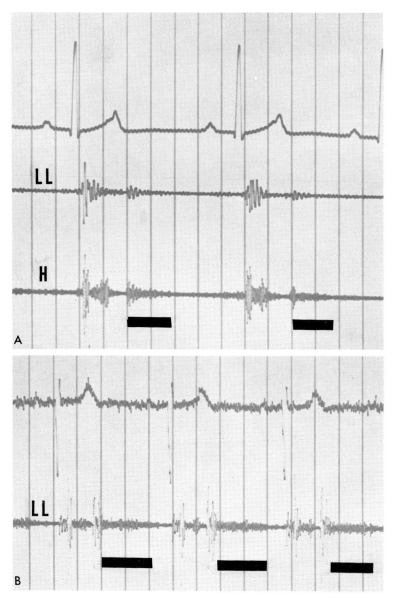

FIGURE 2-15 *A,* Decrescendo diastolic murmur beginning immediately after the second heart sound (black line). The murmur, due to aortic valvular insufficiency, occurred in a Great Dane after prolonged septicemia; a blood culture was positive for *beta* hemolytic *Streptococcus* sp. A systolic murmur was also present.

B, A high-frequency, blowing decrescendo diastolic murmur (black line) was observed over the pulmonic valve in a dog with congenital heart disease (notice negative amplitude in lead II electrocardiogram). No further studies were made on this dog, and the clinical diagnosis of pulmonic stenosis and pulmonic insufficiency could not be proved.

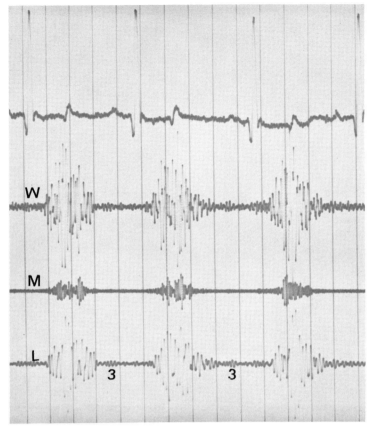

FIGURE 2-16 The diamond-shaped, mixed frequency murmur characteristic of aortic stenosis. This murmur was best auscultated on the cranioventral right thoracic wall. A low-frequency third heart sound is present (3). The high amplitude of the R wave in lead I of the electrocardiogram suggests a left axis deviation which may be associated with left ventricular hypertrophy.

PATENT DUCTUS ARTERIOSUS

A continuous systolic and diastolic "machinery-like" murmur best heard over the aortic-pulmonic valve region is characteristic of a patent ductus arteriosus (PDA). Occasionally it is best heard on the cranial portion of the thoracic wall at the manubrium sterni. Over the remainder of the thorax a systolic murmur similar to that of mitral insufficiency, or no murmur at all, is heard. The distinctive continuous murmur occurs as blood flows from the high-pressure aorta to the low-pressure pulmonary artery, producing turbulence. The murmur is heard in both systole and diastole with late systolic accentuation because of the distance of the ductus from the left ventricle (Fig. 2-18). If pulmonary hypertension is severe, left to right flow diminishes, and the diastolic component can be of decreased intensity or the murmur may disappear (Brody and Prier, 1962). The continuous murmur of a patent ductus arteriosus must be differentiated from other arterio-venous fistulas as well as from rupture of the sinus of Valsalva. In puppies with congenital heart disease and very rapid heart rates, it may be difficult to distinguish a continuous murmur from a loud systolic murmur.

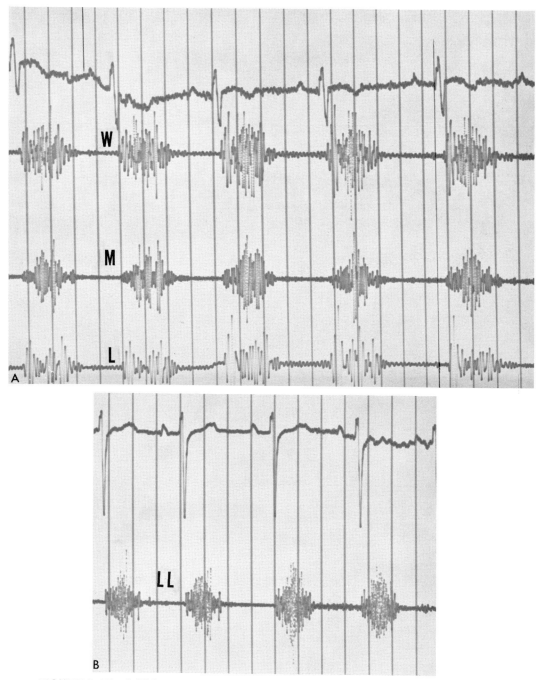

FIGURE 2-17   *A,* This tracing demonstrates the diamond-shaped systolic murmur characteristic of pulmonic stenosis. The negative amplitude of the lead II electrocardiogram occurs with right axis deviation.

B, Similar diamond-shaped murmur recorded at logarithmic frequency (LL) in a dog with pulmonic stenosis.

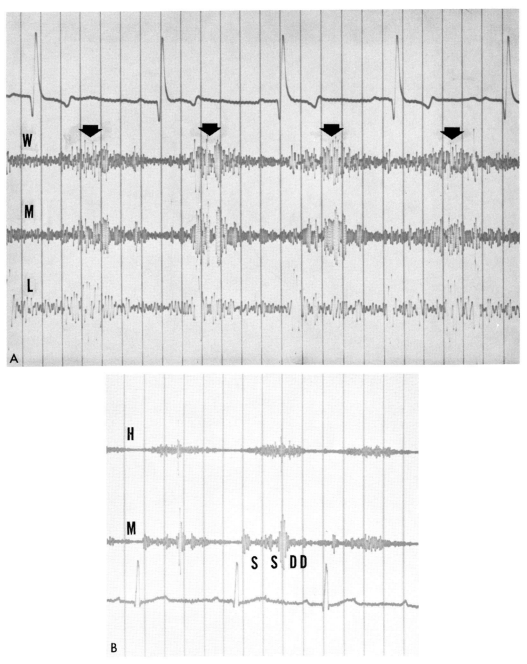

FIGURE 2-18 *A,* Typical continuous "machinery" murmur of patent ductus arteriosus. The late systolic accentuation of the murmur (arrow) gives the impression of a waxing and waning, continuous sound on auscultation. The amplitude of the lead II electrocardiogram recorded simultaneously is greater than 30 mm., a sign frequently observed with patent ductus arteriosus (pattern of left ventricular hypertrophy).

B, If diastole is prolonged, the murmur of patent ductus arteriosus may not be continuous. Notice the late systolic accentuation of the murmur and the obvious systolic (S) and diastolic (D) murmur in this dog whose patent ductus arteriosus was subsequently corrected.

VENTRICULAR SEPTAL DEFECT

A ventricular septal defect (VSD) is characterized by a loud, harsh, mid- to high-frequency holosystolic murmur loudest at the right midthoracic wall which is usually accompanied by a thrill at the point of maximum intensity (Fig. 2-19). A less intense holosystolic murmur similar to that of mitral insufficiency is heard at the area of the mitral valve. The duration and intensity of the murmur may vary considerably (Hamlin, Smetzer, and Smith, 1964). If pulmonary hypertension develops and right ventricular pressures increase significantly, there will be no flow from the left to the right ventricle and no murmur will be heard. Splitting of the second heart sound due to pulmonary hypertension and delayed right ventricular ejection can be associated with ventricular septal defects.

ATRIAL SEPTAL DEFECT AND ANOMALOUS PULMONARY VENOUS DRAINAGE

Auscultatory signs of an atrial septal defect (ASD) are a systolic ejection murmur maximal in the pulmonic area due to increased blood flow across the

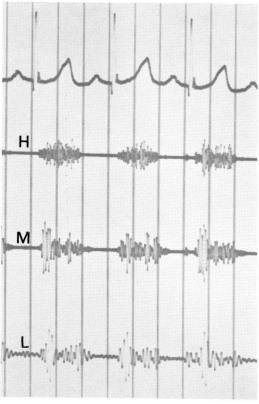

FIGURE 2-19 The holosystolic murmur of mixed frequency (H, M, and L) recorded simultaneously with a lead II electrocardiogram from a dog with a ventricular septal defect. Notice that the murmur begins with the first heart sound and ends abruptly at the second heart sound.

pulmonic valve and constant splitting of the second heart sound (Detweiler and Patterson, 1967) because the pulmonic component of the second heart sound is delayed. An early diastolic murmur may be seen on the phonocardiogram (Hamlin, Smith, and Smetzer, 1963). A high frequency systolic murmur may occur in both anomalous pulmonary venous drainage and atrial septal defects (Detweiler and Patterson, 1967).

ANEMIC MURMURS

Decreased viscosity and increased velocity of blood produce turbulence when the blood hemoglobin level falls below 6 mg. per 100 ml. Anemic murmurs heard on auscultation are usually of low intensity and high frequency and occur during early to mid systole. The murmur, which may be confused with that of mitral insufficiency, usually disappears when the anemia is relieved. Diastolic murmurs have also been reported in association with anemia. (Detweiler and Patterson, 1965). The systolic murmur of anemia is best recognized at the mitral valve area (Fig. 2-20), although one report suggests that the murmur is loudest at the pulmonic or aortic region (Detweiler and Patterson, 1965).

INNOCENT AND FUNCTIONAL MURMURS

Innocent and functional murmurs are produced by increased velocity of blood within the cardiovascular system and by extracardiac factors. Pleural or pericardial effusion, anemia, and fever may be factors in the production of functional murmurs. Pregnancy in humans is occasionally associated with innocent murmurs, but the authors have not observed this phenomenon in pregnant bitches. Truly innocent murmurs, especially in the young dog, may be due to increased velocity of blood flow. These murmurs usually disappear in adult life. If there is uncertainty regarding the origin of a murmur, or whether it is innocent, functional, or pathological, the client should be advised to return the

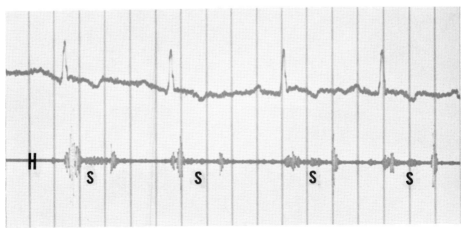

FIGURE 2-20 The anemic murmur is a high-frequency systolic murmur (S) heard on auscultation and observed on the phonocardiogram during early and mid-systole.

dog periodically for examination. The clinician should rule out the common non-cardiac conditions that can produce murmurs, such as anemia, fever, and hyper-thyroidism. It should be kept in mind that often it is impossible to differentiate an innocent from a functional murmur.

Panting will often produce sounds resembling cardiac murmurs. It is difficult to differentiate between a murmur and coarse breathing sounds, and therefore the examiner should attempt to auscultate the thorax with the dog's muzzle held closed. When this cannot be done, of if breathing sounds are still heard, cardiac sounds must be evaluated with caution.

References

Brody, R. S., and Prier, J. E.: Clinico-Pathologic Conference. J. A. V. M. A., 140 (1962): 379.

Butterworth, J. S., Chassin, M. R., McGrath, R., and Reppert, E. H.: Cardiac Ausculta-tion. Grune & Stratton, New York, 1960.

Carmichael, J. A., Liu, S. K., Tashjian, R. J., Radford, G., and Lord, P.: A Case of Canine Subaortic Stenosis and Aortic Valvular Insufficiency, with Particular Reference to Diagnostic Technique. J. Small Anim. Pract., 9 (1968):213.

Detweiler, D. K.: Cardiovascular Diseases in Animals. Encyclopedia of the Cardiovas-cular System (Luisada, Ed.). McGraw-Hill, New York, (1961):27-10.

Detweiler, D. K., and Patterson, D. F.: A Phonograph Record of Heart Sounds and Mur-murs of the Dog. Ann. New York Acad. Sci., 127 (1965):322.

Detweiler, D. K., and Patterson, D. F.: Abnormal Heart Sounds and Murmurs of the Dog. J. Small Anim. Pract., 8 (1967):193.

Ettinger, S. J.: Isoproterenol Treatment of Atrioventricular Block in the Dog. J. A. V. M. A., 154 (1969):398.

Friedberg, C. K.: Diseases of the Heart. 3rd ed. W. B. Saunders Co., Philadelphia, 1966.

Getzen, J. H., and Diamond, E. G.: Saga of the Fourth Heart Sound. Amer. J. Cardiol., 22 (1968):609.

Gould, L., Ettinger, S. J., and Lyon, A. F.: Intensity of the First Heart Sound and Arterial Pulse in Mitral Insufficiency. Dis. Chest, 53 (1968):545.

Hamlin, R. L., Smetzer, D. L., and Smith, C. R.: Interventricular Septal Defect (Roger's Disease) in the Dog. J. A. V. M. A., 145 (1964):331.

Hamlin, R. L., Smith, C. R., and Smetzer, D. L.: Ostium Secundum Type Interatrial Septal Defects in the Dog. J. A. V. M. A., 143 (1963):149.

Luisada, A. A.: From Auscultation to Phonocardiography. C. V. Mosby Co., St. Louis. 1965.

MacCanon, D. M., Bruce, D. W., Lynch, P. R., and Nickerson, J. L.: Mass Excursion Parameters of First Heart Sound Energy. J. App. Physiol., 27 (1969):649.

Patterson, D. F., and Detweiler, D. K.: The Diagnostic Significance of Splitting of the Second Heart Sound in the Dog. Zbt. Vet. Med., 10 (1963):121.

Reynolds, O.: In Cardiovascular Dynamics (Rushmer). 3rd ed. W. B. Saunders Co., Philadelphia, (1970):318.

Sakamoto, T., Kusukawa, R., MacCanon, D. M., and Luisada, A. A.: Hemodynamic Determinants of the Amplitude of the First Heart Sound. Circ. Res., 16 (1965):45.

Tashjian, R. J., and McCoy, J. R.: Acquired Mitral Stenosis Resulting in Left Atrial Dilata-tion with Thrombosis. Cornell Vet., 50 (1960):485.

Van Bogaert, A.: New Concept on the Mechanism of the First Heart Sound. Amer. J. Cardiol., 18 (1966):253.

CHAPTER

3

RADIOGRAPHIC EXAMINATION

TECHNIQUES OF RADIOGRAPHIC EXAMINATION

The radiographic examination is essential for a complete evaluation of the cardiovascular system. The radiographs provide immediate information about the size, shape, and position of the heart and its relation to adjacent structures and are therefore of paramount importance for an understanding of heart disease. The radiograph, as a legal record and objective document, can be stored, reevaluated at any future time, and compared with previous or subsequent radiographs. It therefore provides the opportunity to follow a case over a period of time and to obtain information concerning the development of the disease.

Conditions secondary to cardiac diseases which arise from the close functional and /or anatomical relation of the heart to the great vessels, lung, liver, mediastinum, pericardium, diaphragm, pleural space, or esophagus are often first diagnosed on radiographs. Coexisting diseases unrelated to the heart may also be diagnosed and must be considered as factors in a differential diagnosis concerning the origin of the symptoms. The radiographic findings also act as a guideline in determining the severity of the disease and the therapeutic approach, in evaluating the response to medication, and in predicting the outcome.

Since the information obtained from a radiograph depends on the quality of the picture—a radiograph of poor quality may even be misleading—the factors necessary in obtaining diagnostic radiographs are of primary importance.

To produce thoracic radiographs of good quality in dogs of all sizes, the x-ray machine should fulfill certain minimal requirements. It should be able to generate 100 kvp. at 100 ma. and should have an electric timer capable of at least 1/60 sec. exposure time (Carlson, 1967). However, satisfactory results can be

40

obtained with less powerful equipment provided it is utilized to its fullest capacity and its shortcomings under certain conditions are realized.

Compensating for the voluntary and involuntary movement of the animal is the foremost problem in veterinary radiology. The prevention of respiratory movements is troublesome, and the use of exposure times of 1/60 sec. or less is the usual method of avoiding the resulting blur. Small x-ray units are not capable of delivering enough radiation within short exposure times. The outlines on radiographs exposed for 0.1 sec. or longer are often blurred and of limited diagnostic value. However, in selected cases the animal may be anesthetized, intubated, and hyperventilated, and then the radiograph taken while the respiratory movements are suspended by compressing the rebreathing bag and keeping the lungs inflated.

In large dogs a grid or Potter-Bucky diaphragm should be used to reduce the fog on the radiograph and the resulting loss of contrast, which is caused by scattered radiation. By confining the primary beam to a size and shape that will cover the region to be examined, a further reduction in scattered radiation is achieved. Modern par-speed or high-speed intensifying screens, with the highest practicable definition, should be mounted into the cassettes to achieve short exposure times and good radiographic detail.

To obtain consistent quality and to enable comparison of radiographs which have been made at different stages of a disease, exposure techniques should be standardized. The same type of film, consistent darkroom technique, and identical positioning should be used at all times. The film-tube distance must be kept constant and is preferably at least 91 cm. (36 in.). A greater distance of 120 to 140 cm. (47 to 55 in.) is advantageous in order to minimize enlargement and distortion of the image. However, only large x-ray units are able to compensate for the greater exposure needed if the film-tube distance increases. To maintain uniform density in all radiographs, it is essential in each case to measure the diameter of the thorax with a caliper and to adapt the exposure to the size of the patient according to a technique chart. Allowance must be made for the exposure of obese dogs. The exposures should be made at the same phase of respiration. An exposure made during the expiratory pause offers the advantage of a relatively long period without movement (Wyburn and Lawson, 1967) and is therefore preferable when weak roentgen units are used. However, most of the vascular details are lost, and the lung field is more dense on radiographs made at the expiratory pause than at the end of inspiration. Therefore, we prefer exposures made near the end of inspiration whenever possible. Details on formulating radiographic technique and exposure charts for different types of x-ray machines and the rules for adapting the exposures to the diameter of the patient are available (Carlson, 1967; Douglas and Williamson, 1963; Eastman Kodak, 1968).

Radiographs for cardiac evaluation should include the entire thorax, from about 2 cm. cranial to the first rib to a point just caudal to the first lumbar vertebra. In patients in which a serious cough complicates the cardiac condition, the caudal portion of the cervical trachea should be included on the radiographs in order to evaluate the trachea for possible collapse. The portion of the abdomen included in the radiograph is important for examination of the diaphragm and liver. In the dorsoventral or ventrodorsal position the gas bubble marking the fundus of the stomach provides a sign for identifying the left side. This is helpful in those instances in which the radiograph is labeled incorrectly.

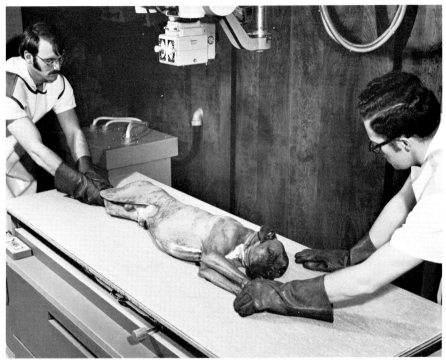

FIGURE 3-1 Positioning of the dog for a recumbent left lateral radiograph. The forelimbs are held parallel and are pulled forward to clear the area of the apical lobes. Care is taken not to rotate the animal. The midpoint of the x-ray beam is centered over the fourth to fifth intercostal space.

A complete and meaningful evaluation of the heart is possible only if the thorax is radiographed in two projections. Frequently, one projection reveals diagnostic information which is missing in the other. Hamlin (1959) considers the dorsoventral radiograph superior to the lateral for assessing enlargement of cardiac chambers.

The importance of consistent positioning in obtaining uniform radiographs has been stressed repeatedly since the original studies by Moritz (1904). For the lateral view the forelimbs must be pulled forward as far as possible to allow an unobstructed view of the cranial lung field and the mediastinum (Figs. 3-1 and 3-2). The dog may be positioned with either the right side or the left side down.

There are few differences between right and left lateral recumbent positions in most dogs. However, it is important to use the same position consistently. The beam should be centered over the fourth to fifth intercostal space, and care should be taken not to rotate the animal because a considerable distortion in the relative positions of the tracheal bifurcation, the great vessels, and the contour of the heart itself may result.

For the *dorsoventral view,* the dog is placed on its sternum (Figs. 3-2 and 3-3). The dorsoventral view is preferable to the ventrodorsal. In the ventrodorsal position the apex of the heart, which is not attached to the sternum, tends to

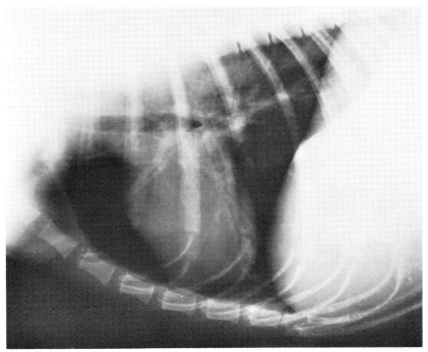

FIGURE 3-2 Left lateral radiograph, normal, 1½-year-old, male Boxer. The radiograph was exposed at full inspiration to obtain optimal contrast between the lung field and the heart and vascular structures. Deep inspiration was forced by holding the dog's nose closed for approximately 30 seconds. Notice the lung tissue separating the heart from the contour of the diaphragm. This dog is of a breed with an intermediate type of thoracic conformation (neither deep nor narrow; see text).

rotate and move according to the law of gravity, resulting in a change in the position and outline of the cardiac silhouette. The differences noticed in the two views can be considerable (see Figs. 3-27 and 3-28).

It is often difficult to obtain perfect dorsoventral radiographs, especially from a dog with a narrow, deep thorax. One should always try to get the cooperation of the patient, because a relaxed, comfortable dog is easier to position, and may even assume the correct position spontaneously. The thoracic vertebrae must be exactly superimposed on the sternebrae. The head should be placed between the forelimbs. The beam is preferably centered over the fifth or sixth intercostal space, which is located approximately at the posterior angle of the scapula. There is usually a tendency to center the beam too far caudally.

If satisfactory dorsoventral positioning cannot be obtained in an anxious or otherwise uncooperative dog, one should not hesitate to tranquilize the animal. If tranquilization is contraindicated, ventrodorsal positioning is sometimes easier to accomplish, and since the distortions created by an incorrect dorsoventral position are more disturbing than a shifting of the heart in the ventrodorsal view, it can be used instead. Subsequent radiographs must be made in the same position.

If the presence of pleural fluid has been suggested on previous radiographs, it might be necessary to radiograph the patient in the standing lateral (Fig. 3-5) or erect position.

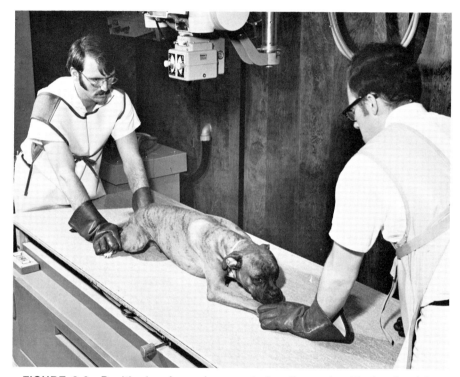

FIGURE 3-3 Positioning for a dorsoventral radiograph with the dog lying on its sternum. The forelimbs are pulled forward and rotated outward slightly so that the scapulae are shifted laterally out of the cranial lung field. This is best accomplished by holding the elbows in slight adduction. By letting the dog rest on its elbows in the front and on its crouching, flexed hindlimbs in the rear, the body is supported comfortably and is prevented from turning to either side. Most dogs tolerate this position better than if the hindlimbs are pulled backward. Great care must be taken to ensure that the sagittal plane of the thorax is exactly vertical and in line with the central x-ray beam. The head is placed between the forelimbs to prevent the caudal neck musculature from obscuring the apices of the lung. The dog should be as relaxed as possible, because tension causes distortion and bending of the spine to one side. Tranquilization is occasionally required. The midpoint of the x-ray beam is centered over the caudal half of the scapulae.

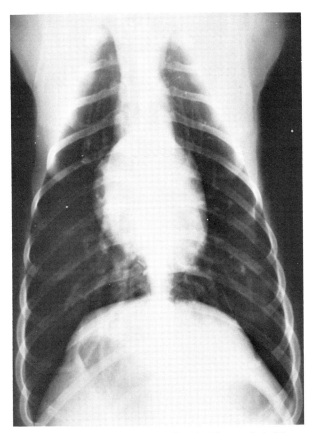

FIGURE 3-4 Dorsoventral radiograph, dog in Figure 3-1. The procedure is the same, and the radiographs are exposed at full inspiration. The lung field is symmetrical, and the sternebrae and spine are superimposed. The entire thorax is included, and the outlines of the diaphragm, the heart, and the aorta are well defined.

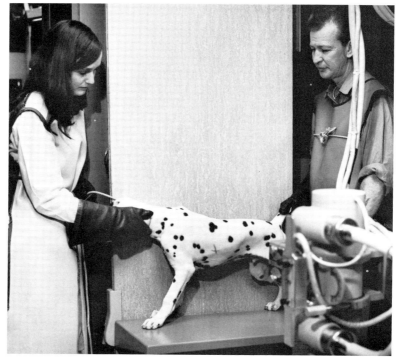

FIGURE 3-5 Positioning of the dog for a standing right lateral radiograph. This position is used if fluid is suspected in the thorax or pericardium. The dog is as close to the vertically positioned roentgen table as possible. The cassette is in the cassette tray of the table and is therefore not seen. Instead of using the table, a cassette holder is employed under most practice conditions. This position could also be used routinely but is impractical. The dog tends to move away from the cassette, and the forelimbs tend to obscure the apical area of the lungs or even other portions of the lungs. The problem of avoiding blurring due to motion is greatly enhanced. A horizontal x-ray beam must be used. The midpoint is centered at the fourth or fifth intercostal space.

THE NORMAL CARDIAC SILHOUETTE

In order to appreciate the diagnostic potentials and limitations of the radiographic examination, it is essential to realize that the radiograph is a momentary, two-dimensional shadow picture of the contracting or expanding three-dimensional heart. The cardiac silhouette is always exaggerated in size. At a film-tube distance of 120 cm., the enlargement of the heart of a dog the size of a German Shepherd will be approximately 6 mm. (Schulze and Nöldner, 1957). At shorter distances the amount of enlargement increases. The projection results in distortion of the cardiac silhouette and in considerable variation in the contour on both the lateral and the dorsoventral views. In the dorsoventral view the heart always appears shortened. The dorsoventral and lateral radiographs must be evaluated side by side, and the final result is obtained by imagining the two views as a three-dimensional object. Familiarity with the normal cardiac anatomy is indispensable for recognition and understanding of pathologic conditions.

The texts on canine anatomy provide basic information about the normal heart (Miller, Christensen, and Evans, 1966). For various reasons, the descriptions gained by conventional anatomic studies from formalinized cadavers are not identical with the radiographic anatomy determined from a living dog (Hamlin, 1960a; Schaller, 1953). The use of standard radiographs of normal animals and of heart models, and the verification of radiographic diagnoses by studying pathologic specimens, facilitate the understanding of thoracic radiographs.

The first detailed study of the radiographic anatomy of the canine heart was published in 1953 by Schaller in Vienna. This study includes a review of earlier publications on canine radiography and contrast studies. In this study the dogs were radiographed in dorsoventral and standing lateral positions, then euthanized and frozen while the same position was maintained. The heart was dissected free, and topographical studies of transverse thoracic sections done at different levels of the frozen cadavers were compared with the previous plain and contrast radiographs of the same animals.

In recent years this basic method has been refined by the use of angiocardiographic techniques, which enable study of the gross morphology of the heart *in vivo*. Hamlin (1960a) identified the cardiac structures which were outlined angiocardiographically by comparing them with anatomical results gained from horizontal sections of canine cadavers. During the last decade cineangiocardiography and angiocardiography using rapid film changers have therefore become favored methods for anatomic and clinical cardiac studies (Buchanan, 1965; Buchanan and Patterson, 1965; Detweiler et al., 1968, Hamlin, 1959, 1960a, 1960b; Patterson and Botts, 1961; Rhodes, Patterson, and Detweiler, 1960, 1963; Tashjian and Albanese, 1960). A textbook on canine angiocardiography and angiography has been published by Canossi et al. (1959). The following presentation is based on these articles and on studies performed at The Animal Medical Center using a rapid biplane roll-film changer, cineangiocardiography, and molds obtained by filling the cardiac chambers with Silastic.

It is easiest to become familiar with the normal cardiac anatomy if the radiographs are always placed on the view box in the same way; this also facilitates the orientation. Since the usual manner of reading and writing is from left to right and from top to bottom of a page, it seems logical to read radiographs in the same way. It is suggested that lateral radiographs be placed on the viewer with the head to the left side. However, consistency in positioning of the radiograph on the viewer is more important than the side to which the head points. The dorsoventral radiograph is always placed on the viewer with the head up and the animal's right side to the interpreter's left. This corresponds to a view of the heart from the ventral side with the patient lying on its back. Postmortem specimens of the dog must also be viewed in this way if the radiographic silhouette is to be compared with the postmortem findings. If a radiograph is unmarked, or if there is evidence that it might have been incorrectly marked as to the right or left side, the positioning can be verified by looking for the gas bubble in the fundus of the stomach, or the density of the spleen; both are normally found on the left side.

Since changes in exposure factors cause variations in radiographic densities, the possibility of underexposure or overexposure should also be considered before the details are evaluated. Wyburn and Lawson (1967) suggest certain criteria for judging the standard of the thoracic radiograph, the most important of which are as follows:

1. The entire bony thorax should be on the radiograph.
2. The proximal front limb should be excluded from the lung field.

3. The outlines of the diaphragm, the heart, and the aorta should be well defined.

4. The ribs should show good bony details.

5. The vascular markings of the lungs should be clearly defined.

6. On the dorsoventral radiograph the density of the spine should be just visible where it is superimposed on the cardiac silhouette.

7. The dorsoventral radiograph should be symmetrical, with the spine directly superimposed on the sternebrae.

8. On the lateral radiograph the costochondral junctions on each side should be on the same level, and the dorsal curvature of the ribs should not extend beyond the spine; this would indicate that the animal had been rotated in either the dorsal or the ventral direction.

Evaluation of the radiograph begins with a study of the structures external to the thorax (Rhodes, Patterson, and Detweiler, 1963). The conformation of the thorax is examined for the presence of anatomical variations and abnormal shapes of the ribs, the spine, and the sternum, such as pectus carinatum, or "chicken breast," and pectus excavatum, a funnel-shaped deformity with the sternum markedly depressed. Bone disease such as secondary nutritional hyperparathyroidism and congenital heart diseases are important causes of thoracic abnormalities in young dogs, where the soft, pliable bones of the ribs, spine, and sternebrae are easily deformed by excessive respiratory movement or enlargement of the heart. Extrathoracic deformities or injuries such as rib fractures also influence the position of the heart within the thorax and may cause respiratory distress. Obesity and emaciation are important factors to consider because of their influence on the size, contour, density, and position of the cardiac silhouette. Fine details of the cardiac contour such as the atrioventricular groove tend to be smoothed by the overlying pericardium and fat pads.

A well-defined configuration of the cardiac silhouette which is considered normal for all dogs does not exist. Considerable variations have been found among dogs of different breeds and body types. Wüller (1953) reported that systematic training increased cardiac size in Greyhounds. In addition, significant differences among successive radiographs of the same animal can occur even if these are made within the same hour. Variations of the silhouette of the normal heart are due to several factors, such as body type or breed, age, respiratory phase and cardiac phase, and positioning of the patient. The primary factors are positioning and variations in conformation of the thorax among the different body types. Furthermore, experience indicates that the change from normal to pathologic is gradual, leaving an intermediate period of indeterminate length during which the normal and diseased hearts appear similar when radiographed. The radiographic interpretation is ambiguous and should be carefully correlated with breed, age, and sex of the patient, history, and clinical and electrocardiographic findings in order to reach a meaningful diagnosis.

In some dorsoventral radiographs the change in thoracic size as well as the position of the diaphragm during respiration tends to alter the position of the cardiac apex. At deep inspiration the apex appears nearer to the midline than at expiration, and the heart is smaller if the inspiration is sustained. In exposures made at 0.05 sec. or less the influence of systole and diastole on shape and positioning becomes noticeable. The left border of the cardiac silhouette looks straighter, the pulmonary artery segment is larger, and the heart is slightly smaller and more sharply delineated at the end of systole than in full diastole. At longer exposure times (0.1 sec. or more), the heart is usually caught in diastole, because the slightly enlarged heart in the diastolic phase effectively blocks the x-ray beam, preventing visualization of the smaller cardiac silhouette in systole. The pulmonary artery segment is less distinct in diastole. A change in the centering of the roentgen beam of one to two intercostal spaces in a cranial or caudal direction changes the size of the lung field as seen in the dorsoventral projection, but the change of the cardiac silhouette is slight. If the beam is centered close to the thoracic inlet, the cardiac silhouette appears shortened (Fig. 3-23).

THE NORMAL LATERAL CARDIAC SILHOUETTE

The conformation of the thorax is evaluated first. In dogs with a narrow, deep thorax, such as Setters (Figs. 3-21 and 3-22), Afghan Hounds, Collies, and Whippets, the cardiac silhouette is more upright than in dogs with a wide, shallow thorax (Fig. 3-19), such as Beagles and Boston Terriers. In the latter body type the heart looks wider and occupies a relatively greater portion of the thorax than it does in dogs with a narrow thorax, such as the Setter. Young animals, up to about 3 months of age, have relatively rounder hearts than adults.

In the lateral projection, the cardiac silhouette has three borders: the dorsal, or base of the heart; the cranial, or right border; and the caudal, or left border. To facilitate the orientation on the radiograph the anatomical situation is shown in a schematic drawing showing the heart *in situ* (Fig. 3-6). In Figures 3-7 and 3-8 the outlines of structures of the right and left heart have been drawn into a normal cardiac silhouette to show their location and contribution to the cardiac outline. The cranial border is located near the third rib, and the caudal border extends to about the eighth rib. For evaluating the dorsal border, which is the most complex of the three and is composed of the densities of the right and left atria and the main pulmonary arteries and veins, the position of the trachea is important. The long axis of the trachea and the thoracic spine form an angle at the thoracic inlet and then diverge caudally. This angle is wider in dogs with narrow, deep thoracic conformation than it is in dogs with a wide, shallow thorax. In certain small breeds such as the Yorkshire Terrier and the Boston Terrier, the trachea runs almost parallel with the spine.

The caudal extremity of the trachea bends slightly ventrally as it bifurcates into the main bronchi and forms the carina. This bend may be absent in young dogs and in adults with wide thoracic conformation. The air-filled, round structure which lies over the base of the heart represents the end-on view of the common origin of the left apical and left cardiac bronchi. The tracheal bifurcation or carina is an important reference point for the assessment of cardiac enlargement and position. In normal dogs the bifurcation is located between the fifth and sixth ribs. It is slightly offset caudally within the cardiac silhouette, thus dividing the heart into a large cranial area (about three-fifths of the cardiac silhouette) including the right ventricle ventrally and the right atrium, main pulmonary artery, and ascending aorta dorsally, and a smaller caudal portion (about two-fifths of the cardiac silhouette) containing the left ventricle and atrium (see Fig. 3-9).

The curve formed by the cranial border of the cardiac silhouette is normally located at the level of the third intercostal space. The ventral and middle portions of the cranial border are consistently formed by the right ventricular wall and the right auricle. The most dorsal portion, which joins the ventral outline of the cranial vena cava, is formed by various structures; in some cases it is the aortic arch, in a few cases the conus arteriosus of the main pulmonary artery, and in the majority

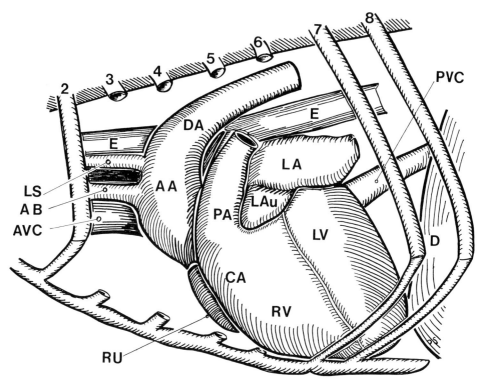

FIGURE 3-6 Schematic drawing of the topography of the canine heart and thorax seen from the left side after removal of the left thoracic wall. The drawing was made after photography of a cadaver frozen in the upright position. (From Schaller, 1953, courtesy of Karger, Basel/New York.)

LS—Left subclavian artery; AB—brachiocephalic artery; AVC—cranial vena cava; E—esophagus; RU—right auricle; AA—aortic arch; DA—descending aorta; RV—right ventricle; CA—conus arteriosus, or right ventricular outflow tract; PA—pulmonary artery; LAu—left auricle; LA—left atrium; LV—left ventricle; PVC—caudal vena cava; D—diaphragm; numbers 2 through 8 refer to the respective ribs.

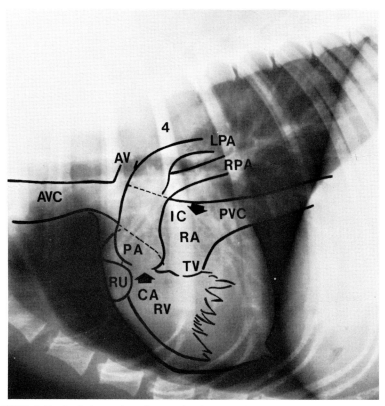

FIGURE 3-7   Left lateral radiograph, dog in Figure 3-2. Tracing delineates the structures of the right heart. The details for the tracing were obtained from angio-cardiograms.

AVC – Cranial vena cava; AV – junction of the azygos vein with the AVC; RU – right auricle; RV – right ventricle; CA – conus arteriosus, or right ventricular out-flow tract, extending to the tricuspid valve (arrow); PA – main pulmonary artery; LPA – left pulmonary artery; RPA – right pulmonary artery; RA – right atrium, divided dorsally by the intervenous crest, IC; arrow caudal to IC points at foramen ovale; PVC – caudal vena cava; 4 – fourth rib.

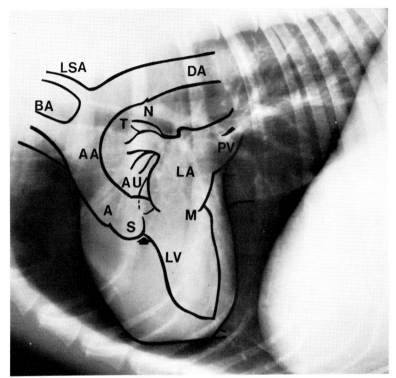

FIGURE 3-8 Lateral radiograph, dog in Figure 3-2. Tracing delineates the structures of the left heart. The details for the tracing were obtained from angiocardiograms.

BA–Brachiocephalic artery; LSA–left subclavian artery; AA–aortic arch; A–ascending aorta; S–sinus of Valsalva (arrow points at aortic valve); AU–small portion of the left auricle; T–tracheal bifurcation; N–notch in the descending aorta, DA, indicating the area of the ligamentum arteriosum; LV–left ventricle; M–mitral valve; LA–left atrium; PV–pulmonary veins.

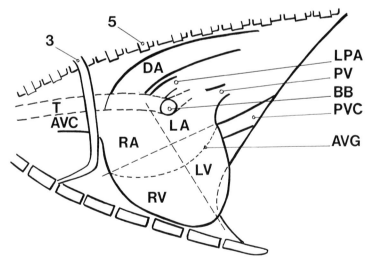

FIGURE 3-9 Schematic drawing showing division of the cardiac silhouette into right and left heart by an apicobasilar line.

T–Trachea; AVC–cranial vena cava; RA–right atrium; RV–right ventricle; LA–left atrium; LV–left ventricle; DA–descending aorta; LPA–left pulmonary artery; PV–pulmonary veins; BB–bronchial bifurcation, common origin of the left apical and cardiac lobar bronchi; PVC–caudal vena cava; AVG–atrioventricular groove; numbers 3 and 5 indicate respective ribs.

of cases the right atrium. The cranial vena cava joins the atrium, forming a slight inward curve called the cranial "waist." The angle at the cranial waist varies according to the inclination of the heart. It is more acute in dogs with upright hearts, such as Setters, and is more obtuse in dogs with greater inclination of the axis of the heart.

As the curved cranial border approaches the sternal outline to run parallel with it, an angle is formed with the sternum which varies according to the inclination of the heart and the size of the right ventricle. This angle is larger in breeds with a narrow thorax, and only a small portion of the cranial border, or none at all, is in contact with the sternum. In breeds with a wide thorax the angle is small, and a greater portion of the cranial border is parallel with the sternum. In the lateral projection the apex of the cardiac silhouette is formed by the interventricular septum. (In the dorsoventral view the apex is formed by the left ventricle.) Fat tissue which accumulates around the apex area or retrosternally often obscures the cranial border as it joins the apex, and it may elevate the heart.

The caudal cardiac border is only slightly curved and lies more perpendicular to the long axis of the body than the cranial one. It is formed by the left ventricle and the left atrium. The ventricular outline merges with the diaphragm in those breeds with a wide and short thorax. The distance between the diaphragm and the caudal cardiac border obviously varies with inspiration and expiration. At the base of the heart the left ventricular border curves inward to form the caudal waist as it meets the left atrial contour. The caudal waist corresponds to the atrioventricular groove. The angle at the caudal waist is more obtuse in upright hearts and more acute in hearts with greater inclination. The left atrial outline then extends dorsocaudally and becomes ill-defined as it joins the pulmonary veins.

The caudal vena cava becomes visible at the center of the diaphragm and runs slightly ventrally to the area of the atrioventricular groove. Sometimes its shadow can be followed a short distance within the cardiac silhouette before it widens and joins the right atrium. The dorsal border of the caudal vena cava is approximately at the level of the cardiac waist.

The point at which the aortic shadow separates from the cardiac shadow varies considerably with body type. The aortic arch usually becomes visible at the vertex of the angle of the cranial waist. In some dogs with deep thoracic conformation the aortic arch extends farther cranially than in others and emerges more ventrally from the area of the right auricle, thus forming the most dorsal part of the cranial border. The aorta is fully delineated only after it crosses the trachea and curves dorsally and caudally within the angle formed by the trachea and the spine.

Normally the main pulmonary artery contributes to the cranial border of the heart only in rare cases. The pulmonary artery becomes visible after it bifurcates into right and left branches immediately cranial to the carina. The left diaphragmatic lobar artery passes over the common origin of the left apical and cardiac lobar bronchi and is seen as a density immediately cranial and dorsal to this lucent oval. It can be followed for a variable distance toward the periphery. The right pulmonary artery crosses from left to right under the carina and may be seen end-on as a dense, round or oval structure at the base of the heart. This structure is sometimes mistaken for an enlarged hilar lymph node. Toward the periphery the right diaphragmatic lobar artery is superimposed on the left atrium, often making it difficult or impossible to distinguish this artery from the pulmonary veins as they converge at the left atrium. The veins are normally less dense than the arteries.

THE DORSOVENTRAL CARDIAC SILHOUETTE

Since true dorsoventral radiographs are difficult to obtain, deviations to one side are often unavoidable and may result in significant distortions. Allowance must be made in interpreting the radiographs if the study cannot be repeated, as for example in very sick dogs. If the thorax is rotated clockwise, the left cardiac border and the cardiac apex appear closer to the left thoracic wall than normal. The pulmonary artery segment moves a small distance in the direction of the apex, and the left side of the heart appears rounder, falsely suggesting left ventricular enlargement. If the thorax is rotated counterclockwise, the right cardiac border becomes rounder and appears closer to the thoracic wall than normal, mimicking right ventricular enlargement. The pulmonary artery segment moves into the spinal shadow. The left auricle appears enlarged, and the left ventricular border is straightened.

When a dog is twisted, there may be a true dorsoventral view of the cranial portion of the thorax and a rotational deviation of the caudal portion, or vice versa. With distortion or rotation the diaphragm appears to be extremely asymmetrical. Normally the cupola of the diaphragm lies slightly to the right of the midline, giving the diaphragmatic outline the shape of an egg with the obtuse, round end pointing to the right and the acute end pointing to the left. If the cupola of the diaphragm appears farther toward the left thoracic wall, a rotation in the clockwise direction is indicated. If the cupola seems to approach the right thoracic wall, a counterclockwise rotation is indicated.

The cardiac silhouette as it appears on a dorsoventral radiograph has been compared to a "lopsided egg" (Wyburn and Lawson, 1967) with rounded cranial and right borders and an almost straight left border, giving it the lopsided appearance. The tracings in the radiographs of Figures 3-10, 3-11, 3-12, and 3-13 illustrate the locations of the right and left cardiac structures and their contributions to the cardiac silhouette in the dorsoventral view. As in lateral radiographs, the cardiac silhouette varies greatly according to the thoracic conformation of the individual dog. It normally extends from the third to about the eighth rib. The base of the heart lies in the midline, and the apex is directed more or less markedly to the left of the midline. In breeds with a wide, short thorax such as Basset Hounds and Beagles, the apex points more to the left side than in breeds with a narrow thorax such as Setters, where the longitudinal axis of the heart may be almost parallel to the midsagittal plane (Fig. 3-23).

In some dogs, mainly those of the brachycephalic breeds, the apex may even lie on the right side, giving the impression that the radiograph has been mislabeled or placed on the viewer incorrectly, with its right side to the interpreter's right. The position of the spleen or the gas bubble in the fundus of the stomach helps to rule out erroneous markings on the radiograph.

The dorsoventral radiograph is characterized by extensive superimposition of the heart chambers, great vessels, trachea, and esophagus. In addition, the shortening of the cardiac silhouette is especially pronounced in dogs with a narrow, deep thoracic conformation (Fig. 3-23). The right border of the mediastinum is formed by the cranial vena cava, which merges at an obtuse angle

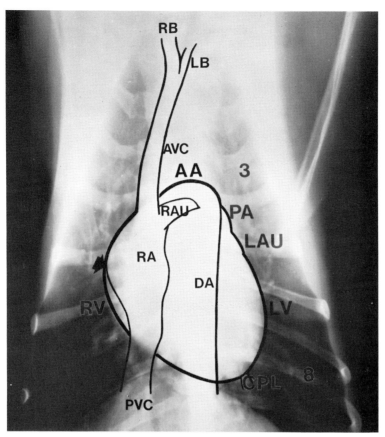

FIGURE 3-10 Dorsoventral radiograph, dog in Figure 3-2. Tracing delineates the right atrium, the caval veins, and the "border-forming" structures. The details for the tracing were obtained from angiocardiograms.

RB—Right brachial vein; LB—left brachial vein, AVC—cranial vena cava; AA—aortic arch; RAU—right auricle; PA—pulmonary artery; LAU—left auricle; arrow points at the separation of the right atrial outline from the right ventricular outline, representing the atrioventricular groove; RV—right ventricle; RA—right atrium; DA—descending aorta; LV—left ventricle; PVC—caudal vena cava; CPL—cardiophrenic ligament; numbers 3 and 8 indicate the respective ribs.

with the cranial border of the right atrium. The right cranial quadrant of the heart is formed by the right atrium and is overlaid caudally by the right ventricle and right pulmonary artery. The atrial border curves medially at about the fourth intercostal space, and from there on the cardiac outline is formed by the right ventricle. The atrioventricular groove may be indicated by a small indentation. As the right ventricular border swings caudomedially, it is interrupted by the caudal vena cava, which traverses the cardiophrenic angle formed by the right cardiac border and the diaphragm. Before reaching the apex, the outline of the right heart ends, sometimes forming a slight notch at the interventricular septum (Figs. 3-10 and 3-11).

The apex of the heart and most of the straight left cardiac border are formed by the left ventricle (Fig. 3-13). The cardiophrenic ligament extends as a thin

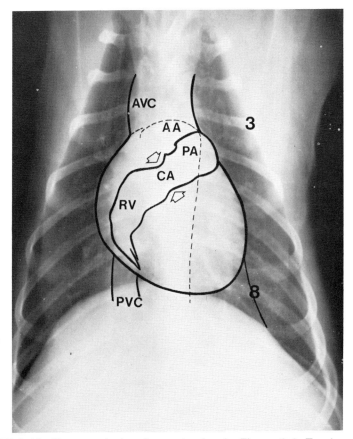

FIGURE 3-11 Dorsoventral radiograph, dog in Figure 3-2. Tracing delineates the right ventricle. Details for the tracing were obtained from angiocardiograms.

AVC—Cranial vena cava; AA—aortic arch; PA—main pulmonary artery, so-called pulmonary artery segment; CA—conus arteriosus, or right ventricular outflow tract; RV—right ventricle; PVC—caudal vena cava; numbers 3 and 8 indicate the respective ribs.

band from the apex to the diaphragm. Near the fourth intercostal space the left ventricular outline terminates, and the left cranial quadrant is formed by the pulmonary artery segment and the right ventricular outflow tract. The left auricle, which lies between the pulmonary artery and the left ventricle, seldom extends beyond the left cranial border in normal dogs. The pulmonary artery segment is the cardiac structure with the greatest degree of pulsation during systole and therefore varies greatly in size on successive radiographs. The medial portion of the pulmonary artery segment merges with the aortic arch.

The contribution of the aortic arch to the cranial cardiac border varies greatly. In some dogs the ascending and descending portions of the aorta are directly superimposed, giving the impression of a narrow aortic arch. In others the ascending and descending portions are not superimposed, and the aortic arch appears wide. In some dogs the arch lies almost totally within the cardiac silhouette. In a small number of dogs with a narrow thorax the arch may be very prominent, extending cranially beyond the cranial border of the heart, which is

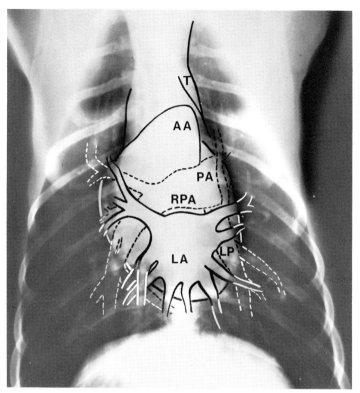

FIGURE 3-12 Dorsoventral radiograph, dog in Figure 3-2. Tracing outlines pulmonary arteries and the confluence of the pulmonary veins at the left atrium. Solid lines represent veins and left atrium; broken lines indicate the pulmonary arteries. Details for the tracings were obtained from angiocardiograms.

T—Thymus, seen only in growing dogs; AA—aortic arch; PA—pulmonary artery; RPA—right pulmonary artery; LP—left pulmonary artery; LA—left atrium.

normally located at the third intercostal space. In radiographs exposed with enough penetration the descending aorta can be seen as an increased density slightly to the left of the spine (Fig. 3-13). In growing dogs the thymus can be seen to the left of the aorta and pulmonary artery as a dense, sail-like structure (Fig. 3-12).

The cranial border of the heart is very complex owing to the varying degree of superimposition of structures such as the aortic arch, brachiocephalic and left subclavian arteries, right auricle, cranial vena cava, and pulmonary artery. The right auricle, which lies at the cranial border, extends a short distance beyond the midline to the left side. It is usually obscured by the aortic arch. The tip of the auricle seldom extends to the left of the aorta.

The brachiocephalic and left subclavian arteries are obscured in the mediastinum. The left subclavian artery lies on the left border of the mediastinum (see Fig. 3-13).

The air-filled trachea contrasts with the dense mediastinal structures and is therefore delineated in radiographs exposed with sufficient penetration. It enters the thoracic cavity at the midline or slightly to the right of it. The thoracic portion

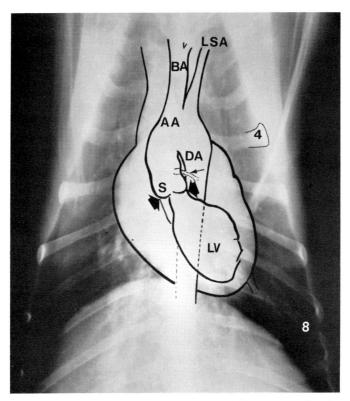

FIGURE 3-13 Dorsoventral radiograph, dog in Figure 3-2. Tracing delineates the structures of the left ventricle and aorta. Details for the tracing were obtained from angiocardiograms.

LSA—Left subclavian artery; BA—brachial artery; AA—aortic arch; DA—descending aorta; S—sinus of Valsalva; large arrows point at the muscular lining of the left ventricular outflow tract; small arrow indicates the origin of the left coronary artery, which is indicated by broken lines; LV—left ventricle; numbers 4 and 8 indicate the respective ribs.

continues to the right of the midline and may bow slightly to the right side as it crosses the aortic arch. The relative positions of the trachea and the esophagus on the right side of the aorta (see Fig. 3-17) are important for the assessment of a persistent right aortic arch. The trachea ends at its bifurcation into the main bronchi, which is also referred to as the carina. The left atrium is located within a caudally opening, acute angle formed by the diaphragmatic bronchi. The left auricle extends to the left and cranially, crossing ventrally to the left stem bronchus and the origin of the left apical and cardiac lobes of the lung. The auricle is normally not visible. The main portion of the left atrium directly overlies the left ventricle (Figs. 3-12 and 3-13).

RELATIVE POSITIONS OF CARDIAC CHAMBERS AND GREAT VESSELS

The three-dimensional arrangement of cardiac chambers and great vessels is difficult to assess from two-dimensional radiographs. There is superimposition of practically all cardiac structures in one or in both projections. The primary

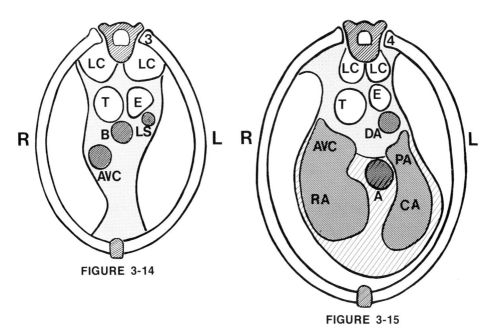

FIGURE 3-14

FIGURE 3-15

FIGURE 3-14 Schematic drawing, section through the thorax at the third rib as seen from the front. (Adapted from Schaller, 1953, courtesy of Karger, Basel/New York.)
  LC—Longus colli muscle; T—trachea; E—esophagus; B—brachiocephalic artery; LS—left subclavian artery; AVC—cranial vena cava; 3—third rib.

FIGURE 3-15 Schematic drawing, section through the thorax at the fourth rib as seen from the front. (Adapted from Schaller, 1953, courtesy of Karger, Basel/New York.)
  LC—Longus colli muscle; T—trachea; E—esophagus; AVC—cranial vena cava; DA—descending aorta; RA—right atrium; PA—pulmonary artery; CA—conus arteriosus; A—ascending aorta; 4—fourth rib.

reasons for this are the asymmetry of the right and left cardiac chambers and the oblique position of the heart within the thoracic cavity. The anatomical positions of the cardiac structures on transverse sections of the thorax at the third, fourth, and fifth ribs are shown in Figures 3-14, 3-15, and 3-16.

Some of the relations as they exist on the *lateral radiograph* are indicated schematically in Figure 3-9. However, the real relationship between right and left ventricles is more complex. A narrow portion of the crescent-shaped right ventricle surrounds the left ventricle laterally and ventrally (see Fig. 3-16). Most of the trabeculae carneae of the right ventricle are located in this lateral extension. They are responsible for the toothed outline of the right ventricle in the lateral angiocardiogram, which serves as a characteristic to distinguish between right and left ventricles in transpositions of the great vessels. The left ventricle and interventricular septum occupy about three-fifths of the total cardiac area. The right atrium is located to the right, cranially and ventrally from the left atrium. The cranial and caudal venae cavae, divided by the intervenous crest, curve ventrally before they join the right atrium (Fig. 3-7). The right auricle extends

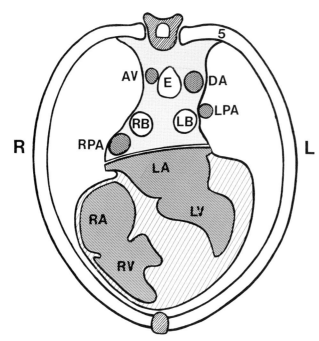

FIGURE 3-16 Schematic drawing, section through the thorax at the fifth rib as seen from the front. (Adapted from Schaller, 1953, courtesy of Karger, Basel/New York.)
AV — Azygos vein; E — esophagus; DA—descending aorta; RPA—right pulmonary artery; RB—right stem bronchus; LB—left stem bronchus; LPA—left pulmonary artery; RA—right atrium; RV—right ventricle; LA—left atrium; LV—left ventricle; 5—fifth rib.

far to the left side and crosses the cranial vena cava ventrally. The right atrium and cranial vena cava surrounds the centrally located sinus of Valsalva and the ascending aortic arch on the right side. The azygos vein, located to the right of the midline, runs almost parallel to the aorta and joins the cranial vena cava. The density of the vein is directly superimposed on the density of the aorta.

The conus arteriosus and the main pulmonary artery arise almost perpendicularly from the right ventricle and cross the ascending aorta on the left side (Fig. 3-6). The bifurcation of the pulmonary artery lies immediately caudal and to the left of the aortic arch. The tricuspid valve appears almost in the center of the lateral cardiac silhouette (Fig. 3-7). The aortic valve is located cranial and to the left of the tricuspid valve. The pulmonic valve lies cranial and ventral to the aortic valve. The mitral valve is located at the fifth intercostal space between the tricuspid valve and the caudal waist and is slightly more dorsal than the tricuspid valve.

On the *dorsoventral projection* the crescent-shaped right ventricle lies to the right and cranial to the left ventricle. The topography of the great vessels, esophagus, and trachea is shown in Figure 3-17 to facilitate the orientation. The right atrium and the cranial and caudal venae cavae are superimposed dorsally on the right ventricle. The left atrium is almost directly superimposed on the left ventricle. Its auricle is squeezed into a narrow space bounded by the pulmonary artery cranially, the left ventricle ventrally, and the pericardium dorsally and laterally. At the cranial border of the silhouette, partially superimposed and followed from right to left, are the cranial vena cava and the right atrium, the trachea, the esophagus, and the aortic arch and the main pulmonary artery (Fig. 3-17). The aortic valve is located in the midline or slightly to the left of the midsagittal plane, and the pulmonic valve is cranial and ventral to it. The aortic arch originates somewhat to the left of the midline, and as it ascends it turns rightward. The descending aorta then returns gradually to the left side.

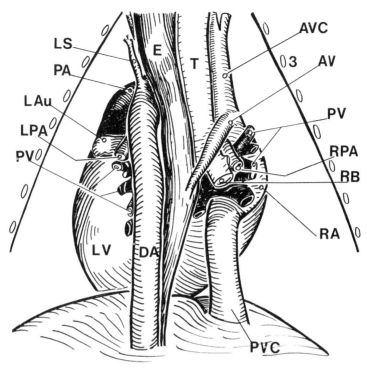

FIGURE 3-17 Schematic drawing of the topography of the canine heart and the structures of the hilar area seen after removal of the lung lobes; dorsal view. Drawing made from photograph of an anatomical specimen obtained by freezing the dog in a standing position. (Adapted from Schaller, 1953. Courtesy of Karger, Basel/New York.)

LS—left subclavian artery; PA—main pulmonary artery; LAu—left auricle; LPA—left pulmonary artery; PV—pulmonary veins; LV—left ventricle; DA—descending aorta; E—esophagus; T—trachea; AVC—cranial vena cava; AV—azygos vein; RPA—right pulmonary artery; RB—right stem bronchus; RA—right atrium; PVC—caudal vena cava; 3—third rib.

THE NORMAL PULMONARY VASCULATURE AND THE NORMAL LUNG FIELD

Because of the close anatomical and functional relationships between heart and pulmonary circulation, the radiographic analysis of the lung field is an integral part of the cardiac examination. Commonly used terms such as "cor pulmonale" and "cardiac lung" reflect the intimate connections between the two organs (Luisada, 1967a). Evaluation of the pulmonary circulation, which is often affected by cardiac diseases, is of primary importance in predicting the clinical course and advising on therapy. Many signs suggesting pulmonary disease are similar or identical to those of cardiac disease. Radiographs reveal the type and degree of pulmonary involvement and are therefore important in determining whether the clinical signs are of pulmonary or cardiac origin.

The vascular markings are the most prominent structures of the lungs. The air-filled alveoli provide a medium of increased lucency against which the dense, blood-filled arteries and veins stand out in bold contrast. The lung is therefore the only organ in which the vasculature is visible on the plain radiograph, and it has been called the "roentgen window" of the body (Sante, 1958). The density of the lung field and the size, shape, and density of the pulmonary arteries and veins are reasonably accurate indicators for detecting arterial and venous hypertension and congestive heart failure. In congenital heart diseases the pulmonary vasculature is often affected. An increased or decreased intrapulmonary blood flow provides a means of recognizing a shunting of blood between the left and right sides of the heart, thus affording basic information as to the type of cardiac defect present.

The degree of contrast between alveoli and vascular structures of normal dogs varies widely with inspiration and expiration, positioning, age of the animal, and radiographic technique. The lung fields of younger dogs are usually more lucent than those of old healthy dogs. Nodular or linear markings of interstitial origin increase the overall density in older animals (Reif and Rhodes, 1966). An underexposed radiograph may simulate a dense lung field, whereas an overexposed one may falsely suggest an extremely lucent lung field as seen with pulmonary emphysema. The density of the descending aorta provides a good standard with which the densities of both the lung field and the intrapulmonary vessels may be compared. Decreased contrast of the lung field as compared with the aorta also results in a loss of contrast between the lung field and its vascular structures. In a normal dog, the density of the intrapulmonary vessels is always less than that of the aorta.

To describe the intrapulmonary vasculature it is advantageous to subdivide the lung into three concentric zones: the central or hilar zone; the middle zone, containing the large bronchial and vascular branches; and the peripheral zone, composed of the parenchyma. The pulmonary arteries and veins are best evaluated in the middle zone. In the periphery the vessels become attenuated and are therefore difficult to evaluate.

The separation of arterial and venous densities is essential for differentiating arterial diseases, such as heartworm disease, from venous engorgement due to passive pulmonary congestion. Arteries and veins are differentiated according to their origin, location, density, and outline (see Figs. 3-12 and 3-30). Most of the pulmonary vascular markings in normal dogs are produced by the arteries. Their course can be more easily followed in large breeds than in small ones. The arteries originate from a point cranial to the tracheal bifurcation (Fig. 3-12). They are denser and better delineated than veins, and they have a slightly greater number of branches. On the dorsoventral radiograph the arteries are located on the lateral side of the bronchial lumen. Small arterial branches are slightly curved in cranial and lateral directions. The veins are recognized by their entry and confluence at the left atrium (Fig. 3-12). They are normally straighter, less dense, and blunter than arteries. Their outlines are not as well defined as those of the arteries. On the lateral radiograph the veins are located ventral and caudal to the apical lobar bronchi. Arteries and veins can be outlined angiocardiographically (see Fig. 5-17).

RADIOGRAPHIC DIAGNOSIS OF CARDIAC ENLARGEMENT

Cardiac disease is manifested radiographically by changes in size, contour, density, and/or position of the cardiac silhouette and great vessels, as well as by extracardiac signs (see pp. 85 to 96). Cardiac enlargement is a cardinal sign of cardiac disease and results from an increase in the volume of blood flowing through the heart or from an increased vascular resistance in the periphery or the lungs. Except in occasional cases, the routine radiograph does not outline a specific cardiac defect and does not show the immediate cause of the disease. The conclusions drawn from a radiograph are indirect and often ambiguous. Enlargement of the cardiac silhouette, for example, can be caused by dilatation; it can result from hypertrophy of the cardiac muscle; or it may be a combination of dilatation and hypertrophy. Cardiac enlargement is therefore either a sign of cardiac compensation (hypertrophy) or a sign of cardiac failure (dilatation) (Fig. 3-29). Other causes of enlargement of the cardiac silhouette are extracardiac masses, pericardial fat pads, pericardial effusion, which is occasionally found in heart disease, and tumors of the hilar area such as aortic body tumors.

A number of conditions, such as arrhythmias, minor valvular disease, or hypertrophy of the cardiac muscle, may not produce changes significant enough to be recognizable on the radiograph. The radiograph may be "blind" even in massive ventricular hypertrophy occurring at the expense of ventricular volume (Hamlin, 1968). Frequently it is the change in contour of the cardiac silhouette caused by enlargement of only one of the great vessels or chambers, rather than the enlargement per se, which suggests a specific diagnosis.

There are three methods of assessing cardiac enlargement radiographically:

1. The *empirical method,* based on experience gained from the evaluation of a great number of cardiac radiographs.

2. The *comparative method,* which uses successive radiographs of the same individual, made with identical technique, to follow a condition through its different stages.

3. The *method of measurement,* based on absolute cardiac and thoracic dimensions or on ratios between cardiac dimensions or between cardiac and thoracic dimensions.

The empirical method is preferred in veterinary medicine. However, extensive experience and thorough knowledge of the normal variations in different breeds are required before meaningful diagnoses can be made. Unless a discriminatory approach is used the results will be subjective and prone to considerable variation and error.

The comparative method is simple and reliable and demonstrates the usefulness of successive standard radiographs in diagnosing a cardiac condition and secondary extracardiac changes. It is, however, limited in application by the likelihood that previous radiographs are unavailable.

The use of absolute measurements and ratios, although desirable, has not become popular in veterinary medicine for reasons that follow.

CARDIAC MENSURATION AND CARDIAC RATIOS

A number of methods have been established for measuring cardiac enlargement in man (Friedberg, 1966; Meschan, 1966). To reduce the magnifying effect of the divergent x-ray beam, standard radiographs are exposed from a distance of 180 cm. (6 ft.) (teleroentgenography), and the dimensions are compared with normal values obtained from nomograms giving the variations of normal cardiac size according to height, weight, body surface area, and sex. The use of relationships between the dimensions of the heart and those of the heart and thorax are of value as a rapid but rough estimation of the cardiac size. However, the usefulness of cardiac mensuration must not be overestimated. Normal ranges of cardiac dimensions are quite large and overlap the pathological ranges to a great degree (Sante, 1958). The correlation of cardiac measurements obtained from plain radiographs with the actual specimen is inaccurate at best, but it is impossible for the physician to obtain more accurate, measurable data regarding cardiac size *in vivo* by any other means (Meschan, 1966).

These methods have thus proved useful in man (Friedberg, 1966); therefore, attempts have been made to adapt these relationships or ratios to the dog. Because of the extreme variation in size of canine hearts according to breed, weight, thoracic configuration, and sex, a correlation of the cardiac size with weight, body surface area, and height is inadequate for use in clinical veterinary medicine.

Schulze and Nöldner (1957) made left lateral radiographs of 1406 dogs from a distance of 120 cm. and established standard ratios between the length (apicobasilar distance) and width of the heart from which cardiac enlargement could be predicted. However, their method has not been applied clinically because the ratios differ from one breed to another. False negative results using this method have been reported (Detweiler and Patterson, 1965). Recently, the use of a planimetric method comparing the surfaces of the thorax and the cardiac silhouette has been advocated (Uhlig & Werner, 1969).

Hamlin (1968) has developed a method using routine dorsoventral radiographs made from a distance of 1 meter (40 in.). Figure 3-18 shows how the measurements are obtained. In a dog with a normal heart, L is approximately equal to R, and LH is about the same size as RH. The sum of LH and RH, the total expanse of both the right and left ventricle from the midline, is equal to less than 65 per cent, or two-thirds, of the total lateral dimension of the thorax, LAT. A, the aortic double density, is always less than half of LC, the distance from the midline to the thoracic wall. The main pulmonary artery segment, MPA, does not protrude in a normal radiograph, and the left auricle, LAu, does not extend beyond the left cardiac border.

In general, reservations concerning the use of cardiac ratios in dogs are similar to those mentioned previously concerning cardiac ratios in man. Ratios give a statistically correct correlation for a large group of individuals; however, the ratios may be incorrect and/or not accurate enough when applied in an individual case. The measurements must also be used with caution because factors such as positioning, body type, mobility of the heart in the thorax, and extracardiac factors influence the results. A slight rotation of the thorax in a clockwise or counterclockwise direction changes the ratio of R to L. The accuracy of the method is diminished by the wide variation of cardiac ratios in normal dogs and by the overlap between normal and pathologic, the distinction between normal and abnormal being arbitrary. The more vertical placement of the heart in dogs with a deep thorax, and its transverse placement in dogs with a short thorax, cause a wide variation of the normal ratios. Elevation of the diaphragm at deep expiration, with ascites, or with advanced pregnancy results in a shifting of the heart and causes the ratios to vary. A shifting of the apex to the left side is quite common with right ventricular enlargement and results in an incorrect ratio be-

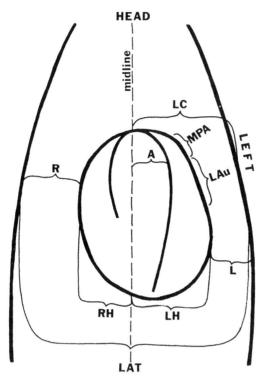

FIGURE 3-18 Diagram for measurements of the thorax and cardiac silhouette in the dog, corresponding to a dorsoventral radiograph examined from the ventral aspect. (From Hamlin, R. L.: J.A.V.M.A., 153 [1968]: 1449.)

M—Midsagittal axis of torso; L—distance between the left ventricular free wall and the left thoracic wall; R—distance between the right ventricular free wall and the right thoracic wall; LH—distance of the leftward expanse of the left ventricle from the midsagittal axis; RH—distance of the rightward expanse of the right ventricle from the midsagittal axis; RH + LH—total distance from the rightward expanse of the right ventricle to the leftward expanse of the left ventricle; LAT—distance between the right and left thoracic walls at the level of the most rightward deviation of the right ventricle and the most leftward deviation of the left ventricle; MPA—pulmonary artery segment; LAu—left auricle; A—width of the aortic double density measured from the midsagittal axis; LC—distance from the intersection of the cranial cardiac contour with the midsagittal axis to the left thoracic wall.

tween R and L, mimicking left ventricular enlargement. The cardiothoracic ratio, $\dfrac{RH + LH}{LAT}$, changes with deep inspiration and expiration. Thoracic deformities, such as funnel chest, make it impossible to use the method. Major disadvantages of the method proposed by Hamlin are that no consideration is given to variations in apicobasilar distance and that only one projection is used.

Moderate enlargement of one or both ventricles is often not indicated. Since only one view is utilized for the measurement, a number of cases are therefore not properly diagnosed.

Regardless of the method used to assess cardiac enlargement in an individual clinical case, the final diagnosis must be based on other signs as well, because cardiac size alone does not necessarily indicate normality or disease. This fact restricts the value of mensuration, whether the results are or are not in close accordance with the specimen.

One hundred thirty-one dogs with cardiovascular disease from which clinical findings, electrocardiograms, phonocardiograms, pressure recordings, angiocardiograms, and/or necropsy results were available were selected at random from our radiographic file. Acquired heart disease was diagnosed in 104 dogs and congenital heart disease in 27 dogs. Where left and/or right heart enlargement was suspected on the basis of measurements, the results were accurate in 107 instances and were either inconclusive or erroneous 91 times when compared with the results of empirically diagnosed right or left ventricular enlargement. Empirical analysis of the cardiac silhouette as seen in lateral and dorsoventral radiographs, combined with assessment of extracardiac signs, was superior for the evaluation of individual cases.

Quantitative methods of determining cardiac size may be advantageous for scientific purposes and statistical analysis of the heart size of homogeneous groups of dogs, as has been shown by Schulze and Nöldner (1957) in normal dogs.

THE EMPIRICAL EVALUATION OF CARDIAC ENLARGEMENT

Both lateral and dorsoventral projections are needed for the assessment of cardiac enlargement. In addition to familiarity with the radiographic appearance of the normal heart, knowledge of the rules governing cardiac enlargement is indispensable. Several articles have been published describing diagnosis of cardiac enlargement (Buchanan, 1968; Carlson, 1967; Detweiler et al., 1968; Hamlin, 1960b, 1968; Rhodes, Patterson, and Detweiler, 1960, 1963; Wyburn and Lawson, 1967).

Generalized cardiac enlargement involving the entire heart is seen with myocardial disease, severe chronic anemia, and infectious or metabolic diseases, and as a result of most of the severe, long-standing valvular diseases. In many cases the normal cardiac silhouette merely seems magnified, because the increase in size has affected all cardiac structures equally. More often, however, the enlargement is disproportionate and results in considerable changes in both the size *and* the contour of the heart. Furthermore, enlargement in only one direction may cause puzzling differences between the cardiac silhouettes seen on the lateral and dorsoventral radiographs. The localized types of enlargement causing changes in the contour of the heart are characteristic of certain diseases and are therefore of great diagnostic value. Although the radiographic signs described are quite significant, they are often not diagnostic in themselves without signs of circulatory failure in the respiratory and abdominal organs and clinical evidence of cardiovascular disease.

Generalized cardiac enlargement must be differentiated from fatty infiltration of the pericardium, pericardial effusion, and peritoneopericardial hernias.

EVALUATION OF GENERALIZED CARDIAC ENLARGEMENT IN THE LATERAL RADIOGRAPH

From the lateral radiograph, cardiac enlargement in the dorsal, cranial, and caudal directions can be evaluated. The outline of a dog's normal heart determined from an early lateral radiograph has been traced on a lateral radiograph made after the dog developed anemia due to chronic external blood loss which resulted in generalized cardiac enlargement (Fig. 3-19).

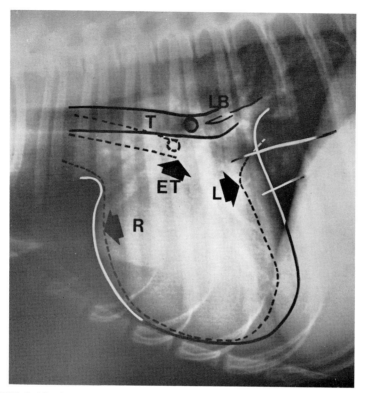

FIGURE 3-19 Left lateral radiograph, 3-year-old, female Beagle. Tracings before and after the heart became enlarged due to intermittent, severe bleeding over a 2-year period. The size of the thorax remained unchanged. The inner, broken lines show the size of the cardiac silhouette at 1 year of age, before the dog became anemic. The outer, solid lines delineate the heart at the age of 3 years.

Arrow R indicates right ventricular enlargement; arrow L indicates left ventricular enlargement; arrow ET points to tracheal elevation. T—Trachea; LB—left stem bronchus, slightly elevated by the left atrium; O with solid line shows location of the common origin of the left apical and cardiac lobar bronchi after cardiac enlargement occurred; O with broken line indicates location of the same structure before enlargement.

Notice that the apex has moved caudally, giving the false impression that the right ventricle has enlarged less than the left ventricle.

The enlarged cardiac silhouette occupies a greater area within the thorax than does the normal cardiac silhouette. However, before assessing the degree of enlargement in an individual case, it is essential to consider the influences of body type, size, and age of the patient; these factors cause considerable variations in normal heart size. Schulze and Nöldner (1957) found that with increasing age the heart tended to become wider and was therefore rounder in appearance.

Cardiac enlargement in the cranial direction, indicating right heart enlargement, can affect the cranial waist in two different ways. If the ventral portion—right ventricular outflow tract—enlarges to a greater extent than the dorsal portion, the cranial border becomes rounder, with the cranial waist being accentuated. If the dorsal portion—right atrium, ascending aortic arch, or pulmonary artery—extends farther cranially than the ventral portion, the right or cranial border is straightened, and the angle formed with the cranial vena cava becomes obtuse; therefore, the cranial waist disappears.

The caudal border is always straighter in the area of the caudal waist, becoming more perpendicular to the long axis of the body. This indicates left ventricular and left atrial enlargement. Extension in the cranial and caudal directions increases the horizontal diameter of the heart. One simple rule which may be helpful in assessing the craniocaudal dimension of the cardiac silhouette in the lateral projection is the number of intercostal spaces between the cranial and caudal borders of the heart. In dogs with a wide thorax, the maximum is about three and one-half intercostal spaces; in dogs with average thoracic configuration and in growing dogs the maximum diameter is about three intercostal spaces; and in dogs with a narrow thorax it approaches two and one-half intercostal spaces. Another rule says that the proportion between apicobasilar distance (distance from cardiac apex to base of the heart at the carina) and the craniocaudal dimension at the base of the heart is about 4:3 (Hamlin, 1960a).

The third and most common type of enlargement occurs in the dorsal direction. The dorsoventral or longitudinal diameter of the heart increases and causes dorsal displacement of the trachea. The angle between the thoracic spine and the trachea becomes more acute, and the ventral curve at the distal end of the trachea disappears. Finally, the trachea may run parallel with the spine. This occurs more easily in dogs with a wide thorax, where the trachea normally forms a more acute angle with the spine, than in those with a narrow thorax. With severe heart enlargement the trachea is in close contact with the spine and appears compressed dorsoventrally.

Since the dorsal displacement of the hilus in dogs with a wide, short thorax such as English Bulldogs is limited by the spine, elongation of the axis of the heart results in shifting of the apex in a caudal and leftward direction. The inclination of the cardiac axis increases, and the caudal border tends to merge extensively with the cupola of the diaphragm.

In those cases in which the right atrium is greatly enlarged, a slight dorsal bulge of the trachea may be noticed cranial to the tracheal bifurcation. Elevation of the caudal trachea and the left stem bronchus indicates left atrial enlargement.

EVALUATION OF CARDIAC ENLARGEMENT IN THE DORSOVENTRAL RADIOGRAPH

A dorsoventral radiograph of the same dog as in Figure 3-19, with the normal cardiac silhouette drawn within the enlarged silhouette, is shown in Figure 3-20.

The enlarged cardiac silhouette occupies a greater area of the thorax than normal. Allowance should be made for variations due to thoracic conformation and phase of respiration. The enlarged cardiac silhouette is usually rounder than normal. The cranial border of the heart may extend slightly more toward the thoracic inlet than in a normal dog. Since the thorax has the form of a funnel with its vertex pointing cranially, it is natural that an enlarged heart would be displaced in a caudal direction where the widening of the thorax provides more space. However, the cupola of the diaphragm and the sternum interfere with this displacement, deflecting the cardiac apex toward the left thoracic wall or occasionally toward the right thoracic wall. The long axis of the heart therefore tends to lie more transversely in a dog with an enlarged heart than in a dog with a normal heart. In a number of cases the enlarged left auricle extends beyond the left cardiac border, appearing as a small, bulging density.

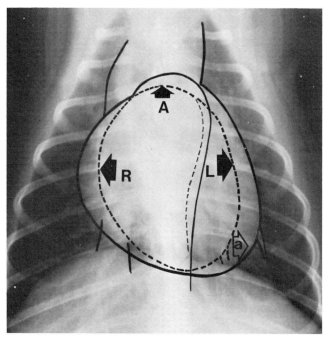

Figure 3-20 Dorsoventral radiograph, dog in Figure 3-19, showing enlargement of the cardiac silhouette as seen in this view. The broken lines show the size of the heart at 1 year of age, prior to enlargement. The solid line shows the heart after enlargement, at 3 years of age.

Arrow R indicates enlargement of the right ventricle; arrow L indicates left ventricular enlargement; arrow A indicates the cranial extension of the aorta due to enlargement; arrow (a) indicates the leftward shifting of the apex, making the enlargement of the left heart look more severe than it really is.

If measurements are used, the cardiothoracic ratio, $\dfrac{LH + RH}{LAT}$, exceeds two-thirds or the total expanse of the cardiac silhouette becomes greater than 65 per cent of the thoracic width. L and R may be nearly equal in generalized cardiac enlargement (Hamlin, 1968).

A decrease in cardiac size is rare. It is seen in growing dogs with achalasia, in which the heart is displaced ventrally by the dilated esophagus. Diminished cardiac size also occurs with malnutrition. In Figures 3-22 and 3-23, a decrease in cardiac size and undercirculation of the lung field are seen in an Irish Setter with adrenocortical hypofunction. Diminished cardiac size is also seen during hypovolemic shock (Gratzl, 1965) (Fig. 17-7*A* and *B*).

THE ENLARGEMENT OF INDIVIDUAL CHAMBERS

Isolated right or left ventricular enlargement is infrequent. Because of the interdependence of the two sides of the heart, a cardiac disease is rarely confined to one chamber as it progresses. The increase in size of one chamber is

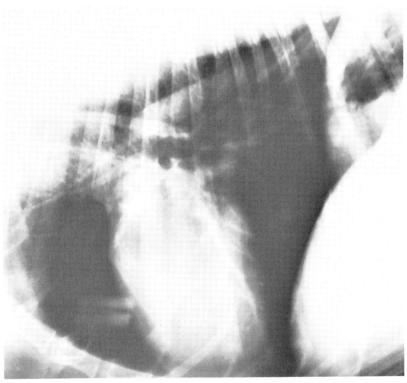

FIGURE 3-21 Left lateral radiograph, 3-year-old, female Irish Setter, illustrating the upright position of the heart in breeds with a narrow, deep thorax.

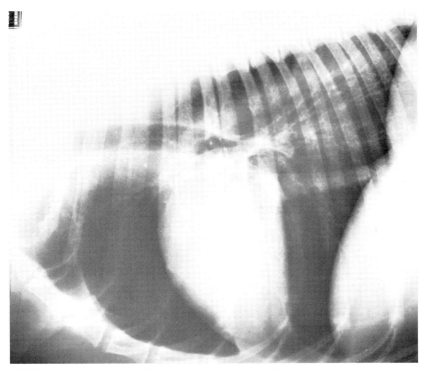

FIGURE 3-22 Left lateral radiograph, dog in Figure 3-21, made 1 year later when the dog was hospitalized for weakness, coughing, and gagging. Hyperkalemia and complete heart block developing into sinoatrial arrest were diagnosed clinically (see Arrhythmias, pp. 302-306) and were attributed to acute hypoadrenocorticism.

Notice the decreased size and more upright position of the heart as compared with Figure 3-21. The lung field is very lucent, and the vascular markings appear as fine structures and are definitely smaller and less dense than in the previous radiograph, indicating reduced pulmonary circulation. The undercirculation of the lungs is due to reduced cardiac output for which the dog tries to compensate by over-inflation of the lungs.

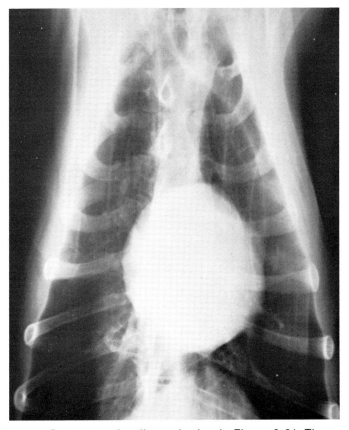

FIGURE 3-23 Dorsoventral radiograph, dog in Figure 3-21. The exposure was made at the same time as was Figure 3-22. The influence of the deep, narrow thoracic configuration on the position of the heart within the thorax and its appearance on the radiograph are accentuated by centering the x-ray beam near the thoracic inlet. Because the heart is upright the x-ray beam penetrates the heart almost parallel to its apicobasilar dimension. Therefore, the cardiac silhouette appears extremely shortened and almost circular.

therefore often accompanied by some degree of enlargement of the opposite chamber and is only a phase in a disease process which tends to culminate in generalized cardiac enlargement.

Care should be taken in differentiating between right and left ventricular enlargement and displacement of the cardiac silhouette which may mimic enlargement of the side to which the displacement occurs. Furthermore, it is possible that excessive enlargement of one chamber induces displacement of the cardiac silhouette to the opposite side. Therefore, the position of the cardiac apex must be evaluated before a final conclusion is made. The cardiophrenic ligament originates near the apex. Therefore, in the rounded heart its position can be used to determine the location of the apex. If this displacement is not considered, an incorrect diagnosis results. Rotation of the heart by unilateral enlargement also does occur, but it is difficult to assess radiographically.

ENLARGEMENT OF THE RIGHT VENTRICLE, RIGHT ATRIUM, AND PULMONARY ARTERY

The right ventricle, right atrium, venae cavae and pulmonary artery comprise a functional unit. Therefore, a condition often affects two or three of these structures in succession, and it is practical to analyze them simultaneously.

Conditions which underlie changes in size or contour are usually related to abnormalities in pulmonary vascular resistance or in the amount of blood volume ejected. If a ventricle must accommodate an increased blood volume, a so-called "volume overload" eventually occurs, resulting in dilatation of the chamber; this, in turn, may be followed by hypertrophy. If a normal volume of blood is ejected against increased resistance, as in pulmonic stenosis, a so-called "pressure overload" occurs and causes ventricular hypertrophy.

In many dogs with right ventricular pressure or volume overload, the concurrent dilatation of the pulmonary artery first suggests the presence of a disease process and may substantiate a diagnosis of right ventricular enlargement. It is especially important to recognize ventricular enlargement when radiographic evidence is minor, as in muscular hypertrophy of the ventricular wall occurring at the expense of end systolic ventricular volume. This occurs in obstruction of the right ventricular outflow tract, such as in pulmonic stenosis, where right ventricular enlargement is often minimal although the actual hypertrophy may be marked (Rhodes, Patterson, and Detweiler, 1963). If cardiac failure ensues, the ventricle dilates regardless of whether pressure or volume overload was the initial cause of failure.

The right ventricle. As the right ventricle increases in size, the cardiac silhouette tends to look rounder and wider than normal in one or usually both projections. The craniocaudal and transverse diameters of the heart increase more than does the apicobasilar distance.

In the *lateral radiograph* (Fig. 3-24) the trachea may be elevated, but the bend at the distal end is usually preserved. Unilateral enlargement of the right ventricle is obvious when the enlarged cardiac area cranial to a line connecting the tracheal bifurcation and the apex is compared with the normal left ventricular area caudal to it. The cranially extended right cardiac border appears straighter than normal if the dorsal portions are primarily involved, or more convex than normal if the ventrally located ventricular outflow tract is enlarged. In the first case the cranial waist disappears, and in the second case it becomes accentuated. The enlarged right ventricle occasionally displaces the apex dorsocaudally, mimicking left ventricular enlargement (Fig. 3-24). If the main pulmonary artery enlarges, it can form the entire dorsal half of the cranial border and causes a broadening of the base of the heart.

In the *dorsoventral radiograph* right ventricular enlargement increases the area of the cardiac silhouette lying to the right of the midline (Fig. 3-25). Consequently, the distance between the thoracic wall and the right cardiac border decreases. Because the position of the greatest rightward extension of the right ventricle varies, the shape of the enlarged chamber also varies, from oblong to triangular. Pronounced enlargement of the right ventricle frequently causes leftward displacement of the cardiac apex; the mobility of the apex in cardiac diseases has been stressed by Hamlin (1960b). The distance between the left cardiac border and the thoracic wall is diminished, and concurrent left ventricular enlargement is falsely suggested. The right apical border becomes more rounded

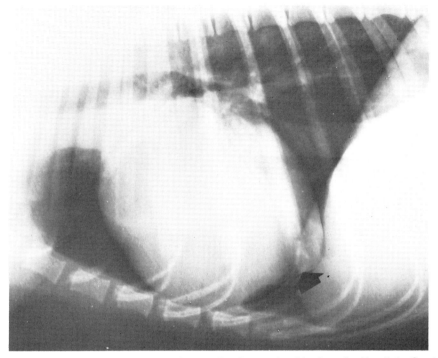

FIGURE 3-24 Left lateral radiograph, 9-month-old, female English Cocker Spaniel with right ventricular enlargement due to pulmonic stenosis. The cardiac silhouette appears rounder than normal due to an increase in width. The trachea is dorsally displaced and runs nearly parallel to the thoracic spine due to an increase in the dorsoventral diameter of the heart. The ventral bend at the caudal extremity is preserved, indicating that the left atrium is not enlarged. The outline of the right heart curves caudodorsally after touching the sternum and ends at a shallow notch near the cardiac apex (arrow). The right ventricular enlargement resulted in a shift of the apex caudodorsally, which might give the false impression that the left ventricle has also enlarged. Notice the rather wide caudal vena cava and the clear lung field.

than normal, and in some cases a small notch is seen as the caudally enlarged right ventricle joins the less involved left ventricle. In other cases the cardio-phrenic ligament serves as a mark to define the apex area (Fig. 3-20).

Radiographic findings in cardiac conditions frequently associated with right ventricular enlargement are summarized in Table 3-1. However, the other factors considered in the evaluation of cardiac conditions, such as age and clinical signs, must always be evaluated in making the differential diagnosis.

The main pulmonary artery. In the *lateral radiograph* the enlarged main pulmonary artery extends cranially and may contribute to the cardiac border (Fig. 18-29).

In the *dorsoventral radiograph* the main pulmonary artery becomes visible as the so-called "pulmonary artery segment" and is located at 1 to 2 o'clock. Enlargement of this structure must be evaluated carefully because its size varies considerably in successive radiographs, depending on the position of the dog and

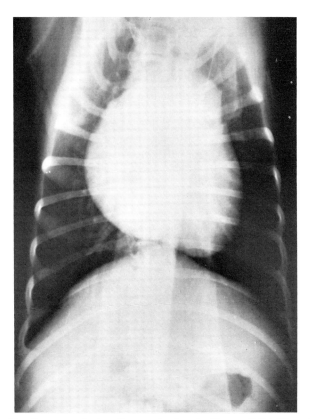

FIGURE 3-25   Dorsoventral radiograph, dog in Figure 3-24. The right side of the cardiac silhouette is definitely rounder and extends farther to the right than normal. There is a well-delineated notch were the enlarged right ventricle joints the inter-ventricular septum. The left ventricular outline appears slightly rounded but is not enlarged. The pulmonary artery segment protrudes leftward and cranially and is typically enlarged, indicating poststenotic dilatation of the main pulmonary artery.

the phase of the cardiac cycle. Marked protrusion of the pulmonary artery is a reliable diagnostic sign for its enlargement due to increased pulmonary blood flow, increased pulmonary arterial pressure (pulmonary hypertension or filling of the arteries with parasites [heartworm disease]), or poststenotic dilatation (Fig. 3-25). In increased pulmonary blood flow (overcirculation with left-to-right shunts), as in patent ductus arteriosus, ventricular septal defect, or atrial septal defect, the main pulmonary artery and the peripheral branches are enlarged. In congenital pulmonic stenosis, a knob-like, poststenotic dilatation occurs, but the peripheral arterial branches are unaffected. A depression at the area of the pulmonary artery segment is seen with tetralogy of Fallot (Buchanan, 1968a) and with other congenital abnormalities in which the pulmonary artery is hypoplastic, such as a hypoplastic right ventricle.

The right atrium.   Enlargement of this structure is difficult to assess. Isolated

TABLE 3-1   COMMON CARDIAC CONDICATIONS ASSOCIATED WITH RIGHT
VENTRICULAR ENLARGEMENT

CONDITION	RADIOGRAPHIC SIGNS
Tricuspid insufficiency	Right atrial enlargement with evidence of systemic congestion such as liver enlargement; sometimes widened cranial and caudal venae cavae; usually dense, congested lung field if tricuspid insufficiency occurs secondary to left ventricular disease
Cor pulmonale[*]	Chronic pulmonary disease such as bronchitis or pulmonary fibrosis; left atrial and left ventricular enlargement with engorgement of pulmonary veins if cor pulmonale is secondary to left heart disease
Dirofilariasis (heartworm disease)	Enlarged pulmonary artery segment; coarse, often extremely enlarged and distorted lobar arteries which may not branch normally and appear pruned instead of tapering toward the periphery; occasionally dilated caudal vena cava; enlarged right atrium
Pulmonic stenosis (uncomplicated)	Usually knob-like protrusion of pulmonary artery segment (post-stenotic dilatation) in lateral or dorsoventral view; normal size of lobar branches; no pulmonary overcirculation; clear lung field
Patent ductus arteriosus	Enlargement of the pulmonary artery segment; pulmonary overcirculation; dense lung field; congestion or edema in long-standing disease; aneurysmal dilatation of the aortic arch to the left; secondary left atrial and left ventricular enlargement. As pulmonary resistance increases the right ventricle becomes hypertrophied
Atrial and ventricular septal defects	Rarely enlargement of the pulmonary artery segment; sometimes overcirculated, dense lung field; secondary enlargement of left atrium and left ventricle
Tetralogy of Fallot	Mainly undercirculated, lucent lung field (cyanosis); pulmonary artery segment usually small but may be normal or even larger than normal. Right ventricular enlargement usually pronounced.

*Cor pulmonale as used here is defined broadly to include any case of right ventricular hypertrophy, strain, or failure caused by disordered pulmonary circulation or secondary to left ventricular failure (Brill, 1958).

right atrial enlargement occurs infrequently in dogs. It is usually associated with tricuspid insufficiency and right heart failure.

In the *lateral radiograph* moderate or severe enlargement of the right auricle can cause disappearance or accentuation of the cranial waist. In extreme atrial enlargement the trachea is sometimes bowed dorsally over the cranial half of the hilus, where it overlies the atrium. The right main stem bronchus may be elevated. Tumors of the heart base or lymph nodes, or disproportionate enlargement of the main pulmonary artery results in a similar displacement of the trachea and should thus be considered in the differential diagnosis (Buchanan, 1968a). Excessive right atrial and right ventricular enlargement occurs occasionally and may mimic pericardial effusion by causing a very large, well-rounded appearance of the cardiac silhouette. In some cases dilatation of the right atrium is accompanied by widening of the cranial and caudal venae cavae. The size of these veins is subject to other influences and therefore does not indicate right atrial enlargement consistently. In well-exposed radiographs the dilated caudal vena cava can be followed within the cardiac silhouette until it widens and disappears as it joins the right atrium. In right heart failure and tricuspid insufficiency, chronic passive venous congestion of the systemic circulation, indicated by liver enlargement, ascites, or pleural effusion, furnishes further indirect evidence for the diagnosis of right atrial dilatation.

In the *dorsoventral radiograph* the enlarged right atrium causes a bulge in the right cranial cardiac silhouette seen at 9 to 11 o'clock. Because the aortic arch overlies the right auricle, it is difficult to assess its relative contribution to the cranial cardiac border.

Quantitative evaluation of right heart enlargement. According to Hamlin (1968), measurements can be used to predict enlargement of individual chambers. In right ventricular enlargement the ratio L/R becomes larger than 2, and the ratio RH/LH becomes larger than 1.5. If the cardiothoracic ratio, $\dfrac{RH + LH}{LAT}$, is greater than 1.5, and if R does not approximate L, then there is further evidence for right ventricular enlargement.

ENLARGEMENT OF LEFT VENTRICLE, LEFT ATRIUM, AND AORTIC ARCH

The rules which govern left ventricular enlargement are basically the same as those mentioned for right ventricular enlargement. The most common left ventricular enlargement, that of mitral insufficiency, represents a combination of primary dilatation and secondary hypertrophy. The increased volume load placed on the ventricle by the valvular insufficiency is appropriately compensated for by dilatation associated with hypertrophy. This mechanism has been well established in man (Dodge and Baxley, 1968), and there is reason to believe that the same is true for dogs (Lord, Carmichael, and Tashjian, 1970).

As in right heart enlargement, the changes in size and contour of the left cardiac structures occur interdependently and should therefore be evaluated simultaneously. Pressure overload in aortic stenosis, to which the ventricle responds with hypertrophy, may cause little or no enlargement of the left cardiac silhouette, as was discussed earlier for pulmonic stenosis. The widened aortic arch calls attention to the underlying condition and suggests the diagnosis. In mitral insufficiency, the diagnosis of mild left ventricular enlargement is made more reliable by the concurrent enlargement of the left atrium.

The left ventricle. In contrast to right ventricular enlargement, left ventricular enlargement, increases the length of the heart axis more than the craniocaudal and transverse diameters of the cardiac silhouette. In early left ventricular enlargement the contour of the cardiac silhouette tends to remain nearly normal, and the condition is therefore not diagnosed. This is in part because the left ventricular outflow tract enlarges first and cannot be evaluated on conventional radiographs; it is obscured by the right ventricle and the pulmonary artery.

In the *lateral radiograph* (Fig. 3-26) the caudal cardiac border is straightened, caudally extended, and more nearly perpendicular to the sternum than normal. The caudal waist becomes less pronounced or disappears completely. The left ventricular border thus continues without visible separation into the ventral border of the left atrium. Therefore, it is difficult to assess the contribution of

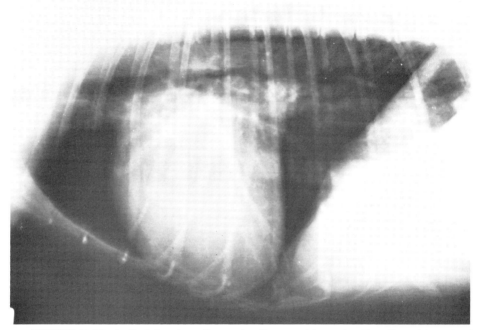

FIGURE 3-26 Left lateral radiograph, 7-year-old, male Poodle with mitral insufficiency, clinical signs of pulmonary congestion, and secondary right heart enlargement. The trachea runs nearly parallel with the spine, and its distal extremity is elevated, indicating cardiac enlargement in the dorsal direction. There is an air-filled structure with an irregular diameter dorsal to the left atrium which represents the left stem bronchus elevated by the enlarged left auricle. The right stem bronchus is seen ventral to the left stem bronchus and runs nearly parallel to it. Its lumen is not compressed dorsoventrally. The left atrium extends caudally, and there is no separation between the enlarged atrium and the dilated pulmonary veins, indicating pulmonary congestion. The caudal waist has become obscured, and there is even a slight bulge at the area. It is difficult to separate the ventricle from the atrium. The left ventricular border is straighter and more perpendicular to the spine than normal. There is also right ventricular enlargement which in this case is probably secondary to left ventricular enlargement.

either chamber to enlargement of the cardiac silhouette in the dorsal direction. The contribution of the atrium is usually underestimated, as can be shown angiocardiographically. The dorsal expansion of the left heart causes elevation of the hilar area. The angle between the trachea and the thoracic spine becomes more acute, or trachea and spine run parallel, and the ventral bend in the distal extremity of the trachea disappears.

In the *dorsoventral radiograph* (Figs. 3-27 and 3-28) the normally straight left cardiac border becomes convex and more like the normal right border. The distance between the left cardiac border and the thoracic wall decreases. The apex may become rounded, and the cardiac area lying to the left of the midsagittal plane increases, as does the distance from the midsagittal line to the widest lateral extension of the left border.

Radiographic findings in cardiac conditions frequently associated with left ventricular enlargement are summarized in Table 3-2. However, the other factors considered in the evaluation of cardiac conditions, such as age and clinical signs, must always be evaluated in making the differential diagnosis.

TABLE 3-2   COMMON CARDIAC CONDITIONS ASSOCIATED WITH LEFT VENTRICULAR ENLARGEMENT

CONDITION	RADIOGRAPHIC SIGNS
Mitral insufficiency	Left atrial enlargement; dorsal displacement of trachea; congestion of pulmonary veins; lung edema associated with right ventricular and generalized cardiac enlargement
Idiopathic cardiomyopathy	Usually generalized cardiac enlargement; congestion of pulmonary veins and ensuing edema
Aortic insufficiency (isolated or associated with aortic stenosis)	Aortic arch dilated; elongated cardiac silhouette extending far cranially into the mediastinum
Aortic stenosis	Prominent aortic arch due to poststenotic dilatation; secondary left atrial enlargement
Patent ductus arteriosus (left ventricular enlargement occurs with ensuing cardiac failure)	Prominent pulmonary artery segment; aneurysmal widening of aortic arch; left atrial and ventricular enlargement; dense, overcirculated lung field; right ventricular enlargement; congestion and edema ensue in longstanding disease
Atrial and ventricular septal defects (secondary enlargement of left ventricle if defect is large enough to cause volume overload)	Right ventricular enlargement; left atrial enlargement; dense, overcirculated lung field; congestion and edema ensue in longstanding, large defects; rarely, widened pulmonary artery segment

The left atrium.   Enlargement of this structure as seen in the *lateral radiograph* (Fig. 3-26) is probably the most frequently diagnosed abnormality of the cardiac contour. Since this almost invariably results from mitral insufficiency, left atrial and left ventricular enlargement usually coexist. Left atrial enlargement is directly responsible for elevation of the trachea. A disproportionate increase in size of the left atrium then elevates all left lobar bronchi which cross over it. The air-filled structure of the common origin of the left apical and cardiac lobar bronchi, which is normally superimposed on the trachea, thus becomes separated from the trachea. The left and right stem bronchi, which are normally superimposed, are forced apart and form a V-shaped structure. In excessive enlargement the central part of the atrium bulges dorsally between the two diaphragmatic bronchi, compressing the left stem bronchus dorsoventrally. The pulmonary veins widen at their junction with the enlarged atrium and appear more dense. For assessing the degree of left atrial enlargement, it is sometimes helpful to consider the distance between the dorsal border of the caudal vena cava and the junction of the left atrium and pulmonary veins. In hearts of normal dogs these structures are separated by only a few millimeters. When the atrium is enlarged and displaced dorsally, the distance may increase to 5 to 10 mm. or more, depending on the size of the patient, the severity of the atrial dilatation, and the degree of right heart involvement.

In the *dorsoventral radiograph* (Figs. 3-27 and 3-28) the left atrium is visible only after moderate to severe enlargement. The enlarged auricle extends beyond the left cardiac border and is visible as a double contour in the cranial half of the left ventricular silhouette. However, in extensive left ventricular enlargement the convex border of the ventricle completely obscures the bulging of the left atrium.

In massive enlargement of the left atrium its central portion is seen in radiographs made with enough penetration as a round, dense mass forcing the main stem bronchi apart. The normally acute angle widens and tends to become obtuse in severe cases. In extreme enlargement the central portion of the left atrium may

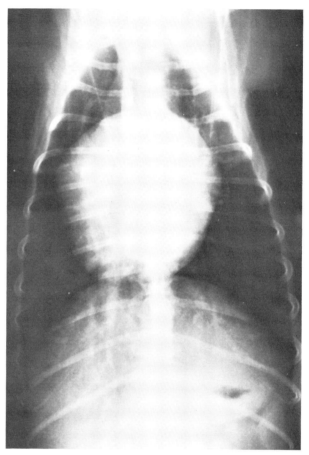

FIGURE 3-27   Dorsoventral radiograph, dog in Figure 3-26. The cardiac silhouette is enlarged due to concurrent left and right ventricular enlargement. The definite bulge of the left cardiac border caudal to the area of the pulmonary artery segment represents the dilated left auricle. Notice the rounded apex. The left ventricular enlargement is not obvious because the apex has shifted to the right side. The moderate right ventricular enlargement also contributes to this impression (compare with Figure 3-28, where the apex has shifted to the left side).

Notice that the lung field appears smaller in this dorsoventral projection than in the ventrodorsal projection in Figure 3-28.

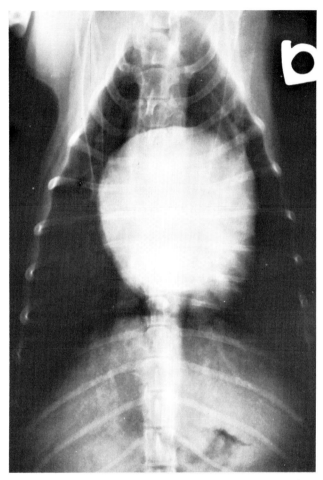

FIGURE 3-28   Ventrodorsal radiograph, dog in Figure 3-26, shown to illustrate the influence of positioning on the shape of the cardiac contour and the location of the apex. Notice that the apex now appears to the left of the midline. The left ventricular enlargement seems more pronounced than in Figure 3-27; however, the right ventricle is smaller than on the dorsoventral radiograph in Figure 3-27, and the left atrial bulge is not as prominent. The change in contour might have been slightly aggravated by the minimal change in the superimposition of the spine and sternum; on this ventrodorsal radiograph the sternum lies slightly to the left of the spine. The location of the apex can be verifield by locating the gas bubble in the stomach, which is always found on the left.

be displaced to the right side, causing a double shadow as it is superimposed on the caudal quadrant of the right ventricular silhouette (Rhodes, Patterson, and Detweiler, 1963). Left atrial enlargement is seen with mitral insufficiency, primary myocardial failure, and atrial fibrillation; it also occurs secondary to left-to-right shunts and aortic stenosis. Mitral stenosis is an extremely rare cause of left atrial enlargement.

The aortic arch.   Because of the wide variation in size and configuration of the aortic arch in normal dogs, the clinical significance of abnormalities is difficult to evaluate. An enlarged aortic arch is seen on both lateral and dorsoventral radiographs as an elliptical protrusion emerging from the cranial and right cardiac borders and extending into the cranial mediastinum. It then curves caudally and continues as the descending aorta. On the lateral radiograph the enlarged aortic arch may create a cranial protrusion in the area normally outlined by the right auricle. In both views the widened aortic arch simulates elongation of the cardiac silhouette. When a patent ductus arteriosus is present, the aortic arch is dilated in an aneurysmal widening and extends farther to the left side than normal. A poststenotic dilatation, as in aortic stenosis, sometimes displaces the trachea markedly to the right.

Quantitative evaluation of left heart enlargement (Hamlin, 1968).   An enlarged left ventricle is suspected if the ratio L/R is less than 0.5 and/or the ratio RH/LH is less than 2/3. At the same time, the cardiothoracic ratio, $\dfrac{RH + LH}{LAT}$, may be greater than 2/3, and L does not approximate R. In aortic stenosis and patent ductus arteriosus the ratio A/LC becomes larger than 0.5. As in the evaluation of the right heart, mild to moderate enlargement of the left heart cannot be diagnosed using measurements.

RECOGNITION OF CARDIAC FAILURE AND EXTRACARDIAC SIGNS OF HEART DISEASE

RECOGNITION OF CARDIAC FAILURE

Radiography is a valuable adjunct in determining the presence of cardiac decompensation. Occasionally radiographic signs compatible with heart failure may be apparent prior to the onset of clinical signs.

The analysis of radiographs consists of four steps:

1. *Detection* of signs compatible with heart failure, which presupposes familiarity with the normal heart and circulation.

2. Accurate *evaluation* of the changes, based on thorough knowledge of hemodynamic and morphologic changes underlying the various cardiac diseases.

3. *Correlation* of the roentgen signs with history, breed, age, sex, and clinical findings.

4. Exercise of *judgment* as to the most probable diagnosis under the circumstances.

Detection of signs of cardiac failure is based on the recognition of cardiac enlargement. Authorities agree that it is the most consistent indication of cardiac

TABLE 3-3   RADIOGRAPHIC SIGNS OF CARDIAC FAILURE

I. *Cardiac signs*	a. *Ventricular enlargement* Dilatation and/or hypertrophy Change in shape and position Differential diagnosis: compensatory dilatation, compensatory hypertrophy b. *Atrial enlargement* Dilatation, degree depending on plasticity and elasticity of wall and atrial pressure Displacement of extracardiac structures
II. *Extracardiac and circulatory signs* 1. *Left heart failure*	a. *Pulmonary signs* Dilated, dense veins indistinctly outlined Distended, prominent arteries Increased interstitial densities (congestion, interstitial edema) Alveolar densities (congestive pulmonary edema, alveolar edema) b. *Pleural signs* Pleural effusion
2. *Right heart failure*	a. Liver enlargement b. Ascites c. Pleural effusion d. Pericardial effusion e. Enlarged cranial and caudal venae cavae

disease (Sante, 1958). However, for a complete evaluation the pulmonary and systemic circulations, as well as the heart, must be included in the examination. Mere assessment of cardiac size is inadequate because cardiac failure and compensatory mechanism may both cause an increase in cardiac size. Furthermore, in instances such as arrhythmias or shock, cardiac failure may ensue with little or no cardiac enlargement. In such cases radiographic signs which indicate failure in the pulmonary or systemic circulation (left or right heart failure) are extremely important. Absence of extracardiac signs of heart failure on a radiograph does not preclude the possibility of cardiac disease. For example, pulmonary edema may be absent in patients dying in cardiogenic shock due to left heart failure (Luisada, 1967b).

The accurate evaluation of the radiographs is based on thorough knowledge of the hemodynamic changes expected when cardiac failure develops. By definition, the signs of cardiac failure ensue when the compensatory mechanisms of the heart become inadequate and the left or the right ventricle or both are unable to accept and expel the venous return throughout the range of physical activity (Friedberg, 1966). Failure of the ventricles follows an increased load (volume or pressure overload) or diminished contractility; quite commonly failure results from a combination of increased load and diminished contractility and leads to an inadequate cardiac output. The heart thus fails to maintain adequate pulmonary or systemic circulation, or both, resulting in pulmonary or systemic signs which can be recognized radiographically (see Table 3-3).

The evaluation of cardiac enlargement leads to different conclusions depending on whether it is due to cardiac hypertrophy, cardiac dilatation, or a combination of both. As has been mentioned earlier, cardiac dilatation and hypertrophy cannot be differentiated on the plain radiograph. Furthermore, false conclusions as to the severity of the disease must not be drawn from actual atrial or ventricular size; for example, left atrial size does not necessarily reflect the degree of mitral valvular insufficiency.

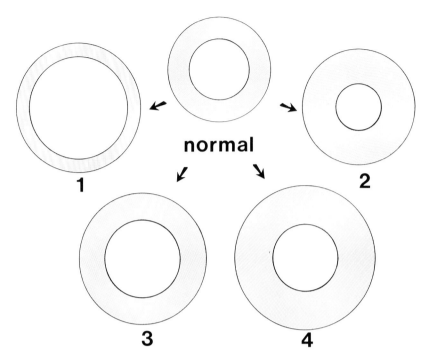

FIGURE 3-29 Diagrams representing the influence of concentric and eccentric dilatation and chronic hypertrophy on the size of the cardiac silhouette. The four possibilities can only be differentiated angiocardiographically. Use of the plain radiograph is limited to the diagnosis of normal cardiac size and enlargement. Therefore, it cannot be determined accurately whether cardiac failure (dilatation) or cardiac compensation (hypertrophy) is responsible for the enlarged silhouette. Furthermore, the presence of concentric hypertrophy cannot be excluded when the cardiac silhouette is of normal size. Therefore, the diagrams reflect the proportions as determined angiocardiographically.

Normal — Represents normal proportions between the muscular wall (shaded ring) and the ventricular lumen (central area). The cardiac silhouette is of normal size.

1 — *Cardiac dilatation* is marked by thinning of the muscular wall and an increase in the ventricular volume. Since the heart muscle becomes stretched in accommodating for the increased volume, the proportions between muscle mass and ventricular volume become unfavorable, and decompensation and cardiac failure eventually result; this is seen, for example, in myocardial disease. Radiographically, the cardiac silhouette is enlarged, and the condition cannot be differentiated from eccentric hypertrophy and mixed eccentric-concentric hypertrophy.

2 — *Concentric hypertrophy* (pure hypertrophy) is marked by an increased muscle mass with no change or often even a decrease in ventricular volume. The cardiac silhouette remains nearly normal in size, and the underlying hypertrophy will be unrecognized on the plain radiograph. Concentric hypertrophy occurs in response to a pressure overload in conditions such as aortic stenosis.

3 — *Eccentric hypertrophy.* The cardiac silhouette looks like a magnified image of the normal heart. The proportion between the mass of the ventricular wall and the ventricular volume has remained normal or near normal. An increase in the muscle mass of the ventricular wall compensates for the increase in volume by a process analogous to normal growth. The radiographically enlarged cardiac silhouette is the result of a compensatory mechanism which allows the heart to respond to an increased volume load without going into failure. Eccentric hypertrophy occurs in mitral insufficiency and cannot be considered a sign of cardiac failure (Grant, Green, and Bunnell, 1965).

Legend continues

Angiocardiography has been used successfully to differentiate dilatation and hypertrophy *in vivo*. By injecting contrast medium into the ventricles, the inner surface of the ventricular walls, which are not seen on the plain film, can be outlined, enabling measurement of the diameter of the ventricular wall or calculation of the ventricular volume.

Studies of left ventricular systolic and diastolic volumes in man and dogs have increased our knowledge of cardiac failure considerably (see Dodge and Baxley, 1968; Grant, Green, and Bunnell, 1965; Grant et al., 1968; Jarmakani et al., 1968). Lord et al. (1970) showed that results obtained in dogs are similar to those obtained in man. Results obtained by angiocardiography, which are important in understanding cardiac enlargement, are summarized as a diagram in Figure 3-29.

EXTRACARDIAC SIGNS OF HEART DISEASE

Pulmonary circulation. Pathologic changes of intrapulmonary vessels are characterized by increased or decreased density and diameter of the vessels, by variations in outline, and by farther extension into the periphery. Because of their subtle nature, many of these changes have gone unnoticed. Only the radiographic changes associated with dirofilariasis have been well described.

The radiographic changes of pulmonary arteries and veins associated with cardiac diseases are summarized in Figure 3-30.

The density of the pulmonary arteries must be evaluated relative to the density of the descending aorta and the pulmonary veins. Due attention must be paid to the background density of the lung field, which is determined by the phase of respiration, by changes in the fluid content in the interstitium or alveoli, and by nodular or linear interstitial opacities caused by present or previous pulmonary disease.

Undercirculation results from decreased pulmonary blood flow. The lung field is more lucent than normal. The arteries and veins appear thin and are sometimes barely visible because of a striking reduction in their size and density. Undercirculation occurs in congenital heart diseases associated with reduced pulmonary blood flow due to right-to-left shunting of blood. Undercirculation is commonly seen with tetralogy of Fallot (Figs. 18-55; 18-56; 18-58) and may also occur with ventricular septal defect or atrial septal defect complicated by pulmonic stenosis. In acquired conditions with decreased cardiac output, such as shock or adrenocortical hypofunction, the lung field may display undercirculation (Fig. 3-22). Overinflation and emphysematous lungs mimic undercirculation owing to the lucent appearance of the lung field.

FIGURE 3-29 *Continued 4—Mixed eccentric-concentric hypertrophy.* The cardiac silhouette looks like a magnified image of the heart with concentric hypertrophy, the difference being that both the size of the cardiac silhouette and the ventricular volume have increased as compared with the normal cardiac silhouette. The proportion between the mass of the ventricular wall and the ventricular volume is in favor of the muscle mass because of hypertrophy of the ventricular wall. Radiographically the heart appears enlarged. Mixed eccentric-concentric hypertrophy occurs in aortic stenosis with concurrent mitral insufficiency, where there is volume overload in addition to pressure overload.

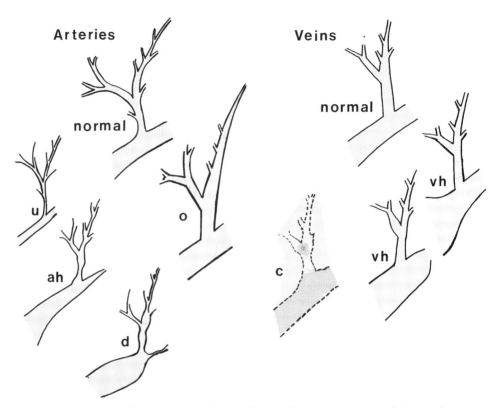

FIGURE 3-30 Diagrams of the radiographic appearance of the pulmonary arteries and veins in normal dogs and in dogs with heart disease.

Arteries—Normally, the arteries are denser and better defined than are the veins. They are often slightly curved craniolaterally, and they have more branches than do the veins.

u—Undercirculation. The arteries are thinner than normal, and their peripheral branches are barely visible in the lung field, which is frequently overinflated when undercirculation is present (see also Fig. 3-22).

o—Overcirculation. The arteries are denser, thicker, and straighter than normal. They also extend farther into the periphery. The lung field becomes denser than normal due to the increased number of vascular densities (see also Fig. 3-31).

ah—Arterial hypertension. The arteries appear denser than normal in the hilar and middle zones of the lungs. Sometimes they are more curved than normal. In the periphery they taper rapidly, and they occasionally have knot-like thickenings as they branch.

d—Hypertension due to dirofilariasis. The hilar and middle portions of the arteries are thickened and often distorted. In the middle zone of the lung field some arteries are pruned. The peripheral branches are thin and distorted and may have knot-like thickenings as they branch.

Veins—Normally, the veins are less dense and not as well delineated as are the arteries. They also appear straighter and coarser than the arteries.

vh—Venous hypertension. The appearance of the pulmonary veins in hypertension varies. In some cases, only the veins in the area of their junction with the left atrium appear dilated, whereas in others the dilatation extends all the way into the periphery, depending on the compensatory interference of reflex mechanisms causing contraction of the venous bed of the pulmonary circulation. The portions of the veins in the middle zone are usually denser than normal, and their opacity may occasionally surpass that of the arteries.

c—Pulmonary congestion. If the fluid which leaks from the arterial capillary bed fails to be resorbed, it accumulates in the perivascular interstitial tissue, resulting in a blurry, hazy outline of the venous structures.

86

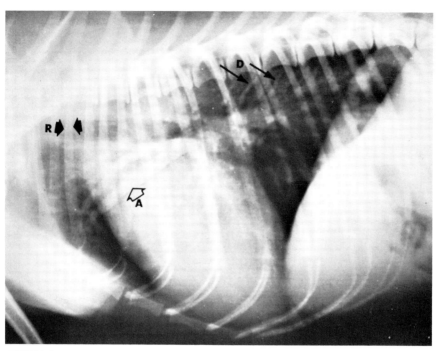

FIGURE 3-31 Left lateral radiograph, 1½-year-old, male Poodle with overcirculation of the lungs due to left-to-right shunting of blood with patent ductus
arteriosus. The apical lobar arteries (arrow A) are dilated, and their diameters exceed
that of the caudal third of the fourth rib (arrow R). Notice that the arteries are located
dorsal to the lucent bands representing the apical lobar bronchi. The lung field
caudal to the heart is denser than normal due to increased vascular densities. The
well-defined, parallel lines in the caudal diaphragmatic lobar area represent dilated
arteries (arrows D), and the less dense bands represent veins. The slight haziness of
the outlines is due to the ensuing interstitial edema, representing congestion. The
cardiac silhouette is enlarged. The cranial border extends farther cranially than
normal due to widening of the aortic arch and dilatation of the conus arteriosus and
the main pulmonary artery. The increased blood flow caused a volume overload of the
left side of the heart, resulting in left atrial dilatation and moderate left ventricular
enlargement.

Overcirculation is caused by an increased pulmonary blood flow. The arteries
and veins are obviously larger, denser, and straighter than normal, and they
extend farther into the periphery. On the lateral radiograph the small peripheral
arteries and veins become visible as straight, parallel lines in the dorsal third of
the diaphragmatic lobe (Fig. 3-31). The arteries in the middle zone of the lung
field appear as dense as or denser than the aorta. The arteries and veins of the
apical lobes are dilated, and their diameter occasionally exceeds that of the caudal
third of the fourth rib, as observed by Buchanan (1968b). Because of the increased
number and density of the intrapulmonary vessels, the lung field appears denser
than normal. Concurrent enlargement of the pulmonary artery segment of the
cardiac silhouette is occasionally seen on dorsoventral radiographs of dogs with
pulmonary overcirculation.

As pulmonary hypertension develops and as interstitial and/or alveolar edema ensue, the vascular structures become blurred, and the signs of over-circulation may no longer be recognized.

Overcirculation occurs in congenital heart diseases associated with left-to-right shunt, such as patent ductus arteriosus (Fig. 3-31), atrial septal defect, or ventricular septal defect. The visibility of the signs described depends on the amount of blood shunted and the duration of the disease.

Overcirculation is also observed with increased cardiac output such as occurs with long-standing, severe anemia. The enlarged vascular structures in over-circulation must be differentiated from purely arterial dilatation, as occurs with dirofilariasis. In overcirculation the arteries are of uniform diameter, they are not distorted, and they taper gradually toward the periphery. Hypervascularity of the lung field can also be due to active congestion in inflammatory pulmonary disease.

Pulmonary hypertension (see Cor Pulmonale, Chapter 16) must be divided into arterial hypertension and venous or postcapillary hypertension. Arterial hypertension results from increased resistance in the arteries, as in dirofilariasis, or from increased resistance in the capillary bed, as in diffuse pulmonary diseases such as pulmonary fibrosis or emphysema. Most often, however, arterial hypertension arises secondarily to venous hypertension.

The radiographic signs of pulmonary arterial hypertension are difficult to evaluate except in dirofilariasis, where there is moderate to excessive widening of the arteries in the hilar and middle zones of the lung field and distortion, thinning, or sudden pruning in the periphery (Fig. 16-6). Arterial hypertension unrelated to dirofilariasis is suggested by widening of the arteries in the hilar and middle zones of the lungs and rapid thinning with uninterrupted outline toward the periphery.

Left heart failure. Venous hypertension in dogs most frequently follows a "backing-up" of blood in the left atrium due to mitral insufficiency and left heart failure. Since pulmonary veins do not have valves, retrograde transmission of pressure waves is facilitated. Arterial hypertension then arises secondarily to venous hypertension. Reflex mechanisms, rather than a purely mechanical trans-mission of the left atrial and venous "back-pressure" to the pulmonary veins and arteries, are considered responsible for secondary pulmonary hypertension (Braun and Stern, 1967).

If radiographs of the lung field can be obtained throughout the development of left heart failure, it becomes apparent that there are several phases of pul-monary involvement in this condition. The initial venous engorgement is followed by interstitial edema and finally by alveolar edema. This subdivision into three phases is arbitrary, and exceptions are frequent. However, the description and the understanding of the radiographic changes are greatly facilitated by a systematic approach.

Pulmonary signs are not apparent in all dogs with left heart failure. The cor-relation between pulmonary vascular signs and clinical findings is sometimes poor. In dogs with obvious left heart failure due to ruptured chordae tendineae, pul-monary vascular signs are often minimal or absent on the radiograph, indicating the compensatory interference of reflex mechanisms.

The radiographic signs of the first phase, in which venous engorgement is the primary sign of left heart failure, include nearly normal lucency of the lung field. The pulmonary veins are distended and appear as dense as or denser than the pulmonary arteries. The venous distention may be confined to the hilar portions of the lung field or may be seen extending into the middle zone. In lateral radiographs a greatly increased number of circular opacities 1 to 3 mm. in diameter become visible in the middle zone of the lung field. These structures represent end on views of dilated peripheral veins.

The second phase, characterized by interstitial edema, ensues as the pulmonary venous pressure rises owing to progressive left heart failure, and the arterial side of the pulmonary circulation becomes affected. Secondary pulmonary arterial hypertension develops, and pulmonary congestion is seen. The density of the lung field increases because of leakage of fluid from the capillaries into the perivascular interstitial tissue. The venous reabsorption of interstitial fluid is diminished, producing interstitial edema or pulmonary congestion (Fig. 3-32). The resulting diffuse, hazy density of the lung field is of the interstitial type (Suter and Chan, 1968). The vascular structures in the middle zone become obscured, and the larger hilar vessels, especially the dense veins, become blurred. This diffuse haziness must be carefully differentiated from apparent increased densities of the lung field resulting from underexposure or an exposure made during the expiratory pause.

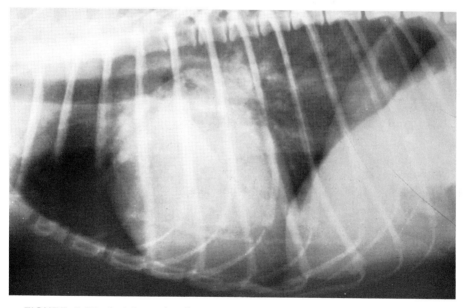

FIGURE 3-32 Left lateral radiograph, 12½-year-old, female Wirehair Fox Terrier with a murmur characteristic of mitral insufficiency and roentgen signs of pulmonary congestion. The distal portion of the trachea is elevated and runs nearly parallel with the thoracic spine. The left stem bronchus, which is visible as a narrow, dark band, is elevated by the enlarged left atrium. Both left and right ventricles are slightly enlarged. The generalized haziness of the lung field fades toward the periphery. An indistinct linear pattern underlies the haziness. The vascular structures are seen only in the hilar zone of the lung field, and their outlines are extremely blurred. The round, blurred densities in the diaphragmatic lobes are end-on views of distended intrapulmonary vessels. The descending aorta is obscured by the increased pulmonary density. The apical lobe is less involved, and the slightly enlarged veins remain visible.

The pulmonary arteries appear denser than normal. A large number of round opacities 1 to 3 mm. in diameter representing end-on views of dilated arteries or veins stand out against the hazy background of the lung field. Since the transudate is confined to the interstitial tissue, fluid does not accumulate in the alveoli, and râles cannot be auscultated during this second phase.

Depending on the compensating potential of the heart, the disease may become stabilized or may progress to pulmonary alveolar edema, the third phase. In a stabilized circulation the congestion results in connective tissue formation and fibrotic changes in the interstitium. The radiographic signs of fibrosis are greatly increased amounts of nonvascular linear densities, discrete polygonal nodules 1 to 2 mm. in diameter (Suter and Chan, 1968), or both. A slight to moderate degree of fibrotic changes is not pathognomonic for chronic congestion. They are regularly observed in older dogs without clinical evidence of current pulmonary or cardiovascular disease (Reif and Rhodes, 1966).

As heart failure progresses into the third phase, fluid begins to exude into the alveoli and leads to pulmonary alveolar edema. During this phase, râles are auscultated clinically. Both cardiac and systemic vascular mechanisms are involved in the development of pulmonary edema (Luisada, 1967b).

Pulmonary edema (Fig. 3-33) is recognized radiographically by an alveolar density characterized as follows (Suter and Chan, 1968):

1. Ill-defined, fluffy margins of the infiltrate fading into the surrounding unaffected lung.

2. Tendency of the infiltrates to coalesce.

3. Presence of "air-bronchograms" and "air-alveolograms" within the infiltrated areas. "Air-bronchograms" refer to the visualization of the air-containing bronchi as radiolucent bands within the lung parenchyma which is filled with transudate. "Air-alveolograms" are small radiolucencies representing groups of air-filled alveoli among the more opaque, fluid-filled alveoli which give the infiltrate a mottled appearance.

4. Central location of the infiltrate, obscuring the cardiac silhouette, and fading of the densities toward the periphery, which is apparently uninvolved.

The characteristics of pulmonary alveolar edema are shown in Figure 3-33. The widened pulmonary arteries remain visible in radiographs made with good penetration, whereas the veins are usually obscured by the edema. Except for the distribution of the infiltrates, pulmonary alveolar edema may be indistinguishable from pulmonary infiltration due to an inflammatory process such as pneumonia, from which it must be differentiated.

Right heart failure.   Right heart failure frequently occurs secondary to left heart failure; therefore, the radiographic signs are those of general cardiac failure and are not pathognomonic for right heart failure. Unless the condition is severe, the radiographic appearance is less obvious than in left heart failure. Since the radiographic signs seen with right heart failure are ambiguous and can also be caused by a large number of extracardiac diseases, careful evaluation of the differential diagnosis is essential.

Marked dilatation, increased density, and distortion of the caudal vena cava are frequent in right heart failure. The enlarged vein can be seen within the cardiac silhouette. The caudal vena cava varies greatly in size with inspiration and expira-

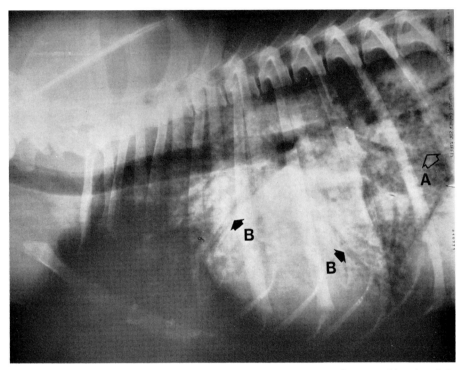

FIGURE 3-33 Left lateral radiograph, 10-year-old, male German Shepherd dog with pulmonary alveolar edema due to left heart failure. The trachea is elevated by the greatly enlarged heart. The left atrium and right and left ventricles are enlarged. The lung field appears mottled due to a large number of patchy densities which tend to coalesce. The dark bands, air-bronchograms (arrows B), represent the air-filled, lucent bronchi which stand out in bold contrast against the denser background of the fluid-filled parenchyma. At arrow A an area of extreme mottling is indicated, representing interdigitation of groups of dense, fluid-filled and lucent, air-filled alveoli referred to as air-alveolograms. The patchy densities are fluffy and are more numerous around the hilar area. The apical lobar area is less involved. The peripheral lobar areas appear overinflated.

tion, and assessment of its true diameter is difficult. Occasionally the junction of the caudal vena cava with the right atrium appears elevated because of the concurrent enlargement of the right ventricle; this sign can be used diagnostically.

Widening of the precardial mediastinum, which is due in part to dilatation of the cranial vena cava, is seen occasionally in right heart failure. On the lateral radiograph the mediastinal silhouette also extends farther ventrally than normal.

Enlargement of the caudal vena cava is usually accompanied by hepatomegaly, congestion of the abdominal organs, and ascites. Blurring of the outlines of the abdominal organs is characteristic of small effusions. Large effusions give the abdomen a ground-glass-like appearance (Fig. 3-34). Since ascites is seen with a large number of extracardiac diseases, careful evaluation of the differential diagnosis as to type and origin of the fluid is required.

Hepatomegaly causes rounding of the lobar borders. Hepatomegaly due to fatty infiltration usually appears less dense than that due to congestion. Liver size is difficult to assess unless enlargement is marked. Since ascites often occurs with hepatomegaly the liver size cannot be evaluated accurately because fluid obscures the details. In such cases a barium swallow is sometimes helpful in outlining the caudal displacement of the stomach by the enlarged liver. If the fluid can be removed and is replaced by gas (air or carbon dioxide), the details of the liver can be visualized by the pneumoperitoneum (Fig. 3-35).

PLEURAL EFFUSION. Transudation of fluid into the pleural space indicates impaired lymphatic drainage due to pulmonary hypertension or, more frequently, elevated systemic venous pressure and is thus seen in both left and right heart failure. Small pleural effusions are found on postmortem examination in 1 per cent of all dogs with right heart failure or combined right and left heart failure (Liu, 1969). Pleural effusion or hydrothorax is an important aid in radiographic diagnosis of heart failure. Small amounts of fluid are difficult to see radiographically unless special positioning is used. According to our experimental results, 50 ml. of fluid in a medium-sized dog or 100 ml. of fluid in a large dog, such as the German Sheperd, are normally not visible either on recumbent or standing lateral radiographs with horizontal beam. On radiographs made with the dog in the erect position these small amounts of fluid might cause the costophrenic angle to appear rounded and somewhat blurred. Amounts of at least 100 ml. of fluid in a medium-sized dog and 200 ml. in a large dog can easily be seen in the standing lateral radiograph; however, they are usually overlooked if the radiograph is made with the dog in the recumbent position. Larger amounts of fluid are seen regardless of positioning; the interlobar fissures are outlined, the lung lobes are retracted from the thoracic wall (Fig. 3-37), and the thorax has a ground-glass-like appearance (Fig. 3-36).

Since pleural effusion may also be seen with conditions such as pleuritis, chylothorax, hemothorax, and tumors, one should be particularly careful in making a differential diagnosis as to its origin. Extreme obesity and a localized accumulation of fat pads at the retrosternal area can mimic pleural effusions, as has been shown by Carlson (1967). An extremely obese dog with a large retrosternal fat pad and pleural effusion due to cardiac failure is shown in Figure 3-38.

PERICARDIAL EFFUSION. Small and moderate pericardial effusions are even more difficult to diagnose than small pleural effusions (see Fig. 3-37). For the diagnostic procedures applied, see Fluoroscopic Examination (pp. 96–98) and Pericarditis (Chapter 15).

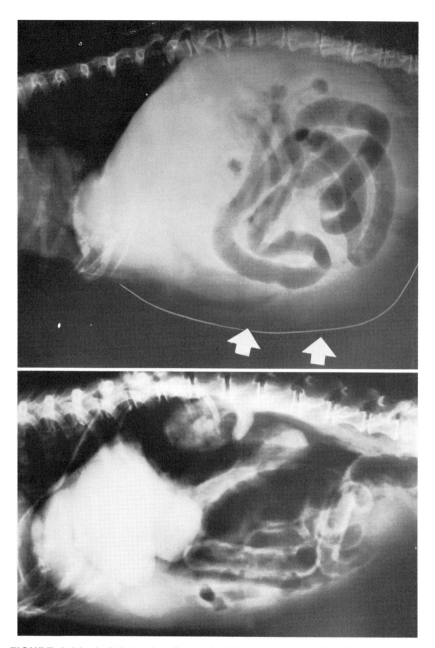

FIGURE 3-34 Left lateral radiograph, 15-year-old, male Dachshund with severe signs of right heart failure. The abdomen is dilated and has a ground-glass appearance. With the exception of some dilated small intestinal loops the details are extremely blurred. The increased density in the cranial abdomen is due to the congested liver; its rounded lobar borders are barely visible in the ventral abdomen. Edema of the abdominal wall and the subcutaneous tissue is indicated by the lack of definition of the abdominal wall and the unusual shape of the prepuce (arrows). Notice that the lung field remained clear.

FIGURE 3-35 Pneumoperitoneum of the dog in Figure 3-34 after removal of 3 liters of fluid from the abdomen by paracentesis and injection of 500 ml. of air. The radiograph was exposed in the left lateral recumbency. Notice the decrease in size of the abdomen. The rounded liver lobes are now well delineated, and the liver enlargement can be better assessed. Some fluid is still present in the ventral abdomen.

93

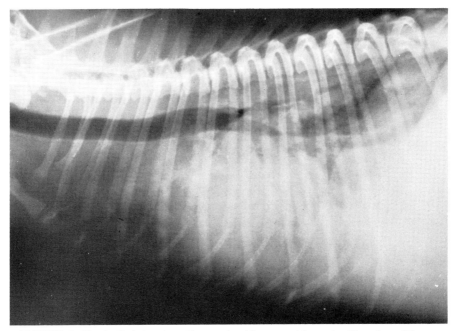

FIGURE 3-36 Left lateral radiograph, 10-year-old, male Beagle with severe clinical signs of right and left heart failure. The density of the thoracic cavity is greatly increased, obscuring the details of the cardiac silhouette and the lungs. The trachea stands out in bold contrast against the density of the lung field and runs nearly parallel with the thoracic spine. The distal extremity of the trachea and the left stem bronchus are elevated, indicating left atrial enlargement. The slight dorsal bend of the trachea cranial to the carina indicates right atrial enlargement. The enlarged right ventricle is obscured by pleural effusion. The cardiac silhouette is displaced caudally. An ill-defined lobar border of the lung is seen in the apical area. The visibility of the air-filled bronchi suggests the presence of pulmonary edema. A standing lateral radiograph with the x-ray beam directed horizontally would be advantageous in demonstrating the thoracic fluid.

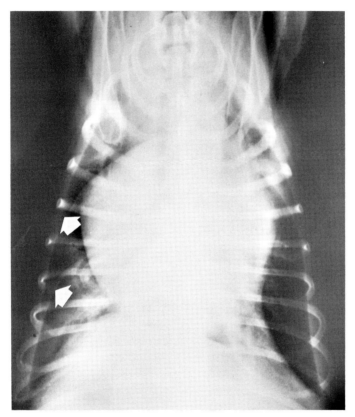

FIGURE 3-37   Dorsoventral radiograph, dog in Figure 3-36. The roentgen signs indicating pleural effusion are much better delineated in the dorsoventral view than on the lateral radiograph. The separation of the lung lobes from the thoracic wall by a layer of fluid is well visualized. The accumulation of fluid in the apical lobar area made these lobes retract caudally. The mediastinum appears widened. The right cardiophrenic angle is typically rounded. The accumulation of fluid in the interlobar fissures is well outlined on the right side of the thorax (arrows).

The cardiac silhouette is greatly enlarged and well rounded, indicating that some pericardial effusion is present in addition to the pleural effusion. The excessively broad cardiophrenic ligament favors the assumption of a pericardial effusion.

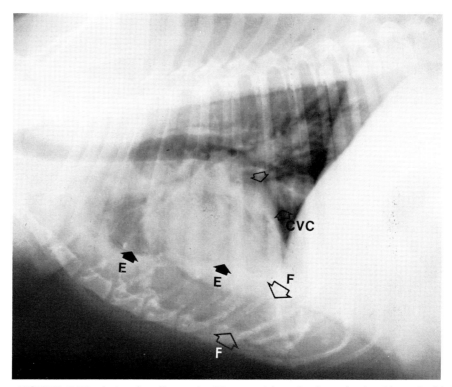

FIGURE 3-38 Lateral radiograph, 12-year-old, male dog of mixed breed which was extremely obese and was unable to walk due to respiratory difficulties and weakness. The thorax appears wider than normal. The heart is separated from the sternum by a lucent pad 3 cm. wide (arrows F) representing a retrosternal fat mass. The retrosternal accumulation of fat must not be confused with pleural effusion, from which it is differentiated by its lesser density. Dorsal to the border of the fat pad there is a second hazy separation of the lobar borders of the lung from a slightly denser area which represents pleural effusion (arrows E).

Both the right and left sides of the heart are enlarged. The cardiac silhouette is ill-defined because of the presence of hazy, patchy densities in the diaphragmatic lobes. These densities indicate pulmonary congestion and edema. Between the arrows a dense, ill-defined structure is seen which is superimposed on the cardiac silhouette. This is the greatly dilated caudal vena cava (CVC), which indicates right heart failure.

SPECIAL TECHNIQUES OF RADIOGRAPHIC EXAMINATION

FLUOROSCOPY

Cardiac fluoroscopy is an important part of the radiographic examination in man (Friedberg, 1966; Meschan, 1966). This technique has been used in veterinary medicine (Pommer, 1935; Wüller, 1953), but it has not assumed the same importance as it has in human medicine. The main reason for the infrequent use of fluoroscopy is the inherent danger of radiation exposure for the examiner and his assistants when a conventional fluoroscopic unit is used.

There are other disadvantages of conventional fluoroscopy. The image cannot be stored. Fluoroscopy is no substitute for plain film radiography. It is easier to evaluate details on a stationary radiograph than from a continuously changing fluoroscopic image. Fifteen to 20 minutes are required for the examiner to adapt to a dark room so that all details of the fluoroscopic image can be evaluated. However, because of lack of time the examiner often neglects proper adaptation to darkness, and in order to compensate for the poor visibility and resolution he tends to use more radiation than would be required after complete adaptation to darkness. This greatly increases the radiation hazard to the examiner and his environment. Unless an image intensifier is available, the use of fluoroscopy should be restricted to the observation of abnormal patterns of motion in the heart or the esophagus.

Image intensification systems increase the brightness of the fluoroscopic image several thousand times, making fluoroscopy far less hazardous. Because of the high cost of these units, however, they are impractical for use in private practice.

Fluoroscopy is essential in cardiac catheterization procedures to control the advancement and location of the tip of the catheter. The combination of image intensification with cineangiography has yielded one of the most rewarding methods of cardiac examination (see Cardiac Catheterization and Angiocardiography (Chapter 5).

In most dogs tranquilization is advisable prior to fluoroscopy. The positioning of the patient depends on the facilities available and on the purpose of the examination. The standing lateral position advocated by Pommer (1935) can be supplemented by other positions in special cases. It is the method of choice in all cases in which pericardial effusion is suspected. Examination with the animal lying on its side, then rotating it around its longitudinal axis, also provides satisfactory results in diagnosing pericardial effusion (Olsson, 1969; Wüller, 1953).

Fluoroscopic examination begins with study of the lung field and mediastinum. The lungs, the diaphragm, and the trachea are carefully evaluated for abnormal motion and for changes in position in dorsoventral and lateral views. Asymmetries are best seen in the dorsoventral view. The heart itself is then evaluated for abnormal size, density, and location, and for rate, rhythm, and amplitude of pulsation.

In some cases an esophagram can be done to outline the position of the esophagus relative to the great vessels and cardiac chambers. For example, with left heart enlargement the contrast-filled esophagus may be indented and in some cases displaced (see The Esophagram, pp. 98–99).

Fluoroscopic examination may assist in making the correct diagnosis of tumors of the hilar area or rare conditions such as aortic or cardiac aneurysm and pericardial rupture and herniation with incarceration of the heart.

Fluoroscopy can be useful in differentiating pericardial effusion from cardiac enlargement, which appear similar radiographically. With pericardial effusion the cardiac silhouette looks globular and tends to appear flattened wherever it touches the thoracic wall. As pericardial fluid accumulates, the cardiac pulsations become dampened or may be absent. Instead of distinct pulsation, undulation is observed. Pericardial effusion is indicated by a difference in pulsation at the dorsal, cranial, and caudal borders of the heart in the standing lateral position; pulsation is barely discernible at the cranial border, is dampened at the caudal border, and is normal at the hilus. In the recumbent position the pulsation or undulation is diminished at the ventral portion of the heart, in contrast with the normal pulsation noticeable at the hilar area. Weak pulsations are also seen in dogs with severe cardiac dilatation and failure and with peritoneopericardial hernias.

If the dog is examined in different positions, such as the standing lateral and erect positions, the pericardial fluid shifts to the dependent part of the pericardium, where the contour of the cardiac silhouette broadens. If free gas is present in the pericardial space owing to gas-forming organisms or previous puncture of the pericardium, a fluid level becomes visible. On both plain radiographs and fluoroscopic examination, only large effusions can be diagnosed. Because small amounts of fluid, as well as considerable cardiac enlargement, are present in many dogs with cardiac failure, differentiation between these two conditions is often impossible.

THE ESOPHAGRAM

Because of the close anatomical relationship of the esophagus to the mediastinal structures, the aorta and its branches, the veins, and the left atrium, enlargement or abnormal arrangement of these structures can be evaluated indirectly by examining the esophagus for indentations, constrictions, or displacement. Since the esophagus is not normally visible on plain radiographs, a barium swallow is necessary for its delineation.

A plain radiograph must be made prior to the administration of contrast medium. Barium sulfate paste (Micropaque or a similar commercial product) or a mixture of barium sulfate with water (equal volumes of each) having the consistency of whipped cream is used for outlining the esophagus.

Radiographs in ventrodorsal and lateral projections must be exposed immediately after the animal has swallowed the contrast medium. The ventrodorsal view can be slightly oblique to avoid superimposition of spine and esophagus, which might otherwise obscure the suspected lesion (Carlson, 1967). Fluoroscopic examination is indicated for study of esophageal function. Minor abnormalities such as small strictures are easily overlooked on radiographs and can only be diagnosed fluoroscopically, but dilatations are usually well outlined on radiographs (Carlson, 1967).

Delineation of a nondilated, normally functioning esophagus to demonstrate a displacement may be difficult because of the minimal amount of barium which adheres to normal esophageal mucosa. In these cases it is necessary to administer contrast medium prior to every examination.

Esophagrams successfully demonstrate the constriction and subsequent cranial dilatation caused by a persistent right aortic arch or an aberrant aortic branch. An esophagram is sometimes necessary to aid in the radiographic diagnosis of heartbase tumors or cardiac enlargement. The contrast study is also helpful in those cases in which pulmonary edema or pleural effusion obscures the details at the base of the heart. Tumors such as chemodectomas, lymphomas, or hemangiosarcomas may cause displacement and indentation of the barium-filled precardial portion of the esophagus. The caudal portion of the esophagus can be displaced by a greatly enlarged left atrium. However, in dogs the esophagram is not used routinely to confirm left atrial enlargement, because the diagnosis can easily be made from a plain radiograph. This differs from the cardiac examination in man, where the esophagram is a routine procedure for demonstrating left atrial enlargement (Friedberg, 1966; Meschan, 1966).

CARDIAC TOMOGRAPHY

Tomography, also called laminagraphy, planigraphy, or body-section technique, is a radiographic technique which is seldom used in veterinary medicine. Tomography enables demonstration of serial planes of the body without interference of superimposed densities. The desired plane is distinguished by blurring out the structures in the superficial and deeper layers. This is achieved by connecting the x-ray tube and the cassette tray by a rod which is fixed at a fulcrum. During exposure the tube and the cassette are moved in opposite directions relative to the fulcrum. The axis of motion and the plane to be examined are thus determined by the fulcrum. The level so determined is the only level of the object which is not blurred out. Details are thus delineated without the use of contrast medium.

Few references to tomography appear in the veterinary literature, although it is a simple and valuable radiographic technique. Geary (1965, 1967) has applied it to examinations of the skull, the spine, and the scapula. He also mentions its usefulness in demonstrating mediastinal densities such as tumors.

At The Animal Medical Center, tomography has been used successfully to study structures of the heart base and also the lung field, mainly the pulmonary vasculature.

Most conventional x-ray units can accommodate a device to make tomograms. The technique is not complicated if the fundamentals are understood. Detailed discussions are available in the medical literature (Andrews, 1936; Jacobi and Paris, 1964; Kiefer, 1943).

For tomography of the hilar area or the lungs, the dog must be anesthetized and intubated. The fulcrum is then set at the level from which a detailed radiograph is to be obtained. The sections can be done longitudinally or transversely, depending on the position of the dog on the roentgen table. Respiratory motion is suspended by first hyperventilating the animal and then mildly compressing the rebreathing bag for about 1 to 2 seconds, during which time the exposure is made.

References

Andrews, J. R.: Planigraphy. Amer. J. Roentgen., 36 (1936): 575.
Braun, K., and Stern, S.: Functional Significance of the Pulmonary Venous System. Amer. J. Cardiol., 20 (1967): 56.
Brill, I. C.: Cor Pulmonale: A Semantic Consideration with Brief Notes on Diagnosis and Treatment. Dis. Chest, 33 (1958): 658.
Buchanan, J. W.: Selective Angiography and Angiocardiography in Dogs with Acquired Cardiovascular Disease. J. Amer. Vet. Radiol. Soc., 6 (1965): 5.

Buchanan, J. W.: Radiology of the Heart. Seminar, 35th Annual Meeting of the American Animal Hospital Association, Las Vegas, Nev. 1968a.

Buchanan, J. W.: Symposium: Thoracic Surgery in the Dog and Cat. III. Patent Ductus Arteriosus and Persistent Right Aortic Arch Surgery in Dogs. J. Small Anim. Pract., 9 (1968b): 409.

Buchanan, J. W., and Patterson, D. F.: Selective Angiography and Angiocardiography in Dogs with Congenital Heart Disease. J. Amer. Vet. Radiol. Soc., 6 (1965): 20.

Canossi, G. C., Dardari, M., Cortesi, M., Brunelli, B., and Pasquinelli, C.: Anatomia Angiografica del Cane. Minerva Medica, Torino, Italy. 1959.

Carlson, W. D.: Veterinary Radiology, 2nd ed. Lea & Febiger, Philadelphia. 1967.

Detweiler, D. K., and Patterson, D. F.: The prevalence and types of cardiovascular disease in dogs. Ann. N. Y. Acad. Sci., 127 (1965): 481.

Detweiler, D. K., Patterson, D. F., Luginbühl, H., Rhodes, W. H., Buchanan, J. W., Knight, D. H., and Hill, J. D.: Diseases of the Cardiovascular System in Canine Medicine. Edited by E. J. Catcott. 1st Catcott ed. American Veterinary Publications, Santa Barbara, Calif. (1968): 559.

Dodge, H. T., and Baxley, W. A.: Hemodynamic Aspects of Heart Failure. Amer. J. Cardiol., 22 (1968): 24.

Douglas, S. W., and Williamson, H. D.: Principles of Veterinary Radiography. Williams & Wilkins Co., Baltimore. 1963.

Friedberg, C. K.: Diseases of the Heart. 3rd ed. W. B. Saunders Co., Philadelphia. 1966.

The Fundamentals of Radiography. 11th ed. Eastman Kodak Company, Rochester, N.Y. 1968.

Geary, J. C.: Tomography — Its Place in Veterinary Radiology. The Newer Knowledge about Dogs. Gaines Research Center, New York. 1965.

Geary, J. C.: Veterinary Tomography. J. Amer. Vet. Radiol. Soc., 8 (1967): 32.

Grant, C., Greene, D. G., and Bunnell, I. L.: Left Ventricular Enlargement and Hypertrophy. A Clinical and Angiocardiographic Study. Amer. J. Med., 39 (1965): 895.

Grant, C., Raphael, M. J., Steiner, R. E., and Goodwin, J. F.: Left Ventricular Volume and Hypertrophy in Outflow Obstruction. Cardiovasc. Res., 4 (1968): 346.

Gratzl, E.: Herzkrankheiten und ihre Diagnostik beim Hund. Berl. Münch. tierärztl. Wschr., 78 (1965): 45.

Hamlin, R. L.: Angiocardiography for the Clinical Diagnosis of Congenital Heart Disease in Small Animals. J. A. V. M. A., 135 (1959): 112.

Hamlin, R. L.: Radiographic Anatomy of the Heart and Great Vessels in Healthy Living Dogs. J. A. V. M. A., 136 (1960a): 265.

Hamlin, R. L.: Radiographic Diagnosis of Heart Disease in Dogs. J. A. V. M. A., 137 (1960b): 458.

Hamlin, R. L.: Analysis of the Cardiac Silhouette in Dorsoventral Radiographs from Dogs with Heart Disease. J. A. V. M. A., 153 (1968): 1446.

Jacobi, C. A., and Paris, D. Q.: X-Ray Technology. 3rd ed. C. V. Mosby Co., St. Louis. 1964.

Jarmakani, M. M., Edwards, S. B., Spach, M. S., Canent, R. V., Capp. M. P., Hagan, M. J., Barb, R. C., and Jain, V.: Left Ventricular Pressure–Volume Characteristics in Congenital Heart Disease. Circulation, 37 (1968): 879.

Kiefer, J.: The General Principles of Body-Section Radiography. Radiog. Clin. Photog., 19 (1943): 2.

Liu, S.-K.: Personal communication. 1969.

Lord, P. F., Carmichael, J. A., and Tashjian, R. J.: Single-Plane Cineangiocardiographic Determinations of Left Ventricular Volume in Normal and Diseased Canine Hearts. Amer. J. Vet. Res., 1970 (in press).

Luisada, A. A.: Symposium on the Pulmonary Heart and the Cardiac Lung (Intro.). Amer. J. Cardiol., 20 (1967a): 1.

Luisada, A. A.: Paroxysmal Pulmonary Edema and the Acute Cardiac Lung. Amer. J. Cardiol., 20 (1967b): 69.

Meschan, I.: Radiology of the Heart. In Roentgen Signs in Clinical Practice. Vol. II. W. B. Saunders Co., Philadelphia. (1966): 1024.

Miller, M. E., Christensen, G. C., and Evans, H. E.: Anatomy of the Dog. W. B. Saunders Co., Philadelphia. 1966.

Moritz, F.: Dtsch. Arch. Klin. Med., 82 (1904-1905): 1. Cited in Schaller, O: Anatomische Grundlagen der Roentgendarstellung des Hundeherzens. 1953.

Olsson, St. E.: Personal communication (1969).

Patterson, D. F., and Botts, R. P.: A Simple Cassett Changer. Small Anim. Clin., 1 (1961): 1.

Patterson, D. F., and Flickinger, G. L.: Subarotic Stenosis in a Boxer. Clinico-Pathologic Conference. J. A. V. M. A., 145 (1964): 363.

Pommer, A.: Die Röntgendiagnostik und Therapie in der Veterinärmedizin. Wien. Tierärztl. Mschr., 22 (1935): 321.

Reif, J. S., and Rhodes, W. H.: The Lungs of Aged Dogs: A Radiographic-Morphologic Correlation. J. Amer. Vet. Radiol. Soc., 7 (1966): 5.

Rhodes, W. H., Patterson, D. F., and Detweiler, D. K.: Radiographic Anatomy of the Canine Heart. Part I. J. A. V. M. A., 137 (1960): 283.

Rhodes, W. H., Patterson, D. F., and Detweiler, D. K.: Radiographic Anatomy of the Canine Heart. Part II. J. A. V. M. A., 143 (1963): 137.

Sante, L. R.: Principles of Roentgenological Interpretation. 11th ed. Edwards Brothers, Inc., Ann Arbor, Mich. 1958.

Schaller, O.: Anatomische Grundlagen der Röntgendarstellung des Hundeherzens. Acta Anat. Separatum, 17 (1953): 273.

Schulze, W., and Nöldner, H.: Röntgenologische Fernaufnahme des Hundeherzens und Versuch ihrer Deutung mit Hilfe einer linearen Messmethode. Arch. Exp. Veterinärmed., 11 (1957): 442.

Suter, P. F., and Chan, K. F.: Disseminated Pulmonary Diseases in Small Animals: A Radiographic Approach to Diagnosis. J. Amer. Vet. Radiol. Soc., 9 (1968): 67.

Tashjian, R. J., and Albanese, N. M.: A Technique of Canine Angiocardiography. J. A. V. M. A., 136 (1960): 359.

Uhlig, K., and Werner, J.: Eine röntgenographische Methode zur Messung der Herzvergrösserung beim Hund. Berl. Münchr. tierärztl. Wschr., 82 (1969): 110.

Wüller, H.: Röntgenologische Untersuchungen über das Hundeherz. Mh. Veterinärmed., 8 (1953): 475.

Wyburn, R. S., and Lawson, D. D.: Simple Radiography as an Aid to the Diagnosis of Heart Disease in the Dog. J. Small Anim. Pract., 8 (1967): 163.

CHAPTER
4

ELECTROCARDIOGRAPHY

It is recognized that normal and abnormal electrocardiographic measurements overlap and that the criteria for the normal electrocardiogram serve only as a guide for the clinician. Deviations from normal in an individual electrocardiogram suggest but are not always diagnostic of heart disease. As additional statistical data become available for the electrocardiograms of dogs of each breed, body type, age, and sex, the data herein may require revision, and "normal" may be more precisely defined. The *value of serial electrocardiograms* from an individual cannot be overemphasized, since serial changes best demonstrate electrocardiographic abnormalities.

CRITERIA FOR THE NORMAL CANINE ELECTROCARDIOGRAM*

Heart rate; 70 to 160 beats/min. for adult dogs; up to 180 beats/min. in toy breeds, and 220 beats/min. for puppies.

Heart rhythm: Normal sinus rhythm; sinus arrhythmia; and wandering sinoatrial pacemaker.

P wave: Up to 0.4 mv. in amplitude; up to 0.04 sec. in duration; always positive in leads II and aVF; positive or isoelectric in lead I.

P–R interval: 0.06 to 0.13 sec. duration.

QRS complex: Mean electrical axis, frontal plane, 40° to 100°.

    Amplitude—Maximum amplitude of R wave 2.5 to 3.0 mv. in leads II, III, and aVF.

    Complex positive in leads II, III, and aVF, negative in lead V_{10}.

    Duration—To 0.05 sec. (0.06 sec. in large breeds).

S–T segment and T wave: S–T segment free of marked coving (repolarization changes).

---

*Derived from personal observations and from sources gratefully acknowledged in the references and cited in the text of the chapter.

102

S–T segment depression not greater than 0.2 mv. in leads II and III and not greater than 0.3 mv. in lead CV_6 LL.

S–T segment elevation not greater than 0.15 mv. in leads II and III.

T wave negative in leads V_{10} and CV_5 RL (except in the Chihuahua).

T wave amplitude not greater than 25 per cent of amplitude of R wave.

BASIC ELECTROCARDIOGRAPHIC CONCEPTS

ELECTROPHYSIOLOGY

The electrocardiogram (ECG) is a graphic record of the voltage produced by cardiac muscle cells during depolarization and repolarization plotted against time (Fig. 4-1). The resting heart muscle cell has an electrical potential of −90 mv. across the cell membrane, the inside of the cell being negative with respect to the exterior. When the cell is stimulated to depolarize, positively charged sodium ions flow into the cell across the semipermeable cell membrane, reversing the polarity of the stimulated portion of the cell membrane. The electrical gradient across the cell wall becomes +30 mv. The muscle cell, when adequately stimulated to depolarize, contracts, probably because calcium diffuses into the myofibrils along with sodium and catalyzes excitation-contraction coupling (Winegrad, 1961).

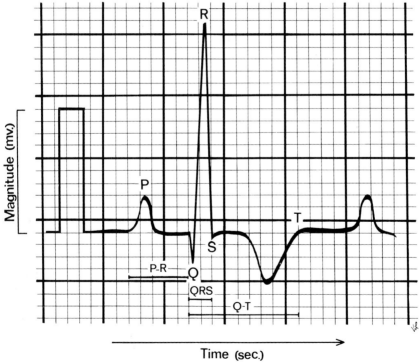

FIGURE 4-1 Schematic representation of lead II electrocardiogram (drawn to scale of 50 mm./sec. paper speed). The standardization impulse, 1 mv., is 10 mm. high on the vertical axis, which represents voltage. Time in seconds is plotted along the horizontal axis. The P-R, QRS, and Q-T intervals, and the P,Q,R,S, and T waves are indicated.

The change in potential which occurs when the electrical gradient across the cell membrane is reversed is registered as a voltage deflection on the electrocardiogram (Fig. 4-2). Potassium begins to diffuse to the outside of the cell during depolarization. When diffusion of potassium ions to the exterior exceeds the influx of sodium, repolarization begins, resulting ultimately in a high concentration of extracellular potassium and intracellular sodium. Repolarization of the heart muscle produces another series of voltage deflections recorded by the electrocardiograph (Fig. 4-2). During the diastolic (resting) phase, sodium returns slowly to the exterior of the cell as potassium returns to the interior.

Random electrical activity is characteristic of brain and most muscular tissue, whereas the electrical activity in the heart is more highly organized. This results from the "functional syncytium" of cardiac muscle, which permits excitation of the entire atrial and/or ventricular mass when one fiber is properly stimulated (Guyton, 1966). Because cardiac muscle is depolarized in such a manner that all electrical charges are summated, an external detector records a single positive or negative charge for depolarization and for repolarization. The electrical activity of the entire heart may thus be determined at an external point, because all the charges at any instant are resolved to one single charge.

MONOPHASIC ACTION POTENTIAL AND SPONTANEOUS DISCHARGE CYCLE. Cardiac ventricular muscle fibers incapable of pacemaker abilities have a monophasic action potential when stimulated. When a stimulus strong enough to raise the resting transmembrane potential (R.P.) to a critical or threshhold potential (T.P.) is applied to a cell, a monphasic action potential representing cellular depolarization is produced (Fig. 4-3A). The rapidly induced action potential of depolarization (phase 0, Fig. 4-3A) is followed by slower cellular repolarization (phases 1 to 3, Fig. 4-3A). The resting transmembrane potential remains at a constant −90 mv. (phase 4, Fig. 4-3A). During phase 0, cellular depolarization and contraction occur, represented by the QRS complex on the simultaneously recorded electrocardiogram. Repolarization, recognized by the S–T segment and T wave on the electrocardiogram, is associated with phases 2 and 3.

The sinoatrial node (S–A node), some atrial fibers, the bundle of His and its branches, and the Purkinje fibers differ from other cardiac tissue because their cells are capable of spontaneous or automatic discharge (Fig. 4-3B). Other atrial

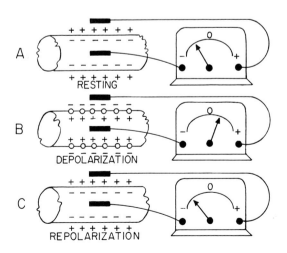

FIGURE 4-2 Stimulation of a cardiac muscle fiber. At the normal resting potential (A), there is a negative electrical charge inside the cell membrane. During depolarization (B) positive charges from outside enter the cell, causing a change in potential which is recorded by the galvanometer. The normal electrical potential is reestablished during repolarization (C). (From Guyton, A. C.: Textbook of Medical Physiology, W. B. Saunders, Philadelphia, 3rd edition, 1966, p. 62.)

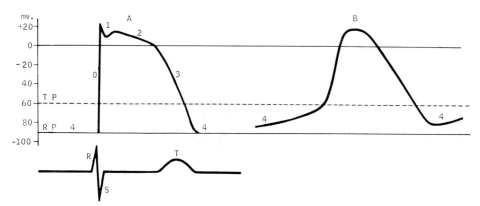

FIGURE 4-3 *A,* Diagrammatic drawing of action potential and electrocardio-gram of cardiac muscle fiber. *B,* Depolarization and action potential of pacemaker fiber. RP—resting membrane potential, TP—threshold potential at which pacemaker spontaneously fires its action potential, O—depolarization with positive overshoot (intrinsic deflection of R wave). 2—plateau, 3 corresponds to T wave, 4—diastole dur-ing which pacemaker undergoes spontaneous slow depolarization until it reaches threshold potential and fires. (From Friedberg, C. K.: Diseases of the Heart, W. B. Saunders, Philadelphia, 3rd edition, 1966, p. 27.)

and ventricular muscle cells are capable of automaticity only in unusual circum-stances (Hoffman, Cranefield, and Wallace, 1966). It has also been demonstrated that there are no automatic fibers in the atrioventricular node (A–V node) and that conduction through the atrioventricular node is both slow and decremental (Hoffman and Cranefield, 1964; Hoffman, 1965). Cells within the heart capable of spontaneous discharge are called pacemaker cells. These cells either act directly as the cardiac pacemaker or have the potential for this action. The fibers with the most rapid rate of spontaneous depolarization of the cell membrane (normally the sinoatrial node) assume the function of the cardiac pacemaker. After repolari-zation is complete (phase 3), there is spontaneous, gradual decay of the trans-membrane potential of pacemaker tissue (phase 4) as electrolytes leak across the semipermeable cell membrane. An action potential representing cellular de-polarization (phase 0) occurs when slow, spontaneous depolarization (phase 4) reaches the threshold potential (Fig. 4-3*B*).

ELECTROCARDIOGRAPHIC THEORIES

Several theories have evolved in an attempt to define the basis of the clinical electrocardiogram. Neither the *local effect theory* nor the *single dipole theory* originally proposed to explain the electrocardiogram is entirely satisfactory. The theory of *local effect* assumed that a lead placed over an anatomic area of the heart measures only the electrical activity of that portion of the heart. In other words, an electrode placed over the left ventricle was thought to record the left ventricular electrocardiographic complex, whereas one placed over the right ventricle would record that of the right ventricle. Evidence now available suggests that this theory is erroneous and can no longer be supported (Grishman, 1968).

The *equivalent generator* or *single dipole theory* assumes that each elec-trically active cell unit acts like a dipole and generates an electrical field within

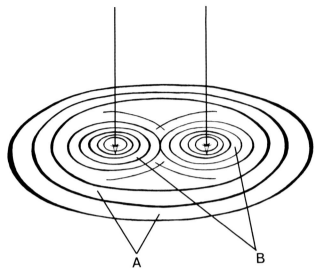

FIGURE 4-4 When two pebbles are dropped into a calm body of water, concentric waves radiate from the two points of entry. If measurements of the waves are made near the site of origin of each wave (*B*), only the force of that one wave is detected. If measurements are made further away (*A*), the forces from both waves are resolved into one effective force. When this principle is applied to the forces of the heart, the theory of the equivalent generator or single effective dipole is described.

the body. In effect, one single dipole which is the equivalent of all the dipoles of the heart is measured at the body's surface. This summation of dipoles is analogous to dropping two pebbles close together into a calm body of water (Fig. 4-4); within a short time the waves produced by each pebble merge, giving the appearance that only one pebble has generated the single wave. The electrical field of the heart appears to arise from an electrical source (dipole) with the positive and negative poles in close proximity, surrounded by fluids and tissues.

The true electrical activity within the heart arises from multiple dipoles (Geselowitz, 1964). The single dipole theory assumes that the multiple dipoles

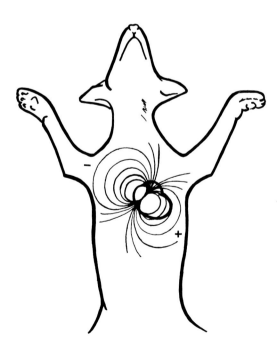

FIGURE 4-5 The single effective dipole generated by the heart is visualized as emerging from the dog's heart as a positive or negative potential radiating over the body. The size and direction of this force, recorded by the electrocardiogram, vary with the orientation of the force to the measuring device (in this case the electrocardiographic lead being recorded).

generated by the heart at a given instant are effectively resolved into a single electrical force before reaching the body surface (Fig. 4-5). Although multipolar components are present, interpretation of the electrocardiogram in terms of a single dipole is considered valid.

THE CARDIAC VECTOR

The measurable properties of a cardiac electrical force or potential are magnitude (size) and direction. The term for a force possessing both magnitude and direction is a *vector;* the vector is represented by an arrow (Fig. 4-6). The length of the arrow is proportional to the magnitude of the force, and the arrowhead indicates the direction of the force. The cardiac vector represents an electrical force of known magnitude and direction determined by the single effective dipole which is the resolution of all the cardiac forces.

An electrocardiographic lead or axis is a hypothetical line drawn between two sites on the body surface where electrodes are placed. The electrocardiographic deflection for any lead is a measurement of the projection of the cardiac vector on that lead. The length of the projection of the cardiac vector on any lead depends on the degree to which the vector is parallel to the lead. For example, consider the projection of the cardiac vector as its shadow on the lead produced by a light source placed perpendicular to the lead (Fig. 4-7). When the vector lies parallel to the lead axis the shadow is the largest possible, producing a large deflection on that lead. When the vector is perpendicular to the lead, only a dot will be cast on the axis, and no deflection is recorded on the lead (Fig. 4-7).

The galvanometer. The basic component of an electrocardiograph, the galvanometer, is a delicate writing instrument suspended within a magnetic field. The string galvanometer was invented by Einthoven and was first used in 1903 to record the electrocardiogram of a man by him. For this major scientific advance, Einthoven received the Nobel Prize in 1924. The string galvanometer required photographic recording of the electrocardiogram. It has never been surpassed in sensitivity, but more recently sensitive, direct-writing galvanometers have been used extensively and have the advantages of much greater ease of operation and portability.

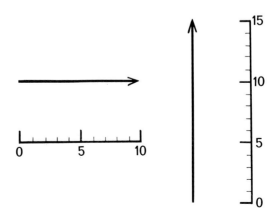

FIGURE 4-6 The arrow represents the cardiac vector. Its length is proportional to the magnitude of the force, and the direction of the arrow represents the direction of the force from the point of origin.

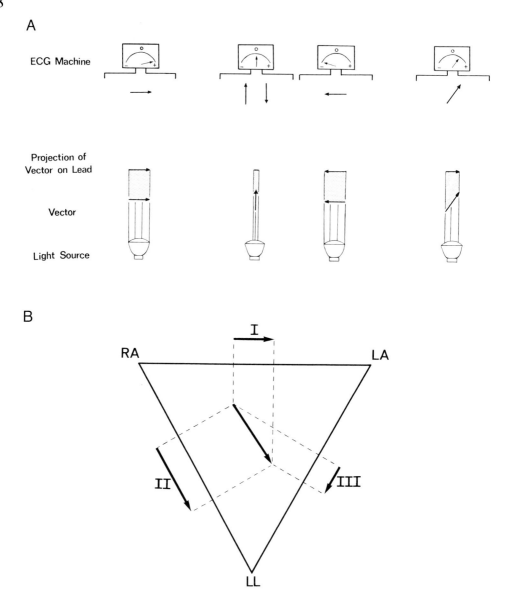

FIGURE 4-7 *A,* The shadow of the cardiac vector projected on an electro-cardiographic lead by a light (energy) source. The vector appears large when it is parallel to the lead. As the angle between the vector and the lead approaches 90°, the projection of the vector on the lead gradually becomes shorter. When the vector is perpendicular to the lead the shadow cast is only a dot, and the electrocardiograph records the force as having zero potential. The direction of the vector toward the positive or negative pole results in a positive or negative deflection, the amplitude of which is directly related to the degree to which the vector is parallel to the lead.

B, It is apparent that when the cardiac vector is projected within a triangle representing the three standard limb leads, the longest vector will be projected on the lead most nearly parallel to the cardiac vector (lead II in this case). Similarly, the shortest vector will be projected on the lead most nearly perpendicular to the cardiac vector (lead III).

The electrical forces produced by the heart are conducted by the electrodes connecting the body surface with the galvanometer. The flow of current causes the writing instrument to move away from the zero potential baseline, resulting in a deflection of the writing instrument. The galvanometer, then, records the heart's electrical activity as its forces are intercepted by electrodes on an arbitrary electrocardiographic lead of the body. Permanent recordings are made by a direct writing instrument such as a heat or ink stylus or by photographing an electrical beam.

The amplitude of a deflection in a recording of any given lead is not the absolute magnitude of the electrical forces being generated by the heart but is rather the projection of the cardiac vector on the given lead. This is so because a deflection which is perpendicular to a lead is recorded in that lead as a dot regardless of the magnitude of the force. A more representative indication of the actual electrical force being generated is seen on the lead which is most nearly parallel to the direction of the force.

The galvanometer records a positive deflection when the cardiac vector is directed toward the positive electrode of the lead being recorded, and a negative deflection when the vector is directed away from the positive electrode. The galvanometer records only a dot or a small deflection when the vector is perpendicular to the lead being recorded (Fig. 4-7).

TECHNIQUES OF ELECTROCARDIOGRAPHY

Methods. Electrocardiographic tracings are satisfactorily recorded with a standard electrocardiograph that measures the cardiac vector recorded on the limb leads (I, II, III), the augmented unipolar leads (aVR, aVL, aVF), and the V lead (exploring thoracic lead). Number 60 alligator clips with the jaws bent slightly open are used as electrodes, instead of the plates used for electrocardiography in man. The clips are fastened securely to the stem of each cable tip (Fig. 4-8) (Ettinger and Tashjian, 1966).

An animal handler familiar with the technique of examination is the most efficient assistant; the owner is a poor assistant, since he rarely restrains the animal properly. The dog is held in right lateral recumbency with its head to the handler's right (Fig. 4-9). The right forearm of the handler rests over the dog's neck, and his right hand holds the forelimbs perpendicular to the torso so that the legs overlie each other. The left arm is placed over the hindquarters, and the left hand holds the hindlimbs extended perpendicular to the body. One or two fingers should separate the limbs so that contact between the electrodes is avoided. Movement of the head or body is restricted using this technique, yet the animal is held firmly and without discomfort. It is essential that the position of the forelimbs is not varied from examination to examination, since even minor changes in forelimb position produce significant changes on the electrocardiogram (Cagan and Barta, 1959; Detweiler and Patterson, 1965; Hill, 1968).

The alligator clip electrodes are attached directly to the animal's skin. The electrode marked RA is attached just proximal to the olecranon on the caudal aspect of the right forelimb, and the electrode marked LA is attached to the same point on the left forelimb. The clips marked RL and LL are likewise attached proximal to the patella on the cranial aspect of the hindlimbs (Fig. 4-10). The V (C) lead is either clipped to the skin over the dorsal midline at the sixth thoracic

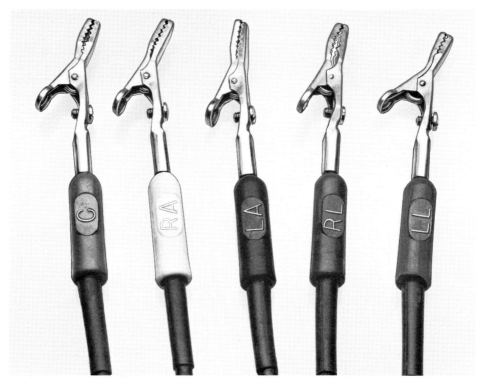

FIGURE 4-8   Alligator clips, No. 60 size, with the jaws bent slightly, make excellent electrodes when they are clipped to the dog's skin. The alligator clips must be securely fastened to the cable tips.

spinous process, where it is the V_{10} lead (Fig. 4-11), or it is used as an exploring lead (see pp. 118-120).

Using a plastic bottle, rubbing alcohol is applied over the alligator clips to moisten the skin and to act as a degreasing agent. A liquid surgical soap such as pHisoHex is rubbed over the skin and electrodes to improve the electrical contact. Alcohol and surgical soap can be mixed together and applied simultaneously if desired. It is not necessary to clip the hair or prepare the skin in any other way. Small dogs and those with thin skin, such as Chihuahuas and Greyhounds, may be uncooperative if the clips are painfully tight. This pressure is alleviated by placing a gauze pad over the skin and attaching the clips over the pad. The pad, clip, and skin are then saturated with alcohol and pHisoHex. Commercial electrode jellies are no better than alcohol and pHisoHex and are often difficult to apply to and remove from the dog's hair.

The electrocardiogram is recorded after the electrodes are attached and moistened. The electrodes must not touch each other or contact the hands of the animal handler. A clean, tight connection between the alligator clips and the cable tips is essential to avoid 60-cycle electrical interference. The cable tips should be scraped clean with sandpaper as often as they become grease-covered, and the alligator clips should be replaced periodically. Needle electrodes can be used in place of alligator clips, although they are not preferred by the authors. Anesthesia or tranquilization is rarely necessary, and most dogs tolerate the procedure well, although excited animals should be muzzled. Hamlin et. al. (1967) found that dogs were calm enough for electrocardiography if they were reassured and held quietly for a few minutes after the electrodes were attached.

Some electrocardiographs require a grounding wire attached to a nearby water pipe or outlet plate. The surface on which the dog is placed must be insulated from the ground. An insulated Formica table is recommended, but a metal table can be used if it is covered with a large piece of rubber sheeting or a woolen blanket.

The various leads are recorded on the standard electrocardiograph by moving the selector switch to the lead desired. The machine automatically establishes correct polarities for the lead chosen.

While each lead is being recorded, a one-millivolt standardization pulse should be made. The standardization pulse should begin from and return to the baseline if it is to be meaningful (Fig. 4-1). The marker button should be used to note the lead being recorded; any marking system recognizable to the clinician is satisfactory. All completed electrocardiograms should be identified immediately

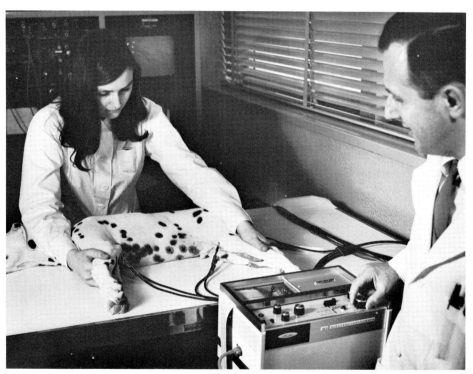

FIGURE 4-9 Position for electrocardiography with the dog held in right lateral recumbency. The legs are held at right angles to the body. The handler keeps the dog in position by placing his right arm over the dog's neck and his left arm over its rump. The clips are attached as in Figures 4-10 and 4-11, and the cable of the electrocardiograph remains on the table so that its weight does not result in a pull on the clips. A standard electrocardiograph, as pictured here, is used for canine electrocardiography.

with the client's name and the dog's case number, the date of the recording, the leads recorded, and the paper speed at which the recordings were made.

The right lateral recumbent position is recommended because much of the empirical electrocardiographic data available in the literature was obtained from dogs in this position. The forelimb position is easily controlled when a dog is in the recumbent position, which adds to the consistency of the recordings. Restraint is often difficult in the prone position, although one investigator (Rubin, 1969) reports otherwise. Use of the sternal position has been advocated by some (Horowitz, Spannier, and Wiggers, 1953; Schulze, Christoph, and Novak, 1957; Gonin, 1962; Crawley and Swenson, 1966; Rubin, 1968) because they feel that the heart is in a more natural physiologic position than it is in when the dog is in lateral recumbency. Regardless of the methods used, the position of the dog's torso and extremities and the placement of electrodes *must not* vary from examination to examination if consistently reproducible recordings are to be obtained and if recordings made at different times are to be compared.

A plexiglass tray with compartments, each containing a metal electrode and a

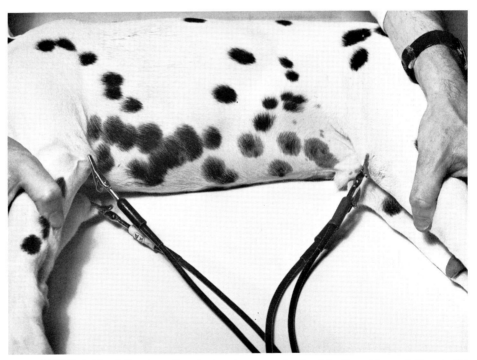

FIGURE 4-10 Alligator clip electrodes are attached to the skin as follows: the RA and LA electrodes just proximal to the right and left olecranons, respectively, and the RL and LL electrodes just proximal to the right and left stifles, respectively. After the electrodes are attached, alcohol and pHisoHex are used to improve electrical contact. To prevent the electrodes from touching, the limbs are separated; alternatively, a piece of paper toweling may be placed between the legs to reduce the likelihood of contact.

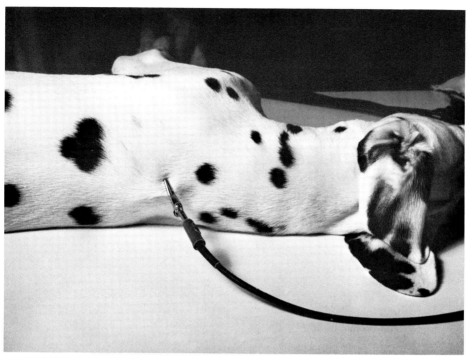

FIGURE 4-11 Viewing the dog from the back, the V_{10} lead (C or V) is attached to the skin at the midline between the scapula at the sixth to seventh thoracic vertebrae. Electrode contact is made with alcohol and pHisoHex.

saline-soaked sponge, has been used to record the electrocardiograms of experimental dogs (Coate, 1967). Recordings are reportedly rapid and accurate and may be made with the dog standing, sitting, or prone.

ELECTROCARDIOGRAPH PAPER AND TIME INTERVALS

Paper made for standard electrocardiographs is divided into large and small squares (Fig. 4-12). Each large one, 5 mm.², is surrounded by a heavy line and encloses 25 smaller, 1-mm. squares. At the standard amplitude, ten small squares (10 mm.) vertically are equal to 1 mv. of electricity (1 cm. deflection = 1 mv.). Time is represented on the horizontal scale of the paper. The length of a large square (5 mm.) represents 0.2 sec. at the slower paper speed, 25 mm./sec., or 0.1 sec. at the more rapid speed, 50 mm./sec. On the border, there are usually vertical lines marking the paper every 75 mm. At the slow paper speed, 25 mm./sec., the time interval between two of these vertical lines is 3 sec., and at 50 mm./sec. it is 1.5 sec. The heart rate is determined by counting the number of ventricular complexes in a 6-sec. period and multiplying by 10. Should the atria and ventricles depolarize asynchronously, separate computations of the atrial and ventricular rates must be made.

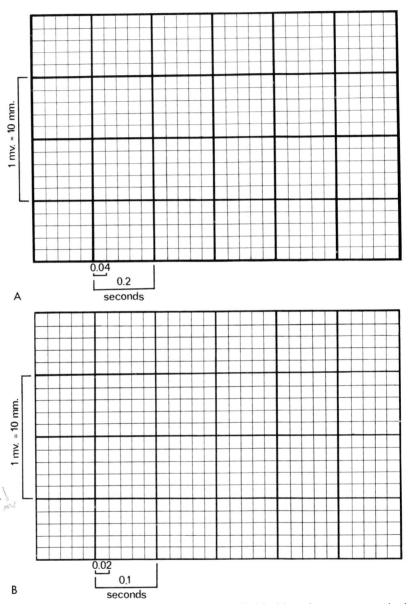

FIGURE 4-12 Electrocardiograph paper is divided into large squares by heavy vertical and horizontal lines at 5-mm. intervals. Within each large square are 25 1-mm.² boxes. *A*, At the standard amplitude of 1 mv. and a paper speed of 25 mm./sec., the smallest box on the scale equals 0.1 mv. On the horizontal scale one small box equals 0.04 sec., and five boxes (the length of the large square) equal 0.2 sec. *B*, At the standard amplitude of 1 mv. and the faster paper speed of 50 mm./sec., the vertical axis is unchanged, each box being equal to 0.1 mv., but on the horizontal scale one small box equals 0.02 sec., and five boxes equal 0.1 sec.

LEADS USED IN ELECTROCARDIOGRAPHY AND VECTORCARDIOGRAPHY

BIPOLAR LEADS

Using Einthoven's three-lead system as modified for the dog, electrodes are placed on the right forelimb (RA), left forelimb (LA), and left hindlimb (LL) (Lannek, 1949) (Fig. 4-13). The right hindlimb electrode (RL) connects the patient to the ground. In lead I, the left forelimb electrode (LA) is the positive terminal, and the right forelimb electrode (RA) is the negative terminal; in lead II the left hindlimb electrode (LL) is the positive terminal and the right forelimb electrode (RA) the negative; and in lead III the left hindlimb electrode (LL) is the positive terminal and the left forelimb electrode (LA) the negative.

Since the limbs act as wire extensions of the electrical field, each electrode is considered to measure the electrical field at the site of attachment of the limb to the torso. The electrodes are considered to be relatively equidistant electrically from the heart and from each other. Thus, in theory, the three standard bipolar limb leads form an equilateral triangle (Einthoven's triangle) with the origin of the cardiac vector, the zero point of the electrical field, at the center point of the triangle (Fig. 4-14).

The three limb lead axes can be redrawn with exactly the same direction, length, and polarity but all passing through zero point at the electrical center of

FIGURE 4-13 Schematic drawing with the left forelimb and right forelimb electrodes connected (lead I), the right forelimb and left hindlimb electrodes connected (lead II), and the left forelimb and left hindlimb electrodes connected (lead III). When the electrodes are connected in this manner, the resulting configuration is the Einthoven triangle (Fig. 4-14). The bottom of the triangle meets in the midabdominal region since in theory the three electrodes are equidistant from the heart.

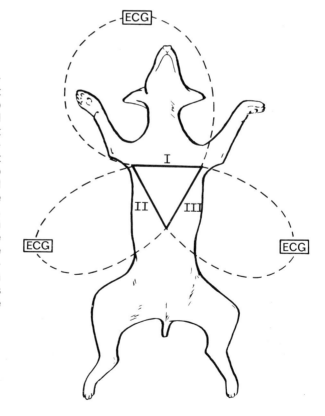

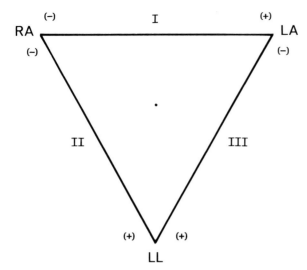

FIGURE 4-14 The Einthoven triangle. When the three limb leads are connected, the center of the triangle represents the origin of cardiac electrical activity. Lead I is a connection between the positive electrode on the LA and the negative electrode on the RA. Lead II connects the negative RA with the positive LL, and lead III connects the negative LA with the positive LL. (LA = left foreleg; RA = right foreleg; LL = left hindlimb.)

the heart, since parallel sides of a parallelogram are of equal length. The figure so obtained is called the triaxial reference system for the standard limb leads (Fig. 4-15). The triaxial system begins and ends at the left forelimb (LA). Thus, the sum of all the vectors must be zero, or:

(1) $$\text{lead I} + \text{lead II} + \text{lead III} = 0.$$

For equation (1) to be valid in a vector system, the voltage amplitude of at least one of the three leads must be negatively directed. In Einthoven's original studies

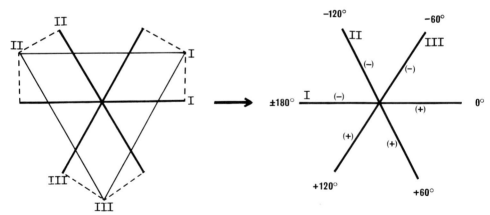

FIGURE 4-15 Triaxial limb leads. By constructing parallelograms for leads I, II, and III, each lead of the Einthoven triangle can be made to intersect the center of the triangle. The three leads now visualized intersecting the center of the triangle are shown in the drawing on the right. A semicircular portion on one side of lead I is numbered from 0° to 180° in a clockwise direction. On the other side of lead I, the semicircle is numbered from 0° to −180° in a counterclockwise direction. The polarity of the leads is determined by the original position of the positive and negative electrodes on the Einthoven triangle (Fig. 4-14).

(1903) this was true for lead II. Since it was desired that the voltage deflections in all three limb leads be upright or positive in the electrocardiogram of the normal man, the polarity of the electrodes in lead II was reversed (Grant, 1957). This, then, is the basis of *Einthoven's law:*

$$\text{lead I} + (-\text{lead II}) + \text{lead III} = 0,$$

or

(2) $$\text{lead I} + \text{lead III} = \text{lead II}.$$

The reversal of polarity in lead II has been utilized consistently in the dog as well as in man. From Einthoven's law (2), the vector of a lead is determined immediately if the other two leads are known; i.e., if lead I + lead III = 4 mv., the amplitude of lead II is 4 mv., and the vector is positively directed.

AUGMENTED UNIPOLAR LIMB LEADS

The unipolar limb leads as introduced by Wilson compared the voltage detected by an exploring electrode placed on one limb to that of the center of the electrical field, which is electrically equivalent to zero. The system was modified and augmented by comparing the electrical activity at one limb to the sum of that

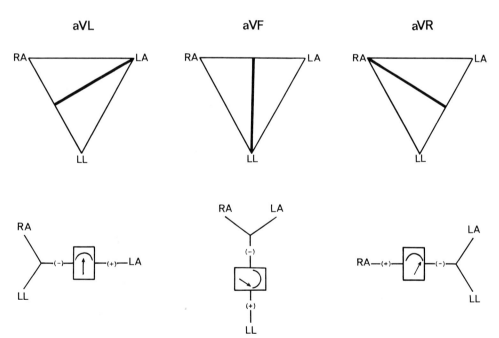

FIGURE 4-16 Augmented limb leads. Lead aVL compares the positive electrode at the LA position and the mean voltage of the RA and LL electrodes. It may be drawn into the Einthoven triangle as shown. Likewise, the voltage at the positive LL electrode is compared with the mean voltage at the RA and LA electrodes (aVF), and the voltage at the positive RA electrode is compared with the mean voltage at the LA and LL electrodes (aVR). LA = left foreleg; RA = right foreleg; LL = left hindlimb.

at the other two (i.e., LL to RA + LA) rather than to the entire field (lead I + [−lead II] + lead III). For each augmented unipolar lead, the voltage at one limb electrode (the positive terminal) is compared with the average voltage across the other two electrodes, which are connected to the negative terminal (Fig. 4-16). In lead aVR the voltage at the positive right forelimb electrode (RA) is compared to the average voltage of the left forelimb (LA) and left hindlimb (LL), connected to the negative electrode; lead aVL likewise compares the voltage at the positive LA electrode to the average voltage of RA and LL at the negative electrode; and lead aVF compares the voltage at the positive LL electrode to the average voltage of RA and LA at the negative electrode. A triaxial unipolar reference system similar to that drawn for leads I, II, and III may be drawn from these relationships (Fig. 4-17).

Thus, six lead axes, I, II, III, aVR, aVL, and aVF, are recorded at different orientations in the frontal plane (head to tail and right to left). When the vectors in any two leads are known, the other four vectors may be determined without difficulty from the Bailey six-axis reference system (Fig. 4-18).

UNIPOLAR PRECORDIAL LEADS

In this system, also developed by Wilson, the positive terminal, the exploring electrode (C or V), is placed on the thorax, and the voltage is compared to the average voltage across the three standard limb leads (theoretically equivalent to zero) at the negative terminal. In man, leads V_1 through V_6 record the electrical activity as measured on the chest at the fourth and fifth intercostal spaces from the sternum to the left mid-axillary line. With these leads, the horizontal or transverse vector (right-to-left and dorsoventral planes) can be estimated (Fig.

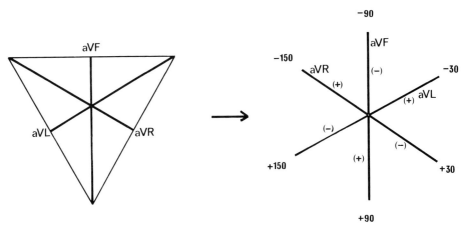

FIGURE 4-17 The augmented unipolar leads are pictured within the Einthoven triangle (left). When the triangle walls are removed, the augmented triaxial leads remain. The outer numbers represent the points of the circle from 0° to 180° and from 0° to −180°. The augmented lead electrode is positive at the point of origin; i.e., aVL is positive on the left forelimb as shown in Figure 4-16.

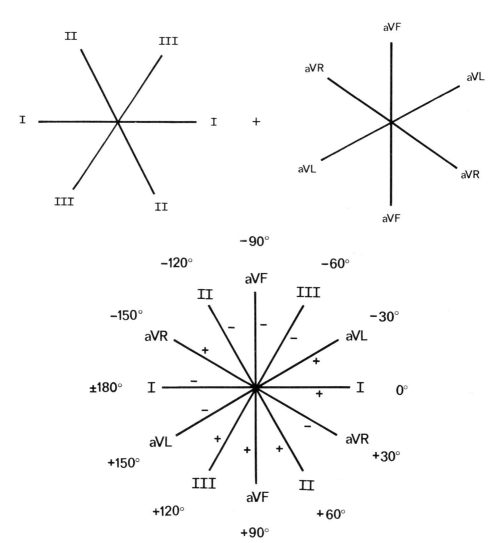

FIGURE 4-18 Bailey six-axis reference system. The upper diagrams represent the limb and augmented limb triaxial leads after being redrawn through the center of the body. When the two diagrams are combined, the Bailey six-axis reference system for the frontal plane results (bottom). The lead axes are marked in 30° increments from 0° to 180° and from 0° to −180°. The six leads are marked with a + at the positive electrode and a − at the negative electrode. Notice that for leads I, II, III, and aVF the polarity and angle of the leads are positive or negative simultaneously. Leads aVR and aVL are positive at the positions of −150° and −30°, respectively, since the positive electrodes for those leads lie in the negative 0° to −180° zone.

4-19). The exploring V leads used in the dog, originally described by Lannek (1949) and modified by Detweiler and Patterson (1965), are:

CV_6 LL — Sixth left intercostal space near the edge of the sternum
CV_6 LU — Sixth left intercostal space at the costochondral junction
CV_5 RL — Fifth right intercostal space near the edge of the sternum
V_{10} — Over the dorsal spinous process of the seventh thoracic vertebra

The unipolar precordial leads are not universally utilized in canine electrocardiography. However, they may provide additional data to suggest a diagnosis of right and left heart enlargement. The V_{10} lead is more popular than the other precordial leads.

ESOPHAGEAL LEAD

An esophageal lead may be used to enlarge and clarify electrocardiographic deflections, particularly when there is doubt as to the presence and/or timing of the P waves. The patient is made to swallow a special flexible lead with an electrode in its tip until the distal tip is over the base of the heart. The esophageal lead is attached to the left forelimb (LA) cable tip, and the machine is set at lead I to record the electrical activity. The limb leads are secured in their usual positions. One of the limb leads should be recorded simultaneously so that the bizarre deflections recorded from the esophageal lead may be correlated with a more familiar limb lead pattern. Multichannel equipment capable of making simultaneous recordings is required for making tracings of this type.

ORTHOGONAL LEADS

Orthogonal lead systems were designed to measure the heart's electrical forces in three dimensions. The three axes required are:
X — Sinistrodextral (left-to-right)
Y — Craniocaudal (head-to-tail)
Z — Dorsoventral (vertebral column to sternum)
By projecting the X, Y, and Z vectors on their axes, the magnitude and direction of the resultant vectors in space are determined (Fig. 4-19). In one uncorrected orthogonal system (Hamlin and Smith, 1960), the axes are as follows:
Lead I provides the sinistrodextral axis, (X);
Lead aVF provides the craniocaudal axis, (Y); and
Lead V_{10} provides the dorsoventral axis, (Z).
These orthogonal leads, derived from anatomical relationships, produce somewhat distorted representation of the true X, Y, and Z axes. More accurate, corrected lead systems were therefore devised (American Heart Association, 1967). Corrected orthogonal lead systems such as the McFee, Schmidt, and Frank systems, designed for use in man, attempt to minimize minor variations such as electrode placement, position of the heart within the thorax, and the nonhomogeneous nature of the body as a conducting medium. The McFee (1961) corrected orthogonal lead system (Fig. 4-20), designed originally for use in the dog, utilizes eleven electrodes placed in the X, Y, and Z planes. Tracings made using this system are reproducible for the same dog when recorded on different

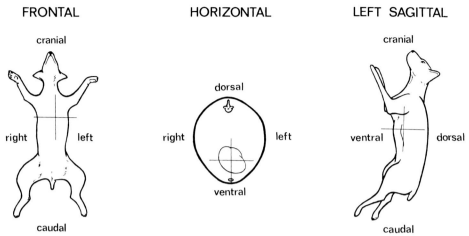

FIGURE 4-19 The frontal, horizontal, and left sagittal planes, The frontal plane represents the XY axes, from left to right (X), and craniad to caudad (Y). The horizontal plane looks into the thorax as if it were open, so that the XZ planes, left to right (X), and dorsal to ventral (Z), are visualized. The left sagittal plane views the dog from the left side standing on his hindlimbs; i.e., the ZY axes, dorsal to ventral (Z), and cranial to caudal (Y).

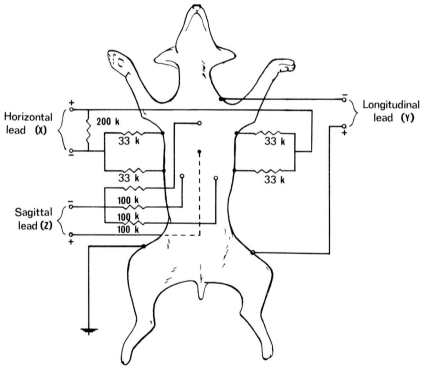

FIGURE 4-20 The McFee orthogonal lead system. A corrected orthogonal lead system designed for the dog utilizes 11 electrodes to measure electrical forces in the X, Y, and Z planes. The specially wired electrodes are placed on the body as demonstrated in the diagram, and the X, Y, and Z leads are recorded simultaneously. This system measures the cardiac vector in three planes more accurately than can the standard ten leads usually used in canine electrocardiography. From McFee, R., and Parungao, A.: Amer. Heart J., 62 (1961): 93.

days and when electrode placement is varied slightly. Again, the positioning of the limbs must be consistent for the most accurate tracings (Hill, 1968).

THE MEAN ELECTRICAL AXIS

For practical purposes in clinical veterinary cardiology, a single determination of the mean electrical axis (MEA), or the average vector (magnitude and direction) for both atrial depolarization and ventricular depolarization, is made in the frontal plane. The mean electrical axis is clinically relevant since it sometimes becomes abnormal with cardiac enlargement. The instantaneous cardiac vectors can be determined from the vectorcardiogram (see pp. 158–167).

The mean electrical axis of ventricular depolarization in the frontal plane (sinistrodextral and craniocaudal) is determined as follows:

1. Choose a complete electrocardiographic complex from any two limb lead recordings. Determine the areas between the baseline and all deflections of the QRS complex for each lead. Then, by adding together the positive and negative values, a numerical value is determined for each lead.

2. The two leads chosen in (1) are found on the Bailey six-axis reference

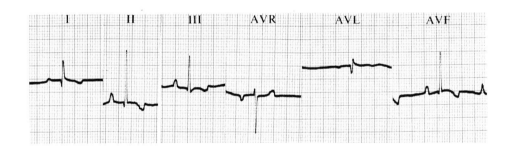

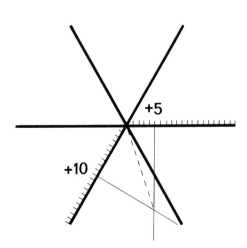

FIGURE 4-21   Mean electrical axis (MEA). *Above,* The six limb leads from a normal dog recorded at paper speed of 50 mm./sec. and standard amplitude of 1 mv. *Below,* Choosing any two of the limb leads (I and III), the positive and negative deflections for each lead are added (I = +5; III = +10). Using the three- or six-axis reference system, perpendicular lines are drawn from the positive or negative point determined for each lead. The perpendicular lines are extended until they meet, and the dotted line drawn from the origin of the reference axis system to the site of their intersection is the mean electrical axis. The mean electrical axis in the frontal plane in this recording from a normal dog is +70°.

system (see p. 119), and the point representing the positive or negative value for the QRS complex in each lead is marked (Fig. 4-21). A perpendicular is drawn from each of the two leads at the points representing the values determined for the QRS complex in (1) (Fig. 4-21). The perpendicular lines from both leads are extended until they intersect (Fig. 4-21).

3. A line drawn from the center of the axis system to the intersection of the two perpendicular lines represents the mean electrical axis for that complex (Fig. 4-21). The mean electrical axis determined using the method described above should vary very little regardless of the pair of limb leads selected. The same method is used to determine the mean electrical axis of atrial depolarization (P wave).

The mean electrical axis can be determined more easily by inspection of the electrocardiogram. Since the electrocardiographic deflection is positive when the cardiac vector moves toward the positive terminal and negative when it is directed toward the negative terminal, an isoelectric or zero deflection (electrocardiographic lead whose area of positivity and negativity under the complex is closest to zero) results when the vector is directed perpendicular to a given lead. Therefore, the mean electrical axis of the heart is approximately perpendicular to the limb lead on the electrocardiogram which is most nearly isoelectric. For example, referring to the Bailey six-axis reference system (see p. 119), if the sum of the areas of positivity and negativity under the QRS complex in lead III is zero, a line perpendicular to the lead is parallel to lead aVR, at $+30°$ or $-150°$. To determine which of the two (i.e., $+30°$ or $-150°$) it is, note whether the deflection on the electrocardiogram is positive or negative for lead aVR. If it is negative the axis is $+30°$; if it is positive, the axis is $-150°$. Using another example, if lead aVL is isoelectric, the perpendicular to lead aVL is $+60°$ or $-120°$, i.e., lead II. Then, if lead II is positive the axis is $+60°$; if it is negative, the axis is $-120°$.

The mean electrical axis of ventricular depolarization in the frontal plane in most normal dogs is between 40° and 100°. An axis less than 40° is compatible with left axis deviation, and an axis over 100° is compatible with and signifies right axis deviation. In either case, deviation of the mean electrical axis from normal warrants a thorough cardiac evaluation (Fig. 4-22). The mean electrical axis does not necessarily correspond to the physical axis of the heart within the body as observed on radiographs.

In a study of normal dogs, the mean electrical axis of ventricular depolarization in the frontal plane was found to be $70° \pm 24.6°$ (Detweiler, 1961). In another study, normal limits for the mean electrical axis in 60 normal dogs with the forelimbs held perpendicular to the body ranged from 45° to 100° (Detweiler and Patterson, 1965). In another study, Yarns and Tashjian (1967) found that the average mean electrical axis in the frontal plane was 72° (35° to 99°) in 14 normal dogs. It has been observed that in dogs with a narrow thorax, such as the Collie, the mean electrical axis in the frontal plane is usually closer to 90°, whereas in dogs with a wide thorax the axis is usually less than 90°. However, there are exceptions, so that the Dachshund, which has a wide thorax, has a mean electrical axis closer to 90° (Gonin, 1962; Hill, 1968). In Gonin's study (1962) the electrical axis changed with position; therefore, tracings recorded with the dog in the prone position had a mean value of 75°, as compared to 66° when the right lateral recumbent position was used.

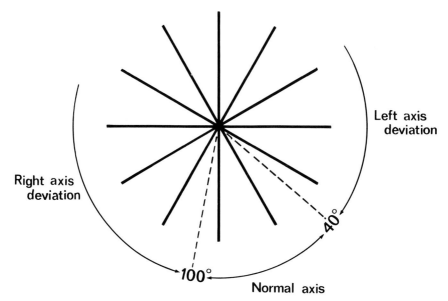

FIGURE 4-22   The normal mean electrical axis in the frontal plane in the dog is from 40° to 100°. A mean electrical axis below 40° is consistent with left axis deviation, and one over 100° is consistent with right axis deviation.

THE CARDIAC CONDUCTION SYSTEM AND THE ELECTROCARDIOGRAM

The cardiac conduction system is composed of specialized cardiac tissue that normally conducts electrical impulses through the heart. This system consists of the sinoatrial (S-A) node, the interatrial bundles, the atrioventricular (A-V) node, the common bundle of His, the right and left branches of the bundle of His, and the Purkinje fibers (Fig. 4-23). With the exception of the atrioventricular node, the cardiac conduction system consists entirely of specialized muscle tissue which spreads the wave of excitation more rapidly than can the myocardium. Conduction is both slow and decremental through the atrioventricular node (Hoffman, 1965), permitting completion of atrial excitation and enabling the ventricle to fill with blood before it contracts.

The P wave of the electrocardiogram represents atrial depolarization, or the spread of excitation from the sinoatrial node through the atrial musculature to the atrioventricular node. The sinoatrial node is located at the junction of the right atrium and the cranial vena cava and lies less than 1 mm. below the epicardium (James, 1962). The P-R segment of the electrocardiogram is the isoelectric or zero potential period that follows the P wave, reflecting the delay of the cardiac impulse at the atrioventricular node. The atrioventricular node lies above the septal leaflet of the tricuspid valve just anterior to the ostium of the coronary sinus (James, 1964). The period from the beginning of the P wave to the end of the P-R segment, i.e., the beginning of the QRS complex, is called the P-R interval.

After a delay in the atrioventricular node, the impulse passes directly to the common bundle of His. Transmission through the common bundle of His, the

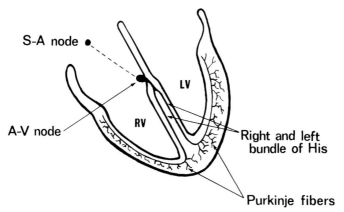

FIGURE 4-23 Cardiac conduction system. The normal impulse in the heart arises from the sinoatrial (S–A) node in the right atrium. The impulses are conducted through specialized tissue in the atrium to the atrioventricular node (A–V). After emerging from the atrioventricular node, the impulse travels briefly through the common bundle of His and then through the right and left branches of the bundle of His to the Purkinje fibers and the ventricular myocardium.

right and left branches of the bundle of His, and the Purkinje fibers results in activation of all areas of the ventricles. When the impulse reaches the ventricular myocardium, depolarization of the cardiac muscle occurs. The electrical phenomenon reflected by the QRS complex of the electrocardiogram is depolarization of the ventricles.

The S-T segment and the T wave of the electrocardiogram represent ventricular repolarization. The S-T segment represents the period of slow repolarization of the ventricles, and the T wave indicates the period of more rapid repolarization. Repolarization of the atria normally occurs during the QRS complex but is usually not seen on the electrocardiogram because its small electrical potential is obliterated by that of ventricular depolarization.

The heart is innervated by both the sympathetic and parasympathetic nervous systems (Fig. 4-24). These are not considered part of the cardiac conduction

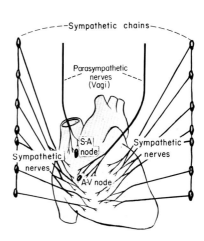

FIGURE 4-24 Cardiac nerves. (From Guyton, A. A.: Textbook of Medical Physiology, W. B. Saunders, Philadelphia, 3rd edition, 1966, p. 187.)

system, but they do influence the heart rate and the conduction of electrical impulses. Stimulation of the sympathetic nerves increases both the heart rate and the force of contraction. Sympathetic stimulation results in the release of norepinephrine at the nerve endings, producing both positive chronotropic (increased rate of contraction) and positive inotropic (increased force of contraction) effects. Increased permeability of the cell membrane to both sodium and calcium is suggested as the mechanism through which norepinephrine acts (Guyton, 1966). Parasympathetic nervous stimulation mediated through the vagal nerves results in release of acetylcholine at the vagal nerve endings. This results in a decrease in the rate of discharge of the sinoatrial node and a diminished rate of transmission of impulses through the atrioventricular node. The mechanism of action of acetylcholine is thought to be hyperpolarization of the cell by allowing increased permeability of the cell membrane to potassium (Guyton, 1966).

THE NORMAL ELECTROCARDIOGRAM

The electrocardiographic deflections must be measured accurately and consistently, since the differences between normal and abnormal are often slight. Measurements of amplitude, on the vertical axis, should be made from the top (or bottom) of the isoelectric baseline to the top (or the bottom) of the wave. Time measurements begin with the first deviation from the isoelectric line and end when the wave first returns to the isoelectric line.

Heart rate.   The range of heart rates in normal dogs at the time of examination is from 70 to 160 beats/min. (180 beats/min. in miniature breeds). In two studies, heart rates ranged from 67 to 214 beats/min. (mean, 122 beats/min.) (Lannek, 1949) and from 86 to 185 beats/min. (mean, 139 beats/min.) (Hamlin et al., 1967). In puppies from 2 to 6 months of age the range was from 88 to 214 beats/min. (mean, 144 beats/min.) (Lannek, 1949). The heart rate in puppies under 2 months old usually exceeds 200 beats/min. In adult dogs, heart rates above 160 beats/min. (180 beats/min. in miniature breeds) are classified as tachycardias, and those below 70 beats/min. are termed bradycardias.

The *P wave* is the first deflection on the electrocardiogram after the isoelectric pause indicating electrical diastole (Fig. 4-25). It should always be positive in leads II and aVF, and it should be isoelectric or positive in Lead I. It may be negative in leads III, aVR, aVL, CV_5 RL, and V_{10} (Detweiler and Patterson, 1965). The first half of the P wave represents right atrial activation, whereas left atrial activation is recorded during the second half. This is so because the spread of atrial excitation begins in the upper portion of the right atrium at the sinoatrial node and then spreads across the atrium depolarizing the left atrium. The maximum normal amplitude of the P wave in any limb lead is 0.4 mv. One author reported the maximum amplitude of the P wave during inspiration as 0.13 mv. in lead I, 0.42 mv. in lead II, and 0.38 mv. in lead III (Lannek, 1949), and in another report the mean amplitude did not exceed 0.3 mv. in any lead in 107 dogs (Burman, Panagopoulos, and Kahn, 1966). Yarns and Tashjian (1967) reported an average P-wave amplitude of 0.30 mv. (0.15 mv. to 0.50 mv.) in lead II. The amplitude of the P wave may increase with an increase in heart rate. Vagal influences within the sinoatrial node account for variations in the amplitude of the P wave from beat to beat (Lalich, Cohen, and Walker, 1941), and it is not

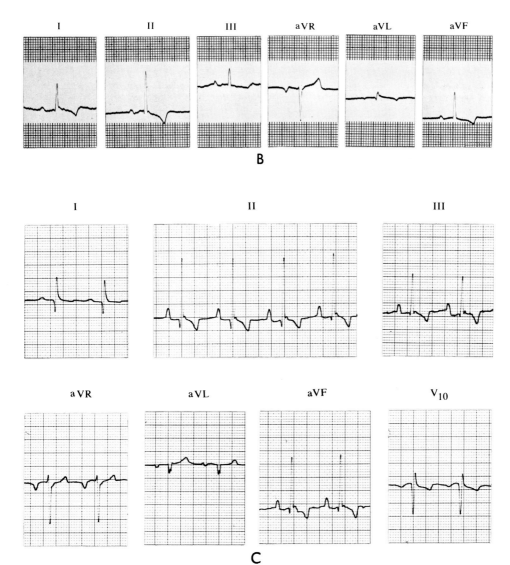

FIGURE 4-25 *Continued*

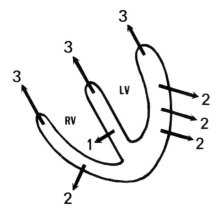

FIGURE 4-26 Ventricular activation. Ventricular depolarization begins in the interventricular septal region, with the initial forces directed rightward (1). The free walls and apex then depolarize, producing the major forces with a leftward direction (2). Terminally, the basal portions of the ventricles and interventricular septum depolarize in such a manner as to produce either a small rightward or leftward force (3). After Hamlin, R. L., and Smith, C. R.: *Am. J. Vet. Res.*, 21 (1960): 702.

in three smooth, transitional phases: initial, main, and terminal. First, the vector is directed from left to right in the interventricular septum. Then it moves from the endocardium to the epicardium, depolarizing the free (lateral) ventricular walls, and finally it moves basally in the upper walls and septum (ventricular outflow tracts). These phases are normally 0.01 sec., 0.025 to 0.035 sec., and 0.01 sec. in duration, respectively (Hamlin and Smith, 1960; Hellerstein and Hamlin, 1960).

The initial vector is oriented rightward, craniad, and ventrad (see pp. 160–161). Therefore, leads I and V_{10} should each have a Q wave, since a negative wave indicates a rightward (lead I) and ventrad (lead V_{10}) force. The Q wave in leads II and aVF represents cranially directed initial forces but should not be of longer duration than 0.01 sec. The initial vector is directed cranially for only a short period prior to turning caudad (see pp. 160–161). If a Q wave is present in older dogs in leads I, II, III, and aVF, and if its amplitude is greater than 0.5 mv. in lead II, it is probably abnormal. Lannek (1949) reports a maximum limit of -1.3 mv. in lead II, but this appears to be excessive for most normal dogs.

The main portion of the QRS complex reflects depolarization of the left and right ventricular free walls. Because the mass of the left ventricle is so much greater than that of the right ventricle, the main electrocardiographic deflection results primarily from depolarization of the left ventricular wall. Thus, in the normal dog the main portion of the QRS complex is directed to the left, caudad, and ventrad, producing an R wave in leads I, II, III, and aVF (leftward and caudad) and a Q wave in lead V_{10} (ventrad).

The terminal force of the QRS complex occurs when the dorsal basal (apicobasilar) region of the heart is depolarized. The direction of the terminal force may be either rightward or leftward, depending on the extent to which the basal region of the left ventricle lies to the right of the midline. If the dorsal basal region of the heart remains electrically on the left side of the thorax, an S wave will not appear in lead I. If part of the dorsal basal region lies electrically to the right side of the thorax, there will be a small S wave in leads I, II, III, and aVF. In normal dogs, there is usually no S wave in lead I, and it may also be absent in lead II (Lannek, 1949). Lead V_{10} should always have a Qr complex, the small r wave representing the terminal dorsal basal depolarization of the heart.

The mean direction of the QRS complex is leftward, caudad, and ventrad. The mean frontal plane electrical axis of the QRS complex is considered normal when it falls between 40° and 100° (see pp. 122–124). In the authors' experience, prolongation of the QRS complex beyond 0.05 sec. in small and medium breeds and 0.06 sec. in large breeds indicates delayed ventricular depolarization. This occurs in association with left ventricular hypertrophy, bundle branch block, formation of premature ventricular ectopic beats, and aberrantly conducted beats. Others report the maximum normal duration of the QRS complex as 0.07 sec. (Detweiler and Patterson, 1965), and 0.08 sec. (Crawley and Swenson, 1966). Lannek (1949) reports the maximal normal duration as 0.06 sec. in light breeds and 0.07 sec. in medium and heavy breeds. In 107 anesthetized dogs, the average duration of the widest QRS complex was 0.045 ± 0.024 sec. in lead II (Burman, Panagopoulos, and Kahn, 1966).

The maximum amplitude of the QRS complex after addition of all positive (R) and negative (Q and S) deflections is not known. However, the upper limit for the normal amplitude of the R wave is 2.5 mv.; an amplitude above 3.0 mv. is always abnormal. Abnormally tall R waves suggest ventricular enlargement. R waves of amplitude less than 0.5 mv. in leads I, II, and III are considered abnormally small (Detweiler et al., 1968b). Diminished amplitudes of the electrocardiographic complexes suggests pericardial and/or pleural effusion, thoracic neoplasia, or other disease conditions resulting in increased mass within the thoracic cavity. This diagnosis can be made only if ventricular complexes are diminished in all leads, including the V leads.

Occasionally the QRS complex is nearly isoelectric in all six limb leads. In this case, the heart is referred to as being horizontally positioned, and the electrical axis is indeterminate in the frontal plane. In such instances, normal values for mean frontal plane electrical axis and wave amplitudes cannot be applied. Interval durations are not altered, however, and the values previously noted may be applied.

The S–T segment and T wave.   This portion of the electrocardiogram represents ventricular repolarization (Fig. 4-25). The S–T segment, which represents the slower phase of repolarization, begins with the end of the ventricular complex (J or junctional point) and ends with the first deflection of the T wave. The T wave represents the most rapid period of ventricular repolarization. It ends when the wave returns to the isoelectric baseline. The S–T segment and T wave should be examined for depression or elevation from the baseline and for changes in the normal contour. The S–T segment is normally isoelectric or slightly concave or convex. In the dog, the polarity of the S–T segment and T wave need not be the same as that of the QRS complex, as is usually the case in man. It is essential to emphasize that criteria established for changes of the S–T segment and T wave in man should not be transferred empirically to canine electrocardiography. T waves are most accurately interpreted when compared with previous tracings from the same patient. In a study of 107 dogs (Burman, Panagopoulos, and Kahn, 1966), negative T waves occurred in lead II in 60 per cent of the dogs and in lead III in 56 per cent of the dogs. In leads aVR, aVL, and aVF, 56 per cent, 58 per cent, and 42 per cent of the dogs, respectively, had positive T waves. In 218 electrocardiograms from 24 normal dogs, there was a Q wave and a negative T wave in 78 per cent of the recordings of lead I and an S wave and positive T wave in 75 per cent of the recordings of lead III (Lalich, Cohen, and Walker, 1941). If the amplitude of the T wave is greater than 25 per cent of that of the R wave (Q wave if it is deeper), left ventricular enlargement may be suspected.

If the T wave is positive in leads V_{10} and CV_5 RL, right ventricular hypertrophy is suggested, although the Chihuahua may be an exception to this rule (Detweiler and Patterson, 1965). Ischemia should be suspected if depression or elevation of the S–T segment is excessive. Abnormal deviations of the S–T segment are: depression of -0.2 mv. or elevation of 0.15 mv. in leads II and III; depression of -0.3 mv. in lead CV_6 LL; or elevation of 0.3 mv. in leads CV_6 LL and CV_6 LU (Detweiler and Patterson, 1965).

A representative sampling of normal electrocardiographic data derived by others is presented in Table 4-1.

TABLE 4-1 NORMAL ELECTROCARDIOGRAPHIC VALUES AS DETERMINED BY SEVERAL AUTHORS*

A. From Lannek, N.: A Clinical and Experimental Study on the Electrocardiogram in Dogs. Thesis, Stockholm, 1949. Reported by Detweiler, D. K.: Cardiovascular Disease in Animals. In *Cardiology:* An Encyclopedia of the Cardiovascular System. (A. A. Luisada, Editor) Volume V, McGraw-Hill, New York (1961): 27-10.

LEAD	AMPLITUDES (mv.)						INTERVALS (sec.)		
	P	Q	R	S	S–Tj	T	P–R	QRS	Q–T
I	0.070 ±0.064	0.522 ±0.388	0.778 ±0.480	0.184 ±0.180	0.016 ±0.036	−0.072 ±0.140	0.096 ±0.019	0.035 ±0.007	0.167 ±0.018
II	0.242 ±0.116	0.682 ±0.454	2.406 ±0.876	0.318 ±0.258	−0.036 ±0.052	−0.146 ±0.336	0.098 ±0.016	0.041 ±0.008	0.176 ±0.018
III	0.180 ±0.112	0.428 ±0.268	1.890 ±0.760	0.432 ±0.330	−0.036 ±0.048	−0.030 ±0.310	0.099 ±0.017	0.041 ±0.008	0.177 ±0.018
CR_6LU	0.350 ±0.114	0.570 ±0.370	4.246 ±1.438	0.528 ±0.406	−0.062 ±0.092	0.370 ±0.554	0.100 ±0.018	0.047 ±0.009	0.194 ±0.022
CR_6LL	0.334 ±0.100	0.406 ±0.276	4.766 ±1.348	0.726 ±0.540	−0.022 ±0.108	0.588 ±0.570	0.102 ±0.019	0.045 ±0.007	0.192 ±0.021
CR_5RL	0.164 ±0.100	— —	2.598 ±1.206	1.236 ±0.766	0.006 ±0.086	0.724 ±0.480	0.104 ±0.021	0.038 ±0.007	0.191 ±0.019

B. From Crawley, G. J., and Swenson, M. J.: Vet. Med., 61 (1966): 363.

WAVE		LEADS (mm.)			
		I	II	III	aVF
Q	Average Range	4.15 0.5-12.0	2.51 0.5-7.75	1.68 0.5-5.25	1.46 0.5-5.0
R	Average Range	6.95 1.5-15.0	19.20 3.0-33.0	15.78 5.0-31.0	18.42 8.0-33.0
S	Average Range	1.84 0.25-12.0	4.42 0.5-17.0	4.91 0.5-16.0	5.10 0.5-20.0

	DURATION (sec.)		
	PR	QRS	QT
Average Range	0.105 0.06-0.18	0.052 0.03-0.08	0.230 0.18-0.28

C. Burman, S. O., Panagopoulos, P., and Kahn, S.: J. Thorac. Cardiovasc. Surg., 51 (1966): 379.

WAVE		LEADS (mm.)					
		I	II	III	aVR	aVL	aVF
P	Mean	+0.44	+3.0	+2.5	−1.6	−1.01	+2.91
	S.D. †	0.10	0.10	0.09	0.09	0.15	0.12
Q	Mean	0.27	1.2	1.3	12.6	8.5	1.7
	S.D.	0.10	0.15	0.10	0.46	0.48	0.09
R	Mean	2.2	16.5	14.8	1.10	2.10	16.2
	S.D.	0.50	0.44	0.43	0.30	0.30	0.34
S	Mean	0.08	1.4	1.30	10.2	0.75	1.95
	S.D.	0.09	0.22	0.15	0.33	0.50	0.20
T	Mean	−0.10	−1.10	−1.00	+1.10	+1.12	−0.95
	S.D.	0.20	0.11	0.18	0.23	0.23	0.17

INTERVAL	LEAD (sec.)		
	I	II	III
P–R	0.096 ± 0.024	0.098 ± 0.024	0.099 ± 0.024
QRS	0.037 ± 0.021	0.045 ± 0.024	0.044 ± 0.024
Q–T	0.167 ± 0.054	0.176 ± 0.054	0.177 ± 0.054

†Standard deviation

D. Horowitz, S. A., Spanier, M. R., and Wiggers, H. C.: Proc. Soc. Exp. Biol. Med., 84 (1953): 121.

WAVE		LEADS (mv.)					
		I	II	III	aVR	aVL	aVF
P	Mean	0.17	0.27	0.16	−0.20	0.02	0.19
	S.D.	0.07	0.09	0.11	0.09	0.10	0.11
Q	Mean	0.16	0.17	0.13	0.20	0.11	0.17
	S.D.	0.24	0.17	0.12	0.45	0.18	0.14
R	Mean	1.05	1.77	1.11	0.21	0.41	1.35
	S.D.	0.58	0.48	0.48	0.24	0.40	0.50
S	Mean	0.09	0.09	0.23	1.21	0.30	0.17
	S.D.	0.14	0.18	0.31	1.27	0.10	0.17
T	Mean	0.05	0.18	0.13	−0.11	−0.04	0.13
	S.D.	0.17	0.26	0.23	0.20	0.14	0.23

	P duration	P–R interval	QRS duration	Q–T interval	Weight	Heart rate
Mean	0.07	0.12	0.06	0.21	17.9	121
S.D.	0.02	0.02	0.01	0.02	3.7	19

*The data for leads I, II, III, CR_6LU, CR_6LL, and CR_5RL (Lannek, 1949, reported by Detweiler, 1961) were obtained from dogs in the right lateral recumbent position, with needle electrodes positioned in the proximal limbs in loose subcutaneous tissue. In this study of 230 dogs, 37 were under 7 months of age and 15 were over 7 years. In another study (Crawley and Swenson, 1966), the dogs were anesthetized or tranquilized and placed in a supine position, and the electrocardiograms were recorded using needle electrodes on clipped areas. Crawley and Swenson (1966) have drawn conclusions concerning abnormal electrocardiographic findings derived from the supine position. A study of 107 anesthetized dogs was made in the right lateral recumbent position with needle electrodes placed subcutaneously (Burman, Panagopoulos, and Kahn, 1966). The electrocardiographic standards reported by Horowitz, Spanier, and Wiggers (1953) were obtained from 30 anesthetized dogs in a supine position.

ELECTROCARDIOGRAPHIC ABNORMALITIES CAUSED BY ENLARGEMENT OF THE CARDIAC CHAMBERS

ATRIAL ENLARGEMENT

Atrial depolarization proceeds from the sinoatrial node to the atrioventricular node, activating first the muscle fibers of the right atrium, then those of the left atrium. When the right atrium enlarges because of dilatation or hypertrophy, the distance from the sinoatrial node to the atrioventricular node is increased, as are the magnitude and duration of the right atrial P forces. Since the increase in duration occurs during the period of normal left atrial activation, represented by the second half of the P wave, there is no net prolongation of the P wave. The amplitude of the P wave is increased in leads II, III, and aVF, being greater than 0.4 mv., and the wave is sharply peaked. This configuration of a tall, peaked P wave is termed "P pulmonale" (Fig. 4-27) because of its frequent association with chronic pulmonary disease.

Depression of the P–R segment, produced by large atrial repolarization forces, is called a "T_a" wave and is associated with right atrial enlargement (Lannek, 1949; American Medical Association, 1967) (see fig. 4-36).

When the left atrium dilates, the duration of atrial depolarization increases, but the course of depolarization is unchanged. Left atrial enlargement is indicated on the electrocardiogram as prolongation of the P wave. When prolongation occurs, there is often a notch separating the right atrial portion of the P wave from the left atrial portion. Prolongation of the P wave over 0.04 sec. is called

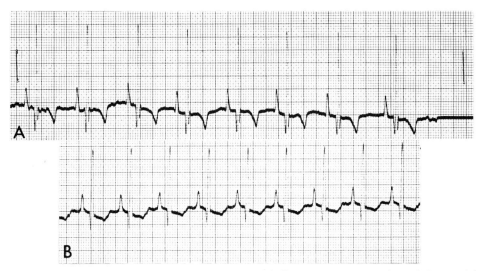

FIGURE 4-27 P pulmonale. Tall, peaked P waves greater than 0.4 mv. in amplitude characterize right atrial enlargement. The P waves in these tracings from dogs with chronic pulmonary disease are markedly enlarged. The tall R waves present in tracing A may indicate left ventricular enlargement. Lead II electrocardiograms.

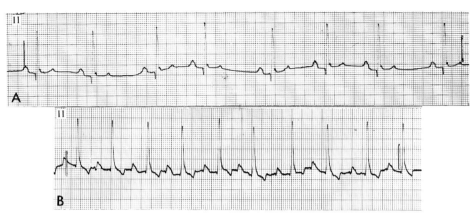

FIGURE 4-28   P mitrale. Enlarged left atria are recognized electrocardiographic-ally by prolongation of the atrial conduction time if the P wave is greater than 0.04 sec.

A, Dog with chronic mitral valvular fibrosis and mitral valvular insufficiency. The duration of the P wave (0.05 sec.) is prolonged. Notching of the P wave seen in this tracing is significant when the duration of the P wave is increased.

B, The P waves in this dog with chronic mitral valvular fibrosis and mitral valvular insufficiency are prolonged to 0.08 sec. Such extreme prolongation is unusual even in dogs with severe mitral valvular insufficiency. The amplitude and duration of the QRS complex are consistent with left ventricular hypertrophy.

"P mitrale" (Fig. 4-28) because of its association with mitral valve disease. Notching of the P wave is insignificant unless it is accompanied by such prolongation.

Biatrial enlargement is diagnosed when P waves are tall, peaked, wide, and notched (Fig. 4-29).

LEFT VENTRICULAR HYPERTROPHY

Left ventricular hypertrophy (LVH) is characterized by exaggeration of the electrical forces of ventricular depolarization. Because the ranges of normal and abnormal often overlap, electrocardiographic findings must be correlated with physical and radiographic findings to determine the degree of left ventricular hypertrophy. In one study, false negative electrocardiographic findings occurred in 69 per cent of dogs known to have left ventricular hypertrophy (Hamlin, 1968). Detweiler et al. (1968a) noted that there are still no adequate criteria for detecting left ventricular hypertrophy electrocardiographically. Therefore, more accurate electrocardiographic criteria are needed for diagnosis of this condition. Analysis of the electrocardiogram for left ventricular hypertrophy is best accomplished by examining the amplitude and duration of the QRS complex, changes of the S–T segment, abnormal wave deflections, and deviations of the mean electrical axis in the frontal plane.

QRS complexes of excessive magnitude occur with left ventricular dilatation and hypertrophy. However, this finding is normal in dogs under 2 years of age with narrow thoracic cavities (Fig. 4-30) and should be disregarded unless the amplitude of the R wave is greater than 3.0 mv. in lead aVF, with an S wave present in that lead (Hamlin, 1968). R waves of amplitude greater than 3.0 mv. in

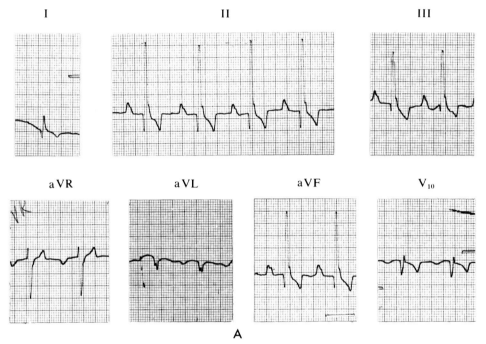

A

FIGURE 4-29 Biatrial enlargement. *A,* The amplitude of the P wave is greater than 0.4 mv. in leads II, III, and aVF and its duration is 0.06 sec. in the same leads, suggesting biatrial enlargement. In addition, the amplitude and duration of the QRS complexes in the other leads, the presence of Q waves in leads I, II, III, and aVF (greater than 0.5 mv. in lead II), and S–T repolarization changes in most leads are consistent with generalized cardiomegaly.

B, This dog with chronic mitral valvular fibrosis and mitral valvular insufficiency had electrocardiographic findings of biatrial enlargement. The increased duration of the P wave beyond 0-04 sec. is recognized in leads II, aVR, aVL, and V_{10}. This demonstrates the value of inspecting all leads if there is a suspicion of cardiac disease.

Illustration continues on opposite page.

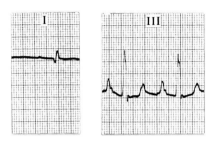

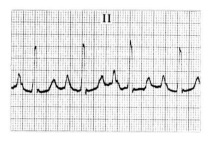

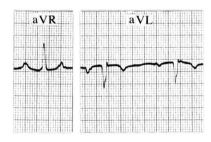

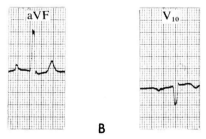

B

FIGURE 4-29 *Continued*

leads II and aVF in puppies are usually associated with patent ductus arteriosus (see page 483). In older dogs, an enlarged left ventricle may be suspected if the amplitude of the R wave in leads II, III, and aVF exceeds 2.5 mv., especially if other electrocardiographic indications of left ventricular hypertrophy are present.

In man, some distinction is made between the electrocardiographic findings of systolic or pressure overload, as occurs with conditions resulting in concentric left ventricular hypertrophy such as aortic stenosis, and diastolic or volume overload, as occurs with conditions resulting in eccentric hypertrophy and dilatation such as mitral insufficiency and patent ductus arteriosus. In pressure overload, R waves in leads III and aVF are small but are larger in lead I (consistent with left axis deviation). In volume overload, the depth of the Q wave and the height of the R wave in leads I, II, and III are increased significantly. This distinction is also recognized in the dog when the electrocardiograms of patent ductus arteriosus, mitral insufficiency, and aortic stenosis are compared (Figs. 4-31 and 4-32). Although abnormalities of the T wave are an important diagnostic aid in man, their value in the dog is unknown.

An increase in the thickness of the left ventricular free wall results in a considerable prolongation of left ventricular depolarization. Therefore, the duration of the QRS complex is frequently increased, exceeding 0.05 sec. However, in dogs of large breeds the duration of the QRS complex must exceed 0.06 sec. before a diagnosis of left ventricular hypertrophy may be considered. Prolongation of the QRS complex may be accompanied by notching or slurring (Fig. 4-31). However, left ventricular hypertrophy cannot be diagnosed on the basis of a slurred or notched QRS complex without evidence of prolongation. *Regardless of the normal duration of the QRS complex, prolongation as compared with previous recording in any individual is highly suggestive of left ventricular hypertrophy if other causes of prolongation, such as ectopic beats, bundle branch block, and aberrant conduction, can be eliminated.* Detweiler et al. (1968a) noted that left bundle branch block may be recorded electrocardiographically in dogs with marked left ventricular hypertrophy. In dogs of the toy and miniature breeds, prolongation of the QRS complex to 0.07 sec., a figure suggested by some as the criterion for left ventricular hypertrophy, is very uncommon.

The increased thickness of the left ventricular free wall occasionally causes a leftward deviation of the mean electrical forces in the frontal plane. If the mean electrical axis in the frontal plane is less than +40°, the electrocardiogram should be examined for other signs of left ventricular hypertrophy (Fig. 4-32). If only leads I and aVF are considered, such an axis deviation is present if the amplitude of the R wave is greater in lead I than in lead aVF (Hamlin, 1968). Hamlin (1968) states that left ventricular hypertrophy should be considered if the amplitude of the S wave is greater than that of the R wave in lead aVF. Since this relationship sometimes occurs with right ventricular hypertrophy, it should not be relied upon as a single electrocardiographic criterion for diagnosing left ventricular hypertrophy. In addition it would occur with *parietal block,* a condition involving abnormal conduction through the left branch of the bundle of His which results in severe left axis deviation.

Other abnormalities of the QRS complex associated with left ventricular hypertrophy are an increase in amplitude of the R wave in lead I to greater than 1.5 mv.; a sum of the amplitudes of the R waves in leads I and aVF greater than 4.0 mv.; and the absence of S waves in lead I (Hamlin, 1968).

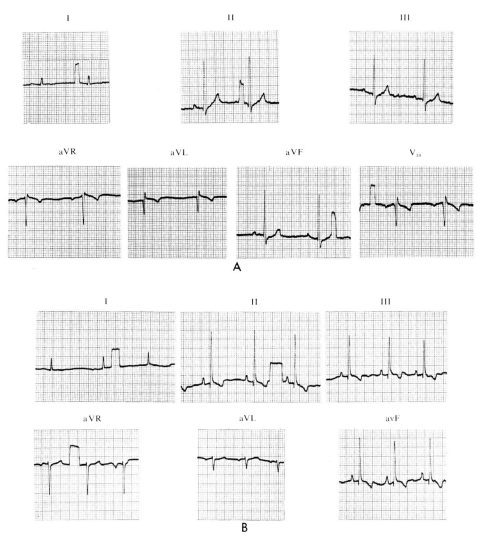

FIGURE 4-30 Tall R waves in normal young dogs. The amplitude of the R wave is often greater than 2.5 mv. in normal dogs under two years of age. (2.6 mv. in lead II of this ECG). However, it rarely exceeds 3.0 mv.

The area under the QRS complex represents the electrical activity generated during ventricular depolarization. Theoretically, the electrical activity of repolarization should be equal to that under the QRS complex. Since electrocardiographic changes during ventricular depolarization suggest hypertrophy, it is reasonable to expect changes during ventricular repolarization as well. When repolarization changes occur in left ventricular hypertrophy, the S-T segment, which is normally isoelectric, sags in a concave direction into the T wave (Fig. 4-31*A* and *C*). Repolarization changes of the S-T segment should be differentiated from the effects of cardiac glycosides or quinidine and from disturbances due to electrolyte imbalances, which also cause electrocardiographic abnormalities.

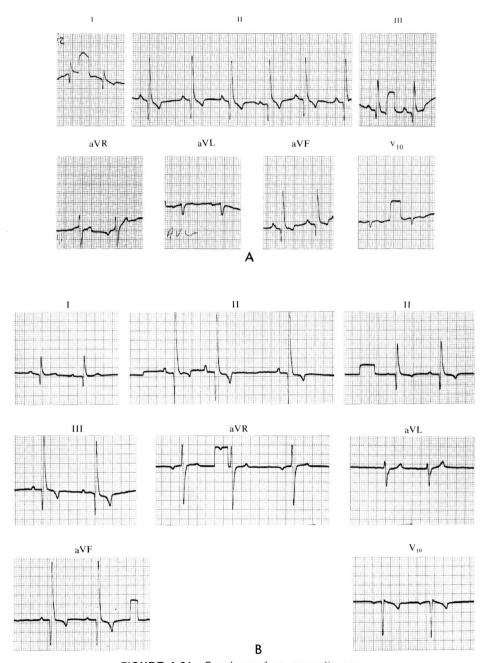

FIGURE 4-31 *See legend on opposite page.*

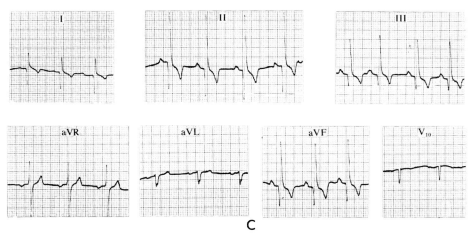

C

FIGURE 4-31 Left ventricular hypertrophy. *A,* Electrocardiogram of a dog with chronic mitral valvular fibrosis and mitral valvular insufficiency. The QRS complex is prolonged to 0.07 sec. (best seen in leads II, III, and aVF). S–T repolarization changes are present in some leads, and P mitrale is seen in leads II, III, and aVF.

B, This dog had markedly enlarged ventricles owing to insufficiency of the mitral and tricuspid valves. The amplitude and duration of the QRS complexes are increased. The amplitude of the R waves is greater than 25 mm. (35 mm. here) in lead II, and the QRS complex is prolonged to 0.07 sec. II at ½ amplitude is also shown.

C, Electrocardiogram of dog with advanced mitral and tricuspid valvular fibrosis. The wide and notched P wave (0.05 sec.), the tall R wave (29 mm.), and wide (0.06 sec.) QRS complexes, as well as S–T repolarization changes in lead II, are consistent with left ventricular hypertrophy. The Q waves in leads II, III, and aVF are deeper than normal (see Fig. 4-36).

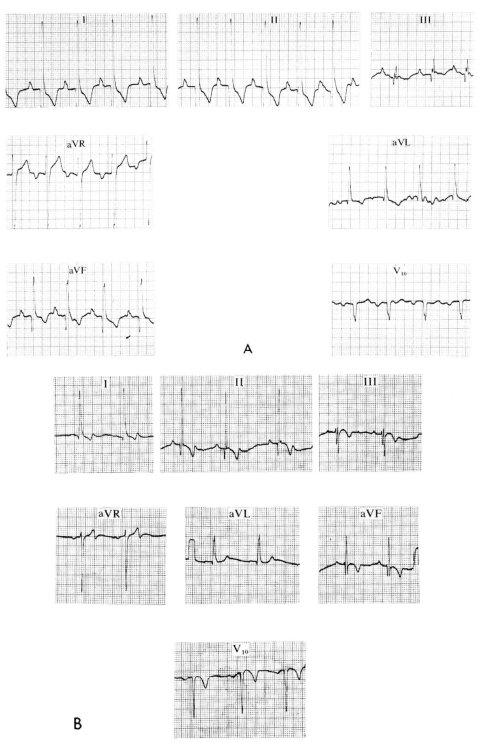

FIGURE 4-32 Left axis deviation. *A,* The mean electrical axis in the frontal plane in this dog with mitral valvular fibrosis is 35°. Notice that the R wave in lead I is tall and positive, as would be expected in left axis deviation. Also present in this tracing are P mitrale, tall and prolonged QRS complexes, and S–T repolarization changes, all of which are consistent with left atrial and left ventricular hypertrophy.

B, In this dog with congenital subaortic stenosis, the mean electrical axis was approximately 20°. Left axis deviation can usually be related to left ventricular hypertrophy.

Abnormalities of the T wave may also suggest left ventricular hypertrophy. If T waves are of very high amplitude, left ventricular hypertrophy or hyperkalemia may be present. T waves of amplitude greater than 25 per cent of that of the R wave in leads II, III, and aVF suggest left ventricular hypertrophy.

RIGHT VENTRICULAR HYPERTROPHY

Right ventricular hypertrophy (RVH) is associated with certain congenital cardiac defects, mitral and/or tricuspid valvular insufficiency, and cor pulmonale, which occurs commonly in heartworm disease. In most cases of acquired right ventricular hypertrophy, the left ventricular mass remains greater than the right ventricular mass. The right ventricular mass predominates only in severe right ventricular hypertrophy due to congenital heart disease.

A consistent finding in right ventricular hypertrophy is a deviation of the mean frontal plane electrical axis beyond 100°. When right ventricular hypertrophy results from acquired heart disease, the mean frontal plane electrical axis usually does not exceed 120° (Fig. 4-33). Heart disease that is associated with more severe right ventricular enlargement may have an axis greater than 120° (Fig. 4-34). When the degree of hypertrophy is minimal, there may be little or no deviation of the mean electrical axis.

When right ventricular enlargement involves the base of the heart or the ventricular outflow tract, as in heartworm disease, S waves may be present in leads I, II, and III. This finding, an $S_1S_2S_3$ pattern, is not often seen in normal dogs but may be observed in dogs with right ventricular hypertrophy (Fig. 4-35). This pattern should also be differentiated from right bundle branch block, an abnormality also associated with S waves in leads I, II, and III (see pp. 149–153).

The left precordial leads suggest the presence of right ventricular hypertrophy when the depth of the S wave is beyond the normal limits (Knight, 1969).

Using leads I and aVF for analysis (Hamlin, 1968), right ventricular enlargement is associated with an S wave of greater amplitude than the R wave in both leads. In other words, right axis deviation is present. In severe right ventricular hypertrophy the S wave in lead aVF is greater than or equal to 2.0 mv., or $\frac{S_1}{R_1}$ and $\frac{S_{aVF}}{R_{aVF}}$ are both greater than 3.0 (Hamlin, 1968).

The presence of a positive T wave in leads CV_5 RL and V_{10} also suggests right ventricular hypertrophy (except in the Chihuahua, when a positive T wave in lead V_{10} is not diagnostic) (Detweiler and Patterson, 1965).

BIVENTRICULAR HYPERTROPHY

Biventricular hypertrophy is difficult to diagnose accurately from the electrocardiogram. The presence of both right and left atrial enlargement, prolonged QRS complexes of high amplitude associated with S–T repolarization changes, and deep Q waves in leads I, II, and III, with the Q wave in lead II being greater than 0.5 mv., are compatible with biventricular hypertrophy (Fig. 4-36).

Text continues on page 149.

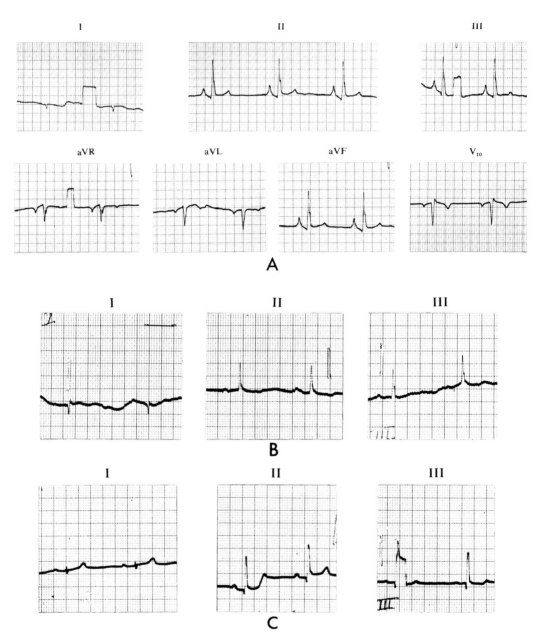

FIGURE 4-33 *See legend on opposite page.*

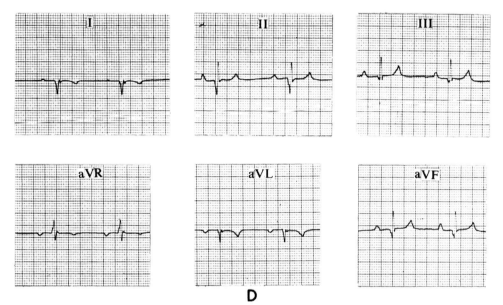

FIGURE 4-33 Right axis deviation. *A,* Dog with acquired tricuspid insufficiency and right ventricular hypertrophy. The mean electrical axis in the frontal plane is 105°. The S wave in lead I is a diagnostic clue suggesting right ventricular hypertrophy. P pulmonale in leads II, III, and aVF supports the diagnosis of right heart disease.

B, Dog with heartworm disease. Prior to destruction of the adult worms, the mean electrical axis in the frontal plane was approximately 115°. The tracing made 100 days later *(C)* demonstrates an axis of 90°, suggesting that the right ventricular mass was returning to normal.

D, The mean electrical axis in the frontal plane was 125° in this dog with chronic pulmonary disease. The prolonged initial phase of depolarization is directed to the right (Q wave in lead I) and cranially (Q wave in lead aVF).

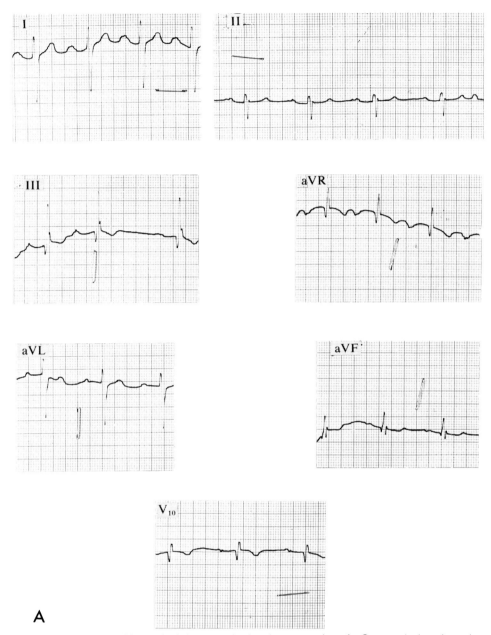

A

FIGURE 4-34   Marked right ventricular hypertrophy. *A,* Congenital pulmonic stenosis in this dog has resulted in deviation of the mean electrical axis in the frontal plane to 170°. In addition, the P wave and QRS complex are prolonged to 0.08 sec. and 0.06 sec., respectively. At necropsy, only congenital valvular pulmonic stenosis was found.

B, Congenital pulmonic stenosis in this dog is consistent with a mean electrical axis in the frontal plane of 135°. P waves are tall and peaked in leads II and aVF. The absence of a terminal R wave (dorsally directed terminal forces) in lead V_{10} is abnormal.

Illustration continues on opposite page.

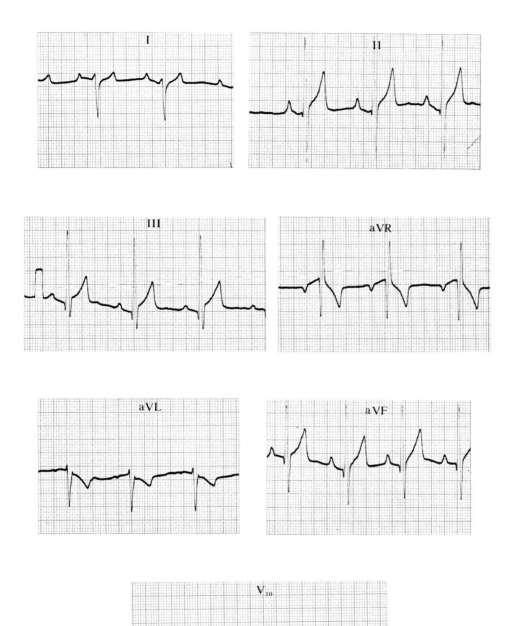

B

Figure 4-34 *Continued*

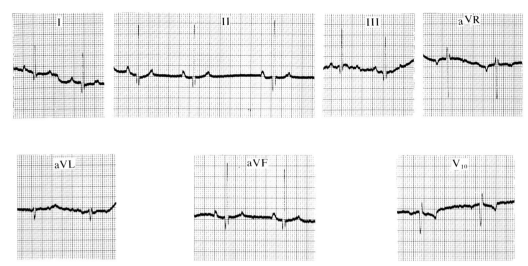

FIGURE 4-35 S_1-S_2-S_3 pattern. This tracing was made from a dog with heartworm disease. The S_1-S_2-S_3 pattern is unusual in normal dogs, and the finding can suggest right ventricular hypertrophy. Such findings warrant further study, especially in areas where heartworms are endemic.

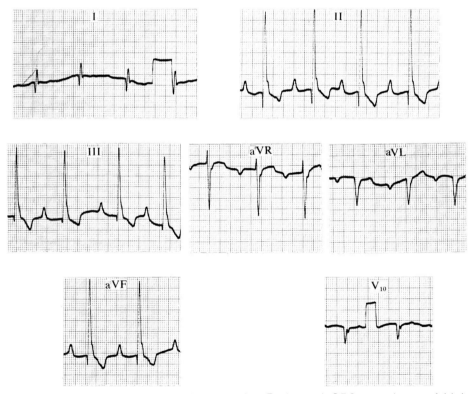

FIGURE 4-36 Biventricular hypertrophy. Prolonged QRS complexes of high amplitude with S–T repolarization changes, Q waves in leads I, II, and III, Q waves deeper than 0.5 mv. in lead II, P pulmonale, and P mitrale are characteristic electrocardiographic findings associated with biventricular hypertrophy. First degree heart block is due to early digitalis intoxication. T_a waves following the tall P waves in leads II, III, and aVF often occur in association with P pulmonale.

BUNDLE BRANCH BLOCK

When conduction through the left or right branch of the bundle of His is disrupted, the electrical impulse is forced to travel through the myocardium. Since the myocardium does not conduct impulses as rapidly as do the specialized conduction tissues, the duration of the QRS complex is prolonged, and the condition is known as bundle branch block. Experimental transection of the right or left branch of the bundle of His in the dog (Scott, 1965) produces electrocardiographic abnormalities similar to those seen clinically in spontaneous right or left bundle branch block.

LEFT BUNDLE BRANCH BLOCK

Section of the left branch of the bundle of His in dogs results in QRS complexes which are positive in leads I, II, III, and aVF (Detweiler, Hubben, and Patterson, 1960; Scott, 1965). The QRS complex is inverted in leads aVR, aVL, and CV_5 LL (Detweiler, Hubben, and Patterson, 1960). All QRS complexes appear normal but are prolonged (Fig. 4-37). In left bundle branch block the initial forces are directed from right to left, but a small Q wave may still be present in lead I, suggesting some left-to-right activation (Detweiler, Hubben, and Patterson, 1960). It has been reported that left bundle branch block is always associated with heart disease in the dog (Detweiler, Hubben, and Patterson, 1960), and we have never seen left bundle branch block in a normal dog. Of six cases of left bundle branch block reported, evidence of myocardial disease was found at necropsy in five (Romagnoli, 1953; Patterson et al., 1961; Buchanan, 1965). Left bundle branch block is occasionally present in dogs with severe left ventricular hypertrophy (Detweiler et al., 1968a).

RIGHT BUNDLE BRANCH BLOCK

Section of the right branch of the bundle of His in dogs produces negative QRS complexes in leads I, II, III, aVL, aVF, CV_6 LL, and CV_6 LU (Detweiler, Hubben, and Patterson, 1960; Scott, 1965). Lead aVL is usually positively directed in the author's experience (see Figs. 4-38 and 4-39). The first portion of the QRS complex need not be abnormal, since conduction through the left side of the heart produces an initially normal pattern. The terminal deflection (Fig. 4-38), during which the slowly inscribed right ventricular depolarization is directed cranially (negative lead aVF) and to the right (negative lead I), is prolonged (Hill, 1968). Hill (1968) reports the presence of an S wave in lead V_{10} in a dog with right bundle branch block. However, this has not been observed in all cases of right bundle branch block seen by the authors and is not an absolute criterion for such a diagnosis. The maximum depolarization time in right bundle branch block observed by us on the vectorcardiogram was 0.08 sec.

Right bundle branch block may occur in normal dogs as an incidental finding. It has also been observed in dogs with right ventricular dilatation (Patterson et al., 1961) and with chronic lung disease. Intermittent right bundle branch block has been observed by us in an otherwise normal dog (Fig. 4-39). The significance of right bundle branch block is not known; however, any dog in which it is recognized should be evaluated for other cardiac abnormalities.

Text continues on page 153.

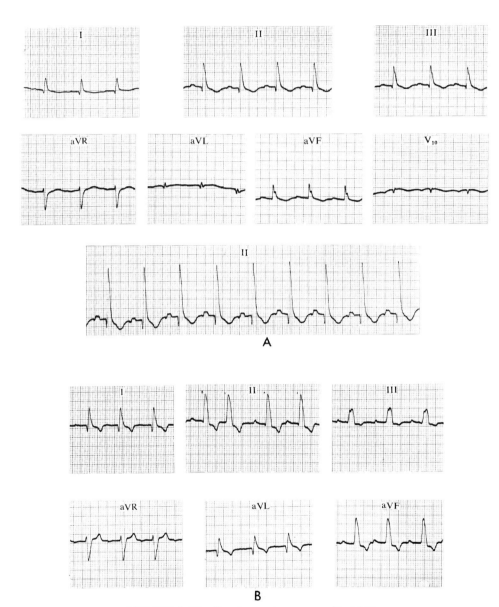

FIGURE 4-37 *See legend on opposite page.*

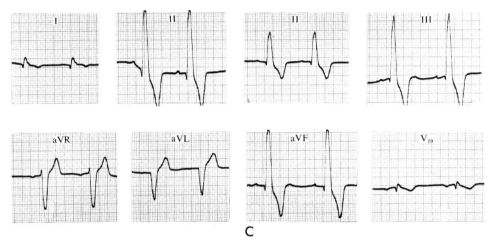

C

FIGURE 4-37 Left bundle branch block. *A,* Electrocardiogram of dog with clinical and radiographic evidence of massive left ventricular and left atrial enlargement. The electrocardiogram is consistent with left ventricular hypertrophy and P mitrale. The width of the QRS complex, which exceeds 0.07 sec., permits a diagnosis of left bundle branch block.

B, A QRS complex 0.08 sec. wide was recorded from a dog with advanced mitral valvular fibrosis. This tracing, consistent with left bundle branch block, is actually an accentuation of the left ventricular hypertrophy pattern. The second complex in lead II is a supraventricular premature beat. (Tracing courtesy of Dr. H. Zweighaft.)

C, Left bundle branch block pattern developed in a dog after surgical intervention for subaortic stenosis. On the electrocardiogram, the small Q wave in lead I suggests that the earliest forces are still directed from left to right. The duration of the QRS complex is 0.10 sec., which is longer than that seen in left bundle branch block associated with left ventricular hypertrophy due to chronic valvular disease.

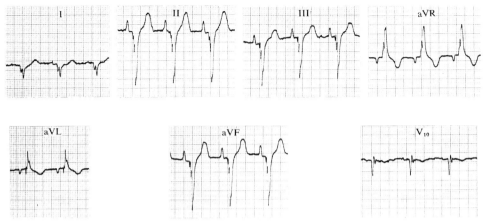

FIGURE 4-38 Right bundle branch block. Electrocardiogram of an otherwise normal dog with right bundle branch block. This electrocardiographic abnormality is characterized by aberrant conduction with negative QRS complexes in leads I, II, III, aVF, and V_{10}. Although this tracing does not demonstrate small R waves in leads I, II, III, and aVF, one may be present (Fig. 4-39). The major forces are late and are directed rightward (prolonged S wave in lead I) and craniad (prolonged S wave in leads II, III, aVF). The QRS complex is prolonged to 0.08 sec., and P pulmonale is present in leads II, III, and aVF. The V_{10} lead demonstrates a terminal S wave indicating a final ventricular force directed ventrally.

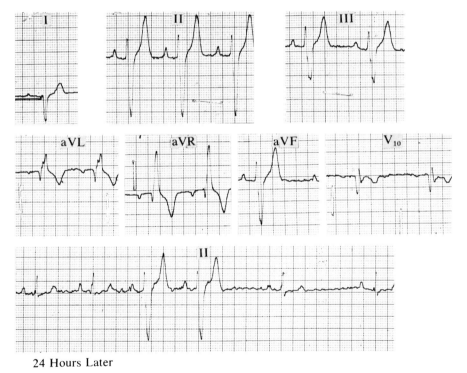

24 Hours Later

FIGURE 4-39 Intermittent right bundle branch block. An electrocardiogram similar to that in Figure 4-38 was recorded in this dog prior to mammary tumor excision. Because of the abnormality another tracing was made the following day (lead II, at bottom). In this strip right bundle branch block occurs intermittently (beats 3 and 4). Since the dog had no other abnormalities contraindicating surgery, the masses were removed without complication.

152

Incomplete right bundle branch block has also been reported (Hill, 1968). In this condition the QRS complex is of normal duration but is negative in leads I, II, III, aVF, CV_6 LL, and CV_6 LU. It is positive in leads aVR, aVL, and CV_5 RL.

ARTIFACTS DUE TO ERRORS IN RECORDING

Technical errors in electrocardiography. A baseline with a regular, saw-tooth appearance suggests interference from 60-cycle alternating current (A–C) (Fig. 4-40). Sixty-cycle interference results from improper grounding or from jamming by electrical lines or machines in the examining area. If 60-cycle interference occurs one should determine whether the machine is properly grounded and should also examine the electrodes to be sure that they are placed on the skin properly and attached firmly to the cable tips. Poor electrode contact with the skin is avoided by applying both alcohol and pHisoHex to the skin and electrodes. For improving the contact, the cable tip and electrodes should be cleaned by frequent scrubbing with steel wool to remove oil and grease that collect. If the interference still occurs in all leads, electrical appliances being used near the patient should be disconnected temporarily. If the technique used is correct and if the interference persists when the examination is conducted in another area of the room, it is likely that the machine is malfunctioning. A broken patient cable may be responsible for 60-cycle interference. To prevent the wires from breaking, it is recommended that the cable not be sharply bent or rolled for storage.

Tremor of the patient, indicated on the electrocardiogram by a fuzzy, irregular baseline, is often encountered in nervous dogs (Fig. 4-41). The owner's reassurance may help to calm the dog, and the veterinarian should attempt to reduce cable tension on the patient by keeping the cable on the table rather than letting it hang off the table, which adds tension to the alligator clip-skin connection.

Irregularities of the baseline of the electrocardiogram are common. Both wandering and irregular baselines can be avoided by improving electrode contact as previously described and by restraining the animal properly during the recording. Heavy breathing may also be responsible for an unstable baseline (Fig. 4-42). When this is done accidentally, the P wave (see polarity) is upright in leads II QRS complex are not recorded, and the complex appears smaller than normal or abnormal (Fig. 4-43).

Reversal of electrode placement. A common technical error made in recording the electrocardiogram is reversal of the right and left forelimb electrodes. When this is done accidentally, the P wave polarity is upright in leads II and III but is negative in lead I, incorrectly indicating a rightward deflection of the P wave (Fig. 4-44). If the electrodes have been so reversed, the recording of lead I must be discarded, but the lead II strip is actually a recording of lead III, and vice versa. Similarly, the recordings of leads aVR and aVL are interchanged. Lead aVF is correct as recorded. Accidental reversal of the hindlimb electrodes has little adverse effect on the electrocardiogram. Reversal of the forelimb electrodes with those of the hindlimbs produces abnormal electrocardiograms, and it is often impossible to obtain any electrical activity in lead I.

Panting and shivering. If the dog pants or shivers during recording of the electrocardiogram, regularly spaced, artifactual waves resembling atrial flutter may be recorded (Fig. 4-45). Since atrial flutter is rare in the dog (see p. 299), any recording suggesting this condition should be carefully scrutinized.

Text continues on page 158.

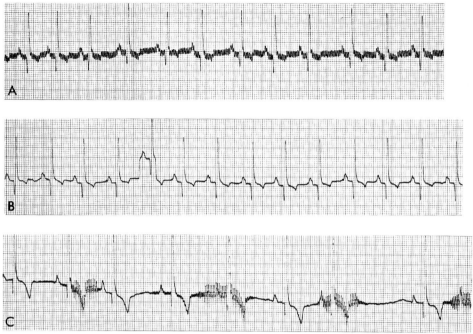

FIGURE 4-40 60-cycle interference. *A,* Electrocardiogram recorded without sufficient conducting media. The small, cyclical, saw-tooth waves represent 60-cycle interference. *B,* Tracing from same dog recorded after the application of greater quantities of pHisoHex and alcohol. *C,* 60-cycle interference produced where the electrodes connected to the patient were intermittently touched by the holder.

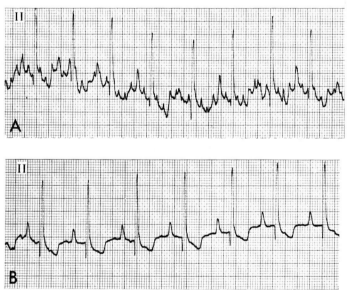

FIGURE 4-41 *A,* Tremor or shivering produces an irregular, wavy baseline on the electrocardiogram. Although most of the complexes are still discernible, it is difficult to obtain measurements. *B,* After the dog was reassured and the technician's hand was placed gently on its thorax, most of the quivering movements stopped, and a much clearer electrocardiogram was recorded. Biatrial and biventricular hypertrophy are suggested by this tracing.

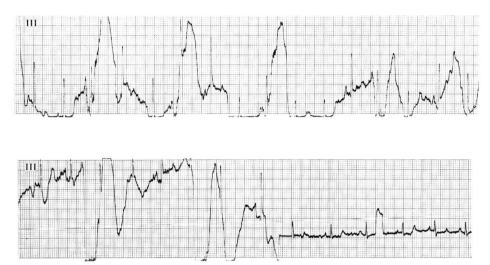

FIGURE 4-42 Artifactual recordings are produced when the dog moves or coughs. The baseline wanders and is irregular. The large excursions result from coughing. By the end of the recording the dog had quieted, and the tracing was clearer.

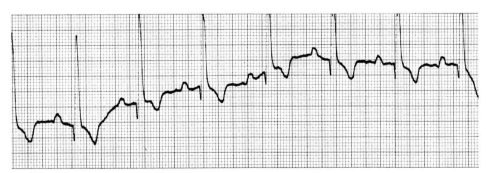

FIGURE 4-43 If the stylus of the electrocardiograph moves too far from the center of the paper, the spike of the QRS complex is cut off at the top or bottom of the graph paper. This results in an artifactually smaller amplitude on the tracing. On this electrocardiogram, the complete, normal complex is followed by progressively smaller R waves recorded as the baseline moves too far from the center.

CORRECT PLACEMENT   INCORRECT PLACEMENT

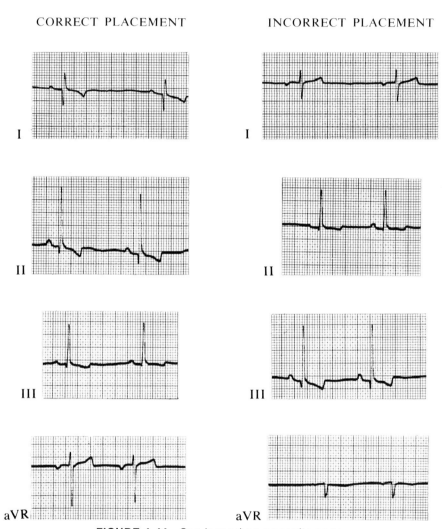

FIGURE 4-44 *See legend on opposite page.*

CORRECT PLACEMENT   INCORRECT PLACEMENT

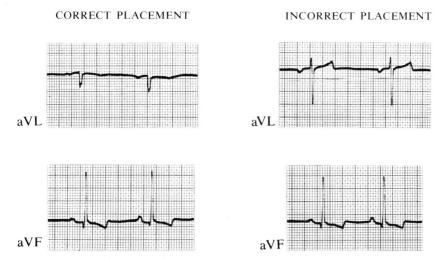

FIGURE 4-44 Electrocardiograms produced when RA and LA electrodes are reversed. When this common technical error occurs, lead I is abnormal; the P wave and QRS complex are negative. When the electrocardiograph is set to record lead II, lead III results, and vice versa, since the machine automatically connects the proper electrodes for the lead selected regardless of misplacement of electrodes. In like manner, leads aVR and aVL are reversed. Lead aVF is correct as recorded. The tracings on the right were recorded with the RA and LA electrodes reversed, and those on the left were recorded with the electrodes properly placed. Reversal of the hindlimb electrodes usually does not grossly distort the electrocardiogram, whereas reversal of both forelimb and hindlimb electrodes results in a grossly deformed electrocardiogram often lacking a lead I.

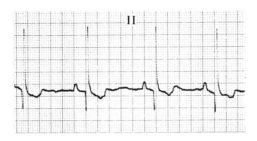

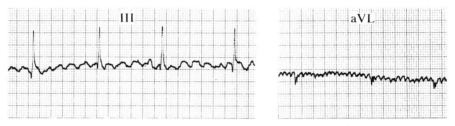

FIGURE 4-45 Artifactual waves resembling atrial flutter. Such artifacts on the baseline are produced when the dog pants or shivers. In this tracing the complexes in lead II are normal, but artifacts are present in the baseline of leads III and aVL. It is important to examine all leads recorded since a normal strip in one lead may then cast doubt on an abnormality thought to be present in another lead.

VECTORCARDIOGRAPHY

The vectorcardiogram (VCG) is another graphic method of describing the electrical activity of the heart. The scalar electrocardiographic tracing plots the magnitude of electrical activity on the vertical axis, and time on the horizontal axis (Fig. 4-1, page 103). In comparison, the vectorcardiogram projects the magnitude and spatial direction of the cardiac vector as visualized in the frontal, horizontal, and sagittal planes of the body (Fig. 4-19, page 121).

The vectorcardiogram is produced when two simultaneously recorded lead axes at right angles to each other are connected to the perpendicular deflecting plates of a cathode ray tube. As the two leads are resolved into one force or vector, the electron beam emitted by the cathode ray tube is displaced. The magnitude and direction of the instantaneous forces are the factors of the direction of the vector and its distance away from the starting point (length).

The mechanics of recording the vectorcardiogram are simple. Two axes are chosen (XY, XZ, or ZY) and are connected simultaneously to the cathode ray tube so that the resultant instantaneous cardiac vectors are displayed on the oscilloscope screen. By adjusting the duration of photographic exposure the entire vectorcardiogram or parts of the vectorcardiogram may be selected for permanent recording. After the desired portions are chosen and identified on the screen, the camera is momentarily activated, and the photographic paper is exposed, the resulting image being exactly the same as the vectorcardiogram observed on the screen.

The vectorcardiogram is thus permanently recorded on a stationary plate of photographic paper. The tracing begins at the dipole center, where the cardiac electrical activity is zero; this point is equivalent to the isoelectric line on the scalar electrocardiogram. The image representing the resolved electrical forces moves to the left or the right and to the top or the bottom of the paper, according to the direction of the force, until a loop or circle is completed, returning to the zero point or isoelectric line. QRS loops which do not close indicate depression or elevation of the S–T segment. The magnitude of the force at any instant is determined by comparing the distance of the image from the dipole center to a previously calibrated setting (25 mm. = 1 mv. is used by the authors). The vector tracing is an unbroken line that can also be divided electronically into small teardrops, each having a predetermined duration. In this text, vectorcardiograms are so recorded that a loop is inscribed in the direction of the narrow or pointed end of the teardrops, each teardrop representing 0.002 sec. movement of the vector since the last teardrop. When the teardrops are close together the conduction of electrical forces is slow, whereas teardrops that are widely spaced indicate rapid movement of the cardiac vector.

The vectorcardiogram is recorded in three planes using the following pairs of axes, as suggested by the American Heart Association (1967):

Frontal plane (XY) – X (sinistrodextral) and Y (craniocaudal)
Horizontal (transverse) plane (XZ) – X (sinistrodextral) and
  Z (ventrodorsal)
Left sagittal plane (ZY) – Z (ventrodorsal) and Y (craniocaudal)

For the vectorcardiogram, the two axes forming each plane must be recorded simultaneously. For each plane, the forces from both axes are resolved into a single force which represents the magnitude and direction of the cardiac vector. The instantaneous forces, represented by teardrops, are recorded for the entire cardiac cycle. The vectorcardiogram is complete when one complete cardiac electrical cycle, i.e., the P, QRS, and T loops, has been recorded.

The vectorcardiogram is advantageous because it is a pictorial representation of the electrocardiographic magnitude, direction, and duration of the heart's electrical forces. In addition, only three scalar orthogonal leads (X, Y, and Z), rather than seven to ten scalar tracings (I, II, III, aVR, aVL, aVF, V_{10}, CV_6 LL, CV_6 LU, and CV_5 RL), need be evaluated to determine the electrical position of the heart in the frontal, horizontal, and sagittal planes. In addition, the scalar X, Y, and Z leads represent corrected orthogonal leads (see pp. 120–122) rather than the anatomically derived limb and thoracic leads.

The vectorcardiogram is simply the electrical resolution of two simultaneously recorded scalar electrocardiographic leads at right angles to each other. The vectorcardiogram may be drawn from the electrocardiogram by inspecting the initial, middle, and terminal forces from two scalar leads and plotting them on the XY, XZ, or ZY axes. Similarly, the electrocardiogram may be determined from the vectorcardiogram. Since the vectorcardiogram represents the two axes of each plane, the instantaneous cardiac vectors may be replotted as scalar X, Y, and Z leads.

Vectorcardiography is a relatively new technique in veterinary cardiology. Thus, the information available is still limited. The data known about the P, QRS, and T loops as determined from the modified orthogonal lead system (leads I, aVF, and V_{10}) and the corrected orthogonal lead system of McFee (X, Y, and Z) are presented. As does the scalar electrocardiogram, the vectorcardiogram varies with thoracic conformation.

THE NORMAL VECTORCARDIOGRAM

The P loop. Using the McFee corrected orthogonal lead system, the P loop is directed leftward, ventrad, and caudad in normal dogs. The mean direction of the P loop in most dogs is between 60° and 90° in the frontal plane (Fig. 4-46).

The QRS loop. The mean direction of the QRS loop is leftward, ventrad, and caudad. The direction of the teardrops in the horizontal and sagittal loops should be counterclockwise, but in the frontal plane it may be either counterclockwise or clockwise. The loop is usually long and thin in the frontal plane, and it occasionally appears as a figure eight. The loop may appear more rounded in the horizontal plane. The initial forces (0.01 sec.) are directed ventrally and to the right. The earliest initial forces may at first be directed craniad but they then move in a caudal direction. The major forces (0.025 to 0.035 sec.) are directed leftward, ventrad, and caudad, and the terminal forces (to 0.01 sec.) move leftward, dorsad, and craniad (see Fig. 4-46).

The T loop. The T loop of the vectorcardiogram varies considerably among individuals. It is usually directed ventrally and just to the right of the midline. In the frontal plane, its direction may be either craniad or caudad (Detweiler and Patterson, 1965) (Fig. 4-46).

LEFT VENTRICULAR HYPERTROPHY

In dogs with left ventricular hypertrophy, the QRS vector loop is longer, wider, and of greater duration than normal (Fig. 4-47). These changes correspond to the increased amplitude and duration of the QRS complex on the scalar electrocardiogram. There is often an increase in the terminal dorsal forces in the QRS loop in the horizontal plane. The vector loops further demonstrate that left ventricular hypertrophy may be regarded as an accentuation of the normal electrocardiogram or vectorcardiogram (Fig. 4-47).

RIGHT VENTRICULAR HYPERTROPHY

Vectorcardiograms indicate pictorially both the degree of right ventricular hypertrophy and the abnormal direction of the cardiac vector. When right ventricular hypertrophy is severe, the vector loops in the frontal and horizontal planes are directed clockwise, the initial forces being leftward, caudad, and ventrad. The middle and terminal segments are directed cranially, to the right, and ventrad or dorsad (or both) (Fig. 4-48). The vectorcardiogram may appear deceptively normal in mild right ventricular hypertrophy, as occurs with mild pulmonic stenosis (Fig. 4-49).

In dogs with either congenital or acquired right ventricular hypertrophy there may be prolongation of the initial forces beyond the 0.01 sec. limit suggested by Hamlin and Smith (1960). If the enlargement is moderate, the initial rightward forces are prolonged beyond 0.01 sec. and may be directed craniad and/or caudad. The middle and terminal portions of the vectorcardiogram are normal (Fig. 4-50). In more severe acquired right ventricular hypertrophy, as occurs with severe heartworm disease, the vector may begin on the left with the major and terminal forces directed rightward (Fig. 4-51).

Text continues on page 166

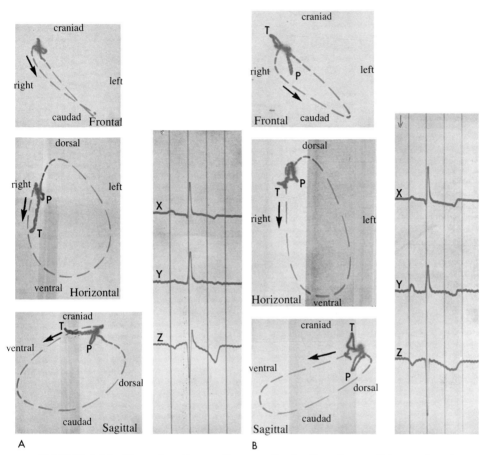

FIGURE 4-46   Normal vectorcardiogram. Scalar time lines = 0.1 sec.; teardrops = 0.002 sec. *A,* Vectorcardiogram, normal dog. The scalar X, Y, and Z leads are recorded, and the resultants of the X and Y leads (frontal plane), X and Z leads (horizontal plane), and Z and Y leads (sagittal plane) are then photographed. In the frontal plane the direction of the teardrops is counterclockwise (arrow). The forces are initially directed rightward and caudad and then turn leftward and caudad. In the horizontal plane the direction is counterclockwise, and the terminal forces are directed dorsally and leftward. The P (small) and T (large) loop are clearly recorded in the horizontal and sagittal planes of this vectorcardiogram.

B, The vectorcardiogram of a normal dog, similar to the vectorcardiogram in *A.* A major difference in the two vectorcardiograms is the orientation of the T loop, which is more cranially directed in this case (frontal and sagittal planes). The P loop, normally directed leftward, caudad, and ventrad, is well produced.

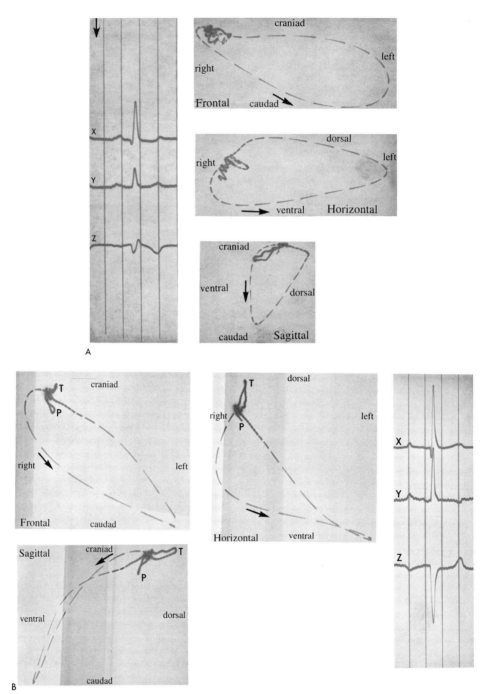

FIGURE 4-47 Left ventricular hypertrophy. Scalar time lines = 0.1 sec.; teardrops = 0.002 sec. *A,* The dog from which this vectorcardiogram was recorded had congenital aortic stenosis. Left axis deviation (frontal plane direction) is indicated because the QRS loop is inscribed almost directly leftward. There is an overall increase in both the duration (0.056 sec.) and magnitude of forces. In the horizontal plane the terminal forces directed dorsally are prolonged.

B, Vectorcardiogram recorded from a dog with advanced mitral and tricuspid valvular insufficiency. The scalar and vectorcardiographic tracings suggest left ventricular hypertrophy by the accentuation of both amplitude and duration of forces. The leftward, caudad, and ventrad direction of the P loop is normal, but the dorsal direction of the T loop is abnormal.

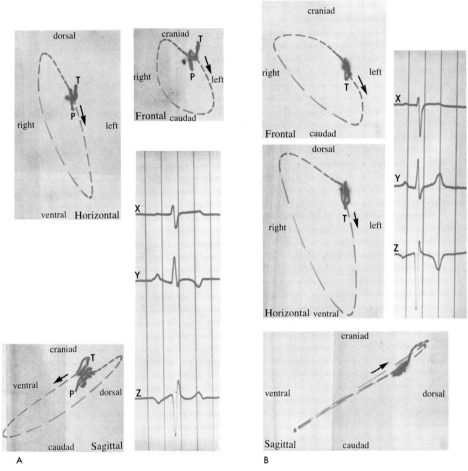

FIGURE 4-48   Right ventricular hypertrophy. Scalar time lines = 0.1 sec.; teardrops = 0.002 sec. *A,* The cardiac vectors indicate right ventricular hypertrophy since the forces are abnormally directed to the right in this dog. The forces in the frontal and horizontal planes originate on the left and follow a clockwise direction to the right. The duration of the QRS complex is not prolonged.

B, The vectorcardiogram recorded from this dog with congenital pulmonic stenosis is similar to that in *A.* One difference is the T wave direction, which is leftward, craniad, and dorsad in *A,* but leftward, caudad, and ventrad in *B.* The significance of the T wave vector in the dog with hypertrophy is not entirely clear.

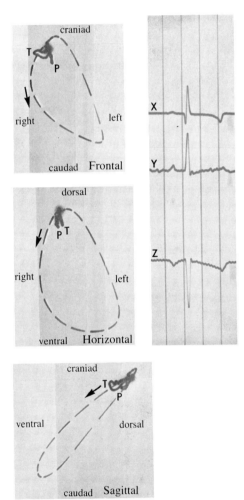

FIGURE 4-49   This apparently normal vectorcardiogram was recorded from a dog with minimal congenital pulmonic stenosis in which the pressure gradient from the right ventricle to the main pulmonary artery determined by cardiac catheterization was 20 mm. Hg. This tracing suggests that the electrocardiogram and vectorcardiogram are not always grossly abnormal in congenital heart disease. Scalar time lines = 0.1 sec.; teardrops = 0.002 sec.

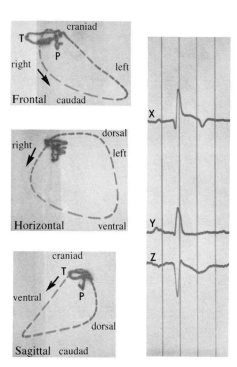

FIGURE 4-50 Prolongation of the initial ventricular forces to the right (0.014 sec.) in this vectorcardiogram is suggestive of acquired right ventricular hypertrophy. A diagnosis of heartworm disease was made from the radiographs and from microscopic examination of blood, and chemotherapy was successful. Scalar time lines = 0.1 sec.; teardrops = 0.002 sec.

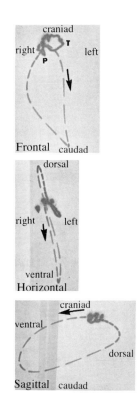

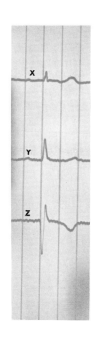

FIGURE 4-51 Acquired right ventricular hypertrophy. The vectorcardiograms of this dog with symptomatic heart worm disease indicate an abnormality in conduction, and right ventricular hypertrophy. In the frontal plane, the forces begin on the left but are directed to the right for approximately half of the period of ventricular depolarization. In the horizontal plane, the second half of the ventricular forces is directed dorsally. In the frontal projection, twice the standard amplitude is used to demonstrate the P and T waves. Scalar time lines = 0.1 sec.; teardrops = 0.002 sec.

BIVENTRICULAR HYPERTROPHY

On the vectorcardiogram, the initial forces are rightward and prolonged, and there is an overall increase in duration and magnitude of all forces (Fig. 4-52).

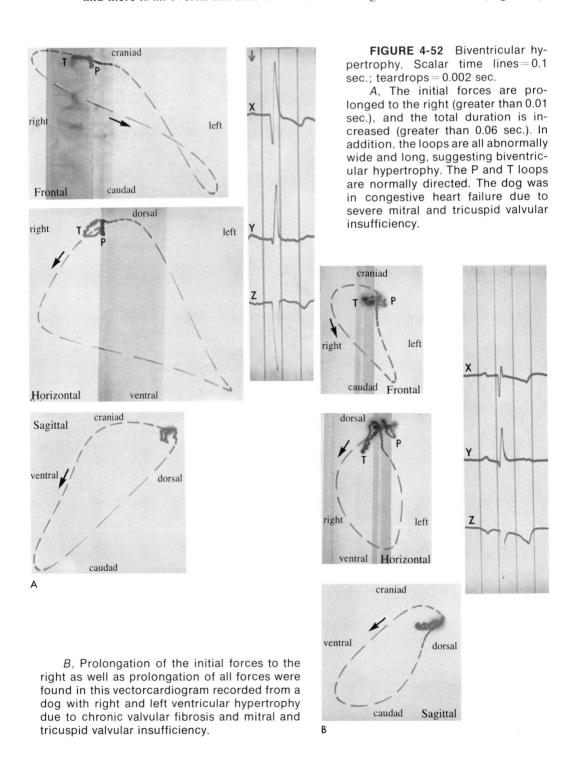

FIGURE 4-52 Biventricular hypertrophy. Scalar time lines = 0.1 sec.; teardrops = 0.002 sec.

A, The initial forces are prolonged to the right (greater than 0.01 sec.), and the total duration is increased (greater than 0.06 sec.). In addition, the loops are all abnormally wide and long, suggesting biventricular hypertrophy. The P and T loops are normally directed. The dog was in congestive heart failure due to severe mitral and tricuspid valvular insufficiency.

B, Prolongation of the initial forces to the right as well as prolongation of all forces were found in this vectorcardiogram recorded from a dog with right and left ventricular hypertrophy due to chronic valvular fibrosis and mitral and tricuspid valvular insufficiency.

RIGHT BUNDLE BRANCH BLOCK

On the vectorcardiogram (Fig. 4-53) the initial forces are leftward, ventrad, and caudad and are followed by prolonged terminal forces (many closely spaced arrows) directed rightward, craniad, and dorsad.

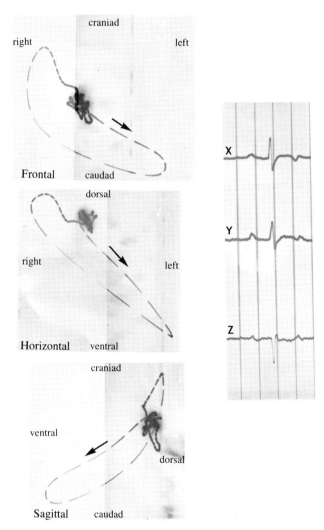

FIGURE 4-53 Right bundle branch block is characterized vectorcardio-graphically by an abnormally prolonged ventricular complex with rightward, dorsal, and cranially directed terminal forces. The vector loop in the horizontal plane is abnormal in its clockwise direction. The many small, closely spaced arrows terminally in all three planes are diagnostic of right bundle branch block. As is often the case in both man and dogs, this dog had no abnormalities other than right bundle branch block. The vectorcardiogram was recorded at twice the standard amplitude to improve visualization of the abnormal terminal forces. Scalar time lines remain at 0.1 sec. and the teardrops at 0.002 sec.

References

American Heart Association: Report of Committee on Electrocardiography. Circulation, 35 (1967): 583.

Bishop, L.: Electrocardiography (A Programmed Course). Warner-Chilcott Laboratories, Morris Plains, New Jersey 1965.

Buchanan, J. W.: Spontaneous Arrhythmias and Conduction Disturbances in Domestic Animals. Ann. New York Acad. Sci., 127 (1965): 224.

Burman, S. O., Panagopoulos, P., and Kahn, S.: The Electrocardiogram of the Normal Dog. J. Thorac. Cardiovasc. Surg., 51 (1966): 379.

Cagan, S., and Barta, E.: Bedingungen des konstanten Elektrokardiogramms beim Hunde. Z. Kreislaufforsch., 48 (1959): 1101.

Coate, W.: A Method for Rapid Electrocardiogram Recording in Unanesthetized Dogs. Lab. Anim. Care, 17 (1967): 247.

Crawley, G. J., and Swenson, M. J.: The Canine Electrocardiogram Prior to and Following Production of Cardiac Lesions. Vet. Med., 61 (1966): 363.

Detweiler, D. K.: Cardiovascular Disease in Animals. In *Cardiology; An Encyclopedia of the Cardiovascular System.* Edited by A. A. Luisada. Vol. V. McGraw-Hill, New York (1961): 27-10.

Detweiler, D. K., Hubben, K., and Patterson, D. F.: Survey of Cardiovascular Disease in Dogs; Preliminary Report on the First 1000 Dogs Screened. Amer. J. Vet. Res., 21 (1960): 329.

Detweiler, D. K., Lunginbühl, H., Buchanan, J. W., and Patterson, D. F.: The Natural History of Acquired Cardiac Disability of the Dog. Ann. N. Y. Acad. Sci., 147 (1968a): 318.

Detweiler, D. K., and Patterson, D. F.: The Prevalence and Types of Cardiovascular Disease in Dogs. Ann. N. Y. Acad. Sci., 127 (1965): 481.

Detweiler, D. K., Patterson, D. F., Lunginbühl, H., Rhodes, W. H., Buchanan, J. W., Knight, D. H., and Hill, J. D.: Diseases of the Cardiovascular System. In *Canine Medicine.* Edited by E. J. Catcott. 1st Catcott Edition. American Veterinary Publications, Inc., Santa Barbara, California (1968b): 589.

Einthoven, W.: The Galvanometric Registration of the Human Electrocardiogram, Likewise a Review of the Use of the Capillary Electrometer in Physiology. Translated in *Classics of Cardiology.* Edited by F. Willius and T. Keys. Vol. 2. H. Schuman, Inc., New York (1941): 722.

Ettinger, S., and Tashjian, R. J.: The How-To of Electrocardiography. Modern Vet. Pract., 47 (1966): 34.

Friedberg, C.: Diseases of the Heart. W. B. Saunders Co., Philadelphia, Pa., 3rd ed., 1966.

Geselowitz, D. B.: Dipole Theory in Electrocardiography. Amer. J. Cardiol., 14 (1964): 301.

Gonin, P.: Ueber die Lage der elektrischen Herzachse beim Hund. Inaugural Dissertation, Bern, 1962.

Grant, R.: Clinical Electrocardiography. McGraw-Hill, New York, 1957.

Grishman, A.: Vectorcardiography — Electrical Basis, Purpose, and Diagnostic Use. Measuring for Medicine, 3 (1968): 1 (Published by Hewlett-Packard, Paramus, New Jersey.).

Guyton, A.: Textbook of Medical Physiology. 3rd ed. W. B. Saunders Co., Philadelphia, Pa., 1966.

Hamlin, R. L.: Electrocardiographic Detection of Ventricular Enlargement in the Dog. J. A. V. M. A., 153 (1968): 1461.

Hamlin, R. L., Olsen, I., Smith, C. R., and Boggs, S.: Clinical Relevancy of Heart Rate in Dogs. J. A. V. M. A., 151 (1967): 60.

Hamlin, R. L., and Smith, C. R.: Anatomical and Physiological Basis for Interpretation of the Electrocardiogram. Amer. J. Vet. Res., 21 (1960): 701.

Hellerstein, H. K., and Hamlin, R. L.: QRS Component of the Spatial Vectorcardiogram and of the Spatial Magnitude and Velocity Electrocardiograms of the Normal Dog. Amer. J. Cardiol., 6 (1960): 1049.

Hill, J. D.: The Significance of the Foreleg Position in the Interpretation of Electrocardiograms and Vectorcardiograms from Research Animals. Amer. Heart J., 75 (1968): 518.

Hill, J. D., Moore, E. N., and Patterson, D. F.: Ventricular Epicardial Activation Studies in Experimental and Spontaneous Right Bundle Branch Block in the Dog. Amer. J. Cardiol., 21 (1968): 232.

Hoffman, B. F.: Atrioventricular Conduction in Mammalian Hearts. Ann. N. Y. Acad. Sci., 127 (1965): 105.

Hoffman, B. F., and Cranefield, P. F.: The Physiological Basis of Cardiac Arrhythmias. Amer. J. Med., 37 (1964): 670.

Hoffman, B. F., Cranefield, P. F., and Wallace, A. C.: Physiologic Basis of Cardiac Arrhythmias (I and II). Mod. Conc. Cardiovasc. Dis., 35 (1966): 103; 107.

Horowitz, S. A., Spanier, M. R., and Wiggers, H. C.: The Electrocardiogram of the Normal Dog. Proc. Soc. Exp. Biol. Med., 84 (1953): 121.

James, T. N.: Anatomy of the A–V Node of the Dog. Anat. Rec., 148 (1964): 15.

James, T. N.: Anatomy of the Sinus Node of the Dog. Anat. Rec., 143 (1962): 251.

Knight, D. H.: Anatomic and Electrocardiographic Correlations of Right Ventricular Hypertrophy in the Dog. Presented at Spring Meeting. Acad. Veterinary Cardiology, Philadelphia, Pa., April 7, 1969.

Lalich, J., Cohen, L., and Walker, G.: The Frequency of Electrocardiographic Variations in Normal Unanesthetized Dogs. Amer. Heart J., 27 (1941): 105.

Lamb, L.: Electrocardiography and Vectorcardiography. W. B. Saunders Co., Philadelphia, Pa., 1965.

Lannek, N.: A Clinical and Experimental Study on the Electrocardiogram in Dogs. Thesis, Stockholm, 1949.

McFee, R., and Parungao, A.: An Orthogonal Lead System for Clinical Electrocardiography. Amer. Heart J., 62 (1961): 93.

Patterson, D. F., Detweiler, D. K., Hubben, K., and Botts, R. P.: Spontaneous Abnormal Cardiac Arrhythmias and Conduction Disturbances in the Dog. Amer. J. Vet. Res., 22 (1961): 355.

Romagnoli, A.: Su di un Caso di Blocco di Branca nel Cane. An. Fac. Med. Vet. Pisa, 6 (1953): 3.

Rubin, G.: Applications of Electrocardiography in Canine Medicine. J. A. V. M. A., 153 (1968): 17.

Rubin, G., Stillwater, Oklahoma: Personal communication. 1969.

Scher, A. M.: Electrical Correlates of the Cardiac Cycle. In *Physiology and Biophysics*. Edited by T. Ruch and H. Patton. W. B. Saunders Co., Philadelphia, Pa. (1965): 565.

Scher, A. M., and Young, A. C.: The Pathway of Ventricular Repolarization in the Dog. Circ. Res., 3 (1956): 461.

Schulze, W., Christoph, H., and Novak, R.: Beitrag zur physiologischen Schwankungsbreite des Elektrokardiograms beim Hund. Arch. Exp. Veterinärmed., 11 (1957): 994.

Scott, R. C.: Left Bundle Branch Block, Part I. Amer. Heart J., 70 (1965): 535.

Winegrad, S.: The Possible Role of Calcium in Excitation-Contraction Coupling of Heart Muscle. Circulation, 24 (1961): 523.

Yarns, D. A., and Tashjian, R. J.: Cardiopulmonary Values in Normal and Heartworm-Infected Dogs. Amer. J. Vet. Res., 28 (1967): 1461.

5

CARDIAC CATHETERIZATION
AND ANGIOCARDIOGRAPHY*

CARDIAC CATHETERIZATION

Physical examination, auscultation, electrocardiography, and radiography can provide a definitive diagnosis in many cardiac disease conditions. In some cases, in which a definitive diagnosis cannot be made or more detailed studies are needed to characterize the condition accurately, specialized hemodynamic studies and contrast radiography are performed. Cardiac catheterization and angiocardiography have become the favored methods for in-depth study of acquired and congenital heart diseases. They are also indispensable tools for research concerning the heart and circulatory system. Without the physiologic data and radiographic findings obtained by cardiac catheterization techniques, human cardiac surgery could not have realized the triumphs it now enjoys.

The first documented cardiac catheterization was done in the horse by Chauveau, and the first intracardiac pressure measurements were done by Chauveau and Marey (1863). In dogs, the technique of passing catheters into the heart or great vessels through the arteries and veins was first performed in 1905 by Bleichroeder (Zimmerman, 1966). In 1929 Forssman successfully guided a ureteral catheter from an arm vein into his own right atrium. However, little attention was paid to cardiac catheterization until Cournand and Ranges (1941) popularized the technique of determining cardiac output by the Fick method, utilizing right ventricular and arterial blood samples and measuring oxygen consumption. Since then, cardiac catheterization has become an increasingly impor-

---

*We are grateful to Dr. P. F. Lord and Dr. J. A. Carmichael for their assistance in the preparation of material for this chapter.

tant technique in cardiology. In 1956 Forssman, Cournand, and Richards received the Nobel Prize for medicine for their pioneering work in this field.

In its broadest sense, cardiac catheterization is used to measure intracardiac and intravascular pressures, as well as the cardiac output and oxygen content of the blood in various heart chambers and peripheral vessels. Indicator dilution studies are useful for cardiac output determinations and for demonstrating the presence and the degree of shunting of blood within the heart (Wood, 1962). Cardiac catheterization is also employed to perform intracardiac electrocardiography, intracardiac phonocardiography, and transvenous pacemaking, and to obtain other hemodynamic measurements such as cardiac contractility, pulmonary and peripheral vascular resistance, and ejection fractions. Angiocardiography and cineangiocardiography, used to visualize normal and pathologic cardiac anatomy, are considered separately (see pp. 189–206).

Because the dog has been favored as a model for cardiovascular studies in experimental medicine and physiology, a great deal of information is available on normal and artificially induced cardiac lesions. In our opinion, there is little doubt that in the future an increasing amount of information acquired by cardiac catheterization will greatly expand that presently available on acquired and congenital heart diseases in the dog.

Cardiac catheterization is a sophisticated subspecialty of cardiology. It is the intention in this chapter to summarize the possibilities and limitations of cardiac catheterization. Those interested in a more complete description are referred to textbooks which deal with the subject of catheterization in greater detail (Rushmer, 1970; Moscovitz et al., 1963; Kory et al., 1965; Friedberg, 1966; Zimmerman, 1966).

Cardiac catheterization should be considered as a collaborative effort between the cardiologist and the radiologist. If the method is to be applied successfully in veterinary medicine, it must be done by a team of specialized doctors. The private practitioner cannot justify the enormous expense for equipment utilized in routine catheterization or angiographic studies. When a case warrants studies that cannot be performed in private practice, the veterinarian should not hesitate to refer the patient to one of the regional veterinary schools or centers with facilities for cardiac catheterization.

A summary of the hemodynamic studies and angiocardiographic procedures during cardiac catheterization is presented in Table 5-1.

LABORATORY EQUIPMENT

In cardiac catheterization, the location of the tip of the catheter must be known at all times. This is most satisfactorily accomplished by the use of an image intensifier (see pp. 96–98) to reduce the radiation exposure that would occur if conventional fluoroscopy were used. An image intensifier and television monitoring system are shown in Figure 5-1.

A multichannel physiologic data recorder and pressure transducers, used for measuring intracardiac pressures and for monitoring the electrocardiogram and other physiologic data, are shown in Figure 5-1. It is essential to monitor the electrocardiogram on the oscilloscope throughout the entire procedure in order to recognize immediately arrhythmias that may result when sensitive areas of the endocardium are touched by the catheter.

TABLE 5-1 SUMMARY OF CATHETERIZATION PROCEDURES USED IN DIAGNOSING THE MOST COMMON CARDIAC DISEASES IN DOGS

HEMODYNAMIC STUDIES

Measurements of the intracardiac pressures should be recorded from all chambers entered during the catheterization procedure. When stenotic lesions are present, pressures on both sides of the stenosis should be recorded simultaneously, or withdrawal pressure tracings may be recorded as the catheter is slowly pulled back across the obstruction. When intracardiac shunts or multiple anomalies are present, simultaneous pressure recordings from different chambers or vessels may be desirable. Simultaneous tracings from the left atrium and pulmonary artery or pulmonary arterial wedge position may help to differentiate left atrial from pulmonary capillary disease.

The cardiac output should be determined whenever possible and compared with normal values (see pp. 210–212).

If left-to-right or right-to-left shunts are suspected in congenital lesions, serial blood samples to determine blood oxygen saturation should be obtained in duplicate from all chambers. Since some shunts result in changes of oxygen saturation in only a portion of the chamber (for example, high ventricular septal defect may be diagnosed by changes in oxygen saturation only in the right ventricular outflow tract), samples should be obtained at different levels within each chamber. Normally, blood oxygen saturation is constant from the right atrium to the main pulmonary artery; thus, an increased oxygen saturation at one level suggests a left-to-right shunt at that level.

ANGIOCARDIOGRAPHY

SUSPECTED DEFECT	POSITION OF ANIMAL	INJECTION SITE FOR SELECTIVE INJECTION (immediate exposure)	OPACIFICATION TIME FOR NONSELECTIVE INJECTION INTO JUGULAR VEIN
Mitral insufficiency	Lateral	Left ventricle via catheter or transthoracic needle	Nonselective procedure not diagnostic
Aortic insufficiency	Lateral	Aorta, supravalvular	Nonselective procedure not diagnostic
Aortic stenosis	Lateral; dorsoventral optional	Left ventricle via catheter or transthoracic needle	5 to 7 sec.
Aortic thrombosis or aortic aneurysm	Lateral; dorsoventral or oblique optional	Aorta, supravalvular	9 to 15 sec.
Tricuspid insufficiency	Lateral	Right ventricle via catheter or transthoracic needle (diagnostic if more than minimal insufficiency)	Nonselective procedure not diagnostic
Dirofilariasis	Lateral and/or dorsoventral	Right ventricle or main pulmonary artery	3 to 5 sec.
Patent ductus arteriosus	Lateral	Aorta, supravalvular via catheter; or left ventricle via transthoracic puncture (exposure after 1 sec.)	5 to 8 sec.
Pulmonic stenosis	Lateral; dorsoventral optional	Right ventricle (conus arteriosus)	2 to 3 sec.
Atrial septal defect (uncomplicated)	Dorsoventral, but no position is fully satisfactory	Left atrium—transseptal if possible; otherwise, main pulmonary artery	Often unsatisfactory; immediate
Ventricular septal defect (uncomplicated)	Lateral; dorsoventral optional	Left ventricle via catheter or transthoracic needle; or main pulmonary artery	Nonselective injection not diagnostic
Tetralogy of Fallot and complicated atrial septal defect or ventricular septal defect with cyanosis	Lateral; dorsoventral optional	Right or left ventricle or both, depending on results of test injection	3 to 5 sec.; usually not diagnostic

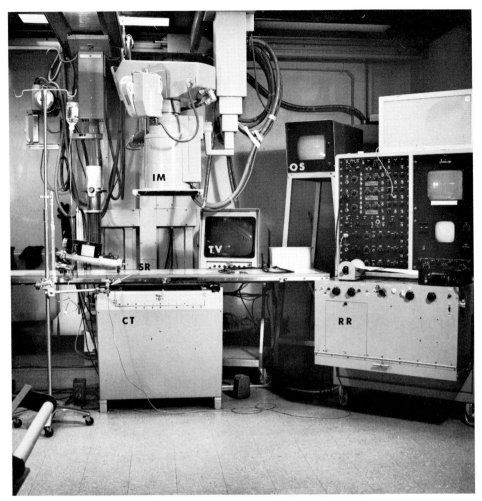

FIGURE 5-1. Equipment of the Elsie Ferguson Laboratories for Comparative Cardiovascular Studies, Caspary Research Institute, The Animal Medical Center, New York, New York.

Cineangiographic unit. IM—image intensifier with closed circuit television camera and 35 mm. cinefluoroscopic movie camera which can expose 7½ to 60 frames per second. TV—television monitor on which the passage and location of the catheters can be followed simultaneously by several persons. CT—catheterization table; table top can be moved horizontally; base contains the x-ray tube, capable of delivering a maximum of 5 ma. at 125 kvp. for fluoroscopy.

Monitoring and recording devices for the catheterization procedure. OS—mobile remote slave oscilloscope which enables continuous monitoring of the ECG and pressure curves during the procedure. RR—8-channel, physiologic research recorder with three ECG-EEG phonoamplifiers, three pressure amplifiers, a multiple-trace cathode ray oscilloscope monitor, and a single-trace cathode ray oscilloscope monitor; the base contains a cathode ray camera with rapid writing attachment for the simultaneous recording of ECG, cardiac pressures, or other variables. SR (white arrow)—a Statham pressure transducer placed near the catheterization table converts the mechanical pressure waves from the cardiac catheters into electrical impulses which are then amplified on the pressure channels of the research recorder (RR).

When cardiac output and blood gas studies are to be performed, specialized equipment is necessary (Fig. 5-2). Equipment for external direct current defibrillation (Fig. 5-3) and therapeutic agents for the treatment of cardiovascular emergencies must be immediately available for use if needed.

Anesthesia equipment for inhalation anesthesia, cardiac catheters, surgical trays, stands for intravenous fluids, and positioning devices are also necessary. A selection of the instruments used for cardiac catheterization is shown in Figure 5-4, and a number of different catheters are shown in Figure 5-5.

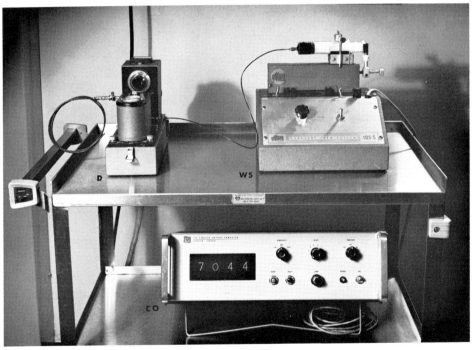

FIGURE 5-2. Optical cardiac output system composed of a constant rate withdrawal system (WS), a cuvette densitometer (D), and a cardiac output computer (CO) to determine the dye dilution curve. The method is based on spectrophotometric measurement of dye dilution. The computer integrates the degree of dye dilution transmitted to it from the spectrophotometer. The cardiac output is then calculated from the readout, which represents the degree of dye dilution as determined by the computer, and the known amount of dye which had been injected into the body.

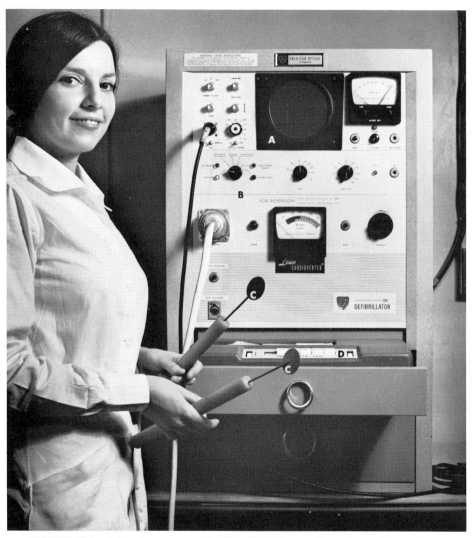

FIGURE 5-3 Intensive care unit. The ECG is monitored continuously on the oscilloscope (A) during or following surgery, cardiac catheterization, or any other procedure with which intensive monitoring is required. If an arrhythmia develops which cannot be controlled medically, cardioversion, defibrillation, or artificial pacing may be accomplished using this unit (B). External cardioversion or defibrillation is performed with insulated paddles (C) placed on each side of the thorax. If the thorax has been opened, defibrillation is performed with the paddles placed directly on the heart. A permanent recording of the ECG can also be obtained using the heat stylus permanent writer (D).

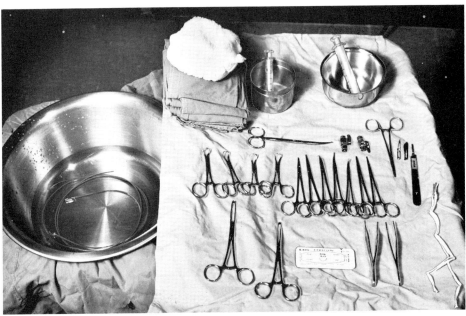

FIGURE 5-4 Surgical tray with instruments required for cardiac catheterization: sterile drapes; gauze sponges; two sponge bowls, the smaller one for contrast medium and the large one for heparinized saline solution used to flush the catheters and to prevent clot formation in the catheters; 5-ml. and 20-ml. glass syringes; fine dissection scissors; two-way stopcocks; a small needle holder; No. 10 and No. 11 Bard-Parker blades with handle; Backhaus towel clamps; at least 6 curved and straight hemostatic forceps; two Allis tissue thumb forceps; 5-0 silk with cardiovascular, atraumatic needle; two Adson thumb forceps; umbilical tape. A large pan containing sterile saline solution is used to store the catheters and to rinse the syringes.

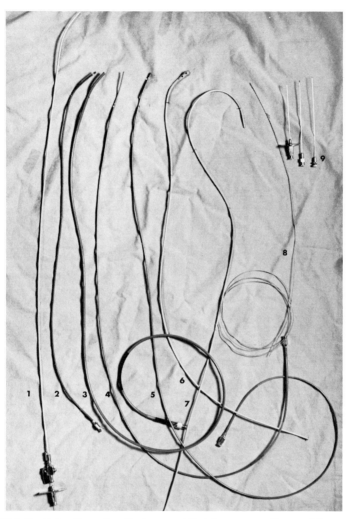

FIGURE 5-5 Selection of catheters and Seldinger needle used for cardiac catheterization and angiocardiography at The Animal Medical Center, New York. (1) Ross transseptal catheter for catheterization of the left atrium and left ventricle by the intravenous route. (2) Goodale-Lubin woven dacron catheter with one end-hole and two laterally opposed eyes. (3) Cournand woven dacron catheter with end-hole only, used mainly for recording intracardiac pressures and taking blood samples. (4) Lehman ventriculography catheter, made of woven dacron, with four eyes 4 cm. from the thin, flexible distal tip. (5) Thin-walled, NIH dacron catheter with a closed distal tip and six round holes near the tip. (6) and (7) Ödman-Ledin (Kifa) catheters with end- and side-holes (6) or with tapered end-hole only (7). The latter catheter, with the preformed, wide curve, is used for measurement of the pulmonary arterial wedge pressure. These catheters are shaped according to the needs of each procedure. (8) Flexible spring guide wire which is used as an adjunct to stiffen and straighten the catheters or in percutaneous catheterization. (9) Seldinger needle for percutaneous puncture of arteries and for percutaneous insertion of catheter.

PREPARATION AND ANESTHESIA

Before beginning a cardiac catheterization, the goals of the procedure must be clearly defined and a protocol written. Provision must be made for dealing with cardiac emergencies such as ventricular fibrillation, cardiac arrest, or the appearance of frequent ectopic beats. Changes in the overall approach because of circumstances that arise during the study should be anticipated as nearly as possible. The results are continuously evaluated during the procedure so that the data recorded are of sufficient quality for interpretation following the procedure.

Because cardiac catheterization is a surgical procedure, the anatomic regions to be penetrated or incised must be clipped, washed, and prepared antiseptically. In almost every situation, veterinary cardiac catheterization requires general anesthesia. Premedication with atropine and a tranquilizer or narcotic agent routinely precedes induction with a short-acting intravenous barbiturate. After endotracheal intubation light anesthesia is maintained with a mixture of halothane or methoxyflurane and nitrous oxide and oxygen. At the low concentration used for this procedure, halothane and methoxyflurane seem to have only minimal effects on blood pressure and respiration. Patients with serious liver or kidney disease or those in heart failure should be induced with a face mask and inhalation anesthetic, since intravenous barbiturates may be contraindicated.

Continuous monitoring of the electrocardiogram to detect complications such as ectopic beats, tachycardia, and ventricular fibrillation should begin immediately after induction and should continue throughout the procedure and the postoperative period until the dog has regained consciousness.

METHODS OF CATHETERIZATION

A number of different methods have been developed for the insertion of catheters into the cardiac chambers. The chambers of the heart are entered either by direct transthoracic cardiac puncture or by advancing catheters through large peripheral veins or arteries. The peripheral vessels are entered by percutaneous needle puncture or by arterial or venous cut-down. A trans-septal catheterization technique has been developed for simultaneous access to the right and left sides of the heart but is seldom needed in canine catheterizations. The choice of the method to be employed depends on the risk involved for the patient, the facilities available, and the inclination of the investigator.

DIRECT CARDIAC PUNCTURE. The easiest but not necessarily the safest or most accurate technique is direct cardiac puncture. It is often difficult to place the needle exactly in the position desired, and its motion may interfere with accurate recordings. Direct puncture of the heart should be performed under light anesthesia or tranquilization if the animal's condition does not preclude their use. For left ventricular puncture, the skin is anesthetized in the lower third of the fifth intercostal space (Fig. 5-6). The needle, attached to a syringe, is passed dorsomedially through the thoracic wall until it touches the ventricular wall; it is then passed into the left ventricular cavity with a short thrust. A brief burst of ectopic beats usually accompanies penetration of the ventricular wall. The arrhythmia should disappear after the needle is left in a fixed position. If the irregularity in cardiac rhythm persists, the needle must be removed immediately. Left ventricular pressures should force bright red, oxygenated blood into the syringe. If the

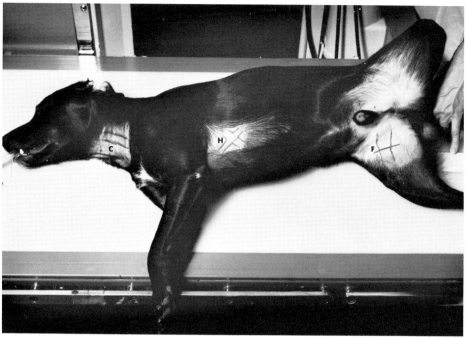

FIGURE 5-6   Dog under general anesthesia placed in lateral recumbency to demonstrate the site for cardiac puncture and the sites for introduction of the catheters for cardiac catheterization. H—Site for left ventricular puncture, ventral third of the fifth intercostal space. C—Site for cervical cut-down or percutaneous catheterization via jugular vein and left carotid artery. F—Site for femoral cut-down and catheterization via the femoral vein and artery.

needle has accidentally penetrated the interventricular septum, unoxygenated, dark red right ventricular blood under considerably low pressure is withdrawn, except when a left to right shunt exists. When a pressure transducer is attached to the needle, damping of the pressure curve suggests that the needle tip has lodged in the ventricular wall or in a papillary muscle. To avoid damaging the left ventricle, commercially available polyethylene catheter and needle combinations may be used. The polyethylene tubing is inserted through the preplaced needle, or a plastic-sheathed needle is used and the needle withdrawn after the left ventricle has been penetrated. Radiographic contrast media may also be injected directly into the left ventricle to determine the position of the needle or for other diagnostic purposes.

The direct puncture technique should be limited to the left ventricle, since right ventricular catheterization via the venous route is performed easily and with little risk. Left ventricular puncture should be limited to use in those dogs in which a more complete cardiac catheterization cannot be performed, or when the aortic valve cannot be crossed during a catheterization procedure. Cardiac tamponade, puncture of the coronary artery branches, pneumothorax, fatal ventricular arrhythmias, and faulty injection of radiopaque dyes into the pericardium and myocardium are complications that can arise when this technique is used.

PERCUTANEOUS TECHNIQUES.   The percutaneous approach, utilizing a needle or catheter through which pressure measurements are made or dye is injected, is especially satisfactory when studying a peripheral rather than a central circulatory anomaly (Ettinger et al., 1968). After percutaneous puncture, thin polyethylene catheters are easily passed through the needle into the vessel or over a previously inserted guide wire. It is difficult to use a large needle for arterial injection unless the needle is to be inserted and then withdrawn immediately. Percutaneous insertion of a Cournand needle which is to remain in place in the femoral artery for several hours has been difficult even in large dogs; therefore, we have discarded it in favor of an arterial cut-down. A polyethylene catheter (Venocath or Intracath) placed in the jugular vein for continuous monitoring of the central venous pressure or for administration of fluids is the most useful application of percutaneous techniques in the dog.

Rising and Lewis (1970) described percutaneous catheterization of the femoral artery using a Cournand needle. Following arterial puncture, a stainless steel guide wire is passed through the needle's lumen, the needle is withdrawn, and a sterile catheter is slipped over the wire and introduced into the artery. The technique is difficult in obese dogs or those with short legs.

CATHETERIZATION BY VENOUS CUT-DOWN.   This technique affords a direct route to the right atrium, right ventricle, main pulmonary artery, and pulmonary arterial wedge positions. The two most commonly utilized sites for venous cut-down are the jugular and femoral veins (Fig. 5-6). If the jugular vein is used, a short cutaneous incision 2 to 3 cm. long (Fig. 5-7) is made in the midcervical

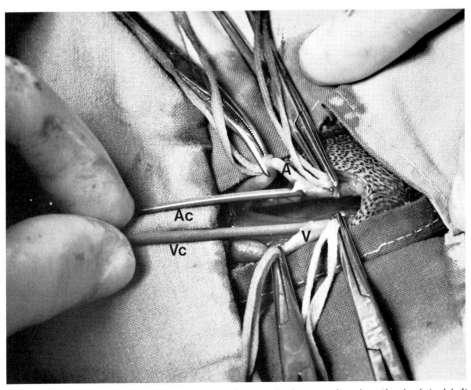

FIGURE 5-7   Surgical cut-down in the cervical area showing the isolated left external jugular vein (V) and the left carotid artery (A). To prevent bleeding, umbilical tape is snuggly fastened just proximal and just distal to the small incisions in the artery and the vein. A large catheter (Vc) is placed in the vein, and a second smaller catheter (Ac) is placed in the carotid artery.

region over the dorsal border of the jugular vein. The vein is carefully dissected free of fascia and adipose tissue for at least 2 to 3 cm. Umbilical tape stay sutures are placed at both ends of the exposed vein and are tightened gently to keep the exposed portion of the vein filled with blood to facilitate venotomy. Silk sutures may be preplaced around the proposed incision to facilitate later closure. A small incision is then made in the vein, the catheter is inserted, and the proximal umbilical ligature is loosened until the catheter is advanced past it. Both umbilical sutures are snugly fastened with hemostats so that blood does not leak out; however, the hemostats should be loose enough to permit movement of the catheter. The catheter, with a three-way stopcock attached to one end, is kept patent by a slow, continuous infusion of heparinized (1 unit/1000 cc.) dextrose and water or normal saline solution. Moistened sterile gauze pads keep the incision site from drying out. The type and size of the catheter depend on the procedure planned (Table 5-2). Under fluoroscopic control, the catheter is carefully advanced to the right atrium, right ventricle, and pulmonary artery. A removable guide wire with a flexible tip located inside the catheter may facilitate passing the catheter through the right ventricular chamber or across the valves.

The other approach commonly used to catheterize the right heart is via the femoral vein. The catheters should be premeasured so that they are neither too long nor too short. If the ends are curved according to the inflow and outflow tracts of the ventricles, passage is facilitated.

TABLE 5-2 CATHETERS USED AT THE ANIMAL MEDICAL CENTER FOR CARDIAC CATHETERIZATION AND ANGIOCARDIOGRAPHY IN THE DOG

TYPE	SIZES	DESCRIPTION AND TIP STYLES	USE
NIH (National Institutes of Health)	5F* to 8F	Closed distal tip with 6 round openings within the first cm. Pediatric types preferred for small and medium-sized dogs.	Angiocardiography, mainly aorta and left ventricle.
Ödman-Ledin (Kifa)	Red—1 Green—2 (Yellow—3 and Grey—4 not used for dogs)	Tubing bought in coils. Length, curves, and tips are shaped according to the proposed procedure. Requires flange or fittings. Is thermoplastic (polyethylene).	Tapered end for percutaneous catheterization. End-hole for measuring of pulmonary wedge pressure. End- *and* side-holes for pressure recordings and left and right ventricular angiocardiography. For contrast injections tip should be tapered.
Goodale-Lubin	5F to 8F	One pair of side-holes close to the open tip. Flexible catheter.	Pressure recordings, angiocardiography, and angiography. Widely used for metabolic studies.
Cournand		End-hole only.	Pressure recordings, withdrawal of blood, determination of pulmonary capillary wedge pressures.
Lehman Ventriculography	5F to 8F	Thin, flexible, blind tip designed to bend at the aortic valve and then to snap into the ventricle. Closed end, 4 side-holes.	Retrograde aortic catheterization and left ventricular angiocardiography. Long tip might keep the holes in the vicinity of the aortic valve cusps.

*F = French sizes.

After the pressure measurements and injections of contrast medium are completed the catheter is slowly withdrawn, clots are massaged from the vein, and the wall is sutured using an atraumatic needle and 5-0 or 6-0 silk. The skin is closed routinely, and a pressure bandage is applied for 24 to 48 hours.

RETROGRADE ARTERIAL CATHETERIZATION OF THE LEFT HEART. The techniques used for left heart catheterization do not differ greatly from venous catheterization, and the two are usually performed simultaneously. The carotid artery or the femoral artery is used (Figs. 5-6 and 5-7). Serious complications such as cerebral thrombosis from embolization, which has occurred in man after transcarotid catheterization (Zimmerman, 1966), are not a serious hazard in dogs; therefore, the transcarotid approach is not contraindicated in dogs. The carotid artery, which lies at the dorsolateral aspect of the trachea, is exposed by bluntly dissecting the loose interstitial and fat tissue dorsomedially from the jugular vein. After the artery is freed for at least 2 cm., a curved hemostat is used to draw the carotid sheath from its position dorsolateral to the trachea to the exterior. The vagus nerve is carefully dissected from the artery, and the artery is freed from the adventitia. Using 6-0 silk, a continuous purse-string suture is preplaced around the area of the planned incision to facilitate closure of the artery after the procedure. Umbilical tape stay sutures are used at both the distal and the proximal ends to secure the vessel before a stab incision is made within the preplaced purse-string suture. The opening can be extended with thumb forceps to permit passing a catheter. A similar technique is employed using the transfemoral approach. A ventriculography, N.I.H. side-hole, or Kifa side- and end-hole catheter is used for left ventricular studies. By controlling the advancement of the catheter under fluoroscopy, the tip can be guided into the descending aorta, the aortic arch, the supravalvular aortic position, or across the aortic valve into the left ventricle. The left atrium can sometimes be entered from the left ventricle by advancing the catheter across the mitral valve. Patency of the catheter is maintained with a heparinized solution of dextrose and water or normal saline.

COMPLICATIONS

Complications arising from cardiac catheterization are divided into minor and major categories. Minor and transient complications do not endanger a patient's life. Brief paroxysms of cardiac arrhythmias frequently occur when the catheter touches sensitive regions of the endocardium. These are of short duration, and since the irregularity usually disappears as soon as the catheter is moved away, antiarrhythmic therapy is not needed. Adequate oxygen saturation decreases the irritability of the endocardium. Difficulties encountered at the incision site can include hematoma formation, seromas, and infections. Intimal damage caused by forcing the catheter into a spastic vessel or a vessel with too small a lumen for the catheter leads to thrombosis and loss of function of the vessel. Clots in the incised vessel almost invariably form during intravascular catheterization. They must be removed by milking the artery or vein before the incision is closed. In some cases it may not be possible to preserve the integrity of the vessels, but this usually does not lead to further problems. To insure that the catheter tip does not break off while in the heart, the catheter must be properly examined prior to its use.

Major complications that may occur during or following catheterization include arrhythmias leading to ventricular fibrillation, accidental perforation of the myocardium and cardiac tamponade (Buchanan and Pyle, 1966), puncture of a vessel wall, damage to the valve leaflets, hemorrhage from an improperly closed incision, and injection of dye into the myocardium with subsequent arrhythmias. For obvious reasons, serious complications and death of the patient are more likely in dogs with advanced cardiovascular diseases. Anesthesia is an inherent risk, especially if prolonged, in patients whose cardiac function and reserves are impaired.

PRESSURE MEASUREMENTS

After the desired vascular compartment has been entered, the needle or catheter is kept patent by a continuous, slow, heparinized infusion, or by inter- mittent flushing with the heparinized solution, or by inserting a blunt stylet within the indwelling needle. To record pressures accurately, the tip of the catheter or needle must be free in the lumen of the vessel. To record pressures, the needle or catheter is attached directly to a pressure transducer, which is based on the prin- ciple of the Wheatstone bridge. Pressure on the gauge produces an imbalance in the Wheatstone bridge, generating a voltage directly proportional to the pressure. This voltage, when amplified by a multichannel physiologic recorder, is observed on an oscilloscope. When the image viewed on the oscilloscope is free of arti- facts, it may be permanently recorded on paper by either photographic or written (heat or ink stylus) methods. When the magnitude of the deflection is compared with that produced by a previously calibrated pressure, the pressure recorded is expressed in mm. Hg. It is often desirable to record two chamber pressures simultaneously for comparison, along with the electrocardiogram, since the elec- trocardiogram assists in timing and the identification of aberrant beats. If a respirator is used, it should be briefly disconnected during the recording to elim- inate respiratory artifacts.

Experience and knowledge of the many difficulties that can arise during the procedure are essential if the results of catheterization studies are to be valid. Pressure tracings must be free of artifacts produced by damping or partial occlu- sion of the catheter by clots, motion of the catheter, or high-frequency interfer- ence (Rushmer, 1970; Moscovitz et al., 1963).

NORMAL INTRACARDIAC PRESSURES

Pressure measurements usually begin with the most distal point in the sys- tem being evaluated, such as the main pulmonary artery or pulmonary arterial wedge position (the most distal point in a branch of the pulmonary artery that can be reached with the catheter tip, where pressure reflects pulmonary venous or left atrial pressure) in the right heart, and the left ventricle or atrium in the left heart. The catheter is then withdrawn gradually and slowly while the pressures within the various chambers are recorded. The normal intracardiac pressures in the canine heart as determined by several investigators are listed in Table 5-3.

Examples of abnormal pressure recordings are included with the discussions of particular cardiac diseases. Normal pressure curves for each cardiac chamber and great vessel are presented in Figures 5-8 through 5-14.

Text continues on page 189.

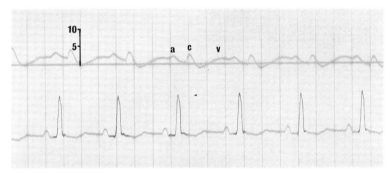

FIGURE 5-8   Right atrial pressure curve. Three low amplitude waves, a, c, and v, characterize the right atrial pressure curve. The "a" wave results from atrial systole, the "c" wave from the bulging of the tricuspid valve into the atrium during ventricular systole, and the "v" wave from filling of the right atrium. The pressure is noted on the scale in mm. Hg. The lead II electrocardiogram was recorded simultaneously.

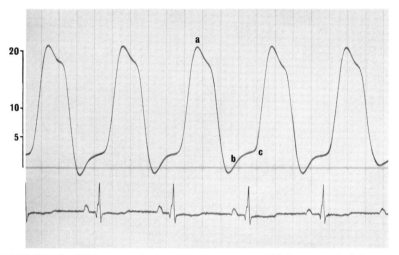

FIGURE 5-9   Right ventricular pressure curve. This normal right ventricular pressure curve and the lead II electrocardiogram were recorded simultaneously. The pressure scale is marked on the tracing in mm. Hg. The right ventricular pressure curve has three important segments: maximal ejection (a), rapid ventricular filling (b), and end-diastolic pressure (c).

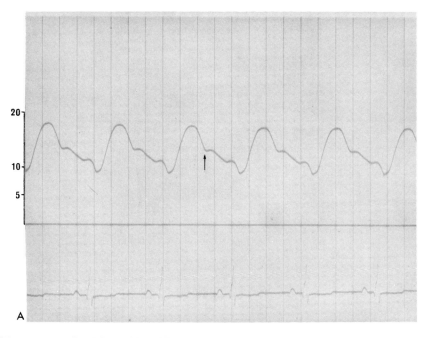

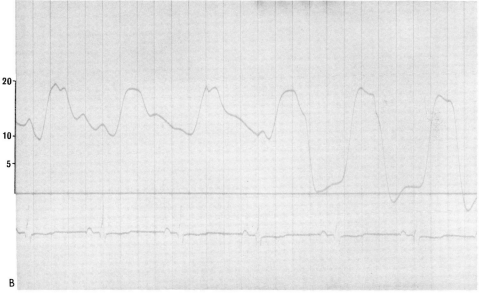

FIGURE 5-10 *A,* Pulmonary artery pressure curve recorded simultaneously with lead II electrocardiogram. The arrow indicates the dicrotic notch, which represents closure of the pulmonic valve; at this time the pulmonary artery pressure no longer exceeds the right ventricular pressure.

B, Continuous pressure recording from the pulmonary artery to the right ventricle. Notice that the peak systolic pressures in the pulmonary artery and the right ventricle are the same, indicating that there is no pressure gradient across the pulmonic valve. The lead II electrocardiogram was recorded simultaneously.

TABLE 5-3 INTRACARDIAC AND VASCULAR PRESSURES IN NORMAL DOGS*

SITE OF MEASUREMENT	SYSTOLIC (mm. Hg)	DIASTOLIC (mm. Hg)	MEAN (mm. Hg)	AUTHOR†
Jugular vein	—	—	0 to 6	Wallace, 1962
Right atrium	—	—	3	Moscovitz et al., 1963
	—	—	4	Ettinger, 1967
Right ventricle	21	2	—	Moscovitz et al., 1963
	<30	—	—	Hamlin, Smetzer, and Smith, 1965
	25 (15 to 40)	4 (0 to 10)	—	Ettinger, 1967
	25 (16 to 35)	0	—	Yarns and Tashjian, 1967
Pulmonary artery	20 to 30	—	—	Wallace, 1962
	21	10	—	Moscovitz, 1963
	24 (15 to 30)	10 (5 to 18)	—	Ettinger, 1967
	20 (15 to 25)	10 (7 to 12)	13 (8 to 16)	Yarns and Tashjian, 1967
Pulmonary arterial wedge	10 (8 to 11)	5 (4 to 6)	7 (6 to 8)	Yarns and Tashjian, 1967
Left atrium	—	—	6	Moscovitz et al., 1963
Left ventricle	108	5	—	Moscovitz et al., 1963
	122 (105 to 160)	4 (0 to 10)	—	Ettinger, 1967
	111 (71 to 157)	0	—	Yarns and Tashjian, 1967
Aorta	108	83	—	Moscovitz et al., 1963
	107 (76 to 155)	86 (66 to 130)	93 (59 to 138)	Yarns and Tashjian, 1967
Femoral artery	140 to 180	—	—	Wallace, 1962
	126 (95 to 150)	84 (65 to 130)	—	Ettinger, 1967

*Variations in normal values among reports may be due in part to the use (or lack of use) of different preanesthetic and anesthetic agents.

†For complete references see page 211.

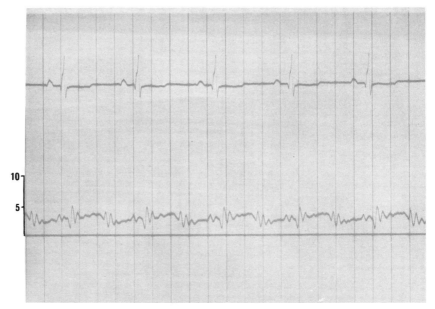

FIGURE 5-11 Pulmonary arterial wedge pressure tracing and lead II electrocardiogram recorded simultaneously. The pulmonary arterial wedge pressure curve is the same as the left atrial pressure curve. An open-ended catheter is used to record this pressure after the catheter is wedged into a distal branch of the pulmonary artery.

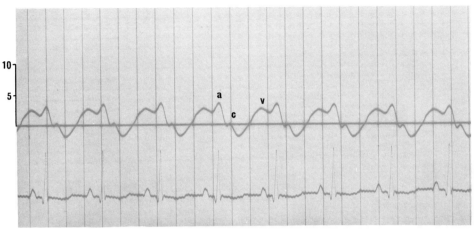

FIGURE 5-12 Left atrial pressure curve and lead II electrocardiogram recorded simultaneously. This left atrial pressure curve was obtained by passing a catheter retrograde from the left ventricle to the left atrium. The a, c, and v waves have the same physiologic meaning as in the right atrial tracing (see Fig. 5-8).

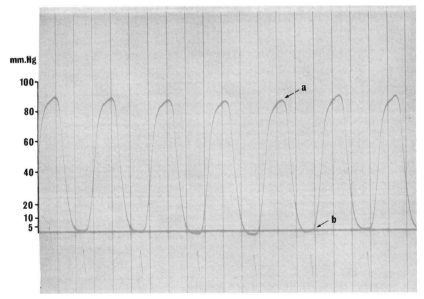

FIGURE 5-13 Left ventricular pressure curve with lead II electrocardiogram recorded simultaneously. This left ventricular pressure curve has two distinctive points of reference, the maximal ejection pressure (a) and the end-diastolic pressure (b).

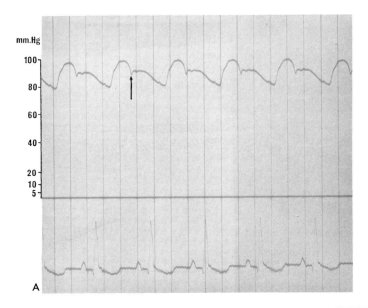

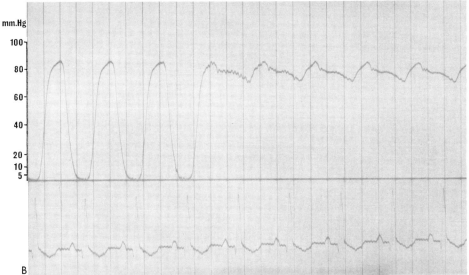

FIGURE 5-14 *A,* Aortic pressure recording and lead II electrocardiogram recorded simultaneously. The arrow indicates the incisura (dicrotic notch) of the aortic pressure curve, which represents closure of the aortic valve, when the aortic pressure falls below left ventricular pressure. *B,* Simultaneously recorded left ventricular withdrawal pressure curve and lead II electrocardiogram. Notice that the systolic pressure in the left ventricle and aorta are the same, indicating that a pressure gradient does not exist across the aortic valve.

ANGIOCARDIOGRAPHY

Angiocardiography refers to the visualization of the heart and great vessels by rapid-sequence serial radiographs made during the passage of contrast medium through the structures of the heart. Angiocardiography provides a unique opportunity for *in vivo* study of the various phases of the cardiac cycle in the different heart chambers. These phases may be studied separately and in relation to each other and to the electrocardiogram, phonocardiogram, and/or intracardiac pressure curves recorded simultaneously (Gribbe, 1964).

Using angiocardiography in patients with cardiac disease, the flow of the contrast medium is followed through a series of radiographs, and shunts, defects in the ventricular or atrial septum, valvular insufficiencies or stenoses and abnormalities of size, shape, or contraction of the cardiac chambers can be visualized. The technique is often more helpful than are other diagnostic methods in determining the location and severity of cardiac lesions, and thus in making specific diagnoses and prognoses (Buchanan and Patterson, 1965). The detailed information obtained is indispensable in performing a number of corrective surgical procedures which have become possible in recent years.

Angiocardiography and cardiac catheterization developed separately for quite some time; the combination of these two techniques has become firmly established only recently as a means of studying the anatomy, physiology, and pathology of the heart *in vivo* (Kieth and Moes, 1966). Intravenous angiocardiography was developed gradually as a diagnostic method in the late 1930's and early 1940's (Steinberg, 1959). Direct injection of a contrast medium into the left ventricle of dogs was reported by Reboul and Racine (1933). The modern technique of selective intracardiac injection of contrast medium was developed for use in man by Chavez, Thorbecker, and Celia (1947).

Image intensification, developed in Germany by Janker (1954), and selective cineangiocardiography have had ever-increasing application in man and also in veterinary medicine. It is an ideal supplement to and frequently a substitute for radiographic cut-film changers.

Over the last 30 years a great deal of information obtained from angiocardiographic studies in experimental dogs has been published in the medical literature. Many of these studies were done to evaluate different techniques of angiocardiography and contrast media. A series of cineangiographic studies concerning the hearts of normal dogs, of puppies, and of dogs under hypothermic conditions was done by Gribbe et al. (1958, 1959, 1961a, 1961b, 1964), who also used angiocardiography for studies of ventricular volume and cardiac output in the dog (1960).

Angiocardiographic techniques were first adapted for use in clinical cases of heart disease in the dog by Hamlin (1959), Tashjian et al. (1959), Hobson (1959), Detweiler, Hubben, and Patterson (1960), Tashjian and Albanese (1960), Hahn (1960), Patterson (1961), and Patterson and Botts (1961). This method was also used to study the anatomy of the canine heart (Hamlin, 1960; Rhodes, Patterson, and Detweiler, 1960 and 1963). An atlas of the anatomy of the heart and the peripheral vessels based on the results of canine angiography and angiocardiography was published by Canossi et al. (1959). The technique has been improved continually and a number of cases of congenital and acquired heart diseases in which angiocardiography was used for diagnosis have been reported in the literature. Buchanan (1965) and Buchanan and Patterson (1965) reviewed the methods of selective and nonselective angiocardiography and their applications to canine cardiology.

METHODS

The methods of angiocardiography can be subdivided into intravenous, nonselective contrast injections and selective procedures in which the contrast medium is injected mechanically through a catheter which has been previously passed into one of the chambers of the heart or the great vessels. Selective angiocardiography is usually part of cardiac catheterization, for which the catheters have already been placed in the heart. The procedure must be carefully planned according to a presumptive diagnosis obtained by conventional clinical examination, electrocardiography, and data obtained from the preceding catheterization. In intracardiac shunts or valvular insufficiencies, the presumptive direction of the blood flow (antegrade or retrograde) and the location of the defect determine the injection site. Angiocardiography is done at the end of the catheterization procedure because the contrast media injected can cause significant hemodynamic changes.

INSTRUMENTS AND EQUIPMENT

Instruments and equipment needed for angiocardiography depend largely on the procedures planned. The procedures are selected according to the type of cardiac disease, the severity of the disease, and the degree of accuracy expected in the study.

The instruments are the same as those used for cardiac catheterization and are shown in Figure 5-4. An image intensification unit, an automatic injector, a rapid film-changer, and a cinefluoroscopic camera or videotape attachment are standard equipment for selective angiocardiography. Some of the equipment is shown in Figure 5-1.

During recent years, great improvements have been made in x-ray equipment developed for angiocardiography, and a great variety of angiocardiographic units are presently available. The various types of equipment developed for human catheterization laboratories are also used successfully in animal catheterizations. For detailed information on angiocardiographic units the reader is referred to textbooks on angiocardiography. Angiocardiographic units are equipped with a generator and tubes which enable multiple exposures, usually from one to 12 per second, to be made within short periods. The units are also equipped with cut-film changers, roll-film changers, or rapid cassette changers which advance the x-ray film automatically. A programming device enables preselection of the total number, the rate, and the timing of the exposures.

The biplane rapid roll-film changer shown in Figure 5-15 is capable of exposing one to 12 radiographs per second simultaneously in two planes. The main advantages of the biplane roll-film changer are that an abnormality that might be overlooked in one plane can be seen in a radiograph made simultaneously at a right angle to the first, and that only one injection of contrast medium is required for the two sets of radiographs.

Because of their versatility, cinefluoroscopic cameras, videotape recordings,

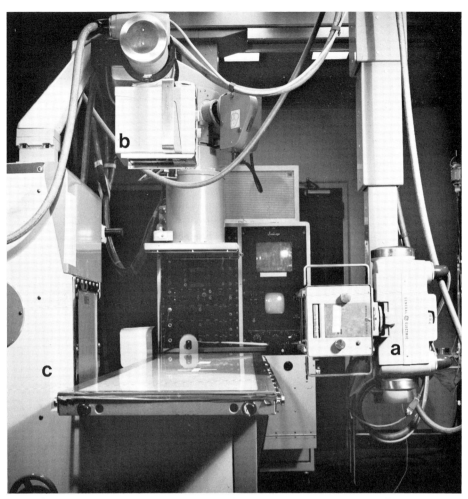

FIGURE 5-15 Biplane x-ray unit with biplane roll-film changer. Tubes a and b are at right angles to each other. They can be activated simultaneously by a fully rectified x-ray generator (maximum, 1600 ma., 160 kvp.) which splits the energy for the tubes at a preset ratio, either 1:1 or 1:2. Radiographs are exposed simultaneously in two different projections. The roll-film changer (c) enables exposure of 1 to 12 radiographs per second. During angiocardiography the top of the catheterization table can be moved from the image intensifier to the roll-film changer without changing the position of the patient.

and regular still cameras have gained increasing popularity among veterinary investigators; however, because of the prohibitive cost of such equipment, its use is limited to specialized institutions.

The lack of sophisticated equipment does not, however, prevent the practitioner from performing angiocardiography in certain situations. It has been shown that diagnostic angiocardiograms can be obtained using the x-ray facilities available in a modern veterinary clinic (Hamlin, 1959; Patterson, 1961; Barrett, 1961; Patterson and Botts, 1961). A primitive cassette changer (or cassette tunnel) can be improvised simply and serves the purpose for which it is designed (Patterson and Botts, 1961). However, a cassette changer is not even necessary, since an angiocardiogram may be obtained by exposing a single cassette at an exactly preselected time following the intravenous injection of contrast medium. Unfortunately, there are serious drawbacks in employing an oversimplified technique. When only a single radiograph is obtained, one of the main advantages of angiocardiography, namely, the comparison of the cardiac chambers at different stages of the heart cycle, is lost. Incomplete or inaccurate diagnoses must be expected owing to superimposition of different chambers and dilution of the contrast medium. The lack of hemodynamic data and blood gas analysis are other serious disadvantages of an oversimplified technique.

For the injection of contrast medium into the jugular vein, an ordinary 2-inch, 16- to 18-gauge needle or one of the many needle-catheter combinations available (Venocath, Bardic Intracath, or Plextrocan) is used.

A wide variety of catheters has been developed for selective angiocardiography. Since cardiac catheterization and angiocardiography are usually done at the same time, the catheters often serve a double purpose. A selection of catheters used at The Animal Medical Center is shown in Figure 5-5.

Catheters have been designed to provide optimal strength, radiopacity, resistance to torsion, and ease of positioning. The outside surface of the catheter must be smooth to minimize intimal damage, and the inside surface must be smooth to guarantee laminar flow of the injected contrast medium. Catheters are usually available in French sizes 5 to 8 (outside diameters 1.68, 2.01, 2.34, and 2.67 mm.). For small dogs, French size 4 catheters are used. The size of the catheter selected for each procedure is dependent upon the size of the vein or artery to be entered, since the catheter must not be forced through the vessel. The greatest possible internal diameter is desirable to guarantee unobstructed flow of the injected contrast medium.

The curves near the tips of the catheters can be preformed, or, if the catheters are thermoplastic, they can be individually adapted to the curves of the cardiac chambers by immersion in hot water (140° to 190° F., depending on the material).

Catheters are also selected according to the arrangement of holes near their tips. For recording intracardiac pressures, catheters with end-holes, side-holes or both are used. For angiocardiography the catheters should have side-holes to diminish the amount of recoil of the tip of the catheter during maximal flow of the contrast medium. Because of this whiplash effect, end-hole catheters are easily displaced and "slap" against the endocardium, causing transient arrhythmias. They also tend to deliver the contrast medium intramurally if they are wedged against the myocardium. End-hole catheters are therefore used mainly for pressure recordings, although they may be used cautiously for intracardiac injections. They are preferentially used for intravascular injections. Different types of catheters and their respective uses are presented in Table 5-2.

Stainless steel spring guide wires are used to straighten catheters during retrograde passage through peripheral vessels. They increase the maneuverability of the catheters, and the flexible spring tip facilitates passage past the valves, especially the aortic valve. These guide wires, originally introduced for use in percutaneous catheterization, consist of closely wound outer springs of stainless steel and central stainless steel wire cores. Both ends of the guide wire are rounded. By having the stiff wire core terminate 3 cm. short of one end of the guide wire, one tip is kept pliable.

CONTRAST MEDIA

Sodium and methylglucamine diatrizoates (Hypaque 50%, Hypaque-M 75%, Renovist 69%, Renografin 76%) are commonly used preparations which are well tolerated by dogs. For hand injections which are done to test the correct location of the tip of the catheters or to outline a suspected defect, Hypaque 75% is diluted with equal amounts of heparinized saline in order to minimize the total dosage of contrast medium. Hypaque-M 75% has been most satisfactory for diagnostic injections because of its high radiographic density and relatively low viscosity, which facilitates injection, and because of the absence of significant secondary reactions. Fisher (1968) provides detailed information concerning iodine content, salt content, and viscosity of the various contrast media at different temperatures.

Negative contrast media such as oxygen (Hobson, 1959) and carbon dioxide (Viamonte, 1963) have been used for selective right heart injections. However, low radiographic contrast and limited applicability have discouraged the use of negative contrast media. Double contrast studies have been done in experimental dogs (Martin, Meredith, and Johnston, 1960).

NONSELECTIVE INTRAVENOUS ANGIOCARDIOGRAPHY

Intravenous angiocardiography may be done by rapid injection of contrast medium through a needle into the jugular or cephalic vein (Hamlin, 1959; Hobson, 1959; Hahn, 1960). A more sophisticated approach is obtained by inserting a catheter into the jugular vein and advancing it into the vena cava or the right atrium (Detweiler, Hubben, and Patterson, 1960; Tashjian et al., 1959; Tashjian and Albanese, 1960; Patterson, 1961).

Advantages of the nonselective procedure are simplicity, speed, use of short-acting anesthesia or none at all, and the minimum of equipment required. Disadvantages are superimposition of the opacified structures (Fig. 5-16A and B), lack of detail due to dilution of the contrast medium as it travels through the heart, difficulty in timing the exposure of the radiographs, and the necessarily slow hand injections. The use of simple devices to serve as cassette changers can overcome some of the disadvantages (Patterson and Botts, 1961). Because of the slow circulation time in congestive heart failure and the prolonged opacification of the right atrium in right atrial dilatation, the details of the heart are frequently obscured, and radiographs are often obtained that are not diagnostic. Therefore, the procedure is often unreliable. Superimposition of the pulmonary artery and the opacified right atrium can be partially overcome by injecting the contrast medium into the caudal vena cava through a jugular catheter or via a catheter inserted into the femoral vein.

Indications for intravenous angiocardiography are abnormalities of the central veins, such as persistent left cranial vena cava or compression of the vein by tumors. Fair to good results can be expected in diagnosing right heart anomalies, such as pulmonic stenosis, and right-to-left shunts, such as patent ductus arteriosus with reversed flow. The outline of tumors of the hilar area or right atrium and the differential diagnosis between pericardial effusion and cardiac enlargement are occasional indications for an intravenous angiogram. Abnormalities of the left side of the heart are rarely outlined satisfactorily (Fig. 5-16b). Residual opacification of the right heart and dilution of the contrast

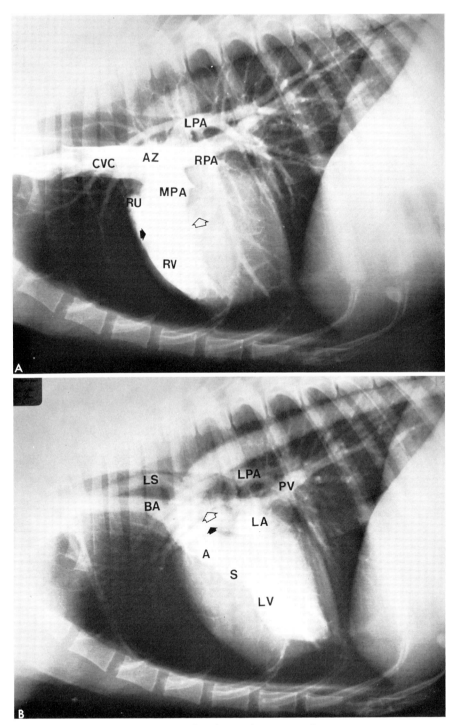

FIGURE 5-16. *See legend on opposite page.*

medium, both common in diseased hearts, make it difficult or impossible to recognize a retrograde flow of contrast medium. The recirculation of contrast medium in left-to-right shunts (atrial septal defects, ventricular septal defects, or patent ductus arteriosus) and regurgitation in valvular insufficiencies (mitral, tricuspid, or aortic insufficiency) are therefore rarely demonstrable with nonselective techniques.

Careful planning of the procedure and experience are important in obtaining diagnostic results. As for selective angiocardiography, a tentative diagnosis should be made before the procedure is done. Intravenous angiocardiography is not a substitute for careful clinical assessment of a case.

Because of the unrest which might follow the rapid injection of contrast medium, tranquilization or anesthesia is recommended except in seriously diseased dogs. An ordinary 2-inch, 16-gauge needle is inserted into the right jugular vein, with the tip of the needle pointing toward the heart. However, catheters should be used whenever possible; they are less prone to slip out of the vein than are needles, and they cause less damage to the endothelium if they remain in place for an extended period. The catheter with the largest possible internal diameter that can easily be passed into the vein should be used, because a wide lumen facilitates rapid injection of the rather viscous contrast medium. The length of the catheter required to reach the right atrium is estimated by the distance from the point of insertion to the fourth rib. In some dogs a small skin incision facilitates venipuncture. Patterson (1961) recommends use of polyethylene tubing with an

FIGURE 5-16   *A,* Left lateral, nonselective angiocardiogram, 1 year old female German Shepherd Dog. Hypaque-M 75% (1 ml./kg. body weight) was rapidly injected by hand into the jugular vein. The exposure was made at the end of the injection. The structures of the right heart are well-outlined by the concentrated contrast medium, but there is some superimposition. The cranial vena cava (CVC) partially obscures the main pulmonary artery (MPA). The cranial portion of the right atrium and the main pulmonary artery are superimposed. The tricuspid valve, which is located approximately at the open arrow, is not outlined. There is partial filling of the right auricle (RU). The pulmonic valve, which is located approximately at the black arrow, is also not outlined. The bifurcation of the main pulmonary artery into the left pulmonary artery (LPA) dorsally and the right pulmonary artery (RPA) ventrally is well-outlined. The small protrusion of contrast medium from the cranial vena cava (CVC) represents the junction of the azygos vein (AZ) with the vena cava.

B, Left lateral, nonselective angiocardiogram of the same dog as above. The exposure was made approximately 7 sec. after the end of the injection. Contrast medium is seen in the left atrium (LA), the left ventricle (LV), and the ascending (A) and descending aorta. Notice the dilution of the contrast medium as it reached the left side of the heart. There is superimposition of the pulmonary vessels on the heart and the aorta. Notice the widening of the base of the aorta into the sinuses of Valsalva (S). The brachiocephalic artery (BA) and the left subclavian artery (LS) are also outlined. Some contrast medium remained in the pulmonary veins of the diaphragmatic lobes (PV), which overlie the right pulmonary artery. The right apical lobar vein (black arrow) and the right apical lobar artery (open arrow) are both visualized. Dorsal to the right apical lobar artery, the left apical lobar vein and the left apical lobar arteries are seen. A small amount of contrast medium is still present in the left pulmonary artery (LPA), from which the left apical lobar artery arises. The small peripheral vascular structures are mostly veins.

outside diameter of 0.128 in. and an internal diameter of 0.085 in. as being suitable for most dogs.

The cephalic vein or the femoral vein, instead of the jugular vein, can be used for the injection; however, the small diameter of these vessels, the tendency for pooling of blood in venous branches, and the greater distance to the heart are serious disadvantages.

The patient is then positioned, and a plain radiograph is made to ensure proper exposure. The lateral recumbent position is usually preferable. If dorsoventral radiographs are required, the use of an intravenous catheter rather than a needle facilitates the injection.

The amount of contrast medium injected depends on its concentration. Concentrations of 1 ml./lb. body weight of 50% Hypaque or 69% Renovist, or 0.5 ml./lb. body weight of 75% Hypaque or 76% Renografin, are considered safe and outline the cardiac structures satisfactorily.

It is advisable to warm the contrast medium to body temperature prior to injection, both to diminish adverse effects due to the low temperature of the solution and to diminish the viscosity. Rapid injection is essential to ensure that the contrast medium is delivered as a concentrated bolus, which in turn provides a good outline of the chambers and vessels.

The exposure times should be as short as possible to prevent blurring due to motion. The timing of the exposure, or preferably the series of exposures, is determined according to the approximate time at which the site of the suspected defect would be opacified. To compensate for the increased density after injection of the contrast medium, the exposure factors are increased by 4 to 6 kvp. over the plain radiographs. According to Tashjian et al. (1959) and Patterson and Botts (1961), the exposures are made 0.5 sec. after injection into the cranial vena cava to outline the right atrium. One to 2 sec. after the injection, the right atrium, right ventricle, and pulmonary artery are all opacified (Fig. 5-16a). At 3 to 5 sec., the pulmonary veins, left atrium, and left ventricle can be seen, and at 6 to 7 sec. (Fig. 5-16b), the contrast medium is in the left ventricle and the thoracic aorta. These times vary greatly in dogs with heart disease. When the lung is bypassed, as in a patent ductus arteriosus with reversed flow, the time of circulation to the left side is decreased. In nearly all other cardiac diseases the circulation time is prolonged. Therefore, the exposure times at which to visualize the left heart in dogs with heart failure should be 9 to 15 sec. after the injection (Patterson and Botts, 1961). Exposures for the demonstration of adult heartworms in the pulmonary artery are made 1.5 to 3.0 sec. after injection into the cephalic or jugular vein (Hobson, 1959; Hahn, 1960). In dogs which have dirofilariasis but are not in heart failure, the circulation time from the right to the left ventricle was 4.5 sec., as compared to 3.3 sec. in normal dogs (Yarns and Tashjian, 1967). Reported injection-exposure intervals vary because of the inconsistent means used to measure these times.

SELECTIVE ANGIOCARDIOGRAPHY

Selective angiocardiography is accomplished by positioning a catheter or needle as near as possible to the defect before the contrast medium is injected. This can be achieved by advancing a catheter retrograde through the arteries or antegrade through the veins into the different cardiac chambers, or by transthoracic puncture of the atria or ventricles.

TRANSTHORACIC PUNCTURE.   Selective angiocardiography by transthoracic left or right ventricular puncture was introduced in veterinary medicine by Hamlin (1959, 1960). Reboul and Racine (1933) had utilized the method in experimental dogs and had proved it superior to intravenous injection of a contrast medium.

The advantages of transthoracic puncture are simplicity, speed, and the need for only a minimum of equipment. Some of the disadvantages of the nonselective procedures are avoided using this technique, and it can be used if selective retrograde catheterization is unsuccessful because of aortic stenosis or vascular spasm in small dogs. After direct ventricular injection, the left ventricle is outlined without superimposition and without undue dilution of the contrast medium. Satisfactory results are obtained in diagnosing aortic stenosis or left-to-right shunts at the ventricular level or beyond, such as in patent ductus arteriosus or ventricular septal defect. Mitral insufficiency can also be demonstrated.

The disadvantages of this technique are mainly the possible complications, the most serious of which are cardiac tamponade due to leakage of blood and/or dye from the ventricle and accidental laceration of branches of a coronary artery. Arrhythmias occur if the needle is inserted too deep and high in the septum, or if faulty injections are made into this area or into the ventricular wall. Ventricular fibrillation and heart block have been repeated in man, and the method is now employed infrequently (Zimmerman, 1966; Braunwald and Gorlin, 1968). Dogs with atrial fibrillation are not candidates for transthoracic puncture because of the inherent high risk of ventricular fibrillation and cardiac standstill. Minor complications are pneumothorax, hemothorax, and transient arrhythmias. Hamlin (1959) noted apnea, premature ventricular contractions, transient cardiac arrest, cardiac tamponade from intrapericardial hemorrhage, hypotension, hyperpnea, and transient vestibular irritation resulting in deviation of the head to either side. However, there were no fatalities in his study, and all complications were transient.

The planning of the procedure and the preparation of the patient are the same as for nonselective intravenous injections. The instruments and the technique have been described previously (see pp. 176–182).

A needle should not remain in the ventricle longer than the time required for a single injection. Therefore, plastic-sheathed needles are preferred because the needle can be removed while the plastic cannula remains in place.

Before transthoracic puncture is done, a test exposure should be made to ensure proper radiographic technique. For the contrast radiographs the exposure must be increased by 4 to 6 kvp.

After puncture the position of the needle is verified by its rhythmic pulsation and by the color of the oxygenated blood flowing through the cannula. The contrast medium is then injected as rapidly as possible, and a radiograph is exposed immediately at the end of the injection.

The dosage of contrast medium is the same as for intravenous injections. If direct ventricular injection is done, a single exposure is sufficient to outline most of the defects which can be visualized using this technique.

SELECTIVE ANGIOCARDIOGRAPHY BY RETROGRADE CARDIAC CATHETERIZATION.   This technique eliminates most of the disadvantages of nonselective intravenous injection of contrast medium and transthoracic cardiac puncture. The procedure is more adaptable than the other techniques, and the results are therefore more consistent. During the preceding catheterization, an evaluation of the hemodynamic changes caused by the defect can be determined from intracardiac pressure recordings, blood gas analysis, and the other data obtained. The details of the defect suspected previously are then visualized using angiocardiography, and a precise diagnosis is made.

The position of the tip of the catheter is continuously under fluoroscopic control, and the location of both the catheter and the suspected defect can be verified before the final angiocardiogram is made by manual injections of small amounts of contrast medium or by pressure recordings. An optimal concentration of contrast medium at the site of the lesion, and therefore detailed cutline of the defect, is thus achieved on the final angiocardiograms. Superimpositions are avoided to a great extent. A retrograde flow of blood such as occurs with valvular insufficiencies or left-to-right shunts can be perfectly demonstrated. For these reasons, and because of its greater safety, selective angiocardiography has superseded the other techniques for use in man.

Disadvantages of this technique are the high cost of the equipment and the expense of the procedure itself.

The instruments and equipment used for selective angiocardiography have been discussed previously (see pp. 171–177). Methods of introducing the catheters, i.e., percutaneously or by performing cut-downs, have also been described earlier (see pp. 178–182).

The catheters used for angiocardiography should have the widest possible bore to allow rapid delivery of the contrast medium. The outer diameter of the catheter is limited by the size of the artery or vein being used. The arteries are frequently affected by spastic constriction, which makes it difficult to use a catheter of adequate size. A French size 4 to 5 catheter is used in small dogs, and in medium-sized to large dogs a French size 6 to 8 catheter is used.

The length of the catheter selected depends on the site of the cut-down and the size of the dog being studied. The shortest possible catheter is preferred because there is less resistance to the injection of contrast medium. For the different types of catheters available, see Table 5-2.

INJECTION SITES. Injections into the cranial or caudal vena cava are usually considered as being nonselective. The disadvantages of these injection sites have been mentioned previously (see pp. 193–196). Vena caval injection is indicated when there is edema of the head and neck (cranial vena caval syndrome) due to tumors of the cranial mediastinum and heart base (thymomas, lymphomas, heartbase tumors, thyroid carcinomas, or abscesses). The cranial vena cava is often displaced to the right side, and injection of contrast medium may help to determine indirectly the cause of compression of the vena cava. Vena caval injection is also required to diagnose congenital anomalies, such as complete or incomplete persistent left cranial vena cava with or without a right cranial vena cava, and complicated atrial septal defects with right-to-left shunts. Injections into the caudal vena cava may be indicated in dirofilariasis with the caval syndrome, or in suspected anomalies of the vein.

Right atrial injections have the same disadvantages as do injections into the cranial vena cava. In congestive heart failure and right atrial enlargement, recognition of details is even more difficult because the prolonged circulation time delays emptying of the atrium. Indications for right atrial injection are atrial tumors, tricuspid stenosis, and complicated atrial septal defects with right-to-left shunting of blood. A left-to-right shunting of blood occurs with uncomplicated atrial septal defects, and these defects are not outlined by right atrial injections because the pressure is normally slightly higher in the left atrium than in the right.

Right ventricular injection of contrast medium is routine for verification of tricuspid insufficiency and pulmonic stenosis. Normal angiocardiograms of selective right ventricular injections are shown in Figures 5-17A and 5-17B. In cyanotic dogs in which a right-to-left shunt at the ventricular level or beyond is suspected, as in tetralogy of Fallot, or complicated ventricular septal defect, right ventricular injection is also indicated. The pulmonary vasculature and left atrium can also be outlined by right ventricular injection, and this site is used for the demonstration of adult heartworms and the secondary changes occurring with heartworm disease. In patent ductus arteriosus with reversed flow, selective pulmonary artery injection is preferable to right ventricular injection.

During the right ventricular injection of contrast medium, some regurgitation into the atrium occurs almost invariably, because the position of the catheter across the valve produces a mild tricuspid insufficiency. Therefore, caution must be exercised in making a diagnosis of tricuspid insufficiency. Since a left-to-right shunting of blood usually accompanies ventricular septal defects, these defects usually cannot be outlined by a right ventricular injection; however, if cineangiocardiography is employed, such a shunt may be visualized as a stream of unopacified blood mixing with the contrast medium in the right ventricle. Because of the normally higher pressure in the left ventricle, shunted blood tends to flow from the left to the right side. If there is doubt as to the direction of flow, a small test injection will usually indicate the direction of the shunt.

Indications for selective pulmonary arterial injections are limited in dogs. They are used specifically to confirm pulmonic insufficiency, to study the pulmonary arteries and veins and the left atrium, and if pulmonary emboli are suspected. According to Buchanan (1965), it is unlikely that the catheter will induce an artificial insufficiency of the pulmonic valve. Pulmonary artery injections can also be used as a substitute for left ventricular injections in those cases in which placing a catheter in the left ventricle is impossible or inopportune. Injection of the contrast medium into the main pulmonary artery in patent ductus arteriosus with reversed flow has the advantages of greater safety and proximity to the ductus which in turn provides better detail.

Left atrial injections are used to verify left-to-right shunting of blood in isolated atrial septal defects. A selective left atrial angiocardiogram of a normal dog is seen in Figure 5-18. Because of the superimposition of large portions of the right and left atria, the defect itself cannot be well visualized. In man this disadvantage is overcome by placing the patient in an oblique position so that the interatrial or interventricular septum is viewed on edge. The presence of contrast in the right atrium confirms the diagnosis. Mitral stenosis, which is the primary indication for left atrial injection in man, is extremely rare in dogs. Another rare indication is a suspected ball thrombus in the left atrium. Occasionally a left atrial injection is made accidentally if a catheter inserted into the right atrium slides through a septal defect into the left atrium. It may be difficult to position the catheter for left atrial injection, and arrhythmias are likely to be produced while the catheter is being advanced through the mitral valve region.

Left ventricular injections are made to demonstrate mitral insufficiency, aortic stenosis, and left-to-right shunts (uncomplicated ventricular septal defect). A selective left ventricular angiocardiogram of a normal dog is presented in

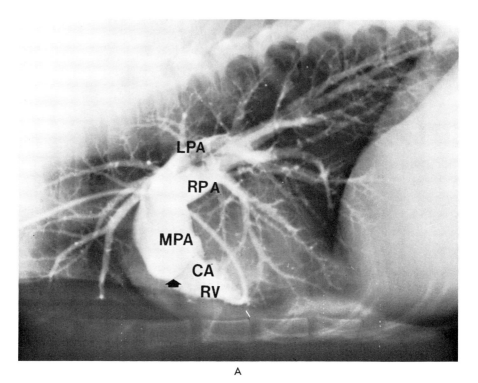

A

FIGURE 5-17 Lateral and dorsoventral angiocardiogram exposed simultaneously using a biplane roll-film changer. Selective right ventricular injection of a normal, 3 year old male dog of mixed breed.

A, Lateral angiocardiogram. The dog was placed in a prone position, and a horizontal beam was used. The angiocardiogram demonstrates that the details of the right ventricle (RV) and main pulmonary artery (MPA) can be outlined much better with a selective than with a nonselective technique (compare with Fig. 5-16). The catheter was inserted into the right ventricle via the jugular vein. The pulmonic valve (arrow) separates the funnel-shaped conus arteriosus (CA) from the main pulmonary artery (MPA). The left and right pulmonary arteries (LPA; RPA) appear closer together than in the exposure made in the lateral position in Figure 5-16, probably because of the greater inclination of the long axis of the heart and the slight rotation which occurs in the prone position. Notice the slight curve of the normally branching peripheral pulmonary arteries.

Illustration continues on opposite page.

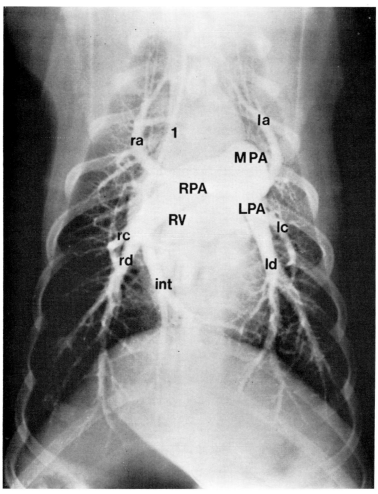

B

FIGURE 5-17 *Continued*
  B, Catheter (1) was passed via the cranial vena cava into the right atrium and
curves medially into the right ventricle (RV). The right pulmonary artery (RPA) is
superimposed on the right ventricle; it branches into the right apical lobar artery
(ra), the right cardiac lobar artery (rc), the right diaphragmatic lobar artery (rd), and
the artery to the intermediate or azygos lobe (int). Because the exposure was made at
the end of systole, the main pulmonary artery (MPA) is very large. The bulge caused
by the main pulmonary artery is also referred to as the pulmonary artery segment of
the cardiac silhouette. The left pulmonary artery (LPA) branches into the left apical
lobar artery (la), the left cardiac lobar artery (lc), and the left diaphragmatic lobar
artery (ld). Notice the slight curvature of the small arterial branches in the diaphragmatic lobar area. In addition, notice that the inclination of the heart can also be
seen in this view. Normally, the right ventricle would be nearly completely obscured
by the right pulmonary artery.

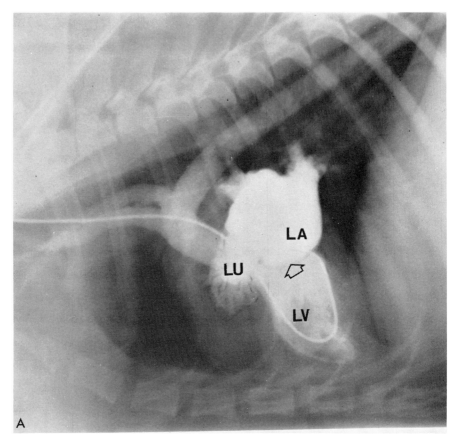

FIGURE 5-18 Right lateral angiocardiogram, selective left atrial injection, clinically normal, 2 year old female dog of mixed breed. The catheter was introduced via the left common carotid artery and was passed retrograde through the aortic valve into the left ventricle and the left atrium. The left atrium (LA) is completely filled with contrast medium, which also fills the left auricle (LU). The inner surface of the left atrium is smooth except for pectinate muscles which are confined to the left auricle and which cause the lucent filling defects. The left atrium is somewhat enlarged, and a small amount of contrast medium outlines the central portions of the pulmonary veins. A moderate amount of contrast medium has passed into the left ventricle (LV) and out into the aorta. Notice that the left auricle is superimposed on the sinus of Valsalva of the aorta. In nonselective angiocardiograms, this lodging of contrast medium in the left auricle can prevent visualization of the sinus of Valsalva.

Figures 5-19*A* and 5-19*B*. Functional mitral insufficiency is likely to occur during injections of contrast medium when ventricular premature contractions are created by the injection. Cineangiocardiography is therefore the preferred method for demonstrating mitral insufficiency, because the heart can be observed during several cycles and because incidental findings such as functional insufficiency during transient arrhythmias are more easily recognized.

Aortic insufficiency is often associated with aortic stenosis. It has also been reported to occur with bacterial endocarditis and ventricular septal defect (Buchanan, 1965). Therefore, a supravalvular aortic injection as well as the ventricular injection is indicated. Aortic root injections are used to demonstrate aortic insufficiency, patent ductus arteriosus, aortic aneurysm or obstruction, and anomalies in the positioning and branching of the aortic arch. It is also used to visualize the coronary arteries (see Fig. 5-19*A*). The term angiography, rather than angiocardiography, should be used in those cases in which the procedure is done to outline peripheral arteries. The correct positioning of the catheter before an aortic injection must be carefully verified to prevent an accidental selective injection into a coronary artery; if a large amount of contrast medium is delivered, this could result in ventricular fibrillation. Selective injection of small amounts of contrast medium into the coronary arteries does not have harmful effects. If a catheter is introduced via the femoral artery in a case of suspected patent ductus arteriosus, the catheter often traverses the open ductus accidentally and a test injection results in opacification of the pulmonary artery instead of a simultaneous outlining of the aorta and pulmonary artery.

COMPLICATIONS IN ANGIOCARDIOGRAPHY

There are two major groups of complications. The first consists of those which arise during surgical intervention as the veins, the arteries, or the heart itself is punctured; or those complications which arise as the catheter is advanced into the cardiac chambers and great vessels. These complications have been mentioned previously (see pp. 182–183).

The second group consists of complications related to the injection of contrast medium. Mechanical damage can result from the jet of the high-pressure injection, from incorrect positioning of the catheter tip, or from whiplash of the catheter tip during the peak rate of flow if catheters without side-holes are used. Rupture of small vessels, bradycardia and hypotension following endocardial or intramyocardial injections of contrast medium, and arrhythmias due to endocardial and myocardial stimulation can also occur. There seem to be no direct, harmful mechanical effects on the heart as a result of high-pressure injection when the catheter is positioned correctly (Friesinger et al., 1965).

Other complications of the second group are related to pharmacodynamic effects of the contrast media. The manifestations and the severity of the complications depend on the chemical properties of the contrast medium, on its osmolarity, on the rate of delivery, on the total dosage administered, and on the condition of the patient. The adverse effects of contrast media presently used are mainly the result of hypertonicity. Allergies are rare; no allergic reaction has been seen in several hundred contrast injections done at The Animal Medical Center to date.

Complications following angiocardiography in man have been carefully analyzed (Braunwald and Swan, 1968), and numerous experiments have been

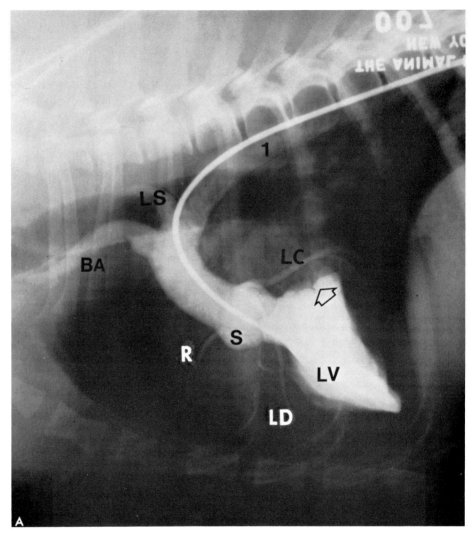

FIGURE 5-19 *A,* Left lateral angiocardiogram, selective left ventricular injection, normal Basset-mixed breed dog of unknown age. Notice the catheter (1), which was advanced retrograde from the femoral artery, through the descending aorta, and into the left ventricle. Both the mitral valve (open arrow) and the aortic valve are closed, and the ventricular outline (LV) is relatively small and well-delineated, indicating that the exposure was made at the beginning of diastole (isometric relaxation). The aortic sinuses of Valsalva (S) are filled with contrast medium. The right coronary artery (R) leaves the cranial sinus. The left coronary artery, which is about twice the size of the right coronary artery, branches almost immediately into the left circumflex coronary artery (LC), lying in the left coronary sulcus, and the left descending branch (LD), lying in or near the left longitudinal sulcus. At the aortic arch, the origin of the larger brachiocephalic artery (BA) is just ventral to the origin of the smaller left subclavian artery (LS). (Angiocardiogram courtesy of Drs. Peter Lord and J. Andrew Carmichael.)

Illustration continues on opposite page.

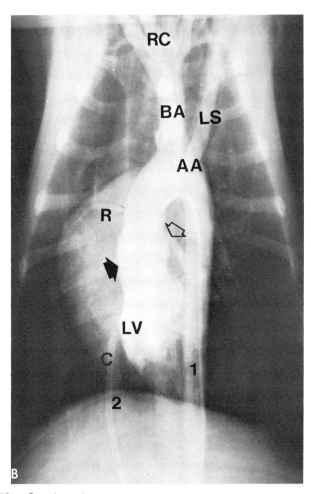

Figure 5-19. *Continued.*

B, Ventrodorsal angiocardiogram, selective left ventricular injection, normal, male Collie-mixed breed dog approximately 1 year old. Notice the catheter (1) which has been advanced retrograde from the femoral artery into the aorta and the left ventricle. A second catheter (2), introduced via the femoral vein, is seen entering the right atrium from the caudal vena cava (C). Hypaque-M 75% (1 ml./kg. body weight) was injected over a period of 1.5 sec. This exposure was made 2 sec. after the beginning of the injection. The left ventricle (LV) is in diastole, and the caudal portion of the ventricle has filled with blood containing no contrast medium which entered from the left atrium. The aortic valve (black arrow) is closed. The left coronary artery (open arrow) originates from the sinus of Valsalva. The right coronary artery (R), which is smaller than the left coronary artery, is barely visible. The brachiocephalic artery (BA) and the left subclavian artery (LS) originate from the aortic arch (AA). The brachiocephalic artery then divides into the right common carotid artery (RC), the left common carotid artery (to the left of RC), and the right subclavian artery (to the right of RC). Abnormalities in the branching of the cranial arteries with or without a persistent right aortic arch are important to recognize because they may cause a localized constriction of the esophagus. The heart has rotated to the right side despite the correct positioning of the thorax; this is due to the normal mobility of the heart. The rotation makes the aortic arch look wider than usual.

done in dogs to determine the underlying mechanisms (Friesinger et al., 1965; Kloster et al., 1967). The results of these experiments show that the increase in plasma volume and the hemodynamic effects are due mainly to hypertonicity; highly concentrated solutions of glucose or sodium chloride exert similar effects. The hypertonicity usually results in a transient marked decrease of the hematocrit level, due in part to shrinkage of the erythrocytes. This reaction is followed by an increase in plasma volume resulting from imbibition of extravascular fluid. The hemodynamic changes following every injection of contrast medium depend on the site of the injection and the dosage of the contrast medium. Friesinger et al. (1965) have shown that left and right ventricular and arterial injections of 1 ml. of Hypaque 90% per kg. of body weight cause peripheral vasodilatation; the peripheral resistance decreases, and the cardiac output increases. When contrast medium was injected into the right ventricle in a dose of up to 3 ml./kg. of body weight, increased pulmonary arterial and right ventricular pressures developed because of impaired pulmonary circulation. The systemic pressures decreased, the cardiac output diminished, and bradycardia and ectopic beats were also regularly encountered. In another study rapid vena caval injection of more than 2 ml./kg. of body weight of Hypaque 90% was followed by sudden death due to pulmonary edema in all experimental dogs (Bernstein et al., 1961).

It has been suggested that partial blockage of the pulmonary vascular bed by aggregated red blood cells may cause these changes (Friesinger, et al., 1965). Studies of the microcirculation after injections of contrast medium have supported this hypothesis (Derrick, et al., 1968).

Selective coronary artery injections have been reported to result first in a decrease and later in an increase in coronary blood flow; myocardial contractility diminishes, and there are striking changes in the electrocardiogram, mainly affecting the T wave (Friesinger, et al., 1965). Central nervous system signs such as apnea for 6 to 10 seconds have been reported (Hamlin 1959; Hahn 1960). According to our experience, vomiting and marked unrest occur in conscious animals. In addition to the aforementioned complications, Hamlin (1959) reported arrhythmias, transient cardiac arrest, hypotension, and transient vestibular irritation following direct intracardiac injections; however, there were no fatalities.

Most of the complications are not serious and are transient. The hemodynamic changes begin to disappear after 2 to 3 minutes. However, catheterization data should not be considered reliable for 12 to 15 minutes after injection of contrast medium. The hemodynamic changes which are harmless in most patients can be serious in dogs with pulmonary disease or incipient heart failure. Special precautions are therefore necessary in those patients. In normal dogs, the excretion of contrast medium begins immediately after the injection. In dogs with impaired renal function, indicated by elevated blood urea nitrogen or creatinine levels, excretion is delayed, and large amounts of contrast medium should therefore not be injected.

The amount of contrast medium injected should be kept low, and careful selection of catheters and positioning of the tip prior to injection are required. Complications must be expected from both nonselective and selective procedures. In all procedures, precise planning, readiness to cope with unexpected situations, and the surgical maxim, "Get in, get done, get out," must be applied to minimize the risk to the dog.

OTHER STUDIES PERFORMED DURING CARDIAC CATHETERIZATION

In addition to pressure recordings and angiocardiography, information about a specific abnormality or the condition of the patient can be obtained by performing special studies during the catheterization procedure, such as blood oxygen analysis and determination of cardiac output. Intracardiac phonocardiography, intracardiac electrocardiography, implanatation of intravenous cardiac pacemakers, and dilution of gaseous indicators such as krypton or hydrogen have not yet been applied routinely in clinical canine cardiac catheterization studies. Discussions of the latter techniques are available in texts on cardiac catheterization in man.

BLOOD OXYGEN AND pH STUDIES

Analysis of the oxygen content of the blood in the cardiac chambers is valuable in determining the presence, size, and direction of intracardiac shunts (Kory, 1965). In addition, oxygen content and saturation and carbon dioxide content of arterial blood can be measured to evaluate pulmonary function. The normal pH of canine blood is 7.4 (range 7.36 to 7.44), and deviations indicate acidosis or alkalosis.

To determine the oxygen saturation of blood, an aliquot is collected anaerobically in heparinized syringes and is quickly removed to the laboratory for oximetry. If the analysis cannot be performed immediately, the syringes should be refrigerated or stored in an ice-water container. Analysis for carbon dioxide can be done by the same method. The Van Slyke manometric technique of blood gas analysis must be performed by a skilled technician, and the results are not available immediately. Therefore the rapid and reliable photoelectric method of oxygen determination is more commonly employed. Fiberoptic intracardiac techniques for determining oxygen saturation of blood provide the most rapid results, but the technique is less suitable because of its expense.

The percentage of oxygen saturation of the blood is a comparison of the actual oxygen content with the potential capacity at the same temperature and barometric pressure:

$$\text{Percent } O_2 \text{ saturation} = \frac{\text{Oxygen content}}{\text{Oxygen capacity}} \times 100$$

It is the partial pressure of oxygen or oxygen tension (pO_2) rather than the percentage of oxygen saturation that determines the capacity of the blood to transfer oxygen to the tissues. The percentage of oxygen saturation is not directly proportional to the partial pressure of oxygen (pO_2). A plot of the pO_2 against the percentage of oxygen saturation demonstrates the relationship between the two at pH 7.4 (Fig. 5-20). An increase in the partial pressure of carbon dioxide (pCO_2) or the acidity of the blood favors oxygen dissociation (Riley, 1965). It is apparent from the S-shaped curve of oxygen dissociation that the pO_2 and the percentage of oxygen saturation are linearly related only between 10 percent and 70 percent oxygen saturation (Fig. 5-20). Above 70 per cent the curve flattens, gradually at first, and then nearly leveling off. Minor deviations at the higher levels of oxygen saturation reflect major changes in the pO_2. Since it is the pO_2 that controls oxygen

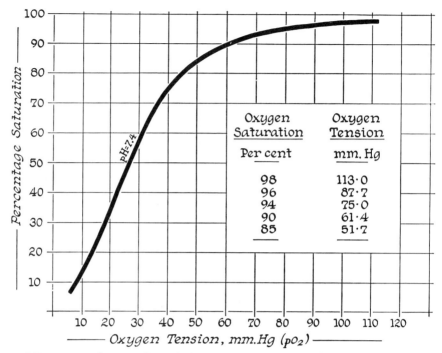

FIGURE 5-20 Oxygen dissociation curve, human blood, pH 7.4. At this pH, the oxygen dissociation curve is S-shaped. When oxygen tension is greater than 60 to 70 mm. Hg, minimal changes in the percentage of oxygen saturation in the blood can reflect large differences in the oxygen tension. (From Friedberg, C. K.: Diseases of the Heart, W. B. Saunders, Philadelphia, 3rd edition, 1966, p. 333.)

TABLE 5-4 OXYGEN SATURATION AND BLOOD GAS VALUES

| | OXYGEN SATURATION | |
SAMPLING SITE	Normal dog* (Percent)	Normal man (Percent)
Anterior vena cava	72 to 75	70 ± 5
Posterior vena cava	68 to 76	80 ± 5
Right atrium	69 to 74.5	75 ± 5
Right ventricle	61 to 76.5	75 ± 5
Pulmonary artery	76.5	75 ± 5
Femoral artery	91	95 to 100

NORMAL BLOOD GAS AND pH IN DOGS	ARTERIAL BLOOD†	VENOUS BLOOD†
pO_2 (mm. Hg)	90 to 100	40
pCO_2 (mm. Hg)	40	45
pH	7.4	7.4

*Data from Detweiler, D. K.: Cardiovascular Diseases in Animals. In Encyclopedia of the Cardiovascular System. Vol. 5 (A. Luisada, ed.) McGraw-Hill, New York. (1961):27-10.

†Data from Sattler, F.: Measuring Ventilation, pH, and Blood Gases in the Surgical Patient. J. A. V. M. A. 154 (1969):511.

diffusion across tissue, such small differences can have vital effects on tissue function.

The oxygen saturation of the blood of the dog being studied should be compared with normal values (Table 5-4). An abrupt increase in the oxygen saturation at any level within the right heart suggests a left-to-right shunt of arterial blood at that level. Similarly, a decrease in the oxygen saturation in the left heart suggests either a right-to-left shunt or a deficiency in the arterialization of the blood in the pulmonary capillaries.

CARDIAC OUTPUT

Cardiac output is defined as the volume of blood ejected by the right or left ventricle in one minute. The cardiac output is often below normal if the heart is affected by a disease that inhibits normal filling or emptying. A pathologically elevated cardiac output is likely to be associated with extracardiac conditions such as anemia and arteriovenous fistulas.

The effects of exercise, anoxia, anesthesia, posture, body temperature, anxiety, sleep, and food on cardiac output have been reviewed by Guyton (1963). Exercise increases the cardiac output. Moderate anoxia increases the cardiac output by reducing the total peripheral resistance, but when anoxia is severe the heart is weakened and cardiac output is diminished. Except for chloroform, anesthesia has no significant effect on cardiac output if the depth is light to moderate. When the plane of anesthesia is deep the cardiac output may be reduced by 25 to 40 per cent. Cardiac output is increased while the patient is lying down, which might explain the beneficial effect of cage rest on patients with congestive heart failure. Ingestion of food, anxiety, and an increase in body temperature result in an increased cardiac output, whereas the cardiac output decreases during sleep.

It has become customary to express cardiac output in terms of body surface area; the resulting ratio is called the *cardiac index*. Use of the cardiac index allows comparison of the cardiac outputs of dogs of different body weights. The cardiac index, expressed in L./min./m.^{2}, is determined as follows (from Guyton, 1963):

$$\text{Cardiac index (L./min./m.}^2) = \frac{\text{Cardiac output (L./min.)}}{\text{Body surface area (m.}^2)} \; ;$$

Body surface area (m.^{2}) = k × body weight [kg.])$^{2/3}$,

where k = 0.112 if body weight > 4 kg.,
and k = 0.101 if body weight < 4 kg.

Table 5-5 gives the body surface area for dogs from 1 to 50 kg. as determined from this formula.

In a detailed study of 145 determinations of cardiac output on 42 normal dogs, Wiggers (1944) found the mean cardiac index to be 2.87 ± 0.44 L./min./m.^{2}. In a study of 12 normal dogs with an average weight of 17.1 kg. (8.2 kg. to 27.2 kg.) in which cardiac output was determined by the indicator-dilution method (see below), the mean cardiac index was 3.50 ± 0.86 L./min./m.^{2} (2.60 to 5.09) (Gould et al., 1970). Haddy et al. (1949) and Haddy and Campbell (1953) reported a mean cardiac output of 3.6 L./min. (22 dogs) and 3.66 L./min. (30 dogs). Yarns and Tashjian (1967) found a cardiac index of 2.7 L./min./m.^{2} (1.8 to 3.7) in six normal dogs.

TABLE 5-5 BODY SURFACE AREA FOR DOGS WEIGHING FROM 1 to 50 KG.

WEIGHT (kg.)	BODY SURFACE AREA (m.²)	WEIGHT (kg.)	BODY SURFACE AREA (m.²)
1	0.101	26	0.983
2	0.160	27	1.008
3	0.210	28	1.032
4	0.254	29	1.057
5	0.327	30	1.081
6	0.369	31	1.105
7	0.409	32	1.129
8	0.448	33	1.152
9	0.484	34	1.175
10	0.519	35	1.198
11	0.554	36	1.221
12	0.587	37	1.243
13	0.619	38	1.266
14	0.650	39	1.288
15	0.681	40	1.310
16	0.711	41	1.331
17	0.740	42	1.353
18	0.769	43	1.374
19	0.797	44	1.396
20	0.825	45	1.417
21	0.852	46	1.438
22	0.879	47	1.458
23	0.905	48	1.479
24	0.931	49	1.499
25	0.957	50	1.520

The minute cardiac volume increases with increasing body weight, yet the cardiac index is of the same order of magnitude for different sizes of dogs (Wiggers, 1944). The cardiac output, cardiac index, total peripheral resistance, stroke volume, heart rate, and circulation time from the right atrium to the femoral artery in 42 dogs in three categories of weight are presented in Table 5-6 (Wiggers, 1944).

In most laboratories the cardiac output is determined by either the Fick principle or the indicator-dilution method.

Using the Fick principle, which was described in 1870, it is assumed that the cardiac output is equal to the amount of oxygen consumed in one minute divided by the arteriovenous oxygen difference. Oxygen consumption is determined by connecting the patient to a basal metabolism unit and measuring the oxygen consumed in one minute. The arteriovenous oxygen difference is determined by measuring the oxygen content of blood before it enters the lungs (mixed venous oxygen content) and after it leaves the lungs (arterial oxygen content). Therefore:

$$\text{Cardiac output (ml./min.)} = \frac{\text{Oxygen consumption (ml./min.)}}{(\text{Arterial } O_2 \text{ content [ml./ml. blood]}) - (\text{Mixed venous } O_2 \text{ content [ml./ml. blood]})}$$

The Fick principle was utilized in 1886 by Grehant and Quinquant to determine the cardiac output in six dogs and later in 1898 by Zuntz and Hagermann in two horses (Guyton, 1963). The Fick method is time-consuming and requires a skilled laboratory technician. Consequently, many laboratories now use the indicator-dilution technique.

The principle of the indicator-dilution technique is that cardiac output is

TABLE 5-6 COMPARISON OF CARDIAC OUTPUT, CARDIAC INDEX, TOTAL PERIPHERAL RESISTANCE, STROKE VOLUME, AND CIRCULATION TIME IN NORMAL DOGS OF DIFFERENT BREEDS*

SIZE OF DOG (kg.)	NO. OF DOGS	NO. OF TESTS	CARDIAC OUTPUT (ml./min.)		CARDIAC INDEX L min./m.^{2} (average)	TOTAL PERIPHERAL RESISTANCE (dynes/sec./ cm.^{5}) (average)	STROKE VOLUME (ml./beat) (average)	HEART RATE (per min.) (average)	CIRCULATION TIME** (sec.) (average)
			(average)	S.D.†					
Extra large (21 to 31)	13	46	2660	±330	2.87	4230	15.8	181	11.5
Large (17 to 20.9)	17	66	2240	±490	2.93	4630	13.8	174	10.2
Medium (10 to 16.9)	12	37	1820	±340	2.75	5570	11.3	161	9.5

*After Wiggers, H.: Cardiac Output and Total Peripheral Resistance Measurements in Dogs. Amer. J. Physiol., 140 (1944):519.

†S.D. = standard deviation

**From right atrium to femoral artery

directly proportional to the degree of dilution of an indicator substance injected into the right side of the heart and then sampled over a period of time at some point downstream. Using indicator substances, blood flow is measured by inducing chemical, electrical, optical, radioactive, or thermal changes in the blood (Kory, 1965).

The photoelectric method employing indocyanine-green dye (Cardiogreen) as an indicator substance has been widely used for cardiac output determinations. A known amount of dye is injected into the right atrium, the right ventricle, or the pulmonary artery, and arterial blood is then withdrawn at any major point downstream. Because of regurgitation of dye into the left atrium in dogs with advanced mitral valvular insufficiency, the aortic root may be preferred as an injection site, with the femoral artery being chosen as the site for sampling the blood. The blood, containing the diluted indicator substance, is withdrawn at a constant rate through a photoelectric densitometer (Fig. 5-2). The amount of light transmitted by the blood is inversely proportional to the concentration of dye. The mean concentration of dye is greater when cardiac output is low. The densitometer produces a concentration curve, the area under which is inversely proportional to the cardiac output. Although the computation of dye dilution may be performed by hand, it may also be done automatically by computer (Fig. 5-2). When the dye is first sensed by the densitometer, a continuous determination is made of the dye concentration (Taylor et al., 1967).

References

Barrett, R. B.: The Rapid Manual Injection Methods of Angiocardiography. Vet. Med., 56 (1961):28.

Bernstein, E. F., Palmer, J. D., Aaberg, T. A., and Davies, R. L.: Studies of the Toxicity of Hypaque 90% Following Rapid Intravenous Injection. Radiology, 76 (1961):88.

Braunwald, E., and Gorlin, R.: Total Population Studied, Procedures Employed, and Incidence of Complications. In *Cooperative Study on Cardiac Catheterization.* Edited by E. Braunwald and H. J. C. Swan. Monograph No. 20. American Heart Association. New York, 1968.

Braunwald, E., and Swan, H. J. C.: Cooperative Study on Cardiac Catherization. Monograph No. 20. American Heart Association, New York, 1968.

Buchanan, J. W.: Selective Angiography and Angiocardiography in Dogs with Acquired
Cardiovascular Disease. J. Amer. Vet. Radiol. Soc., 6 (1965):5.

Buchanan, J. W., and Patterson, D. F.: Selective Angiography and Angiocardiography in
Dogs with Congenital Cardiovascular Disease. J. Amer. Vet. Radiol. Soc., 6 (1965):21.

Buchanan, J. W., and Pyle, R.: Cardiac Tamponade During Catheterization of a Dog with
Congenital Heart Disease. J. A. V. M. A., 149 (1966):1056.

Canossi, G. C., Dardari, M., Cortesi, M., Brunelli, B., and Pasquinelli, C.: Anatomia
Angiografia del Cane. Minerva Medica, Torino, Italy. 1959.

Chauveau, and Marey, E.: Mémoires de l'Académie impériale de Médecine. 26 (1863):
268. Cited in Laszt, L., and Müller, A.: *Ueber den Druckverlauf im linken. Ventrikel.*
Helv. Physiol. Acta., 9 (1951):55.

Chavez, I., Thorbecker, N., and Celia, A.: Direct Intracardiac Angiocardiography: Its
Diagnostic Value. Amer. Heart J., 33 (1947):560.

Cournand, A., and Ranges, H.: Catheterization of the Right Auricle in Man. Proc. Soc.
Exp. Biol. Med., 46 (1941):462.

Derrick, J. R., Brown, R. W., Livanec, G., Bond, T. P., and Mason Guest, M.: Experimental
Effects of Selective Arteriography on the Microcirculation. Amer. J. Surg., 116 (1968):
712.

Detweiler, D. K.: Cardiovascular Diseases in Animals. In *Encyclopedia of the Cardiovascular System.* Vol. 5. Edited by A. Luisada, McGraw-Hill, New York. (1961):27-10.

Detweiler, D. K., Hubben, K., and Patterson, D. F.: Survey on Cardiovascular Disease in
Dogs: Preliminary Report on the First 1000 Dogs Screened. Amer. J. Vet. Res.,
21 (1960):329.

Ettinger, S.: Unpublished observations from seven normal dogs. 1967.

Ettinger, S., Campbell, L., Suter, P., DeAngelis, M., and Butler, H.: Peripheral Arteriovenous Fistula in a Dog. J. A. V. M. A., 153 (1968):1055.

Fick, A.: Sitzungsber. d. phys.-med. In *Diseases of the Heart.* Edited by C. Friedberg. 3rd.
ed. W. B. Saunders Co., Philadelphia, Pa. (1966):307.

Fisher, H. W.: The Choice of Angiographic Contrast Medium, Catheter, and Power Injection. In *Roentgen Techniques in Laboratory Animals.* Edited by B. Felson, W. B.
Saunders Co., Philadelphia, Pa., 1968.

Friedberg, C.: Diseases of the Heart. 3rd ed. W. B. Saunders Co., Philadelphia, Pa. 1966.

Friesinger, G. C., Schaffer, J., Criley, J. M., Gaertener, R. A., and Ross, R. S.: Hemodynamic Consequences of the Injection of Radiopaque Material. Circulation 31 (1965):
730.

Gould, L., Ettinger, S., Carmichael, A., and Lord, P.: Phentolamine and Hemorrhagic
Shock. Angiology, 21 (1970):330.

Gribbe, P.: Cineangiocardiographic Studies of the Heart Action in Different Condition.
Thesis. Stockholm, 1964.

Gribbe, P.: Comparison of the Angiocardiography and the Direct Fick Methods of Determining Cardiac Output. Cardiologia (Basel), 36 (1960): 19.

Gribbe, P., Hirvonen, L., Lind, J., and Wegelius, C.: Cineangiocardiographic Recordings of
the Cycle Changes in Volume of the Left Ventricle. Cardiologia (Basel), 34 (1959):348.

Gribbe, P., Hirvonen, L., Lind, J., and Wegelius, C.: Cineangiocardiographic Observations
in Hypothermic Dogs. Cardiologia (Basel), 39 (1961a):341.

Gribbe, P., Hirvonen, L., and Peltonen, T.: Cineangiocardiographic Studies of Puppies and
Full Grown Dogs. Acta. Physiol. Scand., 51 (1961b):169.

Gribbe, P., Linko, E., Lind, J., and Wegelius, C.: The Events of the Left Side of the Normal
Heart as Studied by Cineradiography. Cardiologia (Basel), 33 (1958):293.

Guyton, A.: Circulatory Physiology: Cardiac Output and Its Regulation. W. B. Saunders
Co., Philadelphia, Pa. 1963.

Haddy, F. J., and Campbell, G. S.: Pulmonary Vascular Resistance in Anesthetized Dogs.
Amer. J. Physiol., 172 (1953):747.

Haddy, F. J., Campbell, G. S., Adams, W. L., and Visscher, M. B.: A Study of Pulmonary
Venous and Arterial Pressures and Other Variables in the Anesthetized Dog by Flexible Catheter Technique. Amer. J. Physiol., 158 (1949):89.

Hahn, A.: Angiocardiography in Canine Dirofilariasis. II. Utilization of a Rapid Film
Changing Technique. J. A. V. M. A., 136 (1960):355.

Hamlin, R. L.: Angiocardiography for the Clinical Diagnosis of Congenital Heart Disease
in Small Animals. J. A. V. M. A., 135 (1959):112.

Hamlin, R. L.: Radiographic Anatomy of the Heart and Great Vessels in Healthy Living
Dogs. J. A. V. M. A., 136 (1960):265.

Hamlin, R. L., Smetzer, D., and Smith, C. R.: Congenital Mitral Insufficiency in the Dog.
J. A. V. M. A., 146 (1965):1088.

Hobson, H.: Angiocardiography in Canine Dirofilariasis. I. J. A. V. M. A., 135 (1959):537.

Janker, R.: Roentgenologische Funktionsdiagnostik. 1954. In Kieth, J. D., and Moes, C. A. F.: Selective Angiocardiography. In *Intravascular Catheterization.* Ed. by H. Zimmerman. 2nd Ed. Charles C Thomas, Springfield, Illinois, 1966.

Kieth, J. D., and Moes, C. A. F.: Selective Angiocardiography. In *Intravascular Catheterization.* Edited by H. Zimmerman, Charles C Thomas, Springfield, Ill. 1966.

Kloster, F. E., Bristow, J. D., Porter, G. A., Judkins, M. P., and Griswold, H. E.: Comparative Hemodynamic Effects of Equiosmolar Injections of Angiographic Contrast Materials. Invest. Radiol., 2 (1967):353.

Kory, R. C., Tsagaris, T. J., and Bustamante, R. A.: A Primer of Cardiac Catheterization. Charles C Thomas, Springfield, Ill. 1965.

Martin, J. F., Meridith, J. R., and Johnston, F. R.: Double Contrast Angiocardiography. Radiology, 74 (1960):947.

Moscovitz, H. L., Donoso, E., Gelb, I. J., and Wilder, R. J.: An Atlas of Hemodynamics of the Cardiovascular System. Grune & Stratton, New York, 1963.

Patterson, D. F.: Angiocardiography. J. Amer. Vet. Radiol. Soc., 1 (1961):26.

Patterson, D. F., and Botts, R. P.: A Simple Cassette Changer. Small Anim. Clin., 1 (1961):1.

Reboul, H., and Racine, M.: Ventriculographie Cardiac Expérimentale. Presse Méd., 37 (1933):763.

Riley, R.: Gas Exchange and Transportation. In *Physiology and Biophysics.* Edited by T. Ruch and H. Patton. W. B. Saunders Co., Philadelphia, Pa. 1965.

Rising, J. L., and Lewis, R. E.: A Technique for Arterial Catheterization in the Dog. Amer. J. Vet. Res., 31 (1970):1309.

Rhodes, W. H., Patterson, D. F., and Detweiler, D. K.: Radiographic Anatomy of the Canine Heart. Part I. J. A. V. M. A., 137 (1960):283.

Rhodes, W. H., Patterson, D. F., and Detweiler, D. K.: Radiographic Anatomy of the Canine Heart. Part II. J. A. V. M. A., 143 (1963):137.

Rushmer, R.: Cardiovascular Dynamics. 3rd ed. W. B. Saunders Co., Philadelphia, Pa. 1970.

Sattler, F.: Measuring Ventilation, pH, and Blood Gases in the Surgical Patient. J. A. V. M. A., 154 (1969):511.

Steinberg, I.: Twenty Years of Angiocardiography. Amer. J. Roentgen., 81 (1959):886.

Tashjian R. J., and Albanese, N. M.: A Technique of Canine Angiocardiography. J. A. V. M. A., 136 (1960):359.

Tashjian, R. J., Hofstra, P. C., Reid, C. F., and Newman, N. N.: Isolated Pulmonic Valvular Stenosis in a Dog. J. A. V. M. A., 135 (1959):94.

Taylor, S. H., MacDonald, H. R., Robinson, M. C., and Sapru, R. P.: Computers in Cardiovascular Investigation. Brit. Heart. J., 29 (1967):352.

Viamonte, M.: CO_2 Angiocardiography in Dogs. J. Amer. Vet. Radiol. Soc., 4 (1963):18.

Wallace, C.: Cardiac Catheterization to Aid in Diagnosis of Cardiovascular Disease. Small Anim. Clin., 2 (1962):324.

Wiggers, H.: Cardiac Output and Total Peripheral Resistance Measurements in Dogs. Amer. J. Physiol., 140 (1944):519.

Wood, E. (Ed.): Symposium on Use of Indicator-Dilution Techniques in the Study of the Circulation. Monograph No. 4. American Heart Association, New York. 1962.

Yarns, D. A., and Tashjian, R. J.: Cardiopulmonary Values in Normal and Heartworm-Infected Dogs. Amer. J. Vet. Res., 28 (1967):1461.

Zimmerman, H.: Intravascular Catheterization. 2nd ed. Charles C Thomas, Springfield, Ill. 1966.

CHAPTER

6

THE RECOGNITION OF CARDIAC DISEASE AND CONGESTIVE HEART FAILURE

The presence of cardiac disease does not necessarily imply that heart failure is also present. Since the two terms, cardiac disease and heart failure, are not synonymous, they should not be used interchangeably.

The Criteria Committee of the New York Heart Association (1966) has provided functional and therapeutic classifications of heart disease for man. The functional classification describes what exercise tolerance a person can bear, and the therapeutic classification describes the limitations that are required in various degrees of heart disease and failure. Since dogs do not limit their own exercise, except in cases of severe heart failure, it has been considered practical by the authors to modify and combine the New York Heart Association's functional and therapeutic classifications to define four phases of cardiac disease. Although clear distinctions between phases II and III are not always obvious, such a classification has been helpful to us in maintaining a uniform method of describing a disease or its course (see Table 6-1).

Specific findings suggesting cardiac disease, but not necessarily heart failure, are as follows (Logue and Hurst, 1970; Detweiler et al., 1968; personal observations):

1. Cardiac enlargement, right-sided, left-sided, or both, as determined by palpation, radiography, and/or electrocardiography.

2. Abnormal cardiac movements such as a left ventricular heave, irregular

TABLE 6-1 PHASES OF CARDIAC DISEASE IN THE DOG*

PHASE	DESCRIPTION
Phase I	Normal activity does not produce undue fatigue, dyspnea, or coughing. Physical activity need not be limited in dogs in this phase of cardiac disease.
Phase II	The dog is comfortable at rest, but ordinary physical activity causes fatigue, dyspnea, or coughing. In these dogs, exercise should be limited moderately; such activities as hunting and long periods of strenuous exercise should be avoided.
Phase III	The dog is comfortable at rest, but minimal exercise may produce fatigue, dyspnea, or coughing. Signs may also develop while the dog is in a recumbent position (orthopnea). Physical activity must be limited; free running and stair climbing should be strictly avoided. Exercise should be limited to short walks and moderate house activity.
Phase IV	Congestive heart failure, dyspnea, and coughing are present even when the dog is at rest. Signs are exaggerated by any physical activity. Total exercise restriction, i.e., absolute cage rest, is essential.

*Modified from Criteria Committee of the New York Heart Association: Functional and Therapeutic Classification of Heart Disease in Man (1966).

precordial movements caused by an irregularly beating heart, and precordial thrills.

3. All diastolic cardiac murmurs and most systolic murmurs (except anemic and low-intensity physiologic murmurs).

4. Abnormal arterial pulsations, including hyperdynamic or hypodynamic pulse, pulse deficits, and gross irregularities of the strength of the pulse.

5. Abnormalities of the cervical veins such as jugular venous distention, a jugular pulse, and cannon "a" waves.

6. Electrocardiographic abnormalities, including left ventricular hypertrophy; right ventricular hypertrophy; left bundle branch block; atrial fibrillation; ectopic supraventricular or ventricular premature contractions occurring singly, in multiples, or as tachycardia; and complete heart block.

7. The presence of diastolic gallop rhythms (third or fourth heart sounds, or both) on auscultation. This finding is usually associated with cardiac failure.

Cardiac disease may be present for an undetermined period of time during which circulatory function remains normal owing to cardiac reserve and compensatory mechanisms. When the heart is no longer able to adapt to increased physiologic demands placed on it, cardiac dysfunction and failure develop. The signs of cardiac disease have been reviewed above. When dysfunction persists, the cardiac output cannot meet the needs of the body's tissues, and other organs are affected increasingly, producing the gross physical signs of congestive heart failure.

CONGESTIVE HEART FAILURE

Congestive heart failure is a clinical syndrome. Physiologically, it is the inability of the heart muscle to maintain an adequate cardiac output—that is, to supply the needs of the body tissues. The changes in pressure and flow of a failing chamber and the compensatory mechanisms that ensue produce the clinical signs of heart failure. The single stimulus for all these changes is the cardiac output which is insufficient for the needs of the body.

It is now recognized that heart failure is a complex alteration of the physiologic homeostatic mechanisms of the heart. Congestive heart failure cannot be simply ascribed to a *backward failure* — that is, an increase in venous pressures behind a failing cardiac chamber. Although it is true that elevated venous pressures are associated with heart failure, such a theory fails to account for the renal mechanism of sodium and water retention or for the diminished perfusion of other organs in the body. The *forward failure* theory, based on the assumption of decreased cardiac output, is likewise incomplete, because it attributes all the signs of congestive heart failure to decreased organ perfusion and the renal retention of sodium and water. If decreased cardiac output alone were responsible for congestive heart failure, one might reasonably expect a shock-like state, with hypotension, rather than a congestive state.

Cardiogenic shock develops after acute cardiac damage and results in arterial hypotension and reduced tissue perfusion. Shock is in part differentiated from heart failure by the fact that heart failure is always congestive. Acute congestive heart failure and shock may develop concurrently, as may be the case with myocardial infarction in man.

When a cardiac chamber fails, its output decreases and the amount of blood remaining within it at the end of systole is increased. The blood pressures in the vessels and chambers behind the failing chamber become elevated. The decreased cardiac output and elevated pressures in the vessels entering the heart stimulate compensatory mechanisms, which in turn result in the clinical signs of congestive heart failure. The compensatory mechanisms include tachycardia, cardiomegaly, arterial and venous vasoconstriction, increased blood volume, and increased venous return. When these homeostatic mechanisms fail to provide the tissue with the necessary blood flow, overt congestive heart failure ensues.

LEFT HEART FAILURE

Left heart failure results from diseases that injure the left atrium, the left ventricle, or both. Included in this category are mitral valvular disease (insufficiency and/or stenosis), aortic valvular disease (insufficiency and/or stenosis), systemic arterial hypertension, coronary artery disease, cardiomyopathies, myocarditis, and those congenital defects involving the left ventricle that are independent of or associated with right ventricular defects.

In left heart failure, ". . . the pulmonary venous pressure rises, not because of a 'backward pressure' but because the venous return, moving in a forward direction, cannot be passed along with normal speed by the failing left chamber" (Friedberg, 1966, p. 277). Increased blood volume (from sodium and water retention) in the pulmonary vascular bed and elevated pulmonary venous and capillary pressures produce changes in pulmonary compliance, vital capacity, and alveolar capillary diffusion which are largely responsible for the signs of left-sided heart failure; these are primarily pulmonary in nature (Friedberg, 1966).

The characteristic pathologic findings are engorged, firm, moist lungs that do not collapse when the thorax is opened. White or blood-tinged frothy fluid is expressed from cut sections of the lung.

CLINICAL SIGNS OF LEFT HEART FAILURE

Cough.   The cough is an early feature of left heart failure in the dog and is usually the most distinctive and alarming feature of the condition. It is best described as low and resonant and usually occurs in paroxysms. It occurs initially at night or in the early morning hours and becomes more frequent as the disease progresses, until it occurs throughout the day. The owner may report that the cough can be elicited whenever the dog becomes excited, drinks water, or pulls on the leash, tightening the collar. White or blood-tinged phlegm is expectorated at the end of the paroxysm; this may be misinterpreted by the owner as a form of vomitus.

Exertional dyspnea.   When carefully questioned, the owner is likely to report that the dog experiences labored breathing during physical exertion. Dogs experiencing dyspnea stop suddenly while exercising. The nares are dilated, and the dog uses the accessory muscles of respiration. With dyspnea of cardiac origin, there is rapid panting or puffing rather than deep, labored breathing. Cardiac dyspnea probably results from increased pulmonary blood volume and elevated pulmonary venous and capillary pressures. It is important to recognize that dyspnea not only is a sign of cardiac disease but can also be related to conditions such as pulmonary diseases, obesity, and acidosis.

Orthopnea.   Orthopnea, a cardinal sign of left-sided heart failure, refers to difficult breathing in the recumbent position. This occurs because the circulating blood volume increases, resulting in increased venous return, pulmonary congestion, and diminished pulmonary compliance (Friedberg, 1966). The dog then unconsciously assumes a semi-sitting position or wakes up.

Paroxysmal dyspnea.   Paroxysmal dyspnea refers to attacks of respiratory distress that occur without apparent cause. In paroxysmal dyspnea, also called *cardiac asthma,* the respiration is wheezing in character, and the signs resemble those of bronchial asthma, which may also be present. Paroxysmal dyspnea may occur at night with respiratory distress, anxiety, sitting up, moving about, and coughing up of mucus. Breathing may be rapid, noisy, and wheezy or bubbling.

The wheezing and other indications of asthma occur because of pulmonary congestion, swelling of the bronchial membranes, and narrowing of the bronchial lumen. The predominant inciting factor is the increased flow of blood to the right heart and lungs. Paroxysmal dyspnea is most common when the dog is in a recumbent position. A cough may occur after the attack but is not a cause of the attack.

Pulmonary edema.   Pulmonary edema refers to the presence of fluid in the pulmonary interstitial spaces and the alveolar luminal spaces. It often occurs as an extension of paroxysmal dyspnea when intense dyspnea, orthopnea, and anxiety develop. Coarse, moist râles are usually obvious even without the use of the stethoscope when pulmonary alveolar edema occurs. The pulmonary fluids may bubble and froth from the mouth and nose, and in severe attacks the dog drowns in its own secretions. The dog becomes cyanotic, and the skin is cold and clammy. The pulse quickly becomes thready. Attacks of pulmonary edema usually subside spontaneously, but the injection of morphine, phlebotomy, and alternating use of tourniquets are often helpful in treating pulmonary edema by reducing the blood volume and thus the venous return to the right heart and lungs (see Chapter 10). Oxygen therapy should also be utilized when pulmonary edema develops.

Cyanosis. Cyanosis is not usually associated with uncomplicated left heart failure. It may occur with acute pulmonary edema, bronchopneumonia, or both, when oxygen cannot enter the fluid-filled alveoli and thus cannot diffuse into the pulmonary capillaries, resulting in arterial unsaturation.

RIGHT HEART FAILURE

In the dog, right heart failure most often develops secondary to left-sided heart failure after pulmonary hypertension has induced a sufficient strain on the right heart. Conditions generally affecting the entire heart, such as myocarditis, arteriovenous fistula, and anemia, result in right heart failure because the right ventricle, the weaker ventricular chamber, is less able than the stronger left ventricle to cope with the additional strain. In addition to left heart failure, diseases affecting the right heart, the pulmonary vessels, or the lungs are also capable of inducing predominant right heart failure. Included in this category are acquired conditions such as tricuspid insufficiency, heartworm disease, neoplasia invading the right heart, cardiac tamponade and pericardial effusion, and the various forms of cor pulmonale. The more common congenital cardiac defects that result primarily in right heart failure are pulmonic stenosis, ventricular septal defect, tetralogy of Fallot, and patent ductus arteriosus.

As right heart failure develops, there is compensatory right ventricular hypertrophy in an attempt to maintain a normal cardiac output regardless of whether the failure is due to elevated pulmonary venocapillary pressures (left heart failure), pulmonary arterial pressure (cor pulmonale), or right ventricular pressure (right heart disease). As the chamber fails, right ventricular end diastolic pressure, right atrial pressure, and central venous pressure all increase. Sodium and water retention occurs, apparently in an attempt to increase the blood volume. As the blood volume is increased, the venous return to the right heart also increases, and the right ventricle is unable to accept the blood and expel it into the pulmonary circulation and left heart. The systemic veins become overloaded, and venous pressures increase. It is this increase in the venous pressures that is responsible for the clinical signs of right heart failure.

Pathologically, right heart failure is characterized by chronic venous congestion resulting in enlarged, firm, and unusually dark-colored abdominal organs, especially the liver, spleen, and kidneys. "Nutmeg liver" is the term used to describe the appearance of that organ after long-standing right heart failure, and venous congestion results in interspersed areas of light and dark color. Hepatic cirrhosis due to fibrous induration is occasionally seen in dogs with chronic right heart failure. Ascites or transudation of edema fluid into the peritoneal cavity is common in right heart failure, and, in the dog, ascites precedes the development of subcutaneous edema. After chronic accumulation of ascitic fluid, the specific gravity of the fluid is eventually increased (greater than 1.018), and red and white blood cells are often present in the fluid. Edema of the gastrointestinal tract and pancreatic congestion also occur with right heart failure. In addition to the chronic passive venous congestion that develops in the abdominal cavity, the brain may be edematous and congested. As the degree of heart failure progresses, subcutaneous, dependent edema develops, followed by edema of the head.

CLINICAL SIGNS OF RIGHT HEART FAILURE

Since right heart failure often develops secondarily to left heart failure, the signs of left heart failure are often also present (see pp. 216-218).

Venous congestion. The superficial veins are distended, and the jugular veins may pulsate, indicating elevation of right atrial and central venous pressures. The retinal veins have been observed to be distended in dogs in advanced heart failure (see p. 11). When venous distention occurs in only one part of the body, a local rather than a systemic cause should be considered. (In heart block and ventricular tachycardia, prominent pulsations of jugular veins may be seen. They result from retrograde transmission of blood from the right atrium into the cervical veins caused by atrial contraction against a closed tricuspid valve, and are called cannon "a" waves.)

Hepatic enlargement and tenderness.   Increased systemic venous pressures result first in chronic passive congestion of the liver and subsequent enlargement of that organ. The spleen becomes clinically enlarged and palpable in the later stages of the disease. Abdominal pain may be elicited owing to the increased tension placed on the liver capsule by the enlarged liver. When pressure is applied to the cranial abdomen, the hepatojugular reflex may be elicited as blood is forced from the liver into the cervical veins, resulting in their distention.

Hepatic function may be disturbed in states of right heart failure, resulting in moderate elevation of the serum glutamic pyruvic transaminase (up to 240 S. F. units), serum glutamic oxaloacetic transaminase, alkaline phosphatase, and urobilinogen levels. Icterus is unusual but may occur. The retention of Bromsulphalein dye (BSP), above 5 per cent after 30 minutes, denotes reduced dye conjugation owing to diminished or delayed hepatic blood flow.

Ascites, hydrothorax, hydropericardium, and subcutaneous edema.   Serous effusions into the peritoneal and thoracic cavities and pericardium, as well as the subcutaneous interstitial tissue, develop as a result of increased portal or capillary hydrostatic pressure. In the dog, as distinguished from man, ascites is common and always precedes subcutaneous edema. Subcutaneous edema due to right heart failure is uncommon and is seen very late in the course of the condition. When it does occur, it is usually bilateral or quadrilateral; the tissues are cold to the touch and pit when digital pressure is applied. Hydrothorax and hydropericardium develop only late in the course of the disease.

Ascites is usually obvious on physical examination. Its presence should immediately suggest the need for a complete differential diagnosis. Ascites results not only from congestive heart failure but also from protein depletion caused by dietary deficiencies, severe parasitism, the malabsorption syndrome, and the nephrotic syndrome. Ascites may also develop in hepatic cirrhosis caused by the presence of lymphatic exudation following portal obstruction and hypoproteinemia. Since ascites is often caused by local abdominal lesions (abdominal neoplasia, infections, or both), the possibility of such conditions must also be evaluated.

Initially, the specific gravity of ascitic fluid caused by congestive heart failure is below 1.018, and the serous effusion is a transudate; but as the ascites becomes chronic the effusate becomes blood-tinged, and the specific gravity is elevated above 1.018. The total protein content of ascitic fluid seems to vary with the etiology of the ascites. Wallace and Hamilton (1962) reported the total protein

TABLE 6-2 TOTAL PROTEIN CONCENTRATIONS IN FLUIDS FROM NORMAL DOGS
AND DOGS IN HEART FAILURE*

FLUID	TOTAL PROTEIN CONCENTRATIONS (Gm/100 cc.)		
	Normal Dogs	Dogs with Mitral Insufficiency	Dogs with Heartworm Disease
Plasma	6.5 to 7.0	4.8	6.0
Ascitic fluid	—	3.0	3.8
Thoracic fluid	—	2.0	2.4
Interstitial fluid	—	0.8	0.5

*Data from Wallace and Hamilton, 1962.

concentrations in plasma, ascitic fluid, thoracic fluid, and interstititial fluid in dogs with mitral insufficiency and heartworm disease (Table 6-2).

It should be stressed that the total protein concentration of ascitic fluid can vary greatly and that many diseases produce ascites. Thus the differential diagnosis of ascites should not be based on the total protein content alone.

Cardiac cachexia. Cardiac cachexia, thought to be due primarily to cellular hypoxia, is the term applied to the obvious malnutrition which may accompany chronic congestive heart failure (Pittman and Cohen, 1964). It is associated with poor appetite, weight loss, malabsorption from the gastrointestinal tract, and a variety of gastrointestinal disturbances. Generalized weakness is often associated with cardiac cachexia. It should be recognized that the nutritional status of the dog in heart failure is probably poor, and attempts must be made to rectify nutritional imbalances. Further, the clinician should remain aware of the fact that a variety of cardiac drugs such as digitalis, diuretics, and sedatives may exacerbate the signs of cardiac cachexia and weakness.

FACTORS RESPONSIBLE FOR PRECIPITATING OR AGGRAVATING CONGESTIVE HEART FAILURE

Dogs with cardiac disease are asymptomatic until the heart's compensatory mechanisms are no longer capable of meeting the body's needs. However, a number of environmental factors may precipitate acute cardiac decompensation. Although it is often impossible to retard the progress of organic heart disease markedly, it is possible to eliminate or avoid certain factors that can precipitate heart failure.

Infections. Infectious processes, especially those involving the respiratory tract, place a distinct burden on the diseased heart. In the presence of cardiac disease, infections should be intensively treated. Prophylactic therapy is occasionally advisable to prevent their occurrence.

Changes in the heart rate and rhythm. A sharp increase in the heart rate can be especially serious, because the increase in rate results in a reduced diastolic filling time and impaired oxygenation and nutrition of the heart muscle. The development of cardiac arrhythmias is associated with decreased cardiac function caused by impaired filling and ineffective contractions.

Sodium loading. Meals or snacks containing moderate to large quantities of sodium may precipitate an acute attack of congestive heart failure; in such cases the body is unable to excrete the sodium, and the subsequent result is the retention of water.

Transfusions. Overloading of the circulatory system and the rapid infusion of fluids, even in normal dogs, may lead to pulmonary edema. In dogs with cardiac disease, overloading is more likely to occur if the infusion contains sodium. Measurement of the central venous pressure is helpful in detecting fluid overloading when the pressure begins to rise sharply during intravenous fluid therapy.

Alterations in environmental heat and humidity. Dogs with cardiac disease are sensitive to fluctuations in both temperature and humidity. A sudden increase in humidity can precipitate heat prostration, because dogs with cardiac disease seem to be unable to regulate heat dissipation as well as normal dogs. In cool environments, less stress is placed on the heart than in hot environments when the same functions are performed. Because of these facts, air conditioning is recommended whenever possible for dogs who seem sensitive to fluctuations in temperature. Similarly, enclosed hair driers or hot air blowers should not be used to dry cardiac patients after baths.

Physical strain. Dogs with advanced cardiac disease are unable to withstand the rigors of prolonged exercise, and some demonstrate exertional dyspnea and fatigue after only minimal exercise. Restriction of exercise should be maintained for these dogs.

Discontinuation of digitalis or diuretics. Dogs which have remained in a satisfactory state of compensation following the formulation of a therapeutic regimen may decompensate if the dosages are altered or if therapy is discontinued.

Other organ disease. Diseases of other parts of the body, such as renal or hepatic dysfunction, anemia, hyperaldosteronism, and pulmonary embolism, may precipitate heart failure by placing further strain on the overburdened heart.

References

Criteria Committee, New York Heart Association: Diseases of the Heart and Blood Vessels—Nomenclature and Criteria for Diagnosis. 6th ed. Little, Brown & Co., Boston. 1966.

Detweiler, D. K., Patterson, D. F., Luginbühl, H., Rhodes, W. H., Buchanan, J. W., Knight, D. H., and Hill, J. D.: Diseases of the Cardiovascular System. In *Canine Medicine.* Edited by E. J. Catcott. 1st Catcott ed. American Veterinary Publications, Inc., Santa Barbara, Calif. (1968):589.

Friedberg, C. F.: Diseases of the Heart. 3rd ed. W. B. Saunders Co., Philadelphia, 1966.

Logue, R. B., and Hurst, J. W.: Etiology and Clinical Recognition of Heart Failure. In *The Heart—Arteries and Veins.* 2nd. ed. Edited by J. W. Hurst and R. B. Logue. Blakiston Division, McGraw-Hill, New York. (1970):434.

Pittman, J. G., and Cohen, P.: The Pathogenesis of Cardiac Cachexia. New England J. Med., 271 (1964):403, 453.

Wallace, C. R., and Hamilton, W. F.: Study of Spontaneous Congestive Heart Failure in the Dog. Circ. Res., 11 (1962):301.

SECTION II

PHARMACOLOGIC AND OTHER THERAPY IN CARDIAC DISEASE

Chapter 7   DIGITALIS AND THE CARDIAC GLYCOSIDES

Chapter 8   ANTIARRHYTHMIC THERAPY

Chapter 9   DIURETICS

Chapter 10   LOW SODIUM DIETS AND OTHER DRUGS AND METHODS INDICATED IN CARDIAC THERAPY

7

DIGITALIS AND THE CARDIAC GLYCOSIDES

Digitalis has been used successfully in the treatment of congestive heart failure and certain cardiac arrhythmias for many years. As the study of cardiac disease and cardiac physiology progresses, so does that of digitalis in an attempt to understand its mode of action and to improve its effectiveness.

Although digitalis cannot be administered without danger of intoxication and iatrogenic death, it should not be avoided because of its lethal or toxic properties. Instead, the veterinarian must be familiar with the pharmacology, metabolism, and excretion rate of the drug, with the indications for its use, and with the clinical and electrocardiographic signs of digitalis intoxication. When it is used properly, digitalis is a most effective therapeutic agent.

Plant extracts containing cardiac glycosides have been used for centuries. Squill was used by the Egyptians about 1500 B.C.; during the Roman Empire it was used as a diuretic, heart tonic, emetic, and rat poison. Digitalis, derived from the purple foxglove (*Digitalis purpurea*), was used first by William Withering (1785) as a treatment for dropsy. In 1799, Ferriar described the cardiac actions of the drug; he regarded its diuretic action as secondary. In this century it has been recognized that the main value of digitalis glycosides is for the treatment of congestive heart failure (Moe and Farah, 1965). In veterinary medicine, the drug was first recorded as a therapeutic agent in the treatment of dropsy in the dog in 1841 (Blaine).

Cardiac glycosides are cultivated as medicinal herbs and as ornamental flowering plants. The leaves contain the greatest proportion of cardiac glycosides. When the leaf is dried, the stalk and midribs are removed, and the leaves are prepared as tablets or in an elixir for administration (Estes and White, 1965).

225

SOURCES OF THE CARDIAC GLYCOSIDES

The leaves of *D. purpurea* are used to produce the glycosides digitoxin, gitoxin, and gitalin (Table 7-1). *Digitalis lanata* leaves yield the glycosides digitoxin, gitoxin, and digoxin (Table 7-1). The glycoside ouabain (G-strophanthin) is a product of the seeds of *Strophanthus gratus* (Table 7-1). Other cardiac glycosides derived from plants include proscillaridin A, from squill (*Urginea maritima*); convallatoxin, from lily of the valley (*Convallaria majalis*); and thevetin, from the yellow oleander (*Thevetia neriifolia*) (Moe and Farah, 1965).

The native cardiac glycosides in the plant are referred to as lanatosides or digilanids. The digilanids of *D. purpurea* (Table 7-1), when subjected to hydrolysis, yield the pure glycosides digitoxin and gitoxin. When *D. lanata* digilanids undergo hydrolysis, the pharmacologically active glycosides yielded are digitoxin, gitoxin, and digoxin (Table 7-1).

In the body, the pure digitalis glycoside, such as digoxin, is hydrolyzed to the pharmacologically active aglycone (genin) and a sugar. Chemically, the basic nucleus of the aglycone belongs to the steroid and sex hormone family (the

TABLE 7-1 BOTANICAL SOURCES AND MAJOR CHEMICAL COMPONENTS OF CARDIAC GLYCOSIDES OF CLINICAL IMPORTANCE[*]

PLANT SOURCE		PRECURSOR GLYCOSIDE	SPLIT OFF BY ENZYMATIC AND MILD ALKALINE HYDROLYSIS [†]	GLYCOSIDE	SPLIT OFF BY ACID HYDROLYSIS [†]	AGLYCONE, OR GENIN
DIGITALIS	*D. purpurea* (leaf)	Purpurea-glycoside A (desacetyl-digilanid A)	Glucose	Digitoxin	Digitoxose (3)	Digitoxigenin
		Purpurea-glycoside B (desacetyl-digilanid B)	Glucose	Gitoxin	Digitoxose (3)	Gitoxigenin
		———		Gitalin	Digitoxose (2)	Gitaligenin (gitoxigenin hydrate)
	D. lanata (leaf)	Lanatoside A (digilanid A)	Glucose + acetic acid	Digitoxin	Digitoxose (3)	Digitoxigenin
		Lanatoside B (digilanid B)	Glucose + acetic acid	Gitoxin	Digitoxose (3)	Gitoxigenin
		Lanatoside C (digilanid C; cedilanid)	Glucose + acetic acid	Digoxin	Digitoxose (3)	Digoxigenin
STROPHANTHUS	*S. Kombé* (seed)	K-strophanthoside	Glucose	K-strophan-thin-β (stro-phanthin)	Glucose + cymarose	Strophanthidin
		K-strophanthoside	Glucose (2)	Cymarin	Cymarose	Strophanthidin
		K-strophanthin-β	Glucose	Cymarin	Cymarose	Strophanthidin
		———	———	Cymarol	Cymarose	Strophanthidol
	S. gratus (seed)	———		Ouabain (G-stro-phanthin)	Rhamnose	Ouabagenin (G-strophan-thidin)
SCILLA (SQUILL)	*Urginea maritima* or *indica* (bulb)	Scillaren A	Glucose	Proscillaridin A	Rhamnose	Scillaridin A

[*]From Moe, G. K., and Farah, A. E.: In The Pharmacologic Basis of Therapeutics, edited by L. S. Goodman and A. Gilman, The MacMillan Company, New York, 3rd ed., 1965.

[†]One mol of sugar or acetic acid is split off, unless the number of mols is otherwise indicated in parentheses.

cyclopentanoperhydrophenanthrene nucleus). The sugar, although not active alone, affects the solubility of the aglycone, thus controlling its potency and toxicity. The aglycones vary in the number and sites of attachment of chemically bound hydroxyl groups, and it is these variations that determine the chemical properties of the glycosides (Rubin, Gross, and Arbeit, 1968).

PHARMACOLOGIC ACTIVITY

Digitalis has at least two modes of action. First, it acts within the heart muscle cell to increase the contractility of actomyosin. Second, by direct stimulation of the vagal nerve and through extravagal effects, digitalis slows the heart rate and delays conduction through the atrioventricular node.

EFFECTS ON CARDIAC CONTRACTILITY

The major pharmacodynamic property of digitalis is its direct positive inotropic effect on the myocardium, i.e., its ability to increase the force of myocardial contraction. The salutary effects of digitalis on cardiac contractility are mediated by an increase in the rate at which ventricular pressure develops. This increase in the rate of rise of ventricular pressure represents an augmentation of the contractile force of the heart. This has been demonstrated during cardiopulmonary bypass in human patients with cardiac disease using a Walton-Brodie strain gauge sutured to the right ventricle, after which a rapid-acting form of digitalis was administered intravenously. A marked increase in contractile force was evident within five minutes (Bloodwell et al., 1960). When a strain gauge had been sewn on the right ventricle of dogs that were not in congestive heart failure but had chronic mitral valvular fibrosis, a nonlinear increase in contractile force was observed after the intravenous administration of ouabain (Gould, Ettinger, and Lyon, 1970). When digitalis intoxication developed, the contractile force of the myocardium diminished, as measured by the strain gauge arch. These findings contrasted with the linear increase in contractility that resulted when two normal dogs were given ouabain. Evidence suggests that this potentiation of contractility occurs because the intracellular cytoplasmic calcium ion concentration is increased during cellular activation (perhaps from the sarcoplasmic reticulum) (Braunwald and Pool, 1968).

In the failing heart, digitalis increases the force of ventricular systole and increases the ventricular diastolic time, resulting in increased cardiac output and decreased venous pressure. Because the tonus of the myocardial fibrils is increased, there is a slight shortening of the fibrils and thus a decrease in the diastolic heart size. The glomerular filtration rate increases, with an improvement in renal circulation, and edema fluid is eliminated (Rubin, Gross, and Arbeit, 1968).

EFFECTS ON CARDIAC RATE AND CONDUCTION

Digitalis reduces the heart rate by central vagal stimulation (cardioinhibition) and also by decreasing the positive chronotropic action (rate of cardiac contraction) of epinephrine and sympathetic nervous stimulation (Mendez, Aceves, and Mendez, 1961; Nadeau and James, 1963). The latter may account for the extravagal action of digitalis, which is important in slowing the heart rate even in dogs which have been treated with atropine. The glycosides suppress atrioventricular conduction and increase the refractory period of atrioventricular transmission. However, digitalis may improve the work capacity of the heart before or without reducing the heart rate. The change in rate is ". . . secondary to the improvement of the circulation and is not the primary therapeutic action of the drug" (Moe and Farah, 1965, p. 674).

Digitalis in low doses increases and at higher dosages depresses electrical excitability and conduction velocity through both the atria and the ventricles. Conduction through the atrioventricular node is slowed by both vagal and extra-vagal effects, as recognized by prolongation of the P-R interval on the electro-cardiogram. Digitalis shortens atrial and ventricular refractory periods but increases functional refractoriness of the atrioventricular node. Increased auto-maticity, or the ability to initiate pacemaker activity anywhere in the heart, is a characteristic effect of digitalis. Thus, even when cellular excitability is depressed by digitalis, automaticity initiates ectopic foci in the ventricle. To demonstrate that the effect of digitalis on the atrioventricular node is a direct as well as a vagal effect, it should be emphasized that high degrees of atrioventricular block induced by digitalis cannot be terminated by either atropine or exercise (Moe and Farah, 1965).

SUMMARY

Digitalis produces a more forceful systole, prolongs diastole, decreases venous pressure, and increases arterial pressure, cardiac output, and stroke volume. Cardiac slowing may accompany these changes.

INDICATIONS FOR DIGITALIS THERAPY

CONGESTIVE HEART FAILURE

The primary indication for digitalis is congestive heart failure caused by failure of one or both ventricles. Digitalis should be used whether the degree of failure is mild or severe. Arrhythmias must be identified, but their presence does not contraindicate digitalis therapy if congestive heart failure is present. The cardiac glycosides are most beneficial when failure has resulted from ventricular overload (i.e., mitral insufficiency, aortic insufficiency); however, regardless of the precipitating factor, treatment with digitalis is indicated until heart failure is abolished.

Digitalis improves cardiac function. After digitalis has been administered to a dog in congestive heart failure and with decreased cardiac function, the dog should be maintained on cardiac glycosides even if it becomes temporarily asymptomatic.

When heart disease is secondary to another disease process, correction of the underlying disease, such as infection, anemia, thyrotoxicosis, or arteriovenous fistula, is essential. In badly damaged hearts, digitalis can be expected to provide only a limited degree of benefit. When the presence of cardiac disease cannot be proved but signs of heart failure persist, a clinical trial of digitalis is indicated.

ARRHYTHMIAS

Digitalis is nearly universally indicated in atrial fibrillation, not only to re-store myocardial efficiency but also to reduce the ventricular rate and to eliminate the pulse deficit. In most instances it should be given at a level sufficient to maintain the heart rate under 160 beats/min.

Atrial and atrioventricular junctional paroxysmal tachycardias are common arrhythmias in dogs. Digitalis reduces the frequency of these arrhythmias, probably by reflex vagal stimulation and by increasing atrioventricular nodal refractoriness. Supraventricular tachycardia is an unusual manifestation of digitalis intoxication, and caution is advised if intoxication is suspected. Ventricular tachycardia and ventricular premature contractions may be contraindications for the use of digitalis because of the danger of inducing ventricular fibrillation. In the presence of ectopic ventricular arrhythmias, the cardiac glycosides must be administered cautiously, and the dog must be monitored electrocardiographically. Although atrial flutter is unusual in the dog, cardiac glycoside therapy would be indicated if it develops.

CONDITIONS IN WHICH DIGITALIS THERAPY IS CONTRAINDICATED OR MAY BE HARMFUL

The only absolute contraindication for digitalis therapy is digitalis intoxication, for continued use of the drug may increase the degree of heart block. In dogs with stable complete heart block of nondigitalis origin and very slow heart rates, digitalis glycosides should be administered only if congestive heart failure is present, and then with care. Ventricular premature contractions and ventricular tachycardia are possible contraindications to digitalis therapy. If these arrhythmias are due to digitalis intoxication, *digitalis must be discontinued immediately.* Since ventricular arrhythmias may indicate increased myocardial irritability owing to decreased cardiac output, digitalis, when properly administered, may reduce the number of ectopic beats by improving myocardial function.

Hypokalemia due to prolonged vomiting, diarrhea, or diuresis is likely to precipitate intoxication when digitalis is administered; it is characterized by weakness, flaccid paralysis, ileus, and hyporeflexia. Therefore potassium must be replaced prior to or in conjunction with glycoside therapy when hypokalemia occurs.

NONINDICATIONS FOR DIGITALIS THERAPY

Digitalis is not indicated for treating tachycardia caused by conditions such as fever, toxemia, infection, and hyperthyroidism unless congestive heart failure is also present. It is also not indicated for treating sinus arrhythmia, sinoatrial block, junctional arrhythmias, or ventricular escape beats unless congestive heart failure is also present. Dogs in shock of noncardiac origin do not benefit by the use of cardiac glycosides. The prophylactic use of digitalis glycosides prior to surgical procedures is not warranted unless the dog is in congestive heart failure or in an incipient failure state. Digitalis has no place in treating a nephritic condition unless congestive heart failure occurs. Caution should be observed when dogs are being treated with calcium salts or with sympathomimetic agents such as ephedrine or epinephrine because the dogs may be sensitive to the addition of digitalis to the therapeutic regimen.

DIGITALIS PREPARATIONS FREQUENTLY USED

1. Powdered digitalis, U.S.P.—ground, whole-leaf digitalis, available in 0.05-Gm. or 0.1-Gm. tablets; also called digitalis leaf. Relatively long-acting preparation.

2. Digitalis tincture, N.F.—1 ml. is equivalent to 0.1 Gm. powdered digitalis leaf. Relatively long-acting preparation.

3. Ouabain injection, U.S.P. (G-strophanthin)—2-ml. vials for injectable intravenous use contain the pure glycoside, 0.25 mg./ml. Rapid-acting preparation.

4. Digitoxin, U.S.P.—pure digitoxin, or mixtures of glycosides of *D. purpurea,* are available in 0.1-mg. and 0.2-mg. tablets and also in the injectable form, 0.2 mg./ml. In theory, 0.1 mg. of digitoxin is equivalent to 0.1 Gm. of powdered digitalis leaf. Relatively long-acting preparation.

5. Digoxin, U.S.P.—glycoside from *D. lanata,* available in 0.125-mg., 0.25-mg., and 0.5-mg. tablets, in elixir form at 0.05 mg./ml., and in 2 cc. vials for injectable use at 0.25 mg./ml. (intravenous or intramuscular). Duration of action is moderate.

6. Lanatoside C, N.F.—the precursor glycoside or digilanid from *D. lanata,* available only for oral use in 0.5-mg. tablets. Duration of action is moderate.

7. Deslanoside, N.F. (Cedilanid-D)—derived from the alkaline hydrolysis of lanatoside C for injectable use, 0.2 mg./ml. Duration of action is moderate.

METABOLISM OF CARDIAC GLYCOSIDES

Since strophanthus, squill, and ouabain are very poorly absorbed from the gastrointestinal tract, they are not administered orally. After intramuscular and subcutaneous injection, the absorption of digitalis glycosides is irregular. Intramuscular injection is accompanied by pain and local tenderness; therefore it is restricted primarily to use in dogs that are difficult to manage. Some cardiac glycosides are readily absorbed from the colon and could be used effectively in suppository form, although this route is rarely chosen. When congestive heart failure and venous congestion of the gastrointestinal tract are present, the rate of absorption is slowed but the amount ultimately absorbed is unchanged (Rubin, Gross, and Arbeit, 1968).

Digitalis accumulates in the body even when a loading dose is not administered. Whether a loading dose or a lower maintenance dosage is given, the amount of digitalis in the body after five days is the same. This is so because a constant percentage of the body's stores of digitalis is excreted daily, so that as more is administered, more is excreted. Therefore, digitalization can be accomplished with or without using a loading dose (see pp. 233-235).

Digoxin has been shown to have an affinity for cardiac muscle. The mean half-life of tritiated digoxin given in one 0.5-mg. dose to dogs was 23 hours in serum and 26 hours in heart muscle. This, then, suggests a direct relationship between the serum concentration and the myocardial concentration (Doherty et al., 1966). Although glycosides are bound to the plasma albumin to varying degrees, this does not explain all the differences in the speed of action of the various drugs.

Because elimination of cardiac glycosides is delayed by severe hepatic or renal damage, the dosage used should be judged accordingly. Excretion of both the unchanged and the degraded glycoside is chiefly through the kidneys. Biliary excretion is negligible in the dog (Moe and Farah, 1965).

DIGITALIZATION

"The digitalization of any patient is a clinical experiment" (Rubin, Gross, and Arbeit, 1968, p. 289). The fundamental principle of digitalization is to administer the drug until the desired therapeutic effect is achieved or until signs of mild intoxication appear. When heart failure is mild, signs of clinical improvement are difficult to assess, and mild states of intoxication are often unavoidable. Also, six to ten days often pass before signs of improvement occur, again making it difficult to avoid mild toxic reactions. In dogs with atrial fibrillation, control and slowing of the ventricular rate, which are easily detected clinically, usually parallel improvement in response to the cardiac glycoside. Similarly, the abolition or reduction of arrhythmias such as ventricular premature contractions is often simultaneous with clinical improvement and satisfactory digitalization.

The veterinarian should be thoroughly familiar with one product each for slow and rapid digitalization (see Tables 7-2 and 7-3) to enable the most accurate and effective use of the glycoside, so that a maximum effect is achieved with a minimum of danger from toxic effects. Although all cardiac glycosides are theoretically similar when used correctly, the authors prefer digoxin tablets for slow digitalization and injectable digoxin or ouabain for rapid digitalization. Above all, *one should not depend upon a fixed dosage rate for the administration of any cardiac glycoside.*

Each product must be assessed individually, occasionally using extremely large or small dosages. Occasionally a dog is examined which for some reason cannot be given even the smallest dosages of a glycoside without showing signs of intoxication. If a dog has a negative response (such as vomiting, diarrhea, or electrocardiographic changes) to even a small dose of a glycoside, another product should be used.

THERAPEUTIC EFFECTS OF DIGITALIS

CLINICAL EFFECTS

The most significant clinical effect of glycoside therapy is alleviation of the cardiac signs (see Chapter 6) of coughing and dyspnea, pulmonary edema and/or congestion, and ascitic fluid and dependent edema, resulting in marked diuresis and weight loss. The dog should be weighed prior to therapy and thereafter at the same time of day to avoid environmental influences. The heart rate is usually reduced, especially if tachycardia or atrial fibrillation was present prior to therapy.

ELECTROCARDIOGRAPHY

Although electrocardiographic changes need not result for digitalization to be complete, electrocardiography is often helpful in recognizing mild or toxic levels of digitalization. In dogs that have a sinus rhythm and that have received adequate levels of digitalis, the P-R interval is often prolonged (Wallace and Hamilton, 1962) from 0.01 to 0.03 sec., and the cardiac rate is often decreased (Ettinger, 1966). It should be stressed that the inotropic and atrioventricular blocking effects of digitalis need not be proportional; thus the effects of digitalis cannot be measured simply by observing atrioventricular conduction changes. (Ogden, Selzer, and Cohen, 1969). Changes in the S-T segment and T wave may also occur during clinical digitalization, and sinus arrhythmia may be accentuated.

Digitalization is effective in controlling or converting arrhythmias for which digitalis therapy is indicated. The ventricular rate in atrial fibrillation should be slowed to the range of 120 to 160 beats/min., the frequency of supraventricular premature contractions should be reduced, and supraventricular tachycardias should be abolished after therapeutic digitalization. When digitalis is indicated for congestive heart failure and ventricular premature contractions or ventricular tachycardia is present, the arrhythmia should be controlled by digitalis or by the association of digitalis and antiarrhythmic agents.

TOXIC EFFECTS OF DIGITALIZATION

CLINICAL EFFECTS

After oral administration, digitalis intoxication begins with anorexia and salivation and progresses to vomiting and diarrhea. When such signs are encountered after the first oral dose, they are usually due to gastrointestinal irritation and may be either disregarded or treated with oral opiates. Neurotoxic effects such as depression, drowsiness, weakness, and seizures are associated with hypokalemia (Lyon and DeGraff, 1963), and all these signs except seizures are commonly associated with the gastrointestinal manifestations of intoxication.

ELECTROCARDIOGRAPHY

Changes in the electrocardiogram vary with the route used for administering the cardiac glycoside. A decreased heart rate and first degree heart block are common when the drug is administered orally. The reduction in heart rate need not, however, be so marked as to produce bradycardia. Second degree atrioventricular block and atrioventricular junctional rhythms develop thereafter, and ventricular premature contractions and ventricular tachycardia (atrioventricular dissociation) usually develop late in the course of intoxication. Although arrhythmias usually develop in the order mentioned, serious electrocardiographic signs of intoxication may occur in almost any sequence.

When the dog is digitalized intravenously, the cardiac glycosides increase automaticity more often than they induce prolongation of atrioventricular conduction time. Therefore arrhythmias such as ventricular premature contractions, ventricular tachycardias, and ventricular fibrillation often develop first, in comparison to the various degrees of atrioventricular block that develop first when oral forms are given. In ten dogs intoxicated with intravenous ouabain, the first signs of intoxication were increased automaticity in eight dogs and prolongation of conduction time in two dogs (Ettinger et al., 1969).

SLOW ORAL DIGITALIZATION (see Table 7-2)

Digitalis is a safe drug to use if the clinician realizes that there is no single digitalizing dose for all dogs. The dosage requirements for each dog depend more on internal factors than on total body weight. Because each dog requires individual attention and monitoring, we feel that the dog should be hospitalized to establish the maintenance requirement for each dog. This also affords the additional benefit of enforced cage rest.

Digitalization may be accomplished in several ways. The most reliable method is to calculate an *approximate* total dose, which is then divided into four equal doses to be administered orally over 36 to 48 hours. The dog's behavior can then be observed closely, and serial electrocardiograms can be recorded. If electrocardiograms are not recorded, the dog should be observed throughout the day and examined carefully twice daily for signs of digitalis intoxication. The dog is brought to mild intoxication, and the daily dosage rate is then reduced to a maintenance level calculated from the total amount of digitalis *used to that point* (not calculated) for digitalization. Maintenance dosage is started 24 hours after the final digitalizing dose unless signs of intoxication persist. If toxic signs continue, digitalis should not be given until the signs have been absent for 24 hours.

The latter method utilizes the loading principle; i.e., more than a daily dose is given to raise the blood level of digitalis rapidly. After five days of loading therapy, however, the blood level of digitalis is no greater than it would be if the drug had been administered in lower daily dosages. As a result, some clinicians prefer to administer a daily maintenance dose from the beginning of therapy. Although toxic reactions are likely to be less severe when the latter method is used, either insufficient or excessive levels of the drug are likely to be administered, and toxic reactions may occur later in therapy (after the fifth to the seventh day) when the dog is not under direct observation by a veterinarian. Since the 48-hour loading dosage is followed by three to five days of maintenance therapy under hospital surveillance, toxic signs are less likely to develop when the dog is sent home. Thus the authors prefer to administer a loading dose in the hospital, followed by three to five days of additional hospital surveillance.

Drugs available for oral use are numerous. In our clinic, digoxin is the glycoside of choice. This drug is preferred to digitoxin or digitalis leaf because of its clinical effectiveness. Digitoxin tablets are not effective by the oral route even in very high doses and do not cause toxic effects for reasons which are not entirely clear, (Ettinger, 1966). Digitoxin often has few salutary effects in dogs with signs of congestive heart failure (Detweiler, 1965).

Digoxin is used orally at the rate of 0.03 to 0.1 mg./lb., divided over the 48-hour period of digitalization (Detweiler, 1965; Ettinger, 1966). The drug is administered until electrocardiographic signs of mild intoxication develop. The dose, based on weight, is at best approximate. *Should signs of intoxication develop before the estimated total dosage has been administered, digitalization is still considered complete, and therapy is discontinued.*

Dogs weighing more than 30 lb. require less digoxin per pound of body weight than do smaller dogs. Therefore, their total dosage is proportionately lower than that for small dogs. For example, a 40-lb. dog may require only $1\frac{1}{2}$ times as much digoxin as a 20-lb. dog, and an 80-lb. dog only twice the amount required for a 20-lb. dog.

TABLE 7-2   RECOMMENDED DOSAGES FOR DIGITALIZATION—ORAL METHOD

PREPARATIONS	TOTAL DIGITALIZING DOSE DIVIDED OVER 48 HOURS (GUIDELINE TO APPROXIMATE DOSAGE)	DAILY MAINTENANCE DOSAGE	COMMENTS
Digoxin, U.S.P.		Approx. 0.01 mg./lb./day*; 1/10 to 1/4 of total required*; 1/8 to 1/5 of total required†	Digitalization complete when clinical or electro-cardiographic intoxication occurs; maintenance dose divided into 2 doses/day; when severe toxic signs occur, they are of brief duration (48 to 96 hours)
0.05 mg./cc. elixir			
0.125 mg. ⎫ tablets*	0.05 to 0.1 mg./lb.*		
0.25 mg. ⎬ tablets	0.03 to 0.1 mg./lb.†		
0.50 mg. ⎭			
Digitoxin, U.S.P.		1/4 of total required‡; 1/8 to 1/5 of total required†	Digitoxin considerably less effective than digoxin for heart failure when both are administered orally in tablet form; toxic reactions very rare, if they occur at all§
0.1 mg. ⎫ tablets	0.2 mg./lb.‡		
0.2 mg. ⎭	0.015 to 0.05 mg./lb.†		
Powdered digitalis, U.S.P. and Digitalis tincture, N.F.		6.4 mg./lb. or more of total required**; 1/8 to 1/5 of total required†	
0.05 Gm. ⎫ tablets	40 mg./lb.**		
0.1 Gm. ⎭	15 to 50 mg./lb.†		
1 cc. tincture equivalent to 0.1 Gm. tablet			

*Recommended by authors.   †Detweiler, 1965.   ‡Ettinger, 1966.   §Hamlin, 1966.   **Wallace and Hamilton, 1962.

It has been reported that higher levels of digoxin than generally administered were necessary to digitalize dogs in congestive heart failure (Ettinger, 1966). Since that time it has become obvious that, although high doses of digoxin are needed, some dogs do not require the highest dosage recommended. However, we have continued to use the approximate total digitalizing dose of 0.1 mg./lb. in small dogs. Electrocardiograms are recorded twice daily for the first 48 hours, and the dog is considered to be digitalized as soon as electrocardiographic signs or clinical signs other than minimal vomiting develop.

Dosages of digitoxin tablets, such as 0.015 to 0.05 mg./lb. total dosage (Detweiler, 1965), and 0.2 mg./lb. body weight (Ettinger, 1966), over 48 hours would seem to be of little value owing to this drug's inert quality in the dog. These dosages do not cause intoxication and are far less effective than digoxin for treating dogs in heart failure. Digitalis leaf is used by some veterinarians. Reports of its efficacy suggest that it be administered at the rate of 40 mg./lb. of body weight total dose, given over 48 hours (Wallace and Hamilton, 1962).

In order to maintain a continuous state of digitalis saturation in the body, a small amount is administered daily to compensate for the amount metabolized or excreted by the body. The daily dose of digitalis to be used should not be the largest dose tolerated, but rather that which maintains the highest degree of cardiac function while relieving signs of congestive heart failure. The daily maintenance dosage is determined only after careful and frequent observation of the dog. The daily level varies with the dog as well as with the form of digitalis being used. When attempting to establish the daily maintenance dose, use is made of the *total dosage required for digitalization, rather than the calculated dose.* For digoxin, approximately one-tenth to one-fourth of the total digitalizing dose is needed daily, administered in two divided doses. This is often approximately 0.01 mg./lb. divided daily. For digitoxin, 25 per cent of the digitalizing dose is given daily. For digitalis leaf, one-eighth to one-fifth of the total dosage used is recommended by Detweiler (1965). The daily maintenance level is increased or reduced as necessary for treatment of problems such as weight change, progressive congestive heart failure, and atrial fibrillation.

RAPID DIGITALIZATION—PARENTERAL ROUTES
(see Table 7-3)

Rapid digitalization is indicated for congestive heart failure with pulmonary edema resulting from acute or chronic cardiac failure, as well as for supraventricular tachycardias. Both the intravenous and the intramuscular routes may be used, but because absorption is irregular and the injections painful, intramuscular administration of cardiac glycosides is used only for digitalizing fractious dogs that do not require intravenous forms. Intravenous infusion produces the most rapid and thus the most effective digitalization in acute states. Since the inherent danger of drug intoxication increases in proportion to the speed with which the drug is effective, intravenous forms are indicated only for severe heart failure. In such cases, electrocardiographic monitoring is essential. Intravenous glycoside therapy should not be attempted in dogs that have received cardiac glycosides in the past ten to 14 days.

Ouabain (G-strophanthin) is the cardiac glycoside preferred by the authors

TABLE 7-3 RAPID DIGITALIZATION—PARENTERAL FORMS*

THERAPEUTIC INDICES	OUABAIN INJECTION, U.S.P.	DIGOXIN INJECTION, U.S.P.
Size of vial	0.5 mg./2 cc.	0.5 mg./2 cc.
Method of administration	Intravenous only	Intravenous or intramuscular (intramuscular causes local pain; if used, preferred site is lumbar muscles)
Total dose	0.02 mg./lb.* 0.01-0.015 mg./lb.†	0.02 mg./lb.* 0.02-0.03 mg./lb.†
Division of dosage	25% to 50% initially, then 25% every 30 min. until intoxication or desired effect is reached	25% to 50% initially, then 25% every 1 to 6 hr. until intoxication or desired effect is reached
Time from administration to onset of effect	3 to 10 min.‡§	5 to 30 min.‡ 10 to 30 min.§
Time from administration to maximum effect	30 min. to 2 hr.‡ 30 min.§	1½ to 5 hr.‡ 1 to 2 hr.§
Maximum duration of intoxication	2 to 6 hr.§	12 to 36 hr.§
Maintenance therapy required	Longer acting glycosides required immediately after treatment to maintain the effect	25% of total dose required for digitalization is given once daily to maintain the effect

*Acetylstrophanthidin is not advised for clinical use because of the rapid onset of its effect (1 to 5 min.) and the danger of inducing fatal arrhythmias. *Recommended by authors. †Detweiler, 1965. ‡Moe and Farah, 1965. §Rubin, Gross, and Arbeit, 1968.

for peracute conditions, and injectable digoxin is preferred for acute but not per-acute heart failure. Both drugs produce a digitalizing effect when approximately 0.02 mg./lb. is administered intravenously as a total dosage. However, because of their different lengths of action, the drugs are administered differently.

The total dosage of ouabain is estimated (0.02 mg./lb.), and 25 to 50 per cent of the total estimated dose is given intravenously immediately. Electrocardiographic monitoring should be continuous during this time. Then 25 per cent of the total calculated dose is given every 30 minutes until digitalization is complete or electrocardiographic disturbances develop. Since the duration of effect of ouabain is so short, the product is not used for maintenance therapy. Instead, maintenance therapy is best achieved using the longer-acting parenteral digoxin or oral glycosides, which are begun immediately after digitalization is completed.

Digoxin is administered intravenously in different ways, depending on the speed of action required. Usually, 25 to 50 per cent of the total calculated dosage is given intravenously, and then 25 per cent more is given every hour until digitalization has occurred. However, if speed is not essential, 25 per cent of the total calculated dose may be given every six hours until the total dosage has been reached. Maintenance doses of injectable digoxin, given once daily, are calculated at 25 per cent of the total digitalizing dose required. Oral maintenance therapy with digoxin may also be utilized. This simply requires an estimation of the oral dosage that would normally be required by a dog of the same size.

For dogs that are difficult to manage, intramuscular digitalization is effected using injectable digoxin. The digitalizing dose is 0.02 mg./lb., divided over 24 to 48 hours. The same precautions are observed as with the oral forms. Once daily injectable maintenance levels are one-fourth to one-sixth of the total digitalizing dosage. If the maintenance dose is to be given orally, it is calculated from the approximate oral dosage given that would have been required to effect digitalization. Because it may cause excessive pain and tenderness, injectable digoxin should be administered in the lumbar muscles.

TREATMENT OF DIGITALIS INTOXICATION

The method of treatment for the overwhelming majority of dogs with digitalis intoxication is to *discontinue all glycoside therapy* until the dog regains its appetite and acts normally and until electrocardiographic abnormalities disappear. If vomiting or diarrhea is excessive, oral opiate preparations or low doses of chlorpromazine or another mild tranquilizer usually provide effective control. After clinical and electrocardiographic signs of digitalis intoxication are controlled, the dog is started on maintenance levels of the glycoside. If intoxication develops in a dog already on a maintenance dosage, the dosage must be reduced accordingly.

Hypokalemia resulting from excessive potassium loss following diuretic therapy, malnutrition, or corticosteroid therapy can precipitate digitalis intoxication. Potassium should be replaced (see p. 252). Diuretics combined with aldosterone inhibitors (see p. 255) have a potassium-sparing effect that may be indicated for long-term therapy if hypokalemia is a problem. For the dog with severe ventricular ectopic arrhythmias (but not atrioventricular nodal conduction disturbances) resulting from potassium depletion, potassium chloride may be administered by *slow* intravenous infusion, giving no more than 40 mEq. diluted in 500 cc. of dextrose in water per day. The electrocardiogram must be monitored frequently for peaking of the T wave, which would suggest hyperkalemia, and serial blood samples should be withdrawn to determine the serum potassium level.

When ectopic impulses occur frequently or continuously as a result of digitalis intoxication, antiarrhythmic therapy may be advisable. The cessation of digitalis therapy is usually sufficient, but if the arrhythmia persists and the dog seems to be in danger of fibrillation, lidocaine or a *beta* blocking agent (propranolol) is indicated (see pp. 245-246 and 266-267).

Ventricular arrhythmias due to digitalis intoxication should not be treated with direct current cardioversion, because this is likely to induce ventricular fibrillation or cardiac standstill in the dog (Katz and Zitnik, 1966).

References

Blaine, D.: Canine Pathology. A Description of the Diseases of Dogs. 4th ed. Longmans, Orme, and Co., London. 1841.

Bloodwell, R. D., Goldberg, L. I., Braunwald, E., Gilbert, J. W., Ross, J., and Morrow, A. G.: Myocardial Contractility in Man. Surg. Forum, 10 (1960):532.

Braunwald, E., and Pool, P. E.: Mechanism of Action of Digitalis Glycosides. (I and II). Mod. Conc. Cardiovasc. Dis., 37 (1968):129.

Detweiler, D. K.: Cardiac Glycosides in the Treatment of Congestive Heart Failure in Dogs. Anim. Hosp., 1 (1965):29.

Doherty, J. E., Perkins, W. H., Gammil, J., Sherwood, J., and Dodd, C.: Tissue Concentration and Turnover of Tritiated Digoxin in Dogs. Amer. J. Cardiol., 17 (1966):47.

Estes, J. W., and White, P. D.: William Withering and the Purple Fox Glove. Sci. Amer., 212 (June, 1965):110.

Ettinger, S.: Therapeutic Digitalization of the Dog in Congestive Heart Failure. J. A. V. M. A., 148 (1966):525.

Ettinger, S., Gould, L., Carmichael, J. A., and Tashjian, R. J.: Phentolamine: Use in Digitalis-Induced Arrhythmias. Amer. Heart J., 77 (1969):636.

Gould, L., Ettinger, S., and Lyon, A.: Pharmacodynamics of Digitalis Glycosides in Heart Failure in Man and Dog. Angiology, (in press) 1970.

Hamlin, R. L.: Ventricular Premature Beats. In *Current Veterinary Therapy 1966-1967*. Edited by R. W. Kirk. W. B. Saunders Co., Philadelphia. (1966):78.

Katz, M. J., and Zitnik, R. S.: Direct Current Shock and Lidocaine in the Treatment of Digitalis-Induced Ventricular Tachycardia. Amer. J. Cardiol., 18 (1966):552.

Lyon, A., and DeGraff, A.: The Neurotoxic Effects of Digitalis. Amer. Heart J., 65 (1963): 839.

Mendez, C., Aceves, J., and Mendez, R.: Inhibition of Adrenergic Cardiac Acceleration by Cardiac Glycosides. J. Pharmacol. Exp. Ther., 131 (1961):191.

Moe, G. K., and Farah, A. E.: Digitalis and Allied Cardiac Glycosides. In *The Pharmacological Basis of Therapeutics*. Edited by L. S. Goodman and A. Gilman. 3rd ed. The Macmillan Co., New York. (1965):665.

Nadeau, R. A., and James, T. A.: Antagonistic Effects on the Sinus Node of Acetyl Strophanthidin and Adrenergic Stimulation. Circ. Res., 13 (1963):388.

Ogden, P. C., Selzer, A., and Cohen, K. E.: The Relationship Between the Inotropic and Dromotropic Effects of Digitalis: The Modulation of these Effects by Autonomic Influences. Amer. Heart. J., 77 (1969):628.

Rubin, I. L., Gross, H., and Arbeit, S. R.: Treatment of Heart Disease in the Adult. Lea & Febiger, Philadelphia. 1968.

Wallace, C. R., and Hamilton, W. F.: Study of Spontaneous Congestive Heart Failure in the Dog. Circ. Res., 11 (1962):301.

Withering, W.: An Account of the Foxglove and Some of Its Medical Uses. 1785. Reprinted in part in *Classics of Cardiology: A Collection of Classic Works on the Heart and Circulation*. Vol. 1. Edited by F. Willius and T. E. Keys. Henry Schuman, Inc., Dover Publications, Inc., New York. (1941).

CHAPTER

8

ANTIARRHYTHMIC THERAPY

QUINIDINE

PHARMACOLOGY

Quinidine is the dextroisomer of quinine. Its major pharmacologic effects are:

1. Depression of myocardial contractility (negative inotrope).
2. Depression of myocardial excitability.
3. Depression of velocity of conduction.
4. Prolongation of the effective refractory period of cardiac muscle and cardiac conduction fibers.
5. Depression of spontaneous discharge of pacemaker tissue.
6. Anticholinergic and antivagal effects.
7. Vasodilation of peripheral arteries and decreased blood pressure.

The depression of myocardial excitability following quinidine administration provides a partial explanation of the drug's ability to abolish or depress formation of ectopic impulses. In addition, the velocity of conduction is uniformly decreased, and this in turn is responsible for prolongation of both the P-R interval and the QRS complex.

Because quinidine causes prolongation of the effective refractory period of cardiac fibers, there is a longer period of time than normal during which the cardiac fibers cannot be excited by an electrical impulse. This important feature effectively abolishes a considerable amount of ectopic activity resulting from repetitive electrical stimulation.

By decreasing the slope of the curve of slow diastolic depolarization (see p. 105), quinidine also reduces the frequency of spontaneous discharge of pacemaker tissue.

239

The antivagal and anticholinergic effects of quinidine prevent cardiac slowing. Thus, despite its general depressant effects on the heart, administration of the drug in therapeutic dosages is likely to result in an increased heart rate. It is likely that the decrease in arterial blood pressure is also partially responsible for the increase in heart rate. After high doses of quinidine are administered, cardiac contractility is markedly decreased, and the previous increase in heart rate is followed by depression of heart rate, conduction, and excitability. Sinoatrial block and prolongation of the Q-T interval and QRS complex then occur. Prolongation of the QRS complex over 25 per cent is considered to be a sign suggesting that toxic levels of quinidine have been administered.

INDICATIONS FOR QUINIDINE THERAPY

Ventricular premature contractions. Ventricular premature contractions are usually a sign of serious cardiac disease (see pp. 280–283). Oral preparations of quinidine are useful if ventricular premature contractions are frequent. When ventricular premature contractions are due to a failing myocardium in a dog that has not been digitalized, digitalis is indicated to treat the arrhythmia; quinidine is withheld because it further depresses contractility. If ventricular premature contractions of nondigitalis origin develop while a dog is receiving cardiac glycosides, quinidine therapy is indicated. Ectopic impulses caused by digitalis intoxication are not usually treated with quinidine preparations (see pp. 237–238).

Ventricular tachycardia. Persistent ventricular tachycardia is a life-threatening arrhythmia that requires intensive therapy. Because intramuscular quinidine requires 30 to 90 minutes before its effect is fully realized, it is not the preferred therapeutic agent. Other therapeutic agents such as lidocaine, procainamide, or direct current cardioversion are preferred. Intramuscular or oral quinidine may be administered at the same time as intravenous lidocaine. The lidocaine temporarily controls the arrhythmia while allowing sufficient time for the quinidine to be effective.

In situations that are not acute, quinidine is employed alone until the desired effect is achieved. In most cases, it is necessary to maintain quinidine therapy for four to six weeks following abolition of the arrhythmia. The electrocardiogram should be recorded periodically after therapy has been discontinued.

Atrial fibrillation. Quinidine is often effective in converting atrial fibrillation to normal sinus rhythm and then in maintaining sinus rhythm in man. However, in veterinary medicine there has not been a high degree of success in converting atrial fibrillation to sinus rhythm with quinidine-type drugs (Detweiler, 1957; Pyle, 1967; Detweiler et al., 1968). Quinidine abolishes atrial fibrillation by decreasing vagal activity and increasing the mean refractory period of the atria, thus reducing the number of atrial wavelets possible (Moe, Rheinboldt, and Abildskov, 1964). Control of the rapid ventricular rate with digitalis prior to attempts at conversion using quinidine is essential. The dose of quinidine should be increased until the desired effect is achieved or until intoxication occurs (see Administration, p. 241). The drug should be discontinued if ventricular premature contractions develop or if the QRS complex is prolonged by more than 25 per cent. In one report, quinidine was administered to nine dogs in atrial fibrillation (Detweiler, 1957); normal sinus rhythm was reestablished in one dog, and transient atrial flutter resulted in two. Figure 11-23 demonstrates the conversion of atrial fibrillation to a sinus rhythm after the oral administration of quinidine.

Other arrhythmias.   Quinidine is sometimes effective for treating paroxysmal supraventricular tachycardia if other methods such as digitalization or carotid sinus pressure fail. Quinidine may be used after digitalization to convert and control atrial flutter, an unusual arrhythmia in the dog.

CONTRAINDICATIONS

Absolute contraindications to quinidine therapy are previous idiosyncratic reactions to the drug and complete atrioventricular block. Quinidine should be used with caution in incomplete atrioventricular block because it may increase the degree of heart block. In congestive heart failure, the indications for its use must be carefully evaluated, because the impaired cardiac contractility would be diminished even more. Quinidine is not the drug of choice to treat arrhythmias of digitalis intoxication, although it may be safely administered along with digitalis (Brandfonbrener, Kjobech, and Cooper, 1968) if there are no signs of digitalis intoxication.

PREPARATIONS AVAILABLE

Quinidine sulfate, U.S.P., is available as tablets or capsules (0.2 Gm. [3 gr.]). It is also available in long-acting tablets (equivalent to 3 gr., Cardioquin, brand of quinidine polygalacturonate; and equivalent to 5 gr., Quinaglute, brand of quinidine gluconate) and in parenteral dosage as quinidine gluconate, injection, U.S.P. 80 mg./cc.).

ABSORPTION AND EXCRETION

Quinidine is completely absorbed from the gastrointestinal tract. Its effect is maximal in one to three hours and persists for six to eight hours. To obtain a cumulative effect it must be administered every two to four hours. When given intramuscularly, the peak effect is reached in 30 to 90 minutes. Quinidine is excreted in the urine within 24 hours (Moe and Abildskov, 1965).

ADMINISTRATION

As is true for the cardiac glycosides, *there is no fixed dosage for quinidine preparations*. Clinical experience suggests that high dosages are necessary if results are to be favorable. Experimental canine studies show that 5 to 10 mg./kg. must be administered to prolong the effective refractory period significantly. At 10 mg./kg. in the dog, a dose greater than that used in man, the threshold of electrical excitability of cardiac tissue is not markedly increased (Moe and Abildskov, 1965).

We have had the best results with quinidine sulfate when 3 to 10 mg./lb. is administered by the oral or intramuscular route.

Oral administration.   The initial oral dosage of quinidine, usually near the lower end of the approximate dosage range of 3 to 10 mg./lb., is followed by a second dose from two to eight hours later, depending upon the urgency of the arrhythmia. When the need is acute, the second and later doses are given every two hours for four or five dosages in order to achieve a cumulative effect. If the arrhythmia persists and intoxication has not occurred, the dosage rate is increased the following day, again giving the drug every two hours for four or five dosages. This schedule is continued until conversion occurs or toxic levels have been administered. After the arrhythmia has been abolished, maintenance dosages are administered. When the urgency is not great, the drug is given every six to eight hours, and the dosage is increased until the desired effect is achieved or until intoxication develops.

Intramuscular administration.   The initial dosage of quinidine is followed by similar doses every two to four hours until the arrhythmia is converted or until signs of intoxication develop. After conversion, oral or intramuscular maintenance therapy is initiated.

Maintenance therapy.   After oral or parenteral therapy has abolished the arrhythmia, quinidine is administered at maintenance levels, usually between 3 and 10 mg./lb., every six to eight hours. In order to reduce the frequency of administration, the long-acting quinidine preparations may be administered every eight to 12 hours, depending on the requirements of the individual dog. The dog should be maintained on quinidine, usually for a minimum of four weeks, and in some cases there is need for permanent maintenance therapy.

SIGNS OF INTOXICATION

Cinchonism is the term for toxic reactions resulting from overdoses of drugs such as quinidine and quinine derived from cinchona bark. Early toxic manifestations of quinidine are usually gastrointestinal and include vomiting and diarrhea. Detweiler (1957) has reported depression, incoordination, and convulsions after the administration of quinidine.

At high dosages, quinidine may produce prolongation of the P-R and Q-T intervals and P wave, as well as changes in the S-T segment of the electrocardiogram. However, the drug need not be discontinued when these electrocardiographic changes occur. When further changes develop, such as prolongation of the QRS complex by 25 per cent or more, the drug should be discontinued lest atrioventricular block, atrial standstill, ventricular tachycardia, or fibrillation result. There is no specific antidote for overdoses of quinidine other than discontinuing the drug and administering symptomatic medical therapy.

If toxic reactions occur when quinidine (or procainamide) alone is used, lower doses of combined quinidine and procainamide may be effective (see Fig. 14-5).

PROCAINAMIDE

After it was shown that procaine elevates the threshold of ventricular muscle to electrical stimulation, efforts were made to develop a similar but longer-acting drug. Procainamide is such a drug; it differs from procaine only in that an amide structure ($-CO \cdot NH-$) has replaced an ester linkage ($-CO \cdot O-$) (Moe and Abildskov, 1965). Chemically, procainamide is p-amino-N(2-diethylaminoethyl) benzamide.

PHARMACOLOGY

The effects of procainamide on the cardiovascular system are similar to those of quinidine. It depresses excitability and slows conduction in the atria and ventricles. At therapeutic levels, cardiac contractility is depressed to a lesser extent than it is with quinidine. As with quinidine, the antivagal and anticholinergic effects of procainamide may produce an increase in the heart rate. When high doses of procainamide are administered, the electrocardiogram indicates prolongation of the QRS complex and P-R and Q-T intervals. Procainamide usually has little effect on blood pressure when administered orally or intramuscularly, but hypotension owing to peripheral vasodilatation may develop when it is administered intravenously.

INDICATIONS

Procainamide, like quinidine, is used to eliminate ventricular premature contractions and ventricular tachycardia. Since ventricular tachycardia is abolished within minutes after intravenous administration of procainamide and within an hour after oral or intramuscular administration, this drug is preferred to quinidine for treating this arrhythmia. The drug is occasionally effective in abolishing digitalis-induced arrhythmias; however, rarely, it may produce ventricular asystole or fibrillation, and newer modalities such as *beta*-adrenergic blocking agents or lidocaine are preferred for the treatment of digitalis-induced ventricular arrhythmias. Procainamide is of limited benefit in treating atrial tachycardia.

CONTRAINDICATIONS

The drug is contraindicated and must be discontinued when complete heart block, prolongation of the QRS complex, or anorexia, nausea, and vomiting develop. Hypotension should be corrected prior to administration of parenteral procainamide, and frequent monitoring is necessary to guard against its development while the drug is being given intravenously. In the presence of atrial fibrillation, the ventricular rate may increase markedly because of the antivagal effects of the medication; therefore previous digitalization to control the ventricular rate is advised.

PREPARATIONS AVAILABLE

Procainamide hydrochloride capsules, U.S.P. (Pronestyl, 250-mg. and 500-mg. capsules), and procainamide hydrochloride injection, U.S.P. (Pronestyl, in 10-ml. vials of 100 mg./ml.), are available for clinical use.

ABSORPTION AND EXCRETION

Procainamide is completely and rapidly absorbed from the gastrointestinal tract, and maximal plasma concentration results in one hour. After intramuscular administration, maximal plasma levels are attained within 15 minutes to one hour. The drug is effective within minutes after intravenous administration. Since plasma levels diminish rapidly, the drug must be administered every four to six hours. Procainamide is excreted primarily by the kidneys and must therefore be used cautiously in dogs with impaired renal function.

ADMINISTRATION

Procainamide may be administered orally, intramuscularly, or intravenously, and the immediate requirements of each dog should be considered in determining the route of administration. Oral forms are not immediately effective but have the marked advantage of increased safety, whereas intravenous forms act rapidly but are more likely to have serious toxic effects than oral forms. Since clinical experience with procainamide is limited, the dosages recommended are based on comparable human dosages which have been used in a limited number of cases.

The human patient is usually given 250 to 500 mg. orally every four to six hours initially, the dosage being increased if the arrhythmia is not abolished. Similar dosages have been used in medium-sized dogs by the authors. In smaller breeds the dosage is initially 125 mg. (approximately half the contents of the 250-mg. capsule); it is increased if the arrhythmia persists and if clinical and electrocardiographic signs of intoxication are absent. Following conversion of the arrhythmia with procainamide, oral maintenance therapy every four to six hours is required.

When a more rapid effect is needed, an intramuscular dosage of 250 to 500 mg. is administered every two hours until the arrhythmia is converted or until intoxication develops. Then an oral maintenance dosage based on the amount of total parenteral procainamide required is administered every four to six hours.

Intravenous therapy should be used only to treat ventricular tachycardia, when ventricular fibrillation seems imminent. Huisman and Teunissen (1963) recommended that procainamide be administered to dogs with ventricular tachycardia at the rate of 100 mg./min., with continuous electrocardiographic monitoring, until conversion or until intoxication develops. Because it is difficult to monitor arterial blood pressure clinically, the dog should be observed carefully for signs of hypotension such as a diminished pulse size and mucous membranes that blanch and fail to return to normal color. Vasopressors such as norepinephrine should be available for immediate intravenous infusion if persistent hypotension develops. In some cases, norepinephrine may be administered simultaneously to combat the effect of hypotension resulting from peripheral vasodilatation and diminished cardiac contractility. After conversion, oral maintenance doses are administered every four to six hours.

SIGNS OF INTOXICATION

Toxic reactions from procainamide are like those of quinidine; the most important are anorexia and vomiting and prolongation of the QRS complex and P-R and Q-T intervals on the electrocardiogram. Ectopic impulses may also be induced. Hypotension is a major toxic reaction to intravenous overdoses of procainamide; when it is present the infusion must be discontinued immediately and corrective therapy instituted. The only specific therapy required for other toxic manifestations is immediate discontinuation of the drug.

LIDOCAINE

PHARMACOLOGY

Lidocaine has been used widely for the management of ventricular arrhythmias because it decreases ventricular excitability and conductivity. Lidocaine, in therapeutic dosages, does not affect myocardial contractility, systemic arterial blood pressure, or the absolute refractory period significantly (Harrison, Sprouse, and Morrow, 1963), although there are some transient depressant effects on these parameters (Constantino, Crockett, and Vasko, 1967). Chemically, lidocaine is diethylaminoacet-2,6-xylidide.

INDICATIONS AND CONTRAINDICATIONS

The drug is effective in controlling ventricular arrhythmias but not atrial arrhythmias. It is useful in treating acute ventricular arrhythmias associated with cardiac surgery, cardiac catheterization, and angiocardiography as well as ventricular arrhythmias resulting from cardiac diseases and digitalis intoxication. It is contraindicated in severe sinoatrial, atrioventricular, and intraventricular block. Excessive prolongation of the P-R interval, the QRS complex, or both necessitates that lidocaine therapy be discontinued.

PREPARATIONS AVAILABLE

Lidocaine is available in many strengths and is often combined with other chemical agents for use as a local anesthetic. For use in cardiology, the intravenous form of lidocaine in 2 per cent solution (Xylocaine *without* epinephrine) is available. It is prepared in 2-cc. and 50-cc. multiple dose vials with 20 mg./cc.

ABSORPTION AND EXCRETION

Lidocaine is a drug with a short duration of activity; it is cleared from the blood stream within 20 minutes. Approximately 90 per cent is metabolized by the liver and is excreted in the urine as free and conjugated phenols. The remaining 10 per cent is excreted by the kidney in unchanged form. For the treatment of ventricular arrhythmias, lidocaine is administered only intravenously because it acts and is metabolized so rapidly.

ADMINISTRATION

The usual dosage of lidocaine is 2 to 4 mg./lb. intravenously over one to two minutes. Continuous electrocardiographic monitoring is essential when lidocaine therapy is undertaken. The duration of its effect may be from ten to 20 minutes, and the drug may be administered every 20 minutes as necessary. The cardiac depressant effect of the drug is less when it is administered intravenously over a period of one minute rather than as a single bolus. A continuous intravenous drip may be used, or it may be given in intermittent dosages intravenously every ten to 20 minutes. Lidocaine is best used in conjunction with other antiarrhythmic agents, such as quinidine, which are administered orally or intramuscularly. In this way the acute ventricular tachycardia may be controlled initially with lidocaine until the other agent takes effect.

For states of digitalis intoxication in dogs, 100 mg. of lidocaine may be given intravenously, followed by a 2 mg./cc. intravenous drip which is continued until the arrhythmia is abolished (Katz and Zitnik, 1966). Quinidine or procainamide should not be used in association with lidocaine for treating digitalis-induced ventricular tachycardia because of their longer duration of action and therefore the possibility of combined intoxication.

SIGNS OF INTOXICATION

Convulsions occur in human beings when 750 mg. of lidocaine is given within one hour, but smaller amounts of this drug have produced convulsions in the dog. If convulsions do occur, they usually subside shortly if lidocaine administration is discontinued. If necessary, ultra-short acting barbiturates may be administered intravenously to control the convulsions.

Endotracheal intubation may be necessary if respiratory arrest follows or if it becomes necessary to administer anesthetic agents if convulsions develop.

DIPHENYLHYDANTOIN

Diphenylhydantoin sodium (Dilantin), chemically 5,5-diphenylhydantoin, has proved effective in treating various arrhythmias in human patients occurring during induction of anesthesia, cardiac catheterization, cardiac surgery, and after cardioversion. The drug also controls digitalis-induced ventricular arrhythmias, but atrial and ventricular arrhythmias not resulting from digitalis intoxication are less well controlled. Diphenylhydantoin has little effect on atrial fibrillation and flutter.

In the treatment of acute arrhythmias, the intravenous route is preferred. Diphenylhydantoin usually acts within five minutes. In man, the dose for a single injection is 5 mg./kg. administered over four to five minutes. Arrhythmias not abolished at this dosage are not likely to be converted at higher doses. After conversion, 100 mg. of diphenylhydantoin is given orally or intramuscularly four times daily (Rubin, Gross, and Arbeit, 1968). Reports are not available on the clinical use of this drug in dogs.

SYNCHRONIZED DIRECT CURRENT ELECTRIC SHOCK

Cardioversion or precordial electric shock is an effective means of controlling some tachycardias. It has not replaced drugs for the treatment of these conditions but rather is often used in conjunction with drug therapy. Also, its high cost and limited applicability preclude its use in most veterinary hospitals.

Using direct current shock, the entire heart is depolarized momentarily, allowing the sinoatrial node to resume its normal pacemaking function. To be effective the shock must be of sufficient current strength, duration, and timing (except in ventricular fibrillation, in which the timing of the shock is inconsequential). On the unit pictured (Fig. 5-3), the duration (2.5 msec.) and timing of the shock (20 msec. after the R wave) are preset, requiring that only current strength be selected. Successive shocks utilizing a greater current are required if the rhythm is not converted. For ventricular fibrillation the largest possible shock (400 watt-seconds) is administered initially. Successful cardioversion of dogs in atrial fibrillation has been reported using shocks between 100 and 275 watt-seconds (Ettinger, 1968).

Cardioversion is indicated for atrial fibrillation, atrial flutter (rare in dogs), and ventricular tachycardia, as well as for supraventricular tachycardia that does not respond to the usual forms of medical therapy.

Cardioversion is contraindicated in arrhythmias resulting from digitalis, quinidine, or procainamide intoxication, because it may induce ventricular fibrillation. It is also not indicated for the treatment of either second or third degree heart block or for occasional ventricular premature contractions.

The dog is prepared for cardioversion by withholding food and water for at least 12 hours prior to shock and by discontinuing digitalis therapy at least 24 hours prior to shock, because fully digitalized dogs may be more likely to develop tachycardias or ventricular fibrillation. In dogs with atrial fibrillation or active ectopic ventricular foci, oral or parenteral quinidine therapy is recommended when possible for 24 hours prior to attempts at cardioversion; otherwise, quinidine should be administered intramuscularly 60 minutes before the shock is to be delivered.

Cardioversion is usually performed while the dog is lightly anesthetized, so that successive shocks can be administered in rapid sequence without inflicting pain.

The dog is clipped on the left and right sides of the thorax near the costochondral arch from the fourth to sixth intercostal spaces to accommodate the paddles. After the dog has been anesthetized and intubated, it is placed on a rubber-covered table in sternal recumbency, and electrocardiographic leads are attached. The clipped sites and the paddles are coated with a layer of electrode jelly, and the paddles are then held firmly against the thoracic walls. After ensuring that *all personnel are away from the table* except for the one or two people holding the paddles, the current strength of the shock is selected. Since not all electrocardiographic machines are protected from the electrical shock, the lead cable may have to be removed from the machine during cardioversion and replaced immediately after. The shock is delivered, and any current remaining in the paddles is released immediately. The electrocardiogram is monitored after the dog relaxes from the brief twitching immediately following the shock. A brief period of ventricular tachycardia often occurs (Fig. 13-22) followed by resumption of sinus rhythm. If cardioversion does not occur, more intense shocks are delivered successively until conversion occurs. If conversion is temporary, or if several high-voltage shocks fail to convert the rhythm, the procedure is discontinued and the dog is permitted to awaken.

Drug therapy following cardioversion varies according to the arrhythmia being treated. Antiarrhythmic therapy is often continued. If atrial fibrillation was the original arrhythmia digitalis is again administered to maintain the maximum positive inotropic effect and to maintain a slow ventricular rate should the arrhythmia return.

References

Brandfonbrener, M., Kjobech, C., and Cooper, E.: The Effect of Digitalization on Quinidine Toxicity. Amer. Heart J., 76 (1968):249.

Constantino, R. T., Crockett, S. E., and Vasko, J. S.: Cardiovascular Effects and Dose-Response of Lidocaine.Circulation, Suppl. to Vol. 35 and 36 (1967):89.

Detweiler, D. K.: Electrocardiographic and Clinical Features of Spontaneous Auricular Fibrillation and Flutter (Tachycardia) in Dogs. Zbl. Veterinärmed., 6 (1957):509.

Detweiler, D. K., Patterson, D. F., Luginbühl. H., Rhodes, W. H., Buchanan, J. W., Knight, D. H., and Hill, J. D.: Diseases of the Cardiovascular System. In *Canine Medicine*. Edited by E. J. Catcott. 1st Catcott ed. American Veterinary Publications, Inc., Santa Barbara, Calif. (1968):589.

Ettinger, S.: Conversion of Atrial Fibrillation Using Direct Current Synchronized Shock. J. A. V. M. A., 152 (1968):41.

Harrison, D. C., Sprouse, J. H., and Morrow, A. G.: The Antiarrhythmic Properties of Lidocaine and Procaine Amide. Clinical and Physiologic Studies of Their Cardiovascular Effects in Man. Circulation, 28 (1963):486.

Huisman, G. H., and Teunissen, G. H. B.: Paroxysmal Ventricular Tachycardia in the Dog. Zbl. Veterinärmed., 10 (1963):273.

Katz, M. J., and Zitnik, R. S.: Direct Current Shock and Lidocaine in the Treatment of Digitalis-Induced Ventricular Tachycardia. Amer. J. Cardiol., 18 (1966):552.

Moe, G. K., and Abildskov, J. A.: Antiarrhythmic Drugs. In *The Pharmacological Basis of Therapeutics*. Edited by L. S. Goodman and A. Gilman. The Macmillan Co., New York. (1965):699.

Moe, G. K., Rheinboldt, W. C., and Abildskov, J. A.: A Computer Model of Atrial Fibrillation. Amer. Heart J., 67 (1964):200.

Pyle, R. L.: Conversion of Atrial Fibrillation with Quinidine Sulfate in a Dog. J. A. V. M. A., 151 (1967):582.

Rubin, I. L., Gross, H., and Arbeit, S. R.: The Treatment of Heart Disease in the Adult. Lea & Febiger, Philadelphia, 1968.

CHAPTER

9

DIURETICS

The primary physiologic functions of the kidney are the removal of waste products and the maintenance of water, electrolyte, and acid-base balance in the body. Briefly, it should be recognized that the kidney functions to maintain water and electrolyte balance first by producing a plasma ultrafiltrate as blood passes through the glomeruli. With the exception of protein and lipids, which do not diffuse across the glomerular membrane, this ultrafiltrate has the same components as the plasma. The ultrafiltrate is then subjected to the active tubular transport of electrolytes and solutes across the cell membrane into the interstitial spaces. Passive diffusion of water and solutes into the interstitial space occurs according to the gradient established by the active transport of sodium and other electrolytes.

The vast majority of sodium cations in the ultrafiltrate, along with the anion chloride, are actively transported from the proximal convoluted tubule into the interstitial space. Water diffuses passively across the cell membrane according to the osmotic gradient established by sodium transport. Sodium and the anion chloride are also actively transported into the interstitial spaces from the loop of Henle, but water does not diffuse freely across the cell membrane at this level. When the filtrate reaches the distal convoluted tubule, sodium continues to be actively transported across the cell membrane, along with chloride.

Potassium, unlike sodium, is completely reabsorbed in the proximal tubule and is then partially secreted into the lumen of the distal tubule. Although all the factors involved in the exchange of potassium and hydrogen for sodium in the distal tubule are uncertain, it is known that both potassium and hydrogen are secreted by cells in the distal tubule, and the exchange of sodium for potassium or hydrogen depends upon the concentrations of sodium, hydrogen, and potassium, as well as on the presence of aldosterone. Aldosterone, an adrenal gland hormone, promotes the exchange of potassium for sodium in the distal tubule, resulting in the conservation of sodium.

Within the tubular cells, carbonic anhydrase catalyzes the equation:

$$CO_2 + H_2O \underset{\text{anhydrase}}{\overset{\text{carbonic}}{\rightleftharpoons}} H_2CO_3 \rightleftharpoons H^+ + HCO_3^-.$$

In the distal tubules the hydrogen ion is exchanged with the sodium ion:

$$H^+ + NaHCO_3 \rightleftharpoons Na^+ + H_2CO_3.$$

Thus sodium is conserved in the distal tubule and is returned to the interstitial fluid as $NaHCO_3$ in exchange for hydrogen. The H_2CO_3 thus produced is then available for regulation of acid-base balance in the kidney or is removed from the body as CO_2 and H_2O.

In addition to the active tubular reabsorption of sodium and other electrolytes, water and solutes diffuse across the cell membranes in response to the osmotic gradient produced by electrolyte movement. It is thus the combination of active tubular transport and passive diffusion that accounts for the reabsorption of electrolytes and water from the ultrafiltrate that passes through the glomerulus.

Renal function is altered in heart failure states; the predominant feature of the alteration is increased sodium and water retention (see Chapter 10). Sodium retention and the subsequent retention of water caused by passive diffusion result from a reduced cardiac output and the subsequent reduction in renal perfusion; also there is an increase in the level of aldosterone, which acts in the distal tubule to increase sodium reabsorption.

When heart failure develops and renal function is altered to the point that there is retention of sodium and water, diuretic agents may be helpful in removing sodium and water from the body. Since a decreased cardiac output initiates salt and water retention, cardiac glycosides should be administered initially to restore normal cardiac function. If glycosides alone are inadequate, diuretics may be added to the therapeutic regimen. The mechanism of action and modes of employment for the diuretic agents most often used for canine heart disease are the basis for the remainder of the chapter.

XANTHINE DERIVATIVES (THEOPHYLLINE AND AMINOPHYLLINE)

The major effects of the xanthine agents are stimulation of the myocardium and relaxation of bronchial smooth muscle. The force of myocardial contraction, pulse rate, and cardiac output are all increased (Ritchie, 1965). Renal blood flow is increased, resulting in an increase in the glomerular filtration rate as a result of increased cardiac output. In addition, aminophylline also appears to inhibit reabsorption of sodium in the renal tubules (Rubin, Gross, and Arbeit, 1968).

When aminophylline or theophylline is given orally, gastric irritation and vomiting, as well as hyperexcitability and tachycardia, may result. These side effects can occur at low therapeutic doses and may require discontinuation of the agent. Because intramuscular injection is associated with local pain, the lumbar muscles are the preferred site for injection. Intravenous administration is not recommended unless the infusion is given very slowly.

Theophylline, a component of a number of drugs, is used alone or in combination with other drugs (see p. 359). Theophylline elixir (80 mg./15 cc. of the elixir) may be used interchangeably with aminophylline tablets (1 tablet = 100 mg.), which are theophylline plus ethylenediamine. The latter is used to increase the absorption of theophylline. The dosage rate for the elixir preparation is 0.2 cc./lb. two to four times daily. For aminophylline tablets, the dose is $\frac{1}{4}$ to 1 tablet given two to four times daily. In the injectable form, 0.25 cc. to 2 cc. of aminophylline (250 mg./cc.) is given, depending on the size of the dog.

The primary indications for the xanthine derivatives in cardiology are cardiac asthma and the cardiac cough (see p. 359). They may also be of value in treating congestive heart failure when used in conjunction with digitalis and other diuretics.

MERCURIALS

The mercurial diuretics act by depressing the active tubular reabsorption of sodium and chloride. Water excretion accompanies the sodium excretion induced by these drugs. The mercurials are mercurated allyl derivatives [R-CH_2-$CH(OY)$-CH_2-Hg-X, where R is the organic radical, OY is a methoxy, ethoxy, or hydroxy group, and X is theophylline in meralluride]. They inhibit tubular reabsorption by liberating ionic mercury, which in turn inhibits the specific enzyme systems responsible for tubular transport of sodium and chloride. The primary site of tubular transport inhibition, according to Mudge (1965), is in the proximal convoluted tubule, but others (Vander et al., 1958; Levitt et al., 1966) suggest that the major action of the mercurial diuretics is on the distal renal tubule.

Mercurial diuretics are potentiated by acidifying salts, whereas their action may be limited in hypochloremic alkalosis. To offset the chloride deficits and the alkalosis, ammonium chloride may enhance the diuretic effect when administered prior to mercurial injection.

The mercurial diuretics are well absorbed parenterally but are incompletely absorbed from the gastrointestinal tract; therefore only injectable forms are used. This restricts the use of mercurials to hospitalized animals or to those dogs seen on an outpatient basis.

Absorption of the mercurials after parenteral administration is rapid, diuresis beginning in one to two hours and reaching its peak effect in six hours (Brest et al., 1968). The mercurials are completely excreted through the kidneys within one day. Mercury poisoning develops only when the drugs are used in dogs with renal insufficiency or with continued, frequent use of the drug. Mercurials are contraindicated in acute renal insufficiency and other uremic or oliguric states, and when there is a known hypersensitivity to mercury.

Mercurials are of great value when instituting therapy for cardiac decompensation in which rapid diuretic action is essential—i.e., when edema, pleural effusion, and ascites are present. In dogs that are unresponsive to oral diuretics, periodic parenteral administration of mercurials may help to relieve fluid retention. The mercurials may also be useful in treating fluid retention resulting from the nephrotic syndrome, glomerulonephritis, and hepatic cirrhosis or portal obstruction (Mudge, 1965).

Most parenteral forms of mercurial diuretics are either irritating or unstable.

We use meralluride (Mercuhydrin), which is available in 1-cc. or 2-cc. vials, with 30 mg. of Hg/cc. It is administered either subcutaneously or intramuscularly at the rate of 1 cc./30 lb. body weight, but using not more than 2 cc. The intravenous route may prove lethal. It may be administered once daily for the first two to three days; thereafter it is discontinued, and oral diuretics are used, or it is administered no more often than once or twice weekly.

THIAZIDES (BENZOTHIADIAZIDE DIURETICS)

The thiazide diuretics are the most commonly employed oral diuretics for treating cardiac edema because they are highly effective, they are well absorbed, and they rarely cause gastric irritation after oral administration. Thiazides are often effective over long periods, and there is little tendency to drug refractoriness. Toxic reactions are uncommon.

It is emphasized by Mudge (1965) that all thiazides have parallel dose-response curves. Thus, if given at equivalent dosages, all thiazide diuretics result in the same amount of chloride diuresis, which correlates directly with the total diuretic effect.

The thiazide diuretics act on the renal tubule to inhibit the reabsorption of sodium and chloride, and thus water, in the proximal convoluted tubule (Mudge, 1965), although Brest et al. (1968) describe their major effect as being in the distal tubule. Sodium concentration in the distal tubule is increased because reabsorption does not occur in the proximal tubule. Marked potassium diuresis occurs when additional sodium is then available in the distal tubule, favoring sodium reabsorption and potassium excretion. The site of action of the thiazides seems to differ from that of the mercurial agents, so that the combination of mercurials and thiazides may result in more intensive diuresis than that resulting when either agent is used alone. Part of the effect of thiazide diuresis is due to the activity of thiazide as a relatively weak carbonic anhydrase inhibitor (see pp. 255–256).

Owing to the exchange of sodium for potassium induced by the thiazide diuretics, marked electrolyte imbalances, resulting in hypokalemia and dilutional

TABLE 9-1 POTASSIUM SUPPLEMENTATION BY FOOD*

FOODS	PORTION SIZE	POTASSIUM (mg.)	SODIUM (mg.)
Fruits			
Grapefruit, raw	1 cup, sections	386	1.0
Oranges	1 medium-sized	366	0.6
Apricots, raw	3 apricots	502	0.7
Bananas	1 medium-sized	630	0.8
Cherries, all types, raw	1 cup, pitted	400	1.5
Dates, dried	1 cup. pitted	1398	1.8
Nuts			
Brazil nuts, shelled	1 cup	938	1.4
Coconut, dried sweetened	1 cup	477	9.9
Pecans, raw	1 cup	454	3.2
Walnuts, English, raw	1 cup	450	2.0

*Modified from Rubin, I. L., et al.: Treatment of Heart Disease in the Adult, Lea & Febiger, Philadelphia, 1968.

TABLE 9-2   DOSAGES OF VARIOUS THIAZIDE DIURETICS

THIAZIDE DIURETIC	TABLET SIZE	TOTAL DAILY
Chlorthiazide		
Diuril	250 mg. and 500 mg. (pediatric syrup has 250 mg./5 cc.)	10 to 20 mg./lb.
Hydrochlorthiazide		
Hydrodiuril		
Oretic	25 mg. and 50 mg.	1 to 2 mg./lb.
Esidrex		
Benzydroflumethiazide		
Naturetin	2.5 mg. and 5 mg.	0.1 to 0.2 mg./lb.
Benuron		

hyponatremia, may occur. Hyponatremia is usually not as serious a problem with thiazides as it is with the mercurials and other more potent diuretics. On the other hand, hypokalemia can induce digitalis intoxication. Cardiac arrhythmias develop when digitalized dogs develop hypokalemia after thiazide therapy. If hypokalemia develops (see Chapter 7), potassium preparations, such as Kay Ciel, Kaon, and Potassium Triplex, or potassium-rich foods that the dog will eat (Table 9-1) should be administered simultaneously with the thiazide. Aldosterone-inhibiting agents such as spironolactone (see p. 255) may spare potassium and can also be used in conjunction with the thiazides when potassium loss is a problem. Enteric-coated combinations of potassium chloride and thiazides are sometimes associated with the development of small bowel ulcerations in man and are not generally recommended for use.

Thiazide diuretics are well absorbed after oral administration. Diuresis begins within one hour and persists for 12 to 24 hours (Brest et al., 1968). Thiazides are initially administered twice daily, and when satisfactory results have been achieved the frequency may be reduced to once daily, using approximately half the original daily dosage (Table 9-2). When possible, occasional thiazide-free days are recommended to assure maintenance of normal potassium levels in the body.

Although some thiazides are available in injectable form, they offer no particular advantage. Thiazides are effective in the doses recommended but have no additional diuretic effect and may result in further electrolyte imbalances when these levels are surpassed.

FUROSEMIDE (LASIX)

Furosemide is an anthranilic acid derivative indicated for edema resulting from cardiac, pulmonary, hepatic, and renal insufficiency. It is especially useful in pulmonary edema because it is effective rapidly. It may also be used when a dog has become refractory to the thiazide and mercurial diuretics.

Furosemide inhibits sodium reabsorption in the proximal and distal convoluted tubules as well as in the loop of Henle. Because the effect of furosemide on the distal tubule does not interfere with aldosterone or carbonic anhydrase inhibitors, these agents may be used concurrently. Furosemide is effective even if glomerular filtration is reduced, a fact that makes it an effective agent in conditions associated with reduced renal flow.

Hypokalemia is reported to be minimal after the administration of furosemide (Becker, Zuschek, and Smith, 1967). Nevertheless, frequent blood electrolyte determinations and serial electrocardiograms are recommended when furosemide is to be used on a long-term basis. Overdoses of the drug may produce marked dehydration and sodium, hydrogen, and chloride depletion, as well as the clinical signs referable to hypokalemia. The occurrence of electrolyte depletion following furosemide therapy is frequent enough to warrant caution when using this drug. This fact does not alter the indications for this agent; rather it suggests the need to be observant for such a possibility.

After intravenous administration of furosemide, diuresis begins within five minutes (slightly longer after intramuscular administration), is maximal within 30 minutes, and persists for two hours. Diuresis begins within one hour after oral administration, the peak response occurs at two hours, and diuresis is complete in six to eight hours.

In the oral form, the dosage rate used by the authors is 1 to 2 mg./lb./dose, given one to three times daily; however, no more than 120 mg./dose is administered regardless of the dog's size. Owing to the potency of furosemide, intermittent rather than continuous therapy is recommended whenever possible. Injectable forms should be reserved for emergency use or when oral treatment is difficult. Parenterally, a dose of 5 to 40 mg. (depending on the size of the dog) is used initially and may be repeated in two hours. If diuresis is inadequate, the dosage is increased until an effective level is reached; then the drug is administered two to three times daily. Simultaneous digitalization and other forms of therapy may be required to treat heart failure.

Because of the rapid effect of furosemide, it is recommended that the drug be given early in the evening so that the dog may urinate prior to the time the owner retires.

One report (Becker, Zuschek, and Smith, 1967) stated that the effective diuretic dosage range of furosemide is from 2.5 to 50 mg./kg. in the dog. Since these figures were obtained from normal dogs rather than from dogs in congestive heart failure, the use of the drug at this high level is not recommended. The drug is packaged for parenteral administration in man in 2-cc. vials containing 10 mg./cc.; it is also available for veterinary use in a concentration of 50 mg./cc., or five times that used in man. Severe electrolyte depletion may result from injudicious use of this product.

ETHACRYNIC ACID (EDECRIN)

Ethacrynic acid is methylene butyryl phenoxyacetic acid. The drug differs chemically from furosemide, but its therapeutic effects are similar; that is, it induces a profound diuresis by affecting sodium and chloride reabsorption in the convoluted tubules and the loop of Henle. Following its use, potassium loss is likely to be marked, as is the development of alkalosis resulting from increased hydrogen loss.

The indications for ethacrynic acid are the same as those for furosemide. Hypokalemia, hypochloremia, and alkalosis are serious side effects, and hypokalemia may induce digitalis intoxication. The speed of action after oral or intra-venous administration is similar to that of furosemide. The dosage schedule for the dog is not known, and the authors have not had any clinical experience with the drug. It is available in 25- and 50-mg. tablets and in lyophilized vials containing 50 mg. of ethacrynic acid, to which 50 cc. of 5 per cent dextrose injection or sodium chloride injection is added prior to injection for reconstitution. Fifty to 200 mg./day orally and 0.5 to 1.0 mg./kg. intravenously are the usual dosage rates in man.

ALDOSTERONE-INHIBITING AGENTS (SPIRONOLACTONES)

Chemical agents that compete with aldosterone, the mineralocorticoid secreted by the adrenal cortex, exert a diuretic effect by inhibiting sodium retention in the distal tubules. Stop flow experiments have demonstrated that spironolactone, a synthetic steroid, is an effective antagonist to the adrenal steroid aldosterone in the distal renal tubules (Vander, Wilde, and Malvin, 1960). In addition to their mild diuretic effect resulting from sodium excretion, the spirono-lactones prevent potassium loss from the distal renal tubules.

Spironolactones are indicated for treatment of edema caused by primary hyperaldosteronism as well as for congestive heart failure states in which aldo-sterone secretion is excessive.

Because diuresis is limited and because three to five days are required to achieve the diuretic effect, the spironolactones are not useful as primary diuretic agents in treating congestive heart failure. However, because of their potassium-sparing effect, they may be used to offset the potassium loss that occurs when thiazides are administered alone.

Spironolactone tablets (25 mg.; Aldactone) are rarely used alone because a more suitable combination of 25 mg. of spironolactone and 25 mg. of hydrochlor-thiazide is available (Aldactazide). This combination is used at the rate normally used for hydrochlorthiazide, 1 to 2 mg./lb./day. It should be administered fre-quently, and when possible it is divided into four equal doses daily. Because the cost of the spironolactones is high, their use is not widespread. Because of the potassium-sparing effect of the spironolactones, hyperkalemic states may be de-tected by taking serial electrocardiograms and blood electrolyte determinations.

CARBONIC ANHYDRASE INHIBITORS (ACETAZOLAMIDE)

Although the carbonic anhydrase-inhibiting agents provide satisfactory diuresis, they are rarely indicated in treating congestive heart failure. They have an undesirable side effect, the development of metabolic acidosis, and the degree of diuresis achieved is no better and possibly less adequate than that obtained using the safer thiazides.

Carbonic anhydrase inhibitors prevent the formation of carbonic acid in the tubule cells and thus prevent dissociation of carbonic acid to hydrogen and bicarbonate. Since hydrogen is not available for exchange with sodium, the sodium is excreted, as is potassium, which is normally exchanged for hydrogen. The sodium and potassium lost carry water with them, thus resulting in an alkaline diuresis.

Acetazolamide (Diamox), available in 250-mg. tablets, is the carbonic anhydrase-inhibiting agent used in man when such an agent is indicated. The dose for dogs is 5 mg./lb. every six hours (Kirk and Bistner, 1969).

References

Becker, W., Zuschek, F., and Smith, G. B.: Report on a New Diuretic-Saluretic Agent — Furosemide. Vet. Med., 62 (1967):760.

Brest, A. N., Seller, R., Onesti, G., Ramirez, O., Swartz, C., and Moyer, J. H.: Clinical Selection of Diuretic Drugs in the Management of Cardiac Edema. Amer. J. Cardiol., 22 (1968):168.

Kirk, R. W., and Bistner, S. I.: Handbook of Veterinary Procedures and Emergency Treatment. W. B. Saunders Co., Philadelphia. 1969.

Levitt, M. F., Goldstein, M. H., Lenz, P. R., and Wedeen, R.: Mercurial Diuretics. Ann. New York. Acad. Sci., 139 (1966):375.

Mudge, G. H.: Diuretics and Other Agents Employed in the Mobilization of Edema Fluid. In *The Pharmacological Basis of Therapeutics*. Edited by L. S. Goodman and A. Gilman. The Macmillan Co., New York. (1965):827.

Ritchie, J. M.: Central Nervous System Stimulants. In *The Pharmacological Basis of Therapeutics*. Edited by L. S. Goodman and A. Gilman. The Macmillan Co., New York. (1965):354.

Rubin, I. L., Gross, H., and Arbeit, S. R.: Treatment of Heart Disease in the Adult. Lea & Febiger, Philadelphia. 1968.

Vander, A. J., Malvin, R. L., Wilde, W. S., and Sullivan, L. P.: Localization of the Site of Action of Mercurial Diuretics by the Stop Flow Technique. Amer. J. Physiol., 195 (1958):558.

Vander, A. J., Wilde, W. S., and Malvin, R. L.: Stop Flow Analysis of Aldosterone and Steroidal Antagonist SC-8109 on Renal Tubular Sodium Kinetics. Proc. Soc. Exp. Biol. Med., 103 (1960):525.

10

LOW SODIUM DIETS AND OTHER DRUGS AND METHODS INDICATED IN CARDIAC THERAPY

LOW SODIUM DIETS

Normal dogs can tolerate the ingestion of large quantities of sodium and water, but dogs with severe heart disease may develop heart failure shortly after being given a salt load. In contrast to the normal dog, these animals are unable to excrete sodium and instead retain fluid, thereby increasing blood and extracellular fluid volumes. Fluid retention is therefore secondary to abnormal sodium retention. Although plasma sodium concentrations are normal or low in dogs in heart failure, total body sodium content is increased.

To explain the sodium retention that occurs with heart failure, Friedberg (1966) reviewed the four most likely mechanisms:

1. Elevation of renal venous pressure.
2. Diminished renal blood flow and renal vasoconstriction.
3. Diminished glomerular filtration and increased filtration fraction.
4. Increased tubular reabsorption of sodium.

Increased renal venous pressures result in decreased sodium and water excretion. The passive congestion of the kidney that develops in congestive heart failure as the venous pressures become elevated may be partially responsible for the sodium retention that occurs. Although it is unlikely that this elevated pressure is the only cause for sodium retention, it seems to contribute to the electrolyte imbalance associated with cardiac disease. Diminished renal blood flow

257

and renal vasoconstriction result directly from decreased cardiac output and the compensatory generalized vasoconstriction responsible for diversion of blood to the most vital organs. The decreased renal blood flow does not result directly in sodium retention; instead, the decreased glomerular filtration rate, increased tubular reabsorption, or both would be the primary mechanism.

It is likely that decreased sodium excretion is a complex interaction between a reduced glomerular filtration rate and a normal to increased rate of tubular reabsorption of sodium. Barger, Rudolph, and Yates (1954) demonstrated that increased tubular reabsorption of sodium and water is the most significant factor in diminished sodium excretion in experimentally induced heart failure in dogs.

One of the major factors influencing increased tubular reabsorption of sodium and water secondary to congestive heart failure is the increased secretion of aldosterone, a hormonal agent produced in the zona glomerulosa of the adrenal cortex. Aldosterone promotes the reabsorption of both sodium and water while increasing the excretion of potassium and hydrogen. Aldosterone levels have been reported as elevated in dogs in spontaneous congestive heart failure as compared with normal dogs (Bojs and Conn, 1965). The increased secretion of aldosterone from the adrenal cortex is related to the renin-angiotensin system, in which the enzyme renin is liberated by the juxtaglomerular cells of the kidney in response to decreased blood volume, decreased renal perfusion pressure, and depletion of salt levels. Renin then acts on angiotensinogen to produce angiotensin I, which is converted in the blood to angiotensin II. The latter, in turn, stimulates the adrenal cortex to secrete aldosterone.

It is considered by some that it is the insufficient cardiac output in congestive heart failure that initiates sodium and water retention (Friedberg, 1966; Genest et al., 1968).

Hamlin, Smith, and Ross (1967) have demonstrated that normal dogs fed a sodium load after a salt-free period excreted nearly all of it within 24 hours. In comparison, dogs with subjective signs of congestive heart failure had after seven days excreted none of a sodium load administered. Another group of dogs not in heart failure but with congenital heart disease or heartworm disease excreted sodium at lower than normal rates from the first to the fifth day and then at maximal rates from the fifth to the seventh day after being fed a salt load. Hamlin, Smith, and Ross (1967) stated that this method is not specific for detecting heart failure but that it may be used in diagnosing hyperaldosteronism, because salt loading when heart failure is not present tests the system's ability to stop secretion of aldosterone. Wallace and Hamilton (1962) have shown that, in normal

TABLE 10-1   APPROXIMATE CALORIC AND SODIUM CONTENT FOR A
CANINE "CARDIAC" DIET*

SIZE DOG	TOTAL CALORIES	TOTAL SODIUM
5 lb.	200	30 mg.
10 lb.	400	60 mg.
25 lb.	875	150 mg.
50 lb.	1500	275 mg.
100 lb.	3000	450 mg.

*Data from Ettinger, S.: Friskies Res. Dig., 3 (3) (1967):1.

TABLE 10-2 SODIUM AND CALORIE CONTENT OF FOODS*

FOOD	AMOUNT	SODIUM (mg.)	CALORIES
Bread, cereals, and potatoes			
Recommended			
Potato	1 (small)	1	70
Polished rice	½ cup	1-10	360
Macaroni	1 cup	1-10	465
Puffed wheat	1 oz.	1-10	100
Spaghetti	1 cup	1-10	355
Not recommended			
Bread	1 slice	200	60
Pretzel	1	275	58
Margarine and oil			
Recommended			
Unsalted margarine	1 tsp.	0-1	50
Vegetable shortening	1 tbsp.	0-1	120
Not recommended			
Mayonnaise	1 tbsp.	60-90	110
Dairy products			
Not recommended			
Milk (regular)	1 cup	122	160
Milk (skim)	1 cup	122	90
Cream cheese	1½ oz.	100-120	160
Cottage cheese	3 oz.	200-300	90
American cheese	1 oz.	200-300	105
Butter	1 tsp.	50	50
Meats, poultry, fish			
Recommended			
Beef (Fresh)	3½ oz.	50	200
Pork (Fresh)	3½ oz.	62	275
Lamb (Fresh)	3½ oz.	84	175
Veal	3½ oz.	67	300
Chicken (no skin)			
Light meat	3½ oz.	64	180
Dark meat	3½ oz.	86	180
Turkey (no skin)			
Light meat	3½ oz.	82	230
Dark meat	3½ oz.	98	230
Not recommended			
Egg	1	70	80
Bacon	2 slices	385	95
Ham (processed)	3 oz.	940	225
Frankfurter	1	560	125
Vegetables (fresh or dietetic canned)			
Recommended			
Asparagus	½ cup	<5	20
Green beans	½ cup	<5	15
Peas	½ cup	<5	55
Green pepper	¼ cup	<5	10
Tomato	1	<5	30
Lettuce	¼ head	<5	15
Corn	½ cup	<5	70
Cucumber	½ cup	<5	<20
Fresh fruits			
Most are low in sodium and are permitted			
Desserts			
Recommended			
Sherbet	½ cup	15-25	120
Not recommended			
Gelatins	½ cup	60-85	50-80
Ice cream	½ cup	60-85	200
Puddings	½ cup	100-200	175

*Modified from Ettinger, S.: Friskies Res. Dig., 3 (3) (1967):1.

TABLE 10-3 GENERAL RULES TO OBSERVE IN PREPARING A LOW-SODIUM DIET*

1. Use NO salts in food or in cooking.
2. Milk products are generally HIGH in sodium.
3. Canned frozen and prepared foods are usually HIGH in sodium.
4. Fresh meats are generally LOW in sodium.
5. All shellfish and prepared fish are HIGH in sodium.
6. DO NOT feed these foods, since they are HIGH in sodium.
   a. Cereals—All breads and cereals are high in sodium except puffed wheat, puffed rice, macaroni, rice, oatmeal, and potatoes.
   b. Snacks—milk, ice cream, puddings, gelatin dessert, salted crackers, baking soda or baking powder products.
   c. High-sodium content meats and fish—luncheon meats, frankfurters, dried beef, sausage, sweetbreads, brains, kidney. Also clams, crabs, scallops, lobster, fish fillets. Cured meats such as ham, bacon, smoked pork, and corned beef. Canned or frozen items, unless marked "SALT FREE."
   d. Cheese and milk—all except unsalted cottage cheese or low-sodium cheddar.
   e. Fats—salted butter or margarine. Fat from salted meats.
   f. Vegetables—fresh artichokes, beets, celery, kale, spinach, chard, and turnips. All canned types, unless salt-free.
   g. Seasoning—all mixed salts.
   h. Condiments—catsup, chili sauce, soy sauce, mustard, horseradish, steak sauce, and prepared dressings.
   i. Miscellaneous—all salted nuts, potato chips, pretzels, olives, relish, pickles, molasses, brown sugar, peanut butter, candy, pudding, and glazed fruits.
   j. Special foods—baby foods, broths, and organ meats should be strictly avoided since salt is a common ingredient in these food preparations.

*Modified from Ettinger, S.: Friskies Res. Dig., 3 (3) (1967):1.

dogs, 90 per cent of the sodium ingested is excreted in the urine within 24 hours, whereas sodium excretion is greatly reduced in dogs with congestive heart failure.

Special diets, low in sodium, are helpful in maintaining sodium balance in the cardiac patient, thus preventing or reducing water retention. Such diets are indicated in all forms of congestive heart failure, regardless of the cause (Pensinger, 1964), as well as when hepatic disease results in ascites. Contraindications to low sodium diets are states of dehydration, debilitation, hyponatremia, and chronic diarrhea (Knapp, 1965). Commercial low sodium diets are preferred because of their balanced nutritional composition but are often refused by the dog. If the dog accepts the diet, it is important to stress to the owner that these diets be fed *without other supplementation.* The canned low sodium diet may be chopped, oven-warmed, or pan-fried without sodium seasoning to make the diet more appealing. When the dog is given snacks containing sodium in addition to the commercial diet, such diets are of little benefit to the patient and may even be harmful. To emphasize the adverse effects of such snacks, it must be recognized that only one pretzel may supply five times the daily sodium allowance of the average toy or miniature dog.

If a home-prepared diet is to be formulated for the cardiac patient, both the daily total sodium intake and the daily total caloric intake for the individual animal must be considered. The cardiac diet requires a high percentage of fat and readily available carbohydrates to supply the caloric needs, as well as protein of high biologic value. The active, older dog may require as much as 30 to 40 calories/lb. of body weight daily. The daily sodium intake per pound should not exceed 6 mg./lb. for small dogs (Table 10-1).

In formulating a low sodium diet (see Tables 10-2 and 10-3), it is best to use fresh meats such as beef or chicken, along with rice or macaroni and/or a vegetable low in sodium as the filler. The diet may be seasoned with small amounts of the following items: lemon, lime, vinegar, honey, maple syrup, onion or garlic powder, oregano, and parsley powder. Salt substitutes are permitted if renal disease is not a problem. A vitamin-mineral supplement should also be given to guarantee nutritional balance when the diet is limited and unvaried. One must be certain, however, that the supplement used does not contain appreciable amounts of sodium.

Many pet owners wish to give snacks. Commercial dog snacks should be strictly avoided because of their high sodium content. They may be replaced with low sodium fillers, such as lettuce and other vegetables listed in the tables, as well as fresh fruit. Matzos (Passover bread) flavored with unsalted margarine and low sodium dietary cookies, available in many bakery shops, are usually well accepted even by fussy dogs, as is unsalted melba toast.

NARCOTIC AGENTS

The use of narcotic agents should be considered only for the temporary treatment of acute congestive heart failure, until the full effects of digitalis and diuretics are realized.

MORPHINE

Injections of morphine may be required in the treatment of acute congestive heart failure. The mode of action of morphine is not completely understood. Vassalle (1961) reported that morphine produces a sympatho-adrenal discharge which then stimulates the *beta*-adrenergic receptors of the myocardium, thereby providing a positive inotropic effect. Morphine has a depressant effect on the respiratory center which interferes with the reflexes responsible for inducing dyspnea and hyperventilation. In addition, morphine-induced peripheral vaso-dilation reduces the load on the heart by reducing venous return. The value of morphine in eliminating restlessness and anxiety in the dog is difficult to assess, but it does provide relief. Vomiting, an unpleasant side effect of the drug, may be prevented by keeping the animal quiet and caged, because vestibular stimulation such as movement increases the frequency of emesis.

Morphine is available in 5-, 8-, 10-, 15-, and 30-mg. tablets and in injectable form prepared in concentrations of 10, 15, 20, and 30 mg./cc. In small dogs, 7.5 mg. (1/8 grain) is injected subcutaneously, and 15 mg. (1/4 grain) is used in large dogs. If vomiting is to occur, it usually does so within five to 15 minutes. Morphine may be repeated in 15 to 30 minutes if its effect is not satisfactory, using about one-half the original dosage. It is occasionally employed several times daily until signs of heart failure are relieved.

Although other narcotic agents, especially Demerol, may be administered in equivalent dosages, the authors find morphine to be the most effective clinically.

CODEINE AND CODEINE DERIVATIVES

Codeine and its derivatives are employed primarily as antitussive agents. Dihydrocodeinone (Hycodan) in tablet (5 mg.) or elixir form (5 mg./tsp.) is widely employed to relieve coughing associated with both cardiac and respiratory conditions. Although its value should not be minimized, it is probably best to attempt suppression of cardiac and respiratory coughs by proper use of digitalis, diuretics, and bronchodilating agents. If these agents are ineffective, narcotic cough suppressants may also be added to the therapeutic regimen.

Dogs react differently to dihydrocodeinone, some becoming lethargic, slow, and depressed and others having no apparent ill effects from similar doses. We use from 1.25 to 10 mg. per dose but recommend that as little as possible be administered. The frequency of administration varies from one to four times daily, again depending on need and individual reactions to the drug. Preparations containing other narcotic cough suppressants may be similarly effective.

PHLEBOTOMY AND TOURNIQUETS

Removal of 50 to 500 cc. of blood by phlebotomy can be life-saving in dogs with acute congestive heart failure and pulmonary edema by reducing both the venous return to the heart and the circulating blood volume. Phlebotomy is difficult to perform in the dog because the patient already in severe respiratory distress *must not* be forcibly restrained. If a needle with a large bore can be introduced into a jugular vein without disturbing the dog, phlebotomy may be performed. The only contraindication to phlebotomy is severe anemia, in which case the blood may be withdrawn and the packed red blood cells reinfused (Orentreich et al., 1968).

When phlebotomy is not possible, tourniquets may be applied on an alternating basis to two limbs at a time. The tourniquets are rotated every 15 to 30 minutes. The effect of the tourniquets is similar to that of phlebotomy—that is, reduction of venous return to the heart. Both phlebotomy and rotating tourniquets are, like morphine, intended for temporary use until cardiac glycosides and potent diuretics are effective.

OXYGEN

In high concentrations (over 50 per cent), oxygen often provides symptomatic relief to the dog in acute congestive heart failure. In general, it is administered by a face mask, if the dog will remain in one place for a period of time, or in oxygen cages, where temperature and humidity control should be available. Intermittent positive pressure respiration may also be of value if the dog will permit intubation and tolerate restraint. Dogs amenable to such treatment are usually preterminal and seldom survive.

When oxygen is not readily available, the use of a fan or air conditioner blowing air directly at the animal often seems to provide some relief from the signs of respiratory distress.

ANTIBIOTIC THERAPY

Because pulmonary edema and congestion provide an excellent environment for bacterial growth, bronchopulmonary infection is frequently associated with heart failure. Therefore, the use of broad-spectrum antibiotics is recommended when fever, leukocytosis, or both accompany congestive heart failure.

ABDOMINAL PARACENTESIS AND THORACOCENTESIS

Abdominal paracentesis is not usually required for the treatment of congestive heart failure. It should be reserved for use in those cases in which dyspnea develops owing to excessive abdominal pressure and in which right heart failure is intractable. Except in emergency situations, it is best to digitalize the patient and administer diuretic agents before resorting to abdominal paracentesis.

If it becomes necessary, the technique should be attempted following micturition to avoid penetrating the bladder. The skin over the linea alba just caudal to the umbilicus is clipped and prepared antiseptically for insertion of a large cannula or needle with a polyethylene catheter. The fluid should be permitted to drain slowly by gravity. A sample of fluid removed from any body cavity should be withdrawn for cellular analysis, chemical analysis, and bacteriologic culture.

In most cases, removal of fluid from the thorax is usually not necessary when pleural effusion complicates congestive heart failure. However, if dyspnea is so severe as to be life-threatening, thoracic puncture must be considered. The puncture site should be determined by radiographic examination. The fluid is ideally removed by draining it into a vacuum container. In emergencies, a large syringe with a three-way stopcock and needle will suffice. In most instances, thoracic fluid of congestive origin can be eliminated by the proper use of cardiac glycosides and diuretics.

THE BELLADONNA ALKALOIDS (ATROPINE)

Atropine reduces secretions produced in the upper and lower respiratory tracts. It also provides bronchial dilatation but does so less effectively than other available drugs. Although expiratory airway resistance decreases after administration of atropine-like drugs, bronchial secretions become viscid and difficult to remove, causing serious danger to the patient.

Atropine-like drugs inhibit salivation, secretion in the respiratory tract, and vagovagal reflexes during anesthesia and surgery. It is this feature that represents the primary indication for the use of atropine in both cardiac and noncardiac patients.

The specific use of atropine in cardiac disease is limited to the treatment of hyperactive carotid sinus reflexes and bradycardia with syncope (see pp. 302–303). The dose of atropine for sinoatrial arrest and atrioventricular block, as well as for a hyperactive carotid sinus reflex, is 0.6 to 2.0 mg. (1/100 to 1/30 gr.) subcutaneously or orally, repeated every two to four hours.

DRUGS AFFECTING THE ADRENERGIC RECEPTOR SITES

Two distinct adrenergic receptor sites, the *alpha-* and *beta-*adrenergic receptors, were proposed by Ahlquist (1948). Stimulation of the *alpha-*adrenergic receptors subserves arteriolar constriction unaccompanied by any primary cardiac action, presumably owing to the lack of *alpha* receptors in the heart. When the *beta*-adrenergic sites are stimulated, peripheral vasodilatation is accompanied by a positive inotropic and chronotropic effect, i.e., an increase in cardiac contractility and heart rate. Selective blockade of the *alpha* receptors produces arteriolar vasodilatation unaccompanied by any primary cardiac effects. In contrast, *beta*-adrenergic blockade is accompanied by a decrease in both cardiac contractility and heart rate.

Drugs that stimulate the adrenergic receptors, i.e., sympathomimetic drugs, are either catecholamines, the basic compound of which is the dihydroxybenzene ring, or noncatecholamines. The ultimate effect of the latter is to effect the release of the catecholamine norepinephrine.

The sympathetic catecholamine response causes an increase in cardiac output. It becomes available in emergency states, and its effects are of sufficient intensity and duration to play a significant role in cardiovascular performance.

ADRENERGIC AGENTS—CATECHOLAMINES

Epinephrine.   The response to epinephrine is generalized adrenergic stimulation, induced by both *alpha*- and *beta*-adrenergic activity. It causes peripheral vasoconstriction (*alpha* effect) at low doses, and vasodilatation and increased cardiac contractility and heart rate (*beta* effect) at higher doses. Epinephrine relaxes bronchial smooth muscle, an important action when it is used to treat allergic reactions. Because intracardiac or intravenous administration may produce ventricular fibrillation, the drug should be given by those routes only in acute, life-threatening emergencies.

Epinephrine is available as a 1:1000 solution for topical use, for inhalation in a 1:100 solution, and as an injectable product in 1:1000 solution.

Norepinephrine.   Norepinephrine is the chemical mediator liberated by the postganglionic adrenergic nerves. It acts primarily to stimulate the *alpha* receptors peripherally and the *beta* receptors in the heart, thus resulting in vasoconstriction and increased cardiac contractility.

Norepinephrine is available as Levophed. Because of its effect in stimulating the *alpha* receptors, norepinephrine is used frequently for the treatment of shock, diluting 4 ml. (1 ml. of 0.2 per cent solution = 1 mg. base) in 1000 ml. of dextrose and water. This is given at the rate of 2 to 4 µg./min. (0.5 to 1 cc.) until the desired effect is achieved. The drug acts for one to two minutes; therefore the degree of *alpha* stimulation is relatively easy to control and maintain. Levophed is also available in 2-ml. vials (0.02 mg. = 200 µg.) for rapid intravenous or intracardiac injection *for cardiac resuscitation only*. The lungs should be thoroughly oxygenated, and further hypotension should be prevented after treatment.

Isoproterenol.   Isoproterenol is a catecholamine that produces an exclusive *beta*-adrenergic response. The main sites of action of the drug are the heart (positive stimulation), the smooth muscle of the bronchi (relaxation), and the peripheral vasculature (dilatation). It is available for injection (Isuprel HCl, 0.2 mg./cc.), inhalation (Isuprel Mistometer, 125 µg./dose), and as sustained-action tablets (Proternol, 15-mg. and 30-mg. tablets). The sublingual forms of Isuprel are not useful in dogs (Ettinger, 1969).

ADRENERGIC AGENTS – NONCATECHOLAMINES

Amphetamine is essentially a central nervous system stimulant; it also induces peripheral *alpha-* and *beta-*adrenergic responses. Blood pressure is increased, but there is no change in cardiac output or heart rate.

Ephedrine is used to treat bronchospasm, Stokes-Adams syndrome, nasal congestion, and allergic disorders. It is also a mydriatic, a pressor agent, and a central nervous system stimulant.

Mephentermine (Wyamine), a pressor agent, produces marked cardiac stimulation, with little change, however, in cardiac output.

Metaraminol (Aramine) is used to treat hypotension.

Methamphetamine is used primarily for central nervous system stimulation and the control of hypotension.

Methoxamine (Vasoxyl) is a pure *alpha-*adrenergic stimulant, increasing blood pressure by peripheral vasoconstriction. It is used for the treatment of hypotension, paroxysmal atrial tachycardia, and congestion and has neither cardiac nor central nervous system effects.

Phenylephrine (Neo-Synephrine) is used to effect nasal decongestion, as a pressor agent, and as a mydriatic. In man, it is also used to control paroxysmal atrial tachycardia. Equipressor doses are 0.8 mg. intravenously, 5 mg. intramuscularly or subcutaneously, or 250 mg. orally.

THERAPEUTIC USES OF ADRENERGIC AGENTS

Cardiac effects. For the treatment of cardiac arrest, Stokes-Adams seizures caused by partial or complete heart block (see pp. 303–308), or ventricular standstill, certain adrenergic drugs are unparalleled. Circulation may often be restored prior to therapy by a strong precordial blow, electrical defibrillation, external cardiac massage, and/or direct stimulation of the myocardium using a needle. Epinephrine or isoproterenol may then help to maintain the cardiac rhythm and output after circulation has been restored.

Epinephrine can be given subcutaneously, intramuscularly, or intravenously. However, because it may induce ventricular fibrillation, other agents such as isoproterenol or norepinephrine are preferred.

For the treatment of cardiac standstill and cardiac arrhythmias (Ettinger, 1969), 0.1 ml. (0.02 mg.) of isoproterenol is administered directly into the heart. If the drug is to be administered by intravenous infusion, 1 mg. (5 cc.) of the drug should be diluted in 200 ml. of 5 per cent dextrose and water, equivalent to 5 μg./ml. The drug may then be administered at the approximate rate of 1 ml./min., so as to maintain a ventricular rate between 80 and 120 beats per minute. If the drug is to be administered by a single intravenous injection, an initial dose of 0.1 ml. (0.02 mg.) may be administered. For the sustained medical treatment of heart block, isoproterenol tablets (Proternol) may be used (see pp. 303–308).

When norepinephrine (Levophed) is used for cardiac arrest, it is administered directly into the heart, injecting 0.25 to 0.75 cc. of the 0.02 per cent solution.

Neither epinephrine nor isoproterenol should be used in the presence of acute heart failure because they increase the heart's oxygen requirements. The heart, already deprived of oxygen when it is failing, would be further stressed by the use of these agents.

Vascular effects. These drugs are used to control hemorrhage and congestion of mucous membranes by positive stimulation of the *alpha* receptor sites. They are used in association with local anesthetics to decrease hemorrhage and to decrease the rate of absorption of the anesthetic. They may help prevent hypotension and shock. Their purpose is to raise blood pressure and therefore provide nutrition to vital organs (Innes and Nickerson, 1965). Norepinephrine (Levophed), mephentermine (Wyamine), and metaraminol (Aramine) provide both cardiac and vascular effects; in comparison, methoxamine (Vasoxyl) and phenylephrine (Neo-Synephrine) have vascular effects only. It should be noted that the rationale of increasing blood pressure by producing peripheral vasoconstriction for the treatment of shock is not universally accepted and that regardless of chemotherapy, volume substitution remains essential.

Cardiac reflex pressor effects. These agents are used to control paroxysmal atrial and junctional tachycardias. Such tachyarrhythmias are treated with phenylephrine (Neo-Synephrine), 0.15 to 0.8 mg. intravenously, or methoxamine (Vasoxyl), 3 to 5 mg. intravenously.

Allergic disorders. For the treatment of acute bronchial asthma, epinephrine and isoproterenol act on the *beta*-adrenergic receptor sites to relieve bronchospasm. Relief often occurs within three to five minutes after 0.2 to 0.5 cc. of epinephrine (1:1000 solution) is administered subcutaneously. Relief is due to decreased bronchospasm, a *beta* effect, and to increased bronchial mucosal vessel constriction, an *alpha* effect, thereby decreasing edema.

ALPHA-ADRENERGIC BLOCKING AGENTS

These drugs prevent responses to adrenergic stimuli mediated through the *alpha* receptors by preventing norepinephrine from attaching to the receptor sites. Two drugs in this category are phenoxybenzamine (Dibenzyline) and phentolamine hydrochloride (Regitine). Although they are occasionally recommended for the treatment of pheochromocytoma and peripheral vascular disease in man, the *alpha*-adrenergic blocking agents have not been utilized for such purposes in the dog. However, they may be utilized in the dog in certain cases of shock and digitalis-induced arrhythmias.

Secondary to volume replacement and in combination with sympathomimetic amines, the *alpha*-adrenergic blocking agents are used occasionally to produce vasodilatation. The theory behind their use is to increase cardiac activity with the sympathomimetic agents while increasing peripheral flow of blood. The danger in using these agents in shock is the marked hypotension that may result. To prevent this, the intravascular volume must be restored, and additional fluids should be available for massive transfusion if necessary.

The intravenous infusion of 5 mg. of phentolamine over 15 minutes, or 0.3 mg./min., has been reported to be successful in treating digitalis-induced arrhythmias in normal dogs (Ettinger et al., 1969).

BETA-ADRENERGIC BLOCKING AGENTS

Propranolol (Inderal) acts to reverse the *beta*-stimulating effects of catecholamines. By counteracting catecholamine action, heart rate is slowed, cardiac output is reduced, and the work of the heart is diminished. Because of the reduction in cardiac output, *beta* blocking agents are contraindicated in the presence of heart failure, because the degree of heart failure may be aggravated. *Beta*-adrenergic blockade occurs at the *beta*-adrenergic receptor sites and therefore does not alter the effects of digitalis, aminophylline, or calcium therapy; these latter agents do not depend upon adrenergic stimulation.

Beta blocking agents may be indicated for the treatment of severe digitalis-induced arrhythmias if therapy is deemed necessary; however, it must be recognized that cardiac output will be diminished. They are also used for slowing the ventricular rate in atrial fibrillation when digitalis is not effective, for treating sinus tachycardia, and in the differential diagnosis of supraventricular tachycardias (by slowing the ventricular rate, the P waves may be visualized). They are contraindicated in congestive heart failure because the condition may be aggravated, in heart block because the degree of block may be increased, and in asthma and obstructive lung disease, where they may precipitate wheezing.

Beta blocking agents are administered by slow intravenous infusion, using 1 to 3 mg., preferably diluted, but the infusion is discontinued when the desired effects have been achieved. The dosage rate for the oral forms in dogs is not known, but 10 to 40 mg. three times daily is used in man.

References

Ahlquist, R. P.: A Study of the Adrenotropic Receptors. Amer. J. Physiol., 153 (1948):586.

Barger, A. C., Rudolph, A. M., and Yates, F. E.: Sodium Retention in Heart Disease. Mod. Conc. Cardiovasc. Dis., 23 (1954):226.

Bojs, G. E., and Conn, H. L.: Distribution of Body Sodium, Potassium, and Water and the Excretion of Aldosterone in Dogs with Spontaneous Heart Failure. Amer. Heart J., 69 (1965):72.

Ettinger, S.: Cardiac Disease—Dietary Control. Friskies Res. Dig., 3 (3) (1967):1.

Ettinger, S.: Isoproterenol Treatment of Atrioventricular Block in the Dog. J. A. V. M. A., 154 (1969):398.

Ettinger, S., Gould, L., Carmichael, J. A., and Tashjian, R. J.: Phentolamine: Use in Digitalis-Induced Arrhythmias. Amer. Heart J., 77 (1969):636.

Friedberg, C.: Diseases of the Heart. 3rd ed. W. B. Saunders Co., Philadelphia. 1966.

Genest, J., Granger, P., DeChamplain, J., and Boucher, R.: Endocrine Factors in Congestive Heart Failure. Amer. J. Cardiol., 22 (1968):35.

Hamlin, R. L., Smith, C. R., and Ross, J. N.: Detection and Quantitation of Subclinical Heart Failure in Dogs. J. A. V. M. A., 150 (1967):1513.

Innes, I. R., and Nickerson, M.: Drugs Acting on Postganglionic Adrenergic Nerve Endings and Structures Innervated by Them (Sympathomimetic Drugs). In *The Pharmacological Basis of Therapeutics*. Edited by L. S. Goodman and A. Gilman. 3rd ed. The Macmillan Co., New York. (1965):477.

Knapp, W. A.: Nutritional Management of Chronic Congestive Heart Failure in the Dog. Proc. 101st Ann. Meeting, A. V. M. A. (1965):148.

Orentreich, N., Ettinger, S., Tashjian, R. J., Stanislowski, E., and Henkin, R.: Intensive Chronic Plasmapheresis in Dogs. Amer. J. Vet. Res., 29 (1968):1929.

Pensinger, R. R.: Dietary Control of Sodium Intake in Spontaneous Congestive Heart Failure in Dogs. Vet. Med., 59 (1964):747.

Vassalle, M.: Role of Catecholamine Release in Morphine Hyperglycemia. Amer. J. Physiol., 200 (1961):530.

Wallace, C. R., and Hamilton, W. F.: Study of Spontaneous Congestive Heart Failure in the Dog. Circ. Res., 11 (1962):301.

SECTION III

ARRHYTHMIAS: DISTURBANCES OF THE CARDIAC RATE AND RHYTHM

Chapter 11   ARRHYTHMIAS: DISTURBANCES OF
THE CARDIAC RATE AND RHYTHM

CHAPTER

11

ARRHYTHMIAS: DISTURBANCES OF THE CARDIAC RATE AND RHYTHM

The majority of arrhythmias were first recognized in man when only leads I, II, and III were used, and most arrhythmias can still be recognized when only these three leads are recorded. In the past two decades most investigators have been concerned with the electrophysiology and etiology of arrhythmias rather

TABLE 11-1   INCIDENCE OF CARDIAC ARRHYTHMIAS IN 95 DOGS FROM 3000
UNSELECTED CONSECUTIVE CASES EXAMINED*

ARRHYTHMIA	NO. OF DOGS
Ventricular premature beats	43
Atrial premature beats	14
Atrial fibrillation	13
Incomplete atrioventricular block	12
Incomplete atrioventricular block with dropped beats	12
Paroxysmal ventricular tachycardia	8
Ventricular parasystole	4
Paroxysmal atrial tachycardia	3
Atrioventricular nodal premature beats	3
Atrioventricular dissociation	3
Atrial flutter	2
Complete heart block	2
Left bundle branch block	2
Right bundle branch block	2
Wolff-Parkinson-White syndrome	1
TOTAL	124

*Data from Patterson et al.: Amer. J. Vet. Res., 22 (1961):355.

TABLE 11-2   DISTURBANCES IN CONDUCTION IN 215 DOGS WITH
CARDIAC ARRHYTHMIAS*

ARRHYTHMIA	NO. OF DOGS
Extrasystoles	
Atrial premature contractions	25
Atrioventricular, with retrograde conduction	23
Atrioventricular, with no retrograde conduction	25
Ventricular premature contraction	66
Heart block	
Grade 1 atrioventricular block	50
Grade 2 atrioventricular block	21
Grade 2 atrioventricular block (Wenckebach block)	11
Complete heart block	6
Sinoatrial standstill	30
Atrial fibrillation	26
Atrial flutter	2
Sinus arrhythmia (non-respiratory)	16
Paroxysmal sinus tachycardia	7
Paroxysmal atrioventricular tachycardia	2
Paroxysmal ventricular tachycardia	2

*Data from Kersten, U., Wintersfeldt, K., and Brass, W.: Tieraerztl. Umsch., 24 (1969):110.

TABLE 11-3   INCIDENCE OF TACHYCARDIA* IN 98 OF 323 DOGS IN WHICH
CIRCULATORY DISTURBANCES WERE SUSPECTED†

TACHYCARDIA	NO. OF DOGS
Continuous sinus tachycardia	85
Paroxysmal sinus tachycardia	1
Atrial flutter	1
Atrial fibrillo-flutter	2
Atrial fibrillation	5
Continuous nodal tachycardia	2
Paroxysmal nodal tachycardia	2
Continuous ventricular tachycardia	1
Paroxysmal ventricular tachycardia	3
Ventricular flutter	1

*Heart rate greater than 160 beats/min.
†Gratzl, E.: Wien. Tieraeztl. Mschr., 47 (1960):281.

than with descriptions of new arrhythmias. Although a few descriptions of arrhythmias appeared in the veterinary literature prior to the introduction of Lannek's thesis in 1949 (Roos, 1924; Roos, 1937; Zanzucchi, 1937; Gyarmati, 1939; Marek, Manninger, and Mòcsy, 1945; Fried, 1949), much of the emphasis on the clinical description of arrhythmias in dogs has appeared since.

Several investigators have reported the incidence of some or all of the arrhythmias recognized in their clinics (Tables 11-1, 11-2, 11-3).

VAGAL ACTIVITY; SINUS RHYTHM; SINUS ARRHYTHMIA; WANDERING PACEMAKER

The sinoatrial (S-A) node, the normal cardiac pacemaker, has the shortest spontaneous discharge cycle of all cardiac pacemaker tissue (see pp. 104–105). Variations of vagal tone are normally responsible for alterations of the cardiac rhythm. An increase in vagal activity results in release of acetylcholine at the nerve ending, which depresses the activity of the sinoatrial node, thereby decreasing the cardiac rate. Similarly, a decrease in vagal activity results in an increased heart rate. If the sinoatrial node is sufficiently depressed by vagal stimulation, other cardiac fibers may assume the pacemaking function. If the entire atrium is depressed, the pacemaker tissue in the area of the junctional atrioventricular (A-V) tissue assumes control. When these fibers are also depressed, the tissue with the next lower threshold, such as the bundle of His or the Purkinje fibers, becomes the pacemaker tissue and assumes the function of cardiac pacing.

A *sinus rhythm* does not vary appreciably in rate from beat to beat, and always originates from the sinoatrial node (Fig. 11-1). Respiration affects vagal tone significantly in dogs. Vagal activity is decreased during inspiration and increased during expiration. When vagal impulses are appreciably diminished during respiration, the heart rate changes continuously but with constant periodicity. If the sinoatrial node remains as the cardiac pacemaker, the rhythmic periodic cardiac rhythm is termed *sinus arrhythmia* (Figs. 11-2 and 11-3). Sinus arrhythmia is unusual in puppies under four weeks of age (Lange, 1937). A continuously changing heart rate caused by shifting of the pacemaker site within the sinoatrial node and/or the atrium is called *wandering pacemaker* (Fig. 11-4). In sinus arrhythmia the configuration of the P wave remains the same, whereas with a wandering pacemaker the configuration of the P wave varies.

Sinus rhythm, sinus arrhythmia, and wandering pacemaker all occur in normal dogs (Figs. 11-1 to 11-4). The presence of sinus arrhythmia often confuses

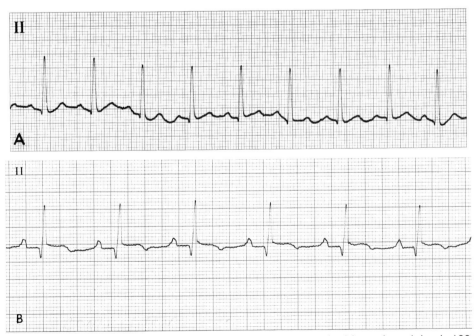

FIGURE 11-1 Normal sinus rhythm. *A,* The heart rate in this toy breed dog is 166 beats/min., and the rhythm is perfectly regular. The electrocardiographic complexes (P to P or R to R) are equidistant, indicating a regular, nonfluctuating rate. *B,* The heart rate in this dog is 136 beats/min., and the rhythm is regular. The complexes are again equidistant.

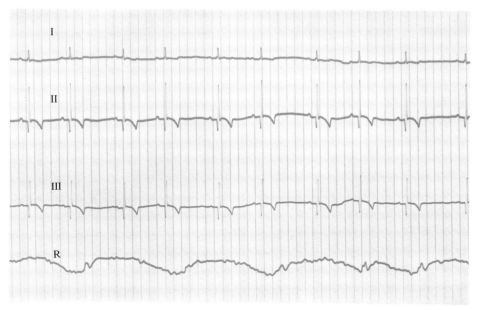

FIGURE 11-2 Respiratory sinus arrhythmia. Leads I, II, and III and the respiration curve (R) were recorded simultaneously. Maximum inspiration occurs at the high points of the respiration curve, and maximum expiration at the low points. Vagal tone is diminished during inspiration, and the heart rate is increased, as indicated by the shorter R to R intervals. Notice that the heart rate is regularly phasic with respiration, a feature of respiratory sinus arrhythmia. Paper speed = 50 mm./sec.; time lines = 0.1 sec.

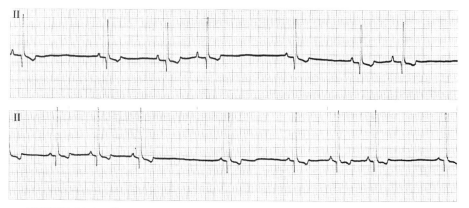

FIGURE 11-3 Sinus arrhythmia. Notice the marked fluctuation in heart rate resulting from respiratory sinus arrhythmia in recordings from two normal dogs. The rate may be described as regularly irregular.

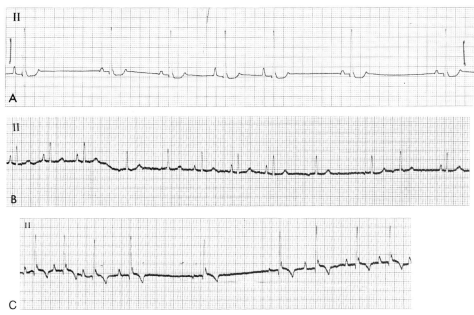

FIGURE 11-4 Wandering pacemaker. *A,* As the heart rate increases owing to decreased vagal tone, the amplitude of the P waves is increased, and the P waves originate from the sinoatrial node. As the heart rate diminishes when vagal tone increases, the form of the P waves changes, in this case becoming smaller as they arise from a pacemaker other than the sinoatrial node. The duration of the P-R interval is constant at 0.10 sec.

B, The wandering pacemaker in this recording is suggested by the slightly negative P waves in some of the complexes. Negative P waves of this nature result from vagal depression of the sinoatrial node and the development of a junctional atrioventricular nodal rhythm.

C, Marked sinus arrhythmia and a wandering pacemaker result in a decreased heart rate (increased R-R interval) and negative P waves in the fifth complex. As the pacemaker returns to the sinoatrial node the rate increases, and positive P waves of varying amplitude result in the sixth and seventh complexes.

measurements made from the electrocardiogram when ectopic impulses are present, thus making their interpretation more difficult. Buchanan (1965) reported that sinus arrhythmia and wandering pacemaker disappear when the heart rate exceeds 120 beats/min. However, this is not always the case; instead, the R-R variation that accompanies sinus arrhythmia may be less pronounced because of the more rapid heart rate.

The application of digital pressure over the pressoreceptor centers, such as the area of the carotid sinus at the bifurcation of the carotid artery, or the eyeball, results in an increase in vagal tone which reduces the heart rate by depressing the sinoatrial node and slowing atrioventricular nodal conduction. Arrhythmias arising from the ventricle are not affected by vagal stimulation, whereas those arising from supraventricular foci (sinoatrial node, atrium, or atrioventricular nodal region) may frequently be slowed or abolished by vagal stimulation. The application of pressure over regions of vagal influence may depress sinoatrial pacemaker tissue, resulting in a lower center assuming the pacemaking function and producing junctional or ventricular escape beats (see pp. 302–303).

CLASSIFICATION OF BEATS ARISING FROM ECTOPIC FOCI (PREMATURE BEATS)

Arrhythmias can be classified and differentiated as follows:

1. *Atrial (supraventricular) beat* — P wave abnormal but positive.

2. *Junctional or atrioventricular nodal (supraventricular) beat* arising from region around the atrioventricular node — P wave negative in leads II, III, and aVF, indicating retrograde conduction of P wave; or no P wave.

3. *Ventricular beat* usually arising from the fibers of the ventricles — QRS complex abnormally wide and unrelated to the P wave, or QRS complex normal but unrelated to the P wave.

Furthermore, atrial, junctional, or ventricular premature beats interrupt the normal sinus rhythm by one of the following different sequences (Fig. 11-5):

Resetting. In resetting, the ectopic beat initiates an entirely new cardiac rhythm. Therefore, the interval from the ectopic P wave to the next P wave is of normal duration.

Resetting with pause. In resetting with pause, the ectopic beat temporarily depresses the sinoatrial node, so that the next sinus beat occurs later in the time sequence than it normally would. The interval between the ectopic P wave and the subsequent sinus P wave is thus longer than the normal P-P interval but less than two normal intervals.

Compensatory pause. The sinus impulse immediately following an ectopic beat may fail to initiate a ventricular beat if the ventricle is still in the absolute refractory period, i.e., the period when no stimulus can be transmitted. As a result, there is a prolonged interval or compensatory pause between the ectopic beat and the next normal sinus beat. Thus, the interval between the normal beats preceding and following the ectopic beat is twice the normal P-P interval.

Interpolation. An interpolated beat is a complete extra beat occurring between two normal beats. The interpolated beat does not interrupt the normal rhythm. These rarely occur in the dog.

Interpolation and compensatory pause are usually associated with ventricular premature contractions, whereas resetting or resetting with pause are more commonly associated with atrial premature contractions and junctional premature contractions.

SUPRAVENTRICULAR PREMATURE CONTRACTIONS (ATRIAL PREMATURE CONTRACTIONS AND JUNCTIONAL PREMATURE CONTRACTIONS)

Atrial premature contractions are characterized electrocardiographically as having premature P waves that occur earlier in time than the normal P wave (Fig. 11-6). The P wave is positive in leads II, III, and aVF. It is different from the normal P wave in size, configuration, or both, because the discharge is from a focus other than the sinoatrial pacemaker. The P wave occurs prematurely but is usually followed by a normal or nearly normal QRS complex, since the pattern of ventricular conduction is usually unaffected. The P-P interval from the previous normal beat to the ectopic beat is shorter than normal. The P-R interval of the ectopic beat may be longer than in normal complexes because the ectopic beat is

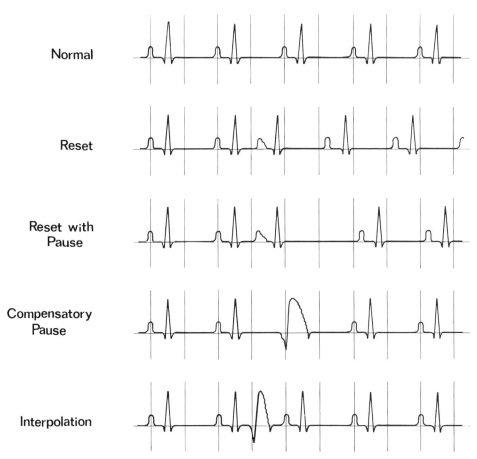

FIGURE 11-5 Schematic representations of normal sinus rhythm and premature complexes. *Normal sinus rhythm.* The heart rate remains constant, and the interval from P to P or from R to R does not change. *Resetting.* An atrial premature contraction (beat 3) resets the sinus rhythm, so that the period from the beginning of the premature P wave to the next normal P wave is equal to exactly one P-P interval. *Resetting with pause.* The atrial premature contraction (beat 3) is followed by a pause greater than one P-P interval but less than two P-P intervals. *Compensatory pause.* The ventricular premature contraction (beat 3) is followed by a compensatory pause; that is, the period from the normal P wave in the beat preceding the ventricular premature contraction to the normal P wave of the beat following the ventricular premature contraction is equivalent to exactly two P-P intervals. The sinus P wave occurs on time, but it is not conducted through the atrioventricular node to the ventricle, which is in a refractory state due to the ventricular premature contraction. *Interpolation.* A ventricular premature contraction (beat 3) occurs between two normal sinus complexes without disrupting normal rhythm. Interpolated beats are unusual in dogs.

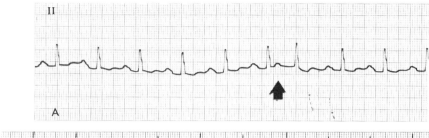

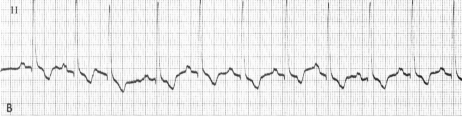

FIGURE 11-6 Atrial premature contractions. *A,* The sinus rhythm in a dog with extreme atrial dilatation (P mitrale) due to chronic mitral valvular fibrosis has been disrupted by an atrial premature contraction (arrow). The atrial premature contraction is characterized by a premature, abnormally shaped P wave, a prolonged P-R interval, and a normal-appearing QRS complex.

B, The aberrant premature P wave in the third complex is superimposed on the end of the previous T wave. The P-R interval is prolonged from 0.10 sec., in the normal complexes, to 0.12 sec. The QRS complex associated with the atrial premature contraction is both of high amplitude and prolonged, consistent with marked left ventricular hypertrophy. In resetting with pause, the pause following the premature beat is approximately 0.42 sec. long; this is greater than one but less than two P-P intervals.

early and because the impulse reaches the atrioventricular node during its relative refractory phase and remains in the atrioventricular node longer (Katz and Pick, 1956). Atrial premature contractions with short P-R intervals are more likely to be followed by aberrant (abnormal) appearing QRS complexes. This is so because early conduction to the ventricles results in an irregular pattern of ventricular depolarization. Atrial premature contractions can be blocked if the atrioventricular node is in a state of absolute refractoriness from a previous contraction; a P wave then occurs early but is not followed by a QRS complex. Atrial premature contractions are usually followed by resetting or resetting with pause rather than by a compensatory pause, since the early aberrant P wave is followed by normal ventricular conduction, allowing enough time for the atrial refractory period to be completed prior to the next normal sinoatrial impulse.

The *salient diagnostic features* of an atrial premature contraction are (after Katz and Pick, 1956):

1. Premature P wave.
2. P wave abnormal in size, configuration, or both.
3. Prolonged P-R interval.
4. QRS-T complex normal or nearly normal (except in unusual cases when conduction is aberrant).

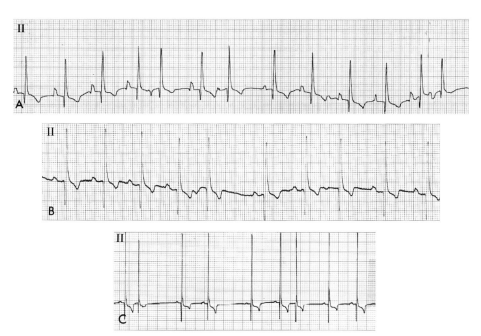

FIGURE 11-7   Junctional premature contractions. *A,* The fifth and thirteenth P waves in this recording are junctional premature contractions since they occur prematurely and are negative. They are followed by normal or nearly normal QRS complexes. The seventh beat is an atrial premature contraction. Both the atrial and junctional premature contractions are followed by resetting with pause.

B, The fifth and eighth beats are junctional premature contractions characterized by premature negative P waves, normal QRS complexes, and resetting with pause. P mitrale and left ventricular hypertrophy are present.

C, Premature QRS complexes which are normal or nearly normal in shape and are not preceded by P waves occur in the second and seventh beats. These are identified as junctional premature contractions, because a P wave is not present and the QRS complex is normal but premature.

Although it is now recognized that the atrioventricular node is not capable of pacemaker activity (Hoffman and Cranefield, 1964), the term "atrioventricular nodal beat" has been used for many years. The term "atrioventricular nodal beat" implies that the fibers near the atrioventricular node have assumed the pacemaker function. The term "junctional beat" may be more appropriate and is used preferentially to "atrioventricular nodal beat."

Junctional premature contractions are characterized electrocardiographically by a premature QRS complex and negative P waves in leads II, III, and aVF (Fig. 11-7), although positive, upright P waves may theoretically occur in these leads if the impulse arises from the region of the coronary sinus. The QRS-T complex usually appears normal. The P-R interval may be shorter than normal since the impulse travels a shorter distance to the atrioventricular node. The P wave is negative because atrial conduction proceeds in a retrograde direction. The P wave may precede, occur during, or follow the QRS complex. This is so because retrograde conduction of the impulse through the atrium is slower than is the forward conduction of the impulse through the ventricle.

The *salient diagnostic features* of junctional or atrioventricular nodal premature contractions are (after Katz and Pick, 1956):

1. Premature QRS-T complex normal in shape.
2. QRS-T complex preceded or followed by an inverted P wave in leads II, III, and aVF or not preceded by a premature P wave.

VENTRICULAR PREMATURE CONTRACTIONS

Ventricular premature contractions may originate from any portion of the ventricle. The closer the ectopic stimulus is to the bundle of His, the more normal the QRS-T complex will appear. Since the impulse of a ventricular premature contraction is conducted through the myocardium, conduction is slower than normal and follows an abnormal pathway. As a result, the characteristic electrocardiographic finding with a ventricular premature contraction is a wide and aberrant ventricular complex (Fig. 11-8). If a ventricular premature contraction arises near the common bundle of His it may be only slightly aberrant in form. Ventricular premature contractions either occur as interpolated beats or are followed by a compensatory pause (Fig. 11-5). Resetting of the cardiac rhythm with or without a short pause at the sinoatrial node is unusual. The sinoatrial node continues to discharge at its normal rate, since impulses arising in the ventricle below the atrioventricular node are not usually conducted retrograde to the

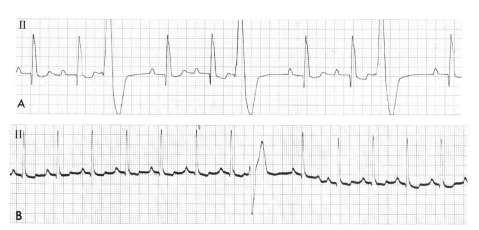

FIGURE 11-8   Ventricular premature contractions. Ventricular premature contractions are characterized by prolonged, aberrant QRS complexes which occur prematurely and are unrelated to a P wave.

A, Two normal sinus beats are followed by a ventricular premature contraction throughout this recording (trigeminal rhythm). The pause from the P wave of the normal beat preceding the ventricular premature contraction to the P wave of the beat following the premature contraction is equal to 1 sec., or two P-P intervals. The "interfered" sinus P wave cannot be seen because it occurs during the period of the ventricular premature contraction, 0.5 sec. following the previous normal P wave. The pause following the ventricular premature contraction is called a compensatory pause. When ventricular premature contractions have the same configuration throughout the recording, they are unifocal in origin. *B,* Ventricular premature contraction followed by a compensatory pause.

atrium. Electrocardiographically, the sinus P wave occurs at its normal interval, often within the bizarre QRS-T complexes, although it may not always be clearly defined if it occurs simultaneously with the QRS complex. The compensatory pause that follows a ventricular premature contraction occurs because the sinus P wave reaches the atrioventricular node while that node is refractory. The refractory state of the atrioventricular node results from partial but incomplete retrograde conduction from the ventricular premature contraction. Therefore, the P waves continue to occur at their regular interval, but the P wave associated with the ventricular premature contraction is not conducted through the refractory atrioventricular node. The interval from the P wave of a normal beat preceding the ventricular premature contraction to the P wave in the next normal cycle following a single ventricular premature contraction is thus exactly that of two normal P-P intervals.

The *salient diagnostic features* of ventricular premature contractions are (after Katz and Pick, 1956):

1. Premature QRS-T complex.
2. Bizarre prolonged QRS complex.
3. P wave unrelated to the abnormal QRS-T complex.

UNIFOCAL, MULTIFOCAL, AND MULTIPLE PREMATURE CONTRACTIONS

Unifocal premature contractions arise from one ectopic focus and are constant or inconstant in form but have P-P (supraventricular premature contractions) or R-R (ventricular contractions) intervals or coupling that remains constant between the normal and ectopic beats (Fig. 11-8). When there is more than one ectopic focus the P-P or R-R intervals vary, and the premature beats which also vary in form are identified as being *multifocal* (Fig. 11-9).

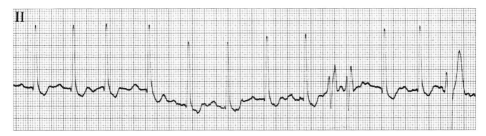

FIGURE 11-9 Multifocal ventricular premature contractions. The ninth, tenth, and thirteenth beats are ventricular premature contractions, but because of the difference in configuration of beats 9 and 10 and beat 13 it may be assumed that the focus of origin for beats 9 and 10 differs from that for beat 13. This suggests at least two sites of origin for the ventricular premature contractions. Beat 3 is a junctional premature contraction.

Premature contractions may occur singly, repetitively, or in varying patterns (Fig. 11-10). Two ectopic beats immediately following a normal beat are termed a *pair*; three are a *run*, and four or more are referred to as a *tachycardia*. *Bigeminy* describes a normal beat followed by a single premature contraction. *Trigeminy* refers to a premature contraction after two normal beats (Fig. 11-8*A*). The terms pairs, runs, and tachycardia, as well as bigeminy and trigeminy, are utilized when referring to atrial, junctional or atrioventricular nodal, and ventricular premature contractions.

Associations.   Atrial premature contractions are usually associated with left atrial dilatation due to chronic mitral valvular insufficiency (Patterson et al., 1961) and may precede atrial fibrillation. However they may result from atrial disease of any origin. Junctional premature beats may also result from chronic mitral valvular insufficiency and from digitalis intoxication, toxic agents, or excessive vagal tone, as well as from increased irritability in the area around the atrioventricular node. Whereas atrial premature contractions rarely occur without atrial disease in the dog, ventricular premature contractions may be associated with drug intoxication, stress or anxiety, cardiac catheterization and surgery, and cardiovascular disease. Ectopic beats are considered serious if they occur frequently, if they are multifocal, or if two or more occur simultaneously. In the early as well as the recent descriptions of ventricular premature contractions in dogs, the presence of ventricular premature contractions is considered pathologic (Lannek, 1949; Detweiler et al., 1968).

Signs.   The dog usually is asymptomatic, although signs such as syncope may accompany frequent premature contractions. When auscultating the heart, one finds that the ectopic contraction occurs early, and a pause follows the premature beat. The intensity of the heart sounds is variable when the ectopic contraction occurs (Fig. 2-11). A pulse deficit may be present.

Treatment.   Treatment is usually not indicated for occasional supraventricular premature contractions. When they occur frequently, atrial disease is usu-

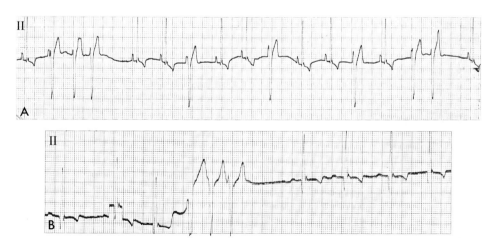

FIGURE 11-10   Multiple ventricular premature contractions. *A*, Ectopic beats may occur singly or in multiples. When two ectopic beats occur together they are termed a pair, and when three occur they are called a run. Paper speed = 25 mm./sec. *B*, A run of ventricular premature contractions interrupts the normal sinus rhythm.

ally present and signs of heart failure are likely to be present. Digitalization is indicated to improve cardiac function by its positive inotropic effect on the ventricular myocardium, and to slow atrioventricular nodal conduction through its vagal and extravagal effects. If ventricular premature contractions are not drug-induced, antiarrhythmic agents may be used (see Chap. 8). In the event of possible digitalis intoxication, digitalis should be *discontinued* when ventricular premature contractions occur. If ventricular premature contractions are a result of decreased myocardial efficiency the cardiac glycosides are indicated. However they should be used in such cases only under strict electrocardiographic supervision.

TACHYCARDIAS

For purposes of classification, heart rate in normal adult dogs should not exceed 160 beats per min. except in toy breeds, in which it may be as high as 180 beats/min. Rates exceeding these are termed tachycardia (paroxysmal or continuous).

When examining an electrocardiographic tracing from a dog with a rapid heart rate, it is often difficult to distinguish the P wave from the previous T wave. Superimposition of T and P waves is suggested if abnormally large T waves are seen (Fig. 11-11). To improve identification of electrocardiographic waves, the paper speed should be increased to 50 or 100 mm./sec. if possible. If all leads are recorded, separation or notching of the combined T and P waves can usually be recognized in at least one lead. An esophageal lead recorded simultaneously with a limb lead would be helpful in evaluating the P wave since the configuration of the P wave on the esophageal lead tracing differs from that observed on the limb lead tracing.

For descriptive purposes, tachycardias may arise from the atrium, from the region of the atrioventricular node, from the bundle of His, or from the ventricle. Since retrograde conduction through the atrioventricular node is unusual (Katz and Pick, 1956), and since the atrioventricular node itself is not capable of pacemaker activity (Hoffman and Cranefield, 1964), it is logical to classify the tachycardias as originating in either supraventricular or ventricular tissue.

SUPRAVENTRICULAR TACHYCARDIA

SINUS TACHYCARDIA. In sinus tachycardia the heart rate exceeds 160 beats/min. (180 beats/min. in dogs of toy breeds) and the P-QRS-T complexes are normal (Fig. 11-12). An important clue to the differentiation of sinus tachycardia from atrial tachycardia is the slight irregularity of the P-P interval in sinus tachycardia. As with any supraventricular tachycardia, the T wave and the P wave may be superimposed if the heart rate is very rapid (Fig. 11-11). Sinus tachycardia may slow with vagal stimulation, such as when pressure is applied to the eyeballs or the carotid sinus, but the rapid rate resumes when the pressure is relieved.

ATRIAL TACHYCARDIA. Atrial tachycardia may be continuous or may begin and end suddenly (paroxysmal atrial tachycardia, PAT). Characteristically, the R-R interval is perfectly regular. With vagal stimulation, paroxysmal atrial tachycardia is usually eliminated entirely or does not change at all. In this arrhythmia

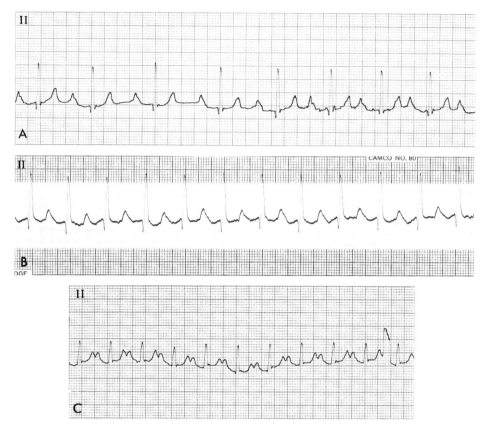

FIGURE 11-11   Superimposition of a P wave and a T wave. *A,* The wide P wave is a result of left atrial dilatation, and the P-R interval of 0.14 sec. indicates first degree heart block resulting from digitalis intoxication. The heart rate is 140 beats/min. *B,* Tracing from the same dog made several months later, when he was presented in heart failure. The heart rate was 200 beats/min.; as a result of decreased diastolic time the T and P waves are superimposed, giving the impression of one large wave between the R waves. *C,* Superimposition of the T and P waves is seen in this tracing from a dog with toxic pyometra. The heart rate is approximately 240 beats/min., and a notch separates the T and P waves.

the P wave differs from the sinus P wave and may also be buried in the previous T wave (Fig. 11-13). Paroxysms of atrial tachycardia are usually broken with vagal stimulation.

PAROXYSMAL ATRIAL TACHYCARDIA WITH BLOCK.   In man, atrial tachycardia with varying degrees of atrioventricular block is often related to digitalis intoxication (Friedberg, 1966). It resembles atrial tachycardia without block in that the rate is rapid; however, the rate is irregular and atrioventricular block occurs. In a two year old German shepherd dog with congenital pulmonic stenosis, paroxysmal atrial tachycardia with block occurred after the rhythm was converted from atrial fibrillation with ouabain (Detweiler, Hubben, and Patterson, 1960). Paroxysmal atrial tachycardia with block is an unusual arrhythmia in the dog.

JUNCTIONAL OR NODAL TACHYCARDIAS.   In this arrhythmia the heart rate

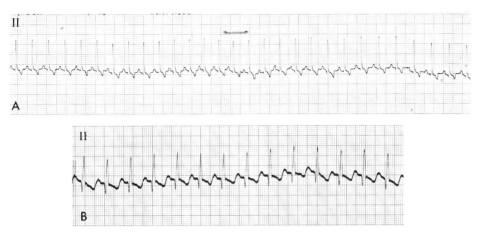

FIGURE 11-12 Sinus tachycardia. *A,* The heart rate is 190 beats/min., and the P wave, QRS complex, and T wave appear normal. This rapid heart rate resulted from excitement. Paper speed = 25 mm./sec. *B,* A heart rate of 250 beats/min. was recorded in this dog with pyometra. The T and P waves are not separated but rather blend into each other as a result of decreased diastolic time.

is rapid and the P wave is negative if it precedes the QRS complex (Fig. 11-14). The P wave may also occur within or following the QRS complex.

It is important to identify the P wave because therapeutic measures are determined according to the point of origin of the ectopic beat. If the P wave is not present and the ectopic beat originates below the atrioventricular node, antiarrhythmic therapy rather than digitalis would be indicated, because digitalis would be likely to aggravate the arrhythmia and it might induce ventricular fibrillation.

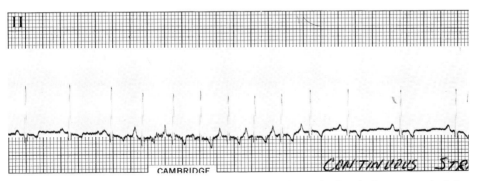

FIGURE 11-13 Atrial tachycardia. A normal sinus rhythm is interrupted at the fourth beat by a rapid burst of atrial beats. The paroxysmal tachycardia stopped spontaneously at the tenth beat, and the rhythm returned to normal. Notice that the configuration of the P waves is different during the run of atrial tachycardia than during normal sinus rhythm. This dog had a history of syncopal episodes which seemed to be related to the atrial tachycardia, both of which subsided after the dog was digitalized.

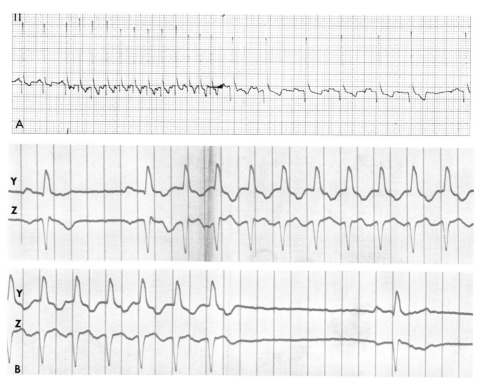

FIGURE 11-14   Junctional tachycardia. *A,* Tracing from a dog with advanced mitral valvular insufficiency and syncopal episodes. The electrocardiogram indicates a rapid burst of beats beginning with the fourth beat. The paroxysmal tachycardia is characterized by QRS complexes which appear nearly normal and are preceded by negative P waves. Normal rhythm resumed at the fifteenth beat; this happened to occur at exactly the time that the paper speed was changed from 25 mm./sec. to 50 mm./sec. (which explains the sudden prolongation of the R-R interval at this point). Notice that the twentieth beat occurs prematurely without a P wave, suggesting an isolated nodal premature contraction. During the paroxysm of junctional tachycardia the heart rate is equivalent to 250 beats/min., and the R-R interval is constant at 0.24 sec.

B, In this continuous tracing of simultaneously recorded Y and Z leads, the normal rhythm is suddenly interrupted by a paroxysm of junctional premature contractions which occur at the rate of 200 beats/min. The premature P waves are reversed in polarity. When the paroxysm ends, there is a long pause between the end of the tachycardia and the next normal sinus beat. This arrhythmia occurred in a dog with symptomatic heartworm disease and heart failure. Paper speed = 100 mm./sec.; time lines = 0.1 sec.

Salient features of supraventricular tachycardia are (after Katz and Pick, 1956):

1. A heart rate over 160 beats/min. (180 beats/min. in the toy breeds) with perfectly regular P waves (sinus tachycardia).
2. P wave abnormal (atrial tachycardia) or absent (junctional tachycardia).
3. QRS complexes of normal duration unless a constant relationship can be shown between the P waves and each aberrant QRS complex.

Associations. Sinus tachycardia occurs in nervous dogs without cardiac disease as well as in dogs with fever, hyperthyroidism, anemia, toxemias, and congestive heart failure. Supraventricular tachycardia (probably sinus in origin) has been observed by the authors in dogs which have ingested soaps containining hexachlorophene and in dogs that have been shocked after biting into an electric cord. Atrial and junctional tachycardias are occasionally produced during cardiac catheterization and surgery. Paroxysmal supraventricular tachycardias are often a sequela to atrial premature contractions resulting from chronic mitral valvular fibrosis. Atrial tachycardia as a sign of cardiac disease has been seen in a dog with aortic body tumor, and in various stages of the treatment of atrial fibrillation (Patterson et al., 1961) as well as in three cases reported by Roos (1937) with infiltration of the atrial walls.

Signs. The pulse rate and heart sounds are rapid and regular, but murmurs are difficult to hear during paroxysmal or persistent supraventricular tachycardias. Syncope, with or without incontinence and convulsions, may occur during paroxysmal atrial tachycardia. In one dog treated by us, over 30 syncopal episodes occurred daily until digitalis therapy was instituted. If prolonged, supraventricular tachycardia may lead to congestive heart failure, especially after soap poisoning and electric shock.

Treatment. Carotid sinus or ocular pressure may terminate attacks of atrial and junctional tachycardia by increasing vagal tone and slowing the sinoatrial pacemaker as well as conduction through the atrioventricular node. The intravenous administration of a cardiac glycoside or vasopressors (such as phenylephrine, 0.8 mg., intravenously; or methoxamine, 5 to 10 mg., intravenously) is effective in the treatment of paroxysmal supraventricular tachycardias in progress, because they induce vagal cardiac stimulation. If direct current cardioversion is available, it is a satisfactory method of resetting a slower sinus rhythm unless the rhythm is paroxysmal atrial tachycardia due to chronic valvular insufficiency (in which case digitalization is indicated). We have used propranolol, a beta adrenergic blocking agent, to convert idiopathic atrial tachycardia in a puppy.

VENTRICULAR TACHYCARDIA AND ATRIOVENTRICULAR DISSOCIATION

When ventricular ectopic beats develop, retrograde impulse conduction to the atrium usually does not occur. Since the sinoatrial node is normal, it continues to discharge independently of the ventricular rhythm, and P waves are regularly produced by atrial depolarization. Since these P waves usually reach the atrioventricular node while it is in a refractory state because of partial retrograde conduction of the ectopic ventricular beat, the P wave does not travel to the ventricle, and it is then termed an *interfered P wave* (Fig. 11-8). When the atrium and ven-

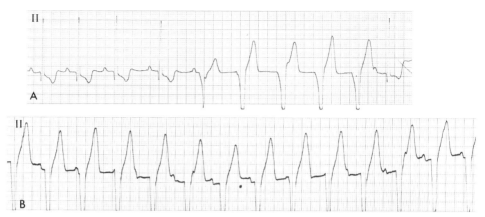

FIGURE 11-15 Ventricular tachycardia. A paroxysm of four or more aberrant ventricular beats interrupting the normal rhythm characterizes ventricular tachycardia. *A,* In this dog with advanced myocardial degeneration, a paroxysm of ventricular tachycardia begins with the fifth beat and continues for five beats until a normal rhythm is resumed. The fifth beat is a fusion beat. *B,* A continuous ventricular tachycardia was recorded from this dog with advanced heart failure due to chronic mitral valvular disease and myocardial degeneration. The P waves, which occur independently of the idioventricular tachycardia, can occasionally be seen. The atrial rate is 143 beats/min.; the ventricular rate is 158 beats/min.

tricle beat at different rates it is likely that a P wave will occasionally reach the atrioventricular node when it is not refractory. This impulse is then conducted through its normal path, thereby depolarizing the ventricle normally. Whereas the previous QRS complexes have been ventricular in origin and therefore aberrant and wide, the sinoatrial impulse conducted through the atrioventricular node and ventricular conduction system produces a normal QRS complex. In other words, for one beat the sinoatrial node has again captured the cardiac rhythm, and the normal beat produced is called a *capture beat* (Fig. 11-16). If the P wave happens to stimulate the ventricular myocardium at the same time that the idioventricular stimulus does, a slightly abnormal QRS-T complex occurs. It is intermediate in form between a capture beat and an idioventricular beat, and the resultant beat is called a *fusion* beat (Fig. 11-16). The timing of a fusion beat is always normal for both atrial and ventricular rhythms, whereas capture beats occur prematurely in ventricular rhythms. Therefore, three different beats may be recognized in ventricular tachycardia or incomplete atrioventricular dissociation: the idioventricular beat, the capture beat, and the fusion beat. The presence of fusion and capture beats verifies both that the ectopic rhythm is ventricular and also that the atrioventricular node has not lost the ability to transmit an impulse from the atrium.

Ventricular tachycardia and atrioventricular dissociation are characterized by the presence of a ventricular pacemaker beating independently of, and faster than, the sinoatrial pacemaker, which also continues to emit impulses, usually interfered P waves (Fig. 11-15). Since widely accepted definitive criteria are not yet available for dogs, the term *atrioventricular dissociation* will be applied to the rhythm if the idioventricular rate is less than 100 beats/min. and is faster than the atrial rate. *Ventricular tachycardia* implies only that the idioventricular rate is greater than 100 beats/min. yet is still faster than the atrial rate. Ventricular capture and fusion beats indicate *incomplete atrioventricular dissociation* because the atrioventricular node is capable of impulse transmission if it is not refractory

(Fig. 11-16) (Ettinger and Buergelt, 1968). If transection (actual or not) of the atrioventricular node prevents atrioventricular impulse conduction, then *complete atrioventricular dissociation* is present. This differs from atrioventricular block in that in atrioventricular block the atrial rate is greater than the ventricular rate, whereas in complete atrioventricular dissociation the ventricular rate exceeds the atrial rate (Katz and Pick, 1956). Atrioventricular dissociation and complete heart

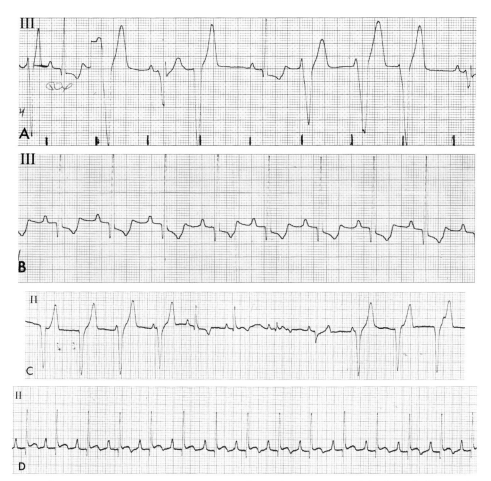

FIGURE 11-16   Ventricular tachycardia with capture and fusion. *A,* The atria and ventricles beat independently of each other in this arrhythmia. The black lines at the bottom of the tracing indicate the atrial rate. Wide, aberrant ventricular beats indicate the idioventricular rhythm (beats 1, 3, 5, 8, and 9). When the P wave arrives at the atrioventricular node when it is not refractory, the impulse captures the ventricle, resulting in a normal QRS complex called a "capture beat" (beats 2 and 6). When the P wave is conducted through the atrioventricular node and depolarizes the ventricle at the same time as does the idioventricular beat, a fusion beat with a configuration between that of the normal capture beat and the idioventricular beat results (beats 4, 7, and 10). *B,* Following the administration of parenteral quinidine sulfate, a normal sinus rhythm resumes. If the idioventricular rate is greater than 100 beats/min., the rhythm is termed ventricular tachycardia. When it is less than 100 beats/min., the rhythm is referred to as atrioventricular dissociation. *C,* The fifth and sixth beats demonstrate ventricular capture, the seventh and eighth ventricular fusion, and the first to fourth and ninth to eleventh represent the dominant ventricular tachycardia. *D,* In most instances, such an arrhythmia should be treated with antiarrhythmic agents to restore a normal sinus rhythm.

block may occur together if two independent pacemakers are present and both are fast enough to prevent the atrioventricular node from emerging from a refractory state. Such a refractory state inhibits atrioventricular conduction and permits the two centers to fire independently of each other.

Isorhythmic dissociation (accrochage and synchrony) can occur with atrioventricular dissociation, ventricular tachycardia, complete heart block, or electrical pacemaking (Ettinger, 1965). In accrochage and synchrony, the atrial rate is affected in some way by the idioventricular pacemaker. In synchrony, the atrial and idioventricular rates are similar for long periods, while the P wave maintains a constant relationship to the QRS complex (Fig. 11-17). In accrochage (Ettinger and Buergelt, 1968) the atrial and ventricular rates are almost identical and the P wave moves in and out of the QRS complex (Fig. 11-18).

A constant ventricular rate (R-R) is a characteristic of atrioventricular dissociation, although frequent ventricular capture beats may produce an irregular ventricular rate (Fig. 11-16).

In supraventricular tachycardias, the impulse usually reaches the atrioventricular node and ventricle when it is receptive to depolarization; the QRS complex is then normal in both duration and configuration. Occasionally, an impulse reaches the ventricles during their relative refractory period; then the QRS complex is likely to be wider than normal and bizarre in configuration because of aberrant conduction. In ventricular rhythms, the depolarization wave from the ectopic ventricular focus spreads through the myocardium, which conducts impulses more slowly than does the Purkinje system. Therefore, the QRS complex is wider than normal in ventricular tachycardias, and the configuration of the QRS complex is abnormal. If the ectopic focus is near the bundle of His, the QRS complex is occasionally of nearly normal duration and configuration.

To differentiate supraventricular tachycardias from ventricular tachycardias, the following points should be considered. Because retrograde conduction from the ventricle to the atrium is unusual, the atrial rate is independent of the ventricular rate in a ventricular tachycardia. In a supraventricular tachycardia the atrial rate is rapid, and the ventricular rate is slower than or the same as the atrial rate. In a ventricular tachycardia, the ventricular rate is more rapid than the atrial rate.

The *salient features* of ventricular tachycardia are (after Katz and Pick, 1956):

1. A series of bizarre, premature beats that are wide in duration and occur in rapid succession.

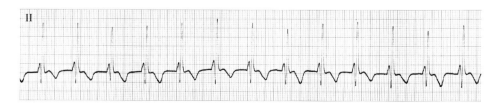

FIGURE 11-17   Atrioventricular dissociation with synchrony. Synchrony is a form of atrioventricular dissociation in which the atrial beat remains in a constant relationship to the QRS complex for prolonged periods of time. In this case the P wave occurred at the beginning of the QRS complex and remained so for minutes.

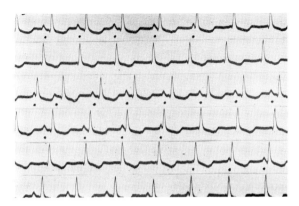

FIGURE 11-18 Atrioventricular dissociation with accrochage. Accrochage is another form of atrioventricular dissociation. In this arrhythmia, the P waves wander in and out of the QRS complex rather than remaining associated with a particular portion of the QRS complex. The dots indicate the location of the P waves when they wander in front of the QRS complex. If the P wave reaches the atrioventricular node early enough to depolarize it, the resultant complex is called a capture beat; it resembles the normal P-QRS complex. Such a beat is seen in the third row, second complex. From Ettinger, S., and Buergelt, C-D.: Am. J. Vet. Res., 29 (1968):1500.

2. The rhythm may be regular or irregular, but upright P waves can be identified at an independent and slower rate.

3. Ventricular capture and fusion beats establish the diagnosis of ventricular tachycardia conclusively.

Associations. Ventricular tachycardia should be considered as a serious cardiac arrhythmia, particularly so because it may occur as a preventricular fibrillation rhythm. Ventricular tachycardia is associated with myocarditis and congestive heart failure. Arteriosclerosis of the smaller coronary arteries, as well as myocardial necrosis and fibrosis, was found at necropsy in four dogs after bouts of paroxysmal ventricular tachycardia (Patterson et al., 1961). Digitalis, quinidine, procainamide, and potassium intoxication can induce ventricular tachycardia, and ventricular tachycardia can occur during, or may be the cause of Stokes-Adams seizures. Although it is uncertain what the actual cause is, emotional disturbances, such as occur occasionally with grooming, may result in ventricular tachycardia. Ventricular tachycardia may develop after precordial electric shock, during cardiac catheterization when sensitive areas of the ventricle are touched, and during some surgical manipulations. The authors have occasionally observed asymptomatic dogs with ventricular tachycardia whose electrocardiograms stabilized after therapy. Although there was no apparent cause for the arrhythmia a presumptive diagnosis of myocarditis was suggested. In one dog which developed paroxysmal ventricular tachycardia in association with hemolytic bacterial infection, the electrocardiogram was normal after the infection subsided (Detweiler, Hubben, and Patterson, 1960).

Signs. Dyspnea, weakness, and collapse are typical signs, and congestive heart failure is sometimes present. Fainting may be reported. Cannon "a" waves are seen in the jugular vein (see p. 8). On auscultation, the intensity of the first heart sound often varies because of variable filling of the ventricle; there is also a continuous or paroxysmal rapid rhythm.

Treatment.   If digitalis, quinidine, or procainamide are being administered, they must be discontinued IMMEDIATELY unless the arrhythmia is known to have another cause or is obviously unrelated to the administration of these agents. Otherwise, antiarrhythmic agents such as quinidine or procainamide (Huisman and Teunissen, 1963; Detweiler et al., 1968) are indicated in treating ventricular tachycardia, as may be lidocaine or diphenylhydantoin, in an attempt to decrease ventricular excitability, prolong the effective refractory period, and slow conduction. When the arrhythmia is acute, intravenous lidocaine or procainamide is most effective in converting the arrhythmia. Quinidine or procainamide is then used orally for maintenance. Direct current shock may be used to reset the cardiac rhythm unless the etiology of the tachycardia is digitalis intoxication, in which case direct current cardioversion should not be employed because it may induce ventricular fibrillation. If congestive heart failure is present and the arrhythmia is considered to be the result of inadequate cardiac output, cardiac glycosides may be considered if they have not been used. A rapid-acting agent such as ouabain may be administered in a small test dose. If the arrhythmia becomes more severe, the glycoside infusion should be stopped immediately until the arrhythmia has been corrected. Ventricular tachycardia due to digitalis intoxication has been corrected successfully with propranolol, a *beta*-adrenergic blocking agent. Isoproterenol is indicated for the treatment of ventricular tachycardia occurring with Stokes-Adams syndrome and complete heart block in the dog, since cardiac pacemakers are generally not immediately available to the practicing veterinarian.

Unlike supraventricular tachycardias, the prognosis for dogs with ventricular tachycardia is very guarded. Ventricular tachycardia with alternating, bidirectional QRS complexes is usually an ominous sign. The prognosis is more favorable if signs of chronic, underlying heart disease are not present and if treatment is instituted immediately.

While conversion of the rhythm to normal is essential, one should attempt to define and correct the condition responsible for causing the arrhythmia (i.e. bacterial endocarditis, toxemia, etc.)

ATRIAL FIBRILLATION

In atrial fibrillation, atrial systole is absent, and the atria remain in a state of diastole (Katz and Pick, 1956). The atrial impulses to the atrioventricular node are rapid, fractionated, and irregular. The ventricular rate is rapid because many impulses excite the atrioventricular node. However, the rapid rate is irregular because some impulses enter the upper portions of the atrioventricular node but fail to emerge, thus making it temporarily refractory to subsequent impulses (Moe and Farah, 1965).

Atrial fibrillation is recognized electrocardiographically by irregularly spaced, normal to slightly aberrant ventricular complexes and the absence of regular P waves, which are replaced by baseline undulations (f waves) (Fig. 11-19). Initially "f" waves can be large (coarse) if the atrial rate is slow, but as the atrial rate increases in speed, the waves become smaller (fine) (Katz and Pick, 1956). Atrial hypertrophy also may increase the size of the "f" waves. Since the electrical orientation of "f" waves is random, they are not necessarily seen most clearly in

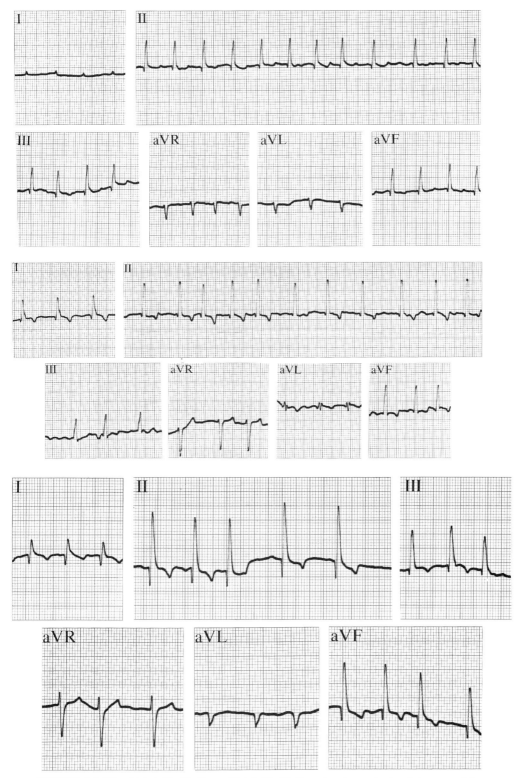

FIGURE 11-19 Atrial fibrillation. Atrial fibrillation is characterized by a rapid, irregular cardiac rate and the absence of P waves on the electrocardiogram. The QRS complexes are normal in configuration, but their duration and amplitude are often increased, suggesting cardiac hypertrophy. The R-R intervals vary, and irregularity of the base line replaces the P waves which normally occur prior to each QRS complex.

293

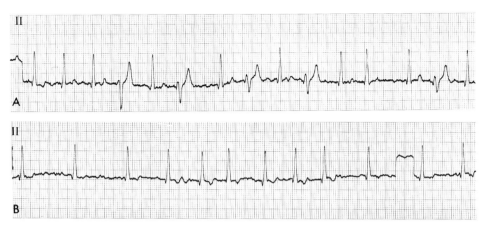

FIGURE 11-20 Atrial fibrillation with ventricular premature contractions. *A,* Atrial fibrillation with multiple unifocal ventricular premature contractions. In this case, the presence of ventricular premature contractions was thought to be the result of diminished cardiac output and congestive heart failure rather than a focal area of inflammation. When cardiac output improved after digitalization, the electrocardiogram was devoid of ventricular premature contractions and showed only atrial fibrillation (*B*).

leads II, III, and aVF as are normal P waves. If atrial fibrillation occurs with complete atrioventricular dissociation, the ventricular rate will be regular. In 22 undigitalized dogs with atrial fibrillation, the atrial rate varied from 430 to 1500 beats/min. (Detweiler, 1957). In the same study the duration of the QRS complex varied from 0.04 to 0.09 sec., averaging 0.064 sec., and seven of the 22 dogs had ventricular premature contractions (Fig. 11-20). When the ventricular rate is very rapid or slow, the marked irregularity in rhythm is difficult to detect on auscultation.

Salient diagnostic features of atrial fibrillation are (after Katz and Pick, 1956):

1. The absence of P waves.
2. The presence of "f" waves that are irregular in spacing, timing, and amplitude.
3. A grossly irregular ventricular rhythm.

Associations. Although atrial fibrillation occurs in a variety of cardiac conditions, it is generally considered to be associated with serious atrial enlargement and pathology. Atrial fibrillation has been reported to occur predominantly in male dogs; in one report (Detweiler, 1957), 82 per cent of the dogs affected were male; in another report (André, 1955) 71 per cent were male.

Of 59 dogs in which atrial fibrillation was diagnosed in our clinics, 75 per cent (45) were male. The arrhythmia was associated with congenital heart disease (patent ductus arteriosus; ventricular septal defect; congenital mitral insufficiency) in 7 per cent (4) of the dogs, and with acquired heart disease in 93 per cent (55). Of the 59 cases, 47 per cent (28) were dogs over 40 lb. in weight (Ettinger, 1969b).

Although the overall incidence of atrial fibrillation within a canine population is low (0.06 per cent of all cases according to Detweiler, 1957; and 0.04 per cent according to Patterson et al., 1961), it is one of the most frequently encountered pathologic cardiac tachyarrhythmias. It occurs most often in the medium-sized and giant breeds. Atrial fibrillation is rare in dogs weighing less than 10 lb., and dogs of medium weight are usually in congestive heart failure at the onset of the arrhythmia (Buchanan, 1965). Buchanan further notes that the giant breeds may have this arrhythmia for many months before congestive heart failure occurs. In our experience the diagnosis of atrial fibrillation in the giant or large breeds is rarely made until the dog shows signs of heart failure, whereas in dogs of the smaller breeds, signs of heart failure, atrial dysrhythmias, and chronic mitral valvular fibrosis are often apparent prior to the onset of atrial fibrillation. This difference is apparently related to the primary etiology of left atrial enlargement. In the smaller breeds it is associated as a further complication of chronic mitral valvular disease, a condition in which clinical signs occur prior to atrial fibrillation. In the larger breeds it is more often associated with idiopathic cardiomyopathy, the signs of which usually develop after atrial fibrillation becomes established.

Atrial fibrillation has been recognized in puppies, but it usually occurs in dogs over six years of age. In older dogs, atrial fibrillation is associated with mitral (and tricuspid) insufficiency and atrial dilatation (Patterson et al., 1961). In younger dogs, atrial fibrillation is associated with idiopathic cardiomyopathy (see pp. 392–400) and congenital heart defects such as patent ductus arteriosus (Fig. 18-4), tricuspid valvular hypoplasia, pulmonic stenosis (Detweiler, 1957), ventricular septal defects, and congenital mitral insufficiency. Although tests for microfilaria were positive in six (29 per cent) of 22 dogs in atrial fibrillation, heartworms were found in only one at necropsy (Detweiler, 1957). One of the 59 dogs seen by us had heartworm disease. The relationship between dirofilariasis and atrial fibrillation is thus unclear.

Signs.   In dogs with atrial fibrillation, signs of left and right heart failure are quite prominent. Syncope, weakness, weight loss and ascites are usually noticed on physical examination. The heart rate is irregular and rapid, and there is a pulse deficit (Fig. 11-21). Heart sounds and any murmurs present are variable in intensity (see pp. 25–26). Atrial fibrillation must be differentiated from ventricular premature contractions, atrial flutter, and paroxysmal ventricular tachycardia.

Treatment.   Because atrial fibrillation in the dog indicates advanced heart disease, a grave prognosis is in order. Therefore medical therapy should be instituted immediately when established atrial fibrillation has been diagnosed. It has been reported (Detweiler, 1957) that death ensues from a few hours to 28 weeks after onset of atrial fibrillation. However the authors have treated several cases successfully for over a year. Although spontaneous conversion from atrial fibrillation to sinus rhythm has not been reported, we have observed paroxysmal atrial fibrillation in several dogs (Fig. 11-22), as has Bonn (1969).

Digitalis is considered the initial treatment of choice for atrial fibrillation. Friedberg (1966) states that it is rare for digitalis to convert atrial fibrillation to sinus rhythm, and that if, in man, conversion to a normal sinus rhythm occurs during digitalis therapy, the arrhythmia converted spontaneously and was paroxysmal rather than established atrial fibrillation. Digitalis slows the ventricular rate through vagal and extravagal influences by increasing the effective refractory period of the atrioventricular transmission system and by increasing the atrial frequency (Moe and Farah, 1965). Therefore, rather than stopping atrial fibrillation, digitalis increases the atrial fibrillating rate but, more significantly, slows the

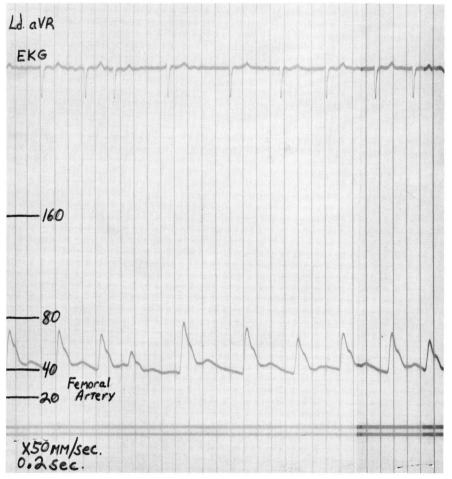

Figure 11-21 Simultaneous recording of electrocardiogram and femoral artery blood pressure curve during atrial fibrillation. The electrocardiogram indicates a rapid, irregular cardiac rate. The blood pressure tracing recorded simultaneously demonstrates the variable amplitude of the pulse generated by each ventricular contraction. The pulse is sometimes so small that a peripheral pulse is not palpable. This results in a pulse deficit when the heart is auscultated simultaneously with palpation of a peripheral artery.

ventricular rate. Digitalis therapy should probably be temporarily discontinued prior to cardioversion to prevent fatal arrhythmias, since cardiac irritability is increased when digitalis and direct current shock are used together (Friedberg, Cohn, and Donoso, 1965). Following cardioversion therapy with digitalis is instituted again.

After the dog has been digitalized and is no longer in heart failure, quinidine, because of its ability to abolish ectopic foci, may be administered in an attempt to restore a normal sinus rhythm. However, there has not been a high rate of successful conversion using this drug in the dog (Detweiler, 1957; Detweiler et al., 1968) although it has occasionally been effective (Detweiler, 1957; Pyle, 1967) (Fig. 11-23). Quinidine should be administered prior to and following cardioversion

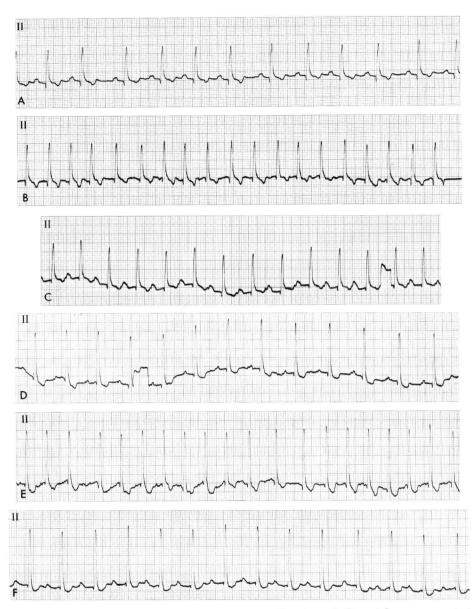

FIGURE 11-22 Paroxysmal atrial fibrillation. Tracings *A*, *B*, and *C* were recorded from a dog with advanced mitral valvular fibrosis. In *A*, sinus rhythm is present, and P mitrale and left ventricular hypertrophy are suggested. Four days later (*B*), the electrocardiogram indicated atrial fibrillation with a ventricular rate of 220 beats/min. Three days after atrial fibrillation developed another electrocardiogram was recorded (*C*), once again revealing a sinus rhythm. The dog had been digitalized prior to the first tracing and was maintained on digoxin throughout the period in which these tracings were made. The only change in therapy was the addition of diuretics after tracing (*A*) was recorded.

Tracings *D*, *E*, and *F* were recorded from another dog in which paroxysmal atrial fibrillation developed. The history and clinical course were the same for this dog as for the dog in tracings *A*, *B*, and *C*.

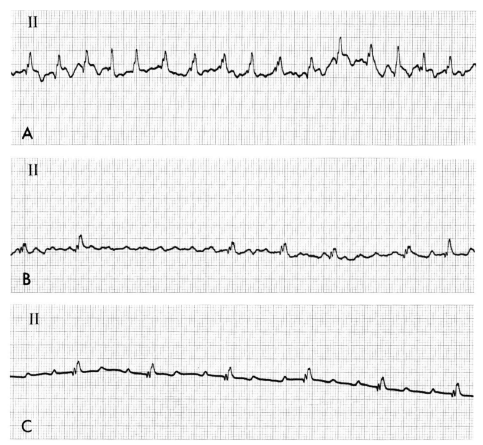

FIGURE 11-23 Conversion of atrial fibrillation by drug therapy. *A,* Atrial fibrillation is characterized by a ventricle beating rapidly and irregularly (280 beats/min.) and by the absence of P waves; it developed in this young dog as a sequela to idiopathic cardiomyopathy. After the dog was digitalized to slow the ventricular rate, digitalis therapy was discontinued. Quinidine was administered orally.

The intermediate rhythm of fibrillo-flutter (*B*) preceded the return of the sinus rhythm (*C*) 12 hours later. Following drug conversion with quinidine, both digoxin and quinidine were administered at maintenance levels.

(see Chap. 8) to prevent ectopic foci from recapturing the rhythm. Although digitalis and quinidine are used therapeutically in man, direct current cardioversion has proved to be rapid and consistently effective in restoring a normal rhythm after atrial fibrillation in man (Friedberg, 1966). It may have some value in dogs but has as yet not been widely utilized (Ettinger, 1968).

Successful cardioversion depolarizes the entire heart momentarily, hopefully allowing the sinoatrial node to resume its normal pacemaking function (Fig. 11-24). An effective shock must be of ample current strength, duration, voltage, and timing. The duration of the impulse, the voltage, and the synchronized timing after the R wave should be preset. The unit used by the authors (Fig. 5-3) is preset to deliver a shock for 2.5 msec. after the R wave. The current strength is hand-selected for each successive shock. In dogs, successful external cardioversion from atrial fibrillation has occurred between 100 and 275 watt-seconds. Im-

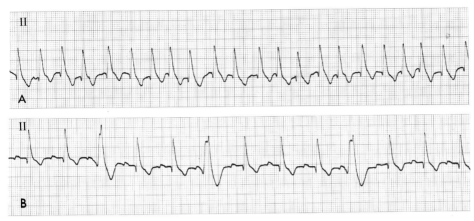

FIGURE 11-24 Conversion of atrial fibrillation to normal sinus rhythm using direct current shock. *A*, Electrocardiogram from a dog in atrial fibrillation with a ventricular rate of 260 beats/min. After treatment with cardiac glycosides to slow the heart rate and to relieve signs of congestive heart failure, cardioversion at 200 watt-seconds was performed. *B*, A normal sinus rhythm with a heart rate of 160 beats/min. was resumed. The third, sixth, and tenth beats are ventricular premature contractions, suggesting an irritable ventricular myocardium.

pulses at 100 watt-seconds are used initially in small dogs, and successive shocks are increased by 50 to 100 watt-seconds each.

Chronic heart failure and atrial fibrillation with cardiac enlargement do not contraindicate attempts at cardioversion. However, the percentage of success may not be high, and relapses are more common in both man and dogs when atrial fibrillation is associated with left atrial enlargement resulting from mitral insufficiency. Although our initial experience with cardioversion in the large breeds was poor, we have had greater success since the smaller electrode paddles were replaced with larger paddles. Cardioversion should be performed only when the patient is properly sedated or anesthetized. In dogs with both atrial fibrillation and congestive heart failure, cardioversion should not be attempted until the congestive heart failure has been controlled and anesthesia is not contraindicated.

ATRIAL FLUTTER

Atrial flutter is an uncommon rhythm in dogs (Clark, Szabuniewicz, and McCrady, 1966) although several cases have been described (Pedini, 1954; Detweiler, 1957; Gratzl, 1960). Detweiler's report also described two cases of atrial flutter that occurred when atrial fibrillation was treated with quinidine. In atrial flutter, P waves, also called flutter waves, are observed. These appear as regular symmetrical waves, which appear to be "saw-toothed." Flutter waves are best seen in leads II, III, and aVF. The ventricles respond in a periodic rhythm to flutter waves, occasionally with a 1:1 response but usually with some degree of atrioventricular block (i.e., 2:1, 3:1, 4:1, etc.). Perhaps the most important consideration in atrial flutter is that artifactual recordings may be mistaken for atrial flutter. Tachypnea, diaphragmatic flutter, hiccups, and tremors, as well as 60-cycle interference, can produce regular rhythmic waves that may be mistaken for atrial flutter (Fig. 4-45).

VENTRICULAR FIBRILLATION

It is important to differentiate ventricular fibrillation from ventricular tachycardia, for both therapeutic and prognostic purposes. The S-T segment and T wave are present on the electrocardiogram in ventricular tachycardia, whereas in ventricular fibrillation there is a complete lack of well-defined QRS complexes (Figs. 11-25, 11-26). The waves of ventricular fibrillation are larger than those of coarse atrial fibrillation. Ventricular fibrillation waves are of low voltage and appear as irregular undulations.

Ineffective twitching which is rapid, irregular, and uncoordinated occurs in ventricular fibrillation. The effect is equivalent to cardiac arrest. Heart sounds, pulse, and blood pressure disappear.

Treatment.   Ventricular fibrillation and cardiac arrest are the cardiac conditions with the gravest significance. Treatment must be instituted immediately and with certainty. Endotracheal intubation for the maintenance of a patent airway is the first consideration after one or more sharp precordial blows and external cardiac massage are begun. The administration of oxygen or continued mouth to

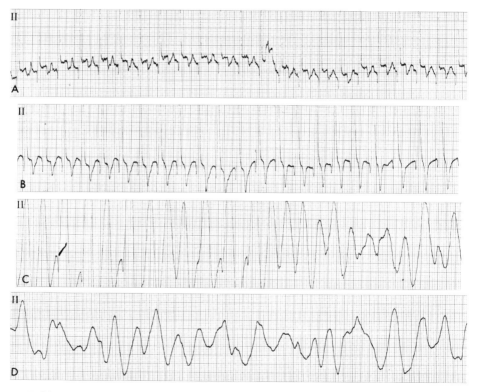

FIGURE 11-25 Ventricular fibrillation. Portions of an electrocardiogram recorded over a period of approximately 1 min. In tracing *A* there is a sinus rhythm and elevation of the S-T segment. Tracing *B* suggests ventricular tachycardia originating from the atrioventricular node or the bundle of His. The rhythm has progressed to ventricular flutter and ventricular fibrillation in tracing *C,* and ventricular fibrillation with a totally irregular baseline and no recognizable wave formation is seen in tracing *D.*

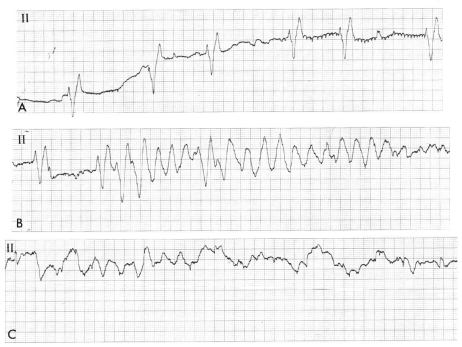

FIGURE 11-26   Ventricular fibrillation. *A,* Electrocardiogram recorded in a terminal state suggests an idioventricular rhythm. *B,* Ventricular flutter has developed. *C,* The irregular undulations of the base line are consistent with ventricular fibrillation.

tube artificial respiration is essential. If a defibrillator is available external defibrillation should be performed immediately using maximum-strength impulses. After intracardiac administration of 0.1 cc. of epinephrine, isoproterenol, or norepinephrine, continuous cardiac massage and artificial respiration are essential until a regular cardiac rate, voluntary respiration, and blood pressure can be restored.

DISTURBANCES IN CARDIAC CONDUCTION

Disturbances in conduction, also known as heart block, are classified as:

1. sinoatrial arrest and sinoatrial block (S-A arrest and S-A block);
2. atrioventricular block (A-V block);
3. bundle branch block (BBB); and
4. short P-R interval with prolonged QRS complex (Wolff-Parkinson-White [WPW] syndrome).

Bundle branch block has been reviewed previously (see pp. 149–153). The Wolff-Parkinson-White syndrome is an unusual condition in the dog but has been described by Patterson et al. (1961).

SINOATRIAL ARREST AND SINOATRIAL BLOCK

Delay or complete omission of the atrial response because of interference with the propagation and/or generation of impulses from the sinoatrial node to the atria produce a pause in the electrocardiogram during which the P wave and the accompanying QRS-T complex do not occur. The duration of the P-P interval is twice or more than twice that of the dominant P-P interval (Fig. 11-27). If the sinoatrial node is depressed, junctional atrioventricular nodal tissue or the ventricular fibers may assume the pacemaking function, generating nodal or ventricular escape beats (Fig. 11-27*B*).

Sinoatrial block is rare and requires differentiation from the frequently recognized sinus arrhythmia and sinoatrial arrest.

Associations.   Sinoatrial arrest or block is usually not clinically significant. It may result from digitalis, quinidine, or procainamide intoxication as well as from excessive vagal stimulation, such as that from ocular or carotid sinus pressure or diseases affecting the sites of vagal influence. Pathologic conditions of the atrial myocardium, such as dilatation or fibrosis, may be related to sinoatrial block. Intermittent sinoatrial arrest is most often observed in brachycephalic breeds as an incidental finding. Delay in cardiac rhythm is regularly related to inspiration and is therefore considered to be an extreme accentuation of sinus arrhythmia. Complete atrial standstill occurs in the presence of marked hyperkalemia (Figs. 17-9 and 17-10).

Signs.   General weakness due to asystole is usually the only clinical sign associated with sinoatrial block (Detweiler, 1952), but syncope with or without Stokes-Adams seizures may occur.

Treatment.   Atropine, epinephrine, or isoproterenol is useful when treatment is indicated to increase the heart rate and speed atrioventricular conduction. If

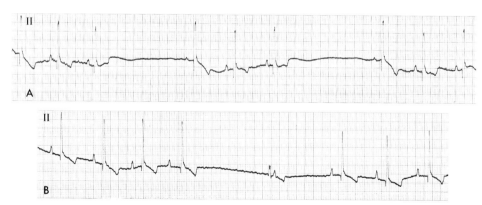

FIGURE 11-27   Sinoatrial arrest. *A,* After every three normal sinus beats occurring approximately 0.46 sec. apart, there is a long pause which is greater than two P-P or R-R intervals. This pause, called sinoatrial arrest, is an accentuation of sinus arrhythmia and occurs commonly in the brachycephalic breeds. This tracing was made from an asymptomatic dog (Boston Terrier) in which the cardiac rhythm was irregular on auscultation. (Courtesy of Dr. E. Baker.) *B,* When sinoatrial arrest is accentuated, the pacemaker tissue with the next lower threshhold is likely to assume the pacemaking function of the heart. After the fourth beat a long pause occurs, and an escape beat is produced. A P wave occurs after the aberrant QRS complex. The beat following the escape beat arises from the sinoatrial node and is therefore normal.

an electrolyte imbalance or a toxic response to a drug is the cause, the inciting agent should be eliminated and treatment administered only as required to increase cardiac conductivity.

ATRIOVENTRICULAR BLOCK

Atrioventricular block defines either partial delay or complete blockage of impulses conducted from the atria to the ventricles.

FIRST-DEGREE ATRIOVENTRICULAR BLOCK (PARTIAL OR INCOMPLETE HEART BLOCK). In first-degree atrioventricular block the P-R interval exceeds 0.13 sec. (Fig. 11-28). Each P wave is followed by a normal QRS-T complex. The cardiac rhythm is normal, and the prolongation of atrioventricular conduction time is properly diagnosed only with an electrocardiogram. When the P-R interval is sufficiently prolonged, the P wave may be superimposed on the preceding T wave; this is also encountered with rapid heart rates. Although first-degree heart block is an electrocardiographic abnormality, it does not necessarily indicate heart disease. It should be noted and correlated with the patient's condition, but disease should be suspected only if a clinical abnormality or drug toxicity is present.

SECOND-DEGREE HEART BLOCK (PARTIAL OR INCOMPLETE HEART BLOCK). In second-degree heart block the P waves and QRS complexes bear a continuous relationship until a ventricular beat is periodically dropped (Fig. 11-29). For example, after seven P-QRS-T complexes, an eighth P wave occurs with no subsequent ventricular complex. In the *Wenckebach* form of second-degree atrioventricular heart block (Fig. 11-29), the P-R interval increases progressively until the atrial impulse fails to emerge from the atrioventricular node; thus, no QRS complex is produced. The R-R interval diminishes while the P-R interval is prolonged. The Wenckebach phenomenon is almost always associated with digitalis intoxication. In *advanced second-degree heart block* (Fig. 11-30), the ventricle responds only to every second, third, or fourth P wave, resulting in 2:1, 3:1, or 4:1 block, respectively. Other forms of advanced second degree heart block may occur, such as 9:5, 5:2, 7:5, etc. Advanced second degree heart block with incomplete atrioventricular dissociation may occur. In such cases the QRS complexes appear normal in configuration and occur at a rate greater than 40 per min. Except when capture beats occur there is no relationship between the P waves and QRS complexes.

THIRD-DEGREE HEART BLOCK (COMPLETE HEART BLOCK). In complete heart block, atrial and ventricular activity are independent but regular, and the P-R intervals are irregular. Because the ventricular complexes bear no constant relationship to the P waves, there is no true P-R interval. More P waves than QRS complexes are usually present because the atrial rate exceeds that of the slow independent ventricular pacemaker (Fig. 11-30), unless atrial fibrillation or ventricular tachycardia occurs. In complete heart block, the QRS complex may be normal or idioventricular, depending on the origin of the ventricular pacemaker — i.e., near the common bundle of His, in the Purkinje system, or in the ventricular myocardium. A slow ventricular rate, under 40 per min., is required for the diagnosis of complete heart block. In the dog, the slow idioventricular rhythm that occurs in complete heart block may be very irregular.

The P-R interval can be used to help distinguish second- from third-degree heart block. The P-R interval following the dropped beat is constant in second-

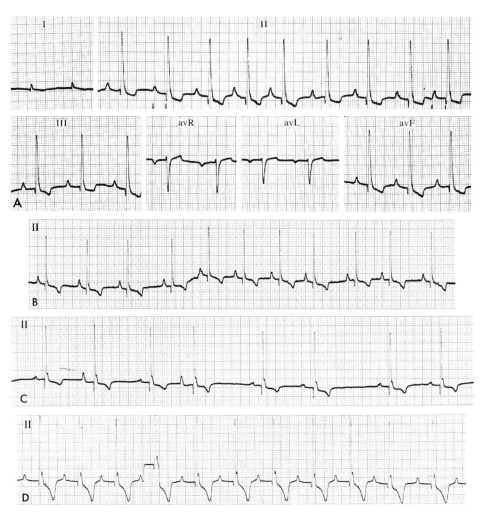

FIGURE 11-28 First degree atrioventricular block (incomplete block). First degree atrioventricular block is characterized by a normal rhythm in which the duration of the P-R interval is greater than 0.13 sec. *A,* The P-R interval is 0.14 sec. and is easily seen in all leads except lead I. Often, however, the P wave and P-R interval are best seen in leads II, III, and aVF. *B,* Tracing from dog with chronic mitral valvular fibrosis and signs of congestive heart failure. Prior to cardiac therapy, the heart rate was 140 beats/min., and the P-R interval was 0.10 sec. *C,* After the dog in *B* showed clinical signs of digitalis intoxication, the heart rate was 90 beats/min., a wandering pacemaker had developed, and the P-R interval was 0.14 sec. in duration, demonstrating mild digitalis intoxication electrocardiographically in the form of first degree heart block. *D,* In another dog, the P-R interval is prolonged to 0.17 sec. as a result of digitalis intoxication.

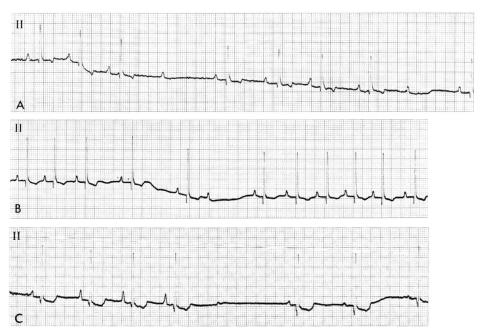

FIGURE 11-29 Second degree atrioventricular block (incomplete heart block). This block is characterized by a normal sequence of electrocardiographic complexes followed by periodic dropping of the QRS complex after a P wave. A, The Wenckebach phenomenon occurs with digitalis intoxication and is characterized by progressive prolongation of the P-R interval until a P wave occurs without a QRS complex. In this tracing the P-R interval progresses as follows: 0.12 sec., 0.12 sec., 0.13 sec., P wave without a QRS complex, etc. B, Second degree atrioventricular block is characterized by normal electrocardiographic complexes until the sixth P wave occurs without a QRS complex. Second degree atrioventricular block in the dog is usually due to digitalis intoxication. C, Second degree atrioventricular block in the dog is often characterized by P waves with variable configurations.

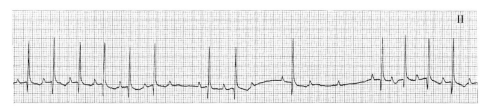

FIGURE 11-30. Advanced second degree atrioventricular block. Various types of second degree heart block are seen in this tracing. The rhythm is normal until the seventh P wave occurs without a QRS complex (7:6 block). The eighth and ninth complexes are complete, but the tenth P wave is not conducted through the atrioventricular node to the ventricle (3:2 block). The eleventh complex is again complete, but the twelfth and thirteenth P waves are not conducted (3:1 block). The fifteenth beat is an atrial premature contraction.

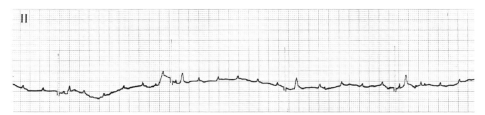

FIGURE 11-31 Third degree heart block. In third degree heart block the P waves occur at one rate, and the QRS complexes occur independently at a slower rate. In this tracing, the P waves are occurring at a rate of approximately 140/min., and the slower idioventricular rate is 26/min. Paper speed = 25 mm./sec.

degree heart block, whereas in third-degree heart block the duration of the P-R interval after the pause varies, since no true relationship between the P wave and the QRS complex exists. At times in advanced second degree heart block there may not be a true relationship between the P wave and the QRS complex.

Associations. Atrioventricular block is associated with many conditions, such as congenital heart lesions (Hamlin, 1966; James and Konde, 1969), toxins from infectious processes (Robertson and Ramy, 1968), and chronic heart disease (Ettinger, 1969a), as well as endocardial and myocardial fibrosis, thoracic masses, surgical cardiac trauma, reflex vagal stimulation, and hypoxia. Digitalis glycosides are probably the most common cause of serious atrioventricular block. Hyperkalemia may be associated with complete heart block as well as with atrial standstill (Figs. 17-9 and 17-10). Buchanan (1965) reported incomplete heart block in dogs with pericardial effusion and heartworms, and Patterson et al. (1961) reported heart block due to a parasitic granuloma near the atrioventricular node. Dear (1970) reported complete heart block with spontaneous reversion to a sinus rhythm in a young dog. In the latter case the condition could not be related to toxic, infectious, or metabolic causes.

Signs. There are no clinical signs associated with first-degree heart block unless the heart block has been produced by digitalis intoxication, in which case vomiting, anorexia, and lethargy are usually recognized first. The intensity of the first heart sound in first-degree heart block may be diminished, since the atrioventricular valves do not close abruptly but rather have time to float into apposition.

Bradycardia and a forceful apical beat denoting increased stroke volume are present with advanced atrioventricular block. Variable degrees of filling of the ventricles produce heart sounds of varying intensity. Low-pitched atrial sounds are heard at the cardiac apex when the atria contract independently of the ventricles (Fig. 2-12). When right atrial systole occurs against a closed tricuspid valve, as often occurs in complete heart block, blood is forced retrograde into the jugular vein, producing a cannon "a" wave. Lifeless, weak dogs are occasionally presented with a history of syncopal seizures with or without convulsions (Stokes-Adams seizures) due to second- and third-degree atrioventricular block (Ettinger, 1969a). Syncope occurs when cerebral ischemia results during the periods of asystole.

Treatment. Therapy is usually not necessary for digitalis-induced heart block, and digitalis must be discontinued *immediately* in all but first-degree heart block. The continued use of digitalis in the presence of first-degree heart block depends on whether symptoms of digitalis intoxication have developed.

Isoproterenol is the drug of choice for the treatment of heart block when clinical signs are present. It increases atrioventricular impulse conduction and ventricular excitability. It is administered either as a 5 μg./cc. intravenous infusion with dextrose and water (1 mg./200 cc.) to effect a ventricular rate of 80 to 120 beats per min. (Ettinger, 1969a), or as a single bolus of 0.05 mg., intravenously (Buchanan et al., 1968) (Fig. 11-32). Isoproterenol is then given every four hours (0.1 to 0.2 mg., intramuscularly or subcutaneously) until rate and rhythm control has been established. Then sustained-action isoproterenol (Proternol) tablets (15 to 30 mg. four to six times a day) are administered. Elixir and sublingual forms of isoproterenol are not recommended for use in treating atrioventricular block in the dog. Atropine, epinephrine, and corticosteroids have been used infrequently since the introduction of isoproterenol. Antiarrhythmic agents accentuate atrioventricular block, as do the digitalis glycosides, which may also increase ectopic

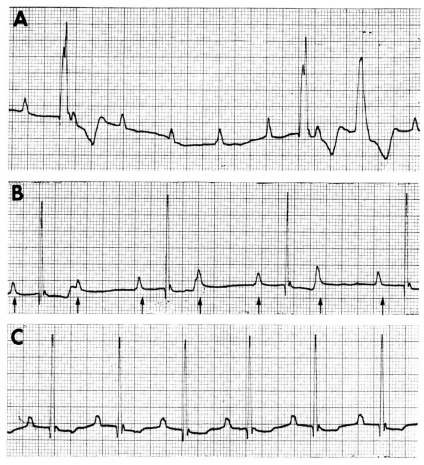

FIGURE 11-32   Heart block and medical therapy. *A,* Complete heart block. The atrial rate is 210/min., and the ventricular rate is 40/min., with a ventricular premature contraction following the second QRS complex. *B,* Forty-eight hours after isoproterenol therapy was initiated, second-degree atrioventricular block with 2:1 conduction is demonstrated by two P waves (arrow) for each successive QRS complex. *C,* Ninety-six hours after therapy was initiated, a normal sinus rhythm returned. *From* Ettinger, S.: J. A. V. M. A., 154 (1969):399.

ventricular irritability. Cardiac glycosides are administered in cases of heart block only when congestive heart failure is intractable (Buchanan et al., 1968). Implantation of a cardiac pacemaker in a dog with complete heart block has been performed successfully (Buchanan et al., 1968).

ARRHYTHMIAS DURING ANESTHESIA AND SURGERY

Arrhythmias are often produced by excessive concentration of anesthetic agents (cyclopropane, halothane, trichlorethylene, and intravenous barbiturates). Anesthetic agents administered in conjunction with catecholamines (such as epinephrine) can precipitate arrhythmias, as can excessive concentrations of carbon dioxide and acidosis. In addition, surgical manipulation of the abdominal viscera, the epiglottis, the adrenal glands, and the bones may stimulate arrhythmias.

In summary, anesthetic and surgical arrhythmias can be controlled by both non-drug and pharmacologic means.

For non-drug correction of arrhythmias:

1. Decrease the concentration of gaseous anesthetics.
2. Eliminate excessive carbon dioxide and increase the oxygen concentration of the anesthetic mixture.
3. Discontinue catecholamine infusion.
4. Discontinue surgical manipulations temporarily.

If these methods fail to diminish the frequency of ectopic impulses, pharmacologic agents may be useful. Lidocaine or procainamide, administered intravenously, are the most commonly used rapid-acting antiarrhythmic drugs. Lidocaine (without epinephrine) is given as a bolus over one to two minutes using an approximate dose of 2 to 4 mg./lb. body weight or less if the arrhythmia is rapidly converted. Procainamide is less desirable because it may induce arterial hypotension. It may be given in doses of 100 mg., waiting approximately 1 min. between doses, until conversion of the arrhythmia occurs or intoxication develops.

References

André, T.: Enlargement of the Heart with Congestive Heart Failure in Dogs. Nord. Vet.-Med., 7 (1955):905.

Buchanan, J. W.: Spontaneous Arrhythmias and Conduction Disturbances in Domestic Animals. Ann. N. Y. Acad. Sci., 127 (1965):224.

Buchanan, J. W., Dear, M. G., Pyle, R. L., and Berg, P.: Medical and Pacemaker Therapy of Complete Heart Block and Congestive Heart Failure in a Dog. J. A. V. M. A., 152 (1968):1099.

Clark, D. R., Szabuniewicz, M., and McCrady, J. D.: Clinical Use of the Electrocardiogram in Animals. Vet. Med., 61 (1966):751, 861, and 973.

Dear, M. G.: Spontaneous Reversion of Complete A-V Block to Sinus Rhythm in the Dog, J. Small., Anim. Pract., 11 (1970):17.

Detweiler, D. K.: Heart Disease in Dogs. Univ. Pa. Bull., Vet. Ext. Quart., 125 (1952):21.

Detweiler, D. K.: Electrocardiographic and Clinical Features of Spontaneous Auricular Fibrillation and Flutter (Tachycardia) in Dogs. Zbl. Veterinaermed., 4 (1957):509.

Detweiler, D. K., Hubben, K., and Patterson, D. F.: Survey of Cardiovascular Disease in Dogs—Preliminary Report on the First 1,000 Dogs Screened. Amer. J. Vet. Res., 21 (1960):329.

Detweiler, D. K., Patterson, D. F., Luginbühl, H., Rhodes, W. H., Buchanan, J. W., Knight, D. H., and Hill, J. D.: Diseases of the Cardiovascular System. In *Canine Medicine*. Edited by E. J. Catcott. 1st Catcott Edition. American Veterinary Publications, Inc., Santa Barbara, California (1968):589.

Ettinger, P.: Synchronization During Electrical Pacing. Amer. Heart J., 70 (1965):110.

Ettinger, S.: Conversion of Spontaneous Atrial Fibrillation in Dogs, Using Direct Current Synchronized Shock. J. A. V. M. A., 152 (1968):41.

Ettinger, S.: Isoproterenol Treatment of Atrioventricular Block in the Dog. J. A. V. M. A., 154 (1969a):398.

Ettinger, S.: Unpublished Observations of Atrial Fibrillation, 1969b.

Ettinger, S., and Buergelt, C. D.: Atrioventricular Dissociation (Incomplete) with Accrochage in a Dog with Ruptured Chordae Tendineae. Amer. J. Vet. Res., 29 (1968):1499.

Fried, K. J.: Fibrillation and Tachysystole of Auricles and Ventricles in Dogs. Cas. Cesk. Vet., 5 (1949):98.

Friedberg, C. K.: Diseases of the Heart. W. B. Saunders, Philadelphia, 1966.

Friedberg, C. K., Cohn, L. J., and Donoso, E.: Arrhythmias Following External Direct-Current Shock. Circulation, Supplement 32 (1965):II-89.

Gratzl, E.: Tachykardien beim Hund, eine klinische und elektrokardiographische Studie. Wien. Tieraerztl. Mschr., 47 (1960):281.

Gyarmati, E.: Klinische elektrokardiographische Untersuchungen beim Hunde. Diss., Budapest, Hungary. 1939.

Hamlin, R.: Heart Block. In *Current Veterinary Therapy 1966—1967*. Edited by R. W. Kirk. W. B. Saunders, Philadelphia, 1966.

Hoffman, B. F., and Cranefield, P. F.: The Physiological Basis of Cardiac Arrhythmias. Amer. J. Med., 37 (1964):670.

Huisman, G. H., and Teunissen, G. H. B.: Paroxysmal Ventricular Tachycardia in the Dog. Zbl. Veterinaermed., 10 (1963):273.

James, T. N., and Konde, W. N.: A Clinicopathologic Study of Heart Block in a Dog, with Remarks Pertinent to the Embryology of the Cardiac Conduction System, Amer. J. Cardiol., 24 (1969):59.

Katz, L. N., and Pick, A.: Clinical Electrocardiography. Part I. The Arrhythmias. Lea & Febiger, Philadelphia, 1956.

Kersten, U., Winterfeldt, K., Brass, W.: Zur Häufigkeit von Herzrhythmusstörungen beim Hund. Tieraerztl. Umsch., 24 (1969):110.

Lange, H.: Über den Eintritt der Atmungsarrhythmie in der ersten Lebenzeit des Hundes. Diss., University of Munich, Munich, Germany. 1937.

Lannek, N.: A Clinical and Experimental Study on the Electrocardiogram in Dogs. Royal Vet. College, Stockholm, Sweden, 1949.

Marek, J., Manninger, R., and Mòcsy, J. F.: Spezielle Pathologie und Therapie der Haustiere. Edited by Fischer, Jena, Germany, 9th ed. 1945.

Moe, G. K., and Farah, A. E.: Digitalis and Allied Cardiac Glycosides. In *The Pharmacological Basis of Therapeutics*. Edited by L. Goodman and A. Gilman. The Macmillan Co., New York, 3rd ed., 1965.

Patterson, D. F., Detweiler, D. K., Hubben, K., and Botts, R. P.: Spontaneous Abnormal Cardiac Arrhythmias and Conduction Disturbances in the Dog (A Clinical and Pathologic Study of 3000 Dogs). Amer. J. Vet. Res., 22 (1961):355.

Pedini, B.: Flutuazione Atriale Pura E Bigeminismo Extrasistolico In Un Cane. Vet. Italiana, 5 (1954):1003.

Pyle, R. L.: Conversion of Atrial Fibrillation with Quinidine Sulfate in a Dog. J. A. V. M. A., 151 (1967):582.

Robertson, B. T., and Ramy, C. T.: Reversible Heart Block in a Dog. J. A. V. M. A., 152 (1968):1110.

Roos, J.: Auricular Fibrillation in the Domestic Animals. Heart, 11 (1924):1.

Roos, J.: Atrioventrikularer Herzrhythmus beim Hund (Paroxysmale Tachycardie mit periodischem Herzstillstand). Tijdschr. Diergeneesk, 64 (1937):969. [Abstract in Wien. Tieraerztl. Mschr., 24 (1938):151.]

Zanzucchi, A.: Le Aritmie Cardiache nel Cane. Richerche di Electrocardiografia Clinica. Profilàssi, 10 (1937):136.

SECTION IV

ACQUIRED AND CONGENITAL HEART DISEASE

Chapter 12 THE INCIDENCE OF HEART DISEASE IN DOGS

Chapter 13 ACQUIRED VALVULAR AND ENDOCARDIAL HEART DISEASE

Chapter 14 ACQUIRED DISEASES OF THE MYOCARDIUM

Chapter 15 DISEASES OF THE PERICARDIUM

Chapter 16 COR PULMONALE

Chapter 17 MISCELLANEOUS CONDITIONS AFFECTING THE CARDIOVASCULAR SYSTEM

Chapter 18 CONGENITAL HEART DISEASES

Chapter 19 SURGICAL CORRECTION OF PATENT DUCTUS ARTERIOSUS AND VASCULAR RING ANOMALIES

12

THE INCIDENCE OF HEART DISEASE IN DOGS

The term heart disease encompasses all morphologic and functional cardiac pathology. Since this text is devoted to the description of clinical cardiac disease, only those pathologic conditions that are known to produce clinical signs are described. However, even this limited number of conditions requires appropriate classification if the diseases are to be presented systematically.

It is generally accepted that cardiac diseases should be classified as acquired or congenital. Heart disease is congenital when an animal is born with a cardiac anomaly resulting from defective embryologic development. This does not imply, however, a genetic basis for the defect. Acquired heart disease refers to any cardiac condition that develops after birth, again without implicating a specific etiologic factor.

Congenital heart diseases are classified according to the anatomic structures involved. In most cases insufficient information precludes classification of acquired heart diseases entirely according to etiology, although such a classification would be desirable for prognostic, differential diagnostic, and therapeutic purposes. Thus, in this text, acquired heart diseases are also classified according to the structures involved—the valves and endocardium, the myocardium, and the pericardium. The disease conditions in these categories are then further subdivided with respect to the lesions, the etiology, and any complications, such as left atrial tear secondary to chronic valvular fibrosis. Primary lung disease (cor pulmonale) and miscellaneous conditions affecting the heart are also included in this classification.

This classification is admittedly arbitrary, and it does not always correlate with the classification adopted by pathologists. It is not always possible to correlate even extensive morphologic myocardial abnormalities with clinical signs of disease (Detweiler et al., 1968b). Furthermore, because cardiac diseases are often atypical and do not always fit into one of the broad categories proposed, a condition can simultaneously display features that are typical of more than one type of disease. Nevertheless, as our knowledge in cardiology increases, new data will help to improve and complete this classification, and real or apparent differences from other classifications, such as those used by the pathologists, will hopefully be eliminated.

The results of clinical surveys of heart disease in dogs vary greatly, depending on factors such as the diagnostic criteria used and the geographic location in which the study has been made.

In one study (Detweiler and Patterson, 1965), heart disease (congenital and acquired) was present in 545 of 4831 dogs (11.3 per cent) examined consecutively at the University of Pennsylvania (Fig. 12-1 and Table 12-1). In addition, heart disease could not be ruled out in 482 other dogs in the group, and 37 dogs had conditions which could lead to heart disease. Of the 545 dogs which had heart disease, 27 (5 per cent) had congenital lesions, and 518 (95 per cent) had acquired lesions. Of the 4831 dogs, 1.4 per cent were in congestive heart failure, and 75 per cent of these had clinical or postmortem evidence of valvular fibrosis and myocardial damage (Detweiler et al., 1968a). The prevalence of cardiovascular lesions recognized clinically by Detweiler et al. (1961) and at necropsy by Jones and Zook (1965) in two different hospitals is shown in Figures 12-2 and 12-3.

At the veterinary college in Hannover, Germany, 1037 dogs were examined over three and three-fourths years because they had a history compatible with heart disease (Kersten, 1968). Heart disease was definitely diagnosed in 745 dogs, or in approximately 5 per cent of all dogs examined in the clinic during this period. In 145 dogs, heart disease could not be ruled out. Congenital heart disease was diagnosed in 2.4 per cent of the dogs with cardiac disease.

In a study done by Taylor and Sittnikow (1968) at the veterinary college in Helsinki, Finland, in 1967, 166 of 4126 dogs examined in the clinic had clinical signs compatible with heart disease. On special cardiac examination, 124 (3 per cent) were found to have definite heart disease, 15 (0.34 per cent) had pulmonary diseases, and the remaining dogs had other diseases. Of the 124 dogs with heart disease, 112 dogs (90.3 per cent) had acquired cardiac lesions, and 12 dogs (9.7 per cent) had congenital heart disease.

The clinical approach to congenital cardiovascular disease differs in many ways from the approach to acquired heart disease. The veterinarian is often sought by the owner of a dog with acquired heart disease because the dog has developed signs of heart failure. On the other hand, congenital disease is often first recognized during routine examination for a health certificate or vaccination, or prior to anesthesia. Thus, the condition is often recognized before signs of heart failure develop.

The methods used to diagnose congenital heart disease also differ from those used in diagnosing acquired disease. In most dogs with acquired disease, the history and physical examination provide a great portion of the information needed for the final diagnosis, and electrocardiography and radiography confirm or amplify the tentative diagnosis. In dogs with congenital heart disease, the physical examination must often be supplemented by a number of special procedures, such as cardiac catheterization and angiocardiography, before a definitive diagnosis can be made.

The specialized studies required to confirm the diagnosis of congenital car-

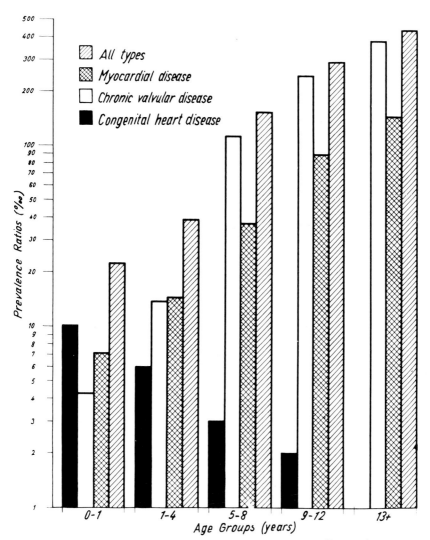

FIGURE 12-1   Prevalence ratios of various types of heart disease by age groups. Data from 4831 dogs. From Detweiler, D. K., and Patterson, D. F.: Ann. N. Y. Acad. Sci., 127 (1965):481.

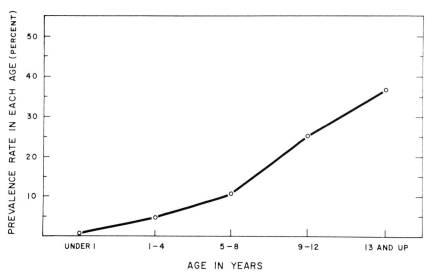

FIGURE 12-2 Prevalence of clinically recognized cardiovascular disease in 3000 dogs. Based on data from Detweiler, D. K., et al.: Amer. J. Public Health, 51 (1961):228. *In* Detweiler, D. K. and Patterson, D. F.: Ann. N. Y. Acad. Sci., 127 (1965): 481.

diac anomalies often require expensive, sophisticated equipment which cannot be justified in private practice. In the description of the conditions, mention is made of these specialized studies, even though they may not be clinically feasible, in order to provide a more complete description of the condition as well as additional information on the pathophysiology of the specific defect.

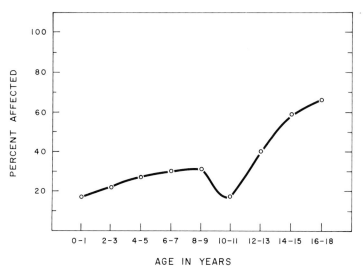

FIGURE 12-3 Age distribution of cardiovascular lesions found at necropsy. From Jones, T. C., and Zook, B. C.: Ann. N. Y. Acad. Sci., 127 (1965):671.

ACQUIRED HEART DISEASE

The prevalence of acquired cardiac disease in dogs is known because clinical and pathologic studies are available from large numbers of dogs (Detweiler et al., 1960; Detweiler et al., 1961; Patterson et al., 1961; Das and Tashjian, 1965; Detweiler and Patterson, 1965; Jones and Zook, 1965; Pensinger, 1965; Detweiler et al., 1968a, 1968b; Kersten, 1968; Pensinger, 1968; Taylor and Sittnikow, 1968). In general, acquired heart disease is recognized in approximately 8 to 10 per cent of a large, randomly selected group of dogs (Detweiler and Patterson, 1965).

Acquired heart disease is most common in dogs over five years of age. Although chronic fibrosis of the atrioventricular valves has been observed in 72 per cent (Detweiler and Patterson, 1965) and 73 per cent (Pensinger, 1965) of dogs with heart disease, other conditions are seen often enough to warrant consideration. Whereas the incidence of heart disease is only slightly greater in male than in female dogs (Detweiler and Patterson, 1965), the incidence of chronic congestive heart failure is two and one-half times greater in males than in females (Detweiler et al., 1961).

The prevalence ratios of acquired and congenital heart diseases in different age groups, as reported by Detweiler and Patterson (1965), are presented in Figure 12-1 and Table 12-1.

In Kersten's study (1968), approximately 5 per cent of the clinic population, or 745 dogs over a period of three and three-fourths years, were recognized as having heart disease. Acquired heart disease was diagnosed in 97.6 per cent of these cases. Myocardial disease was reported in 47.8 per cent of the cases; these dogs did not have murmurs, but cardiac enlargement and electrocardiographic changes such as ventricular premature contractions, conduction disturbances, or disturbances in depolarization and repolarization were present. Valvular disease was diagnosed in 46.1 per cent of the 745 dogs when typical murmurs could be auscultated, and a large number of dogs in this group also had signs of myocardial disease. In 3.7 per cent of the dogs with heart disease, cardiac enlargement was evident on radiographs but there were no other clinical signs.

TABLE 12-1 TYPES OF HEART DISEASE FOUND AMONG 4831 DOGS SCREENED (CLINICAL AND/OR POSTMORTEM DIAGNOSES)*

Congenital heart disease		27
Pulmonic stenosis	6	
Patent ductus arteriosus	5	
Subaortic stenosis	3	
Tetralogy of Fallot	3	
Persistent right aortic arch	2	
Pulmonic stenosis and patent ductus arteriosus	1	
Interventricular septal defect	1	
Incompletely diagnosed	6	
Acquired heart disease		518
Chronic valvular disease	297	
Myocardial disease	68	
Chronic valvular and myocardial disease	94	
Other	59	
Total		545

*From Detweiler, D. K., and Patterson, D. F.: Ann. N. Y. Acad. Sci., *127*:481, 1965.

Of 4126 dogs examined by Taylor and Sittnikow (1968), 112 dogs had acquired heart disease (90.3 per cent of all dogs with heart disease). Of this group of 112 dogs, 48 had myocardial disease, 30 had valvular disease, 14 had both valvular and myocardial disease, and 20 had other heart diseases such as acute heart failure, cor pulmonale, pericardial adhesions, and mediastinal tumors. The high incidence of myocardial disease was attributed to the fact that many of the dogs examined had myocardial disease secondary to other conditions such as uremia or pyometra. Of 38 dogs which were necropsied, valvular disease was found in 16 and myocardial disease in 22.

CONGENITAL HEART DISEASE

Since many puppies die early in the postnatal period or are still-born, the true incidence of congenital heart disease in dogs is unknown. Further, many puppies affected with congenital heart disease die prior to six to eight weeks of age, before they have been examined by a veterinarian, and necropsy examinations are rarely performed on these dogs.

Anderson (1957) reported that 30 per cent of puppies from a Beagle colony died earlier than six weeks of age, and although figures were not given for the incidence of heart disease, such a high postnatal mortality rate probably indicates that some dogs had congenital heart disease. To further demonstrate the likelihood of early postnatal mortality, Patterson (1968) reported that of 36 offspring from test matings of dogs with patent ductus arteriosus, two pups died before one week of age owing to heart failure associated with patent ductus arteriosus. In 15 others with clinical signs of patent ductus arteriosus in which the ductus was not corrected surgically, nine died because of congestive heart failure between two and six weeks of age.

The incidence of congenital cardiac anomalies recognized clinically is considerably less than that of acquired heart disease. Detweiler and Patterson (1965) and Patterson (1965) suggested that congenital lesions occurred in about 0.5 per cent of the 4831 consecutive cases examined by them and Patterson (1968) subsequently increased this figure slightly to 0.68 per cent.

Jones and Zook (1965) recognized 18 cases of congenital disease among 991 canine necropsies. Of the 18 dogs, 15 (83 per cent) were under one year of age.

In dogs examined because of clinical signs referable to heart disease, the incidence of congenital heart disease was 2.4 per cent in one study (Kersten, v. Winterfeldt, and Brass, 1969) and 9.7 per cent in another (Taylor and Sittnikow, 1968).

The incidence of congenital cardiac defects is higher in purebred dogs (8.9 per 1000 cases) than it is in mongrel dogs (2.6 per 1000 cases) (Patterson, 1968). Patterson (1968) also reported that the incidence of a number of congenital defects was higher in certain breeds than in the general population. Patent ductus arteriosus prevailed in Poodles, Pomeranians, and Collies; pulmonic stenosis in the English Bulldog, Chihuahua, and Fox Terrier; tetralogy of Fallot in the Keeshond; subaortic stenosis in the German Shepherd, Boxer, and Newfoundland; and persistent right aortic arch in the German Shepherd and Irish Setter. With the exception of patent ductus arteriosus, which occurs more often in female than in male dogs (2.49 per 1000 vs. 1.45 per 1000), there seems to be no significant sex predisposition for congenital cardiac defects.

TABLE 12-2 CARDIOVASCULAR MALFORMATIONS IN 290 DOGS*

MALFORMATION	NUMBER OF MALFORMATIONS		
	1953-1957 (50 dogs)	1958-1965 (240 dogs)	TOTAL (290 dogs)
Patent ductus arteriosus	14	68	82
Pulmonic stenosis	10	47	57
Aortic stenosis	3	37	40
Persistent right aortic arch	6	17	23
Ventricular septal defect	2	18	20
Tetralogy of Fallot	2	9	11
Ostium secundum atrial septal defect (incl. patent foramen ovale)	1	11	12
Persistent left cranial vena cava	3	10	13
Mitral insufficiency		9	9
Pericardial anomalies:			
Pericardio-diaphragmatic hernia	1	2	3
Absent pericardium		1	1
Incomplete pericardium		1	1
Arterial anomalies:			
Retroesophageal right subclavian artery		1	1
Separate origin of right subclavian			
Artery from ascending aorta		2	2
Ebstein's anomaly of the tricuspid valve	1		1
Tricuspid insufficiency		1	1
Double outlet right ventricle		1	1
Anomalous pulmonary venous drainage		1	1
Conduction disturbance without			
Gross malformations			
Right bundle branch block		2	2
Wolff-Parkinson-White Syndrome		1	1
Arteriovenous fistula		1	1
Incompletely diagnosed	11	31	42
TOTAL†	54	271	325

*From Patterson, D. F.: Circ. Res., 23:171, 1968.
†More than one malformation was found in 32 dogs.

Of 290 dogs with congenital heart disease described by Patterson (1968), a definitive diagnosis was made in 248; 216 dogs had single congenital anomalies, and multiple anomalies were present in 32 dogs (Table 12-2).

From analysis of pedigree, test matings of affected dogs, and chromosomal analysis (Patterson et al., 1966; Patterson, 1968), it has been recognized that certain congenital cardiac anomalies, such as patent ductus arteriosus in the Poodle, valvular pulmonic stenosis in Beagles, and fibrous subaortic stenosis in Newfoundlands, result from specific, genetically determined developmental abnormalities. There is some degree of genetic influence on persistent right aortic arch in the German Shepherd, as well as on persistent left cranial vena cava associated with persistent right aortic arch in this breed. Tetralogy of Fallot is one of a number of congenital cardiac malformations which are genetically determined in the Keeshond breed.

References

Anderson, A. C.: Puppy Production to the Weaning Age. J. A. V. M. A., 130 (1957):151.
Bohn, F. K.: Paroxysmales Vorhofflimmern bei Hunden. Deutsche Tierärztliche Wochenschrift, 76 (1969):198.

Das, K. M., and Tashjian, R. J.: Chronic Mitral Valve Disease in the Dog. Vet. Med., 60 (1965):1209.

Detweiler, D. K., Hubben, K., Patterson, D. F., and Botts, R. P.: Survey of Cardiovascular Disease in Dogs — Preliminary Report on the First 1000 Dogs Screened. Amer. J. Vet. Res., 21 (1960):329.

Detweiler, D. K., Luginbühl, H., Buchanan, J. W., and Patterson, D. F.: The Natural History of Acquired Cardiac Disability of the Dog. Ann. N. Y. Acad. Sci., 147 (1968a): 318.

Detweiler, D. K., and Patterson, D. F.: The Prevalence and Types of Cardiovascular Disease in Dogs. Ann. N. Y. Acad. Sci., 127 (1965):481.

Detweiler, D. K., Patterson, D. F., Hubben, K., and Botts, R. P.: The Prevalence of Spontaneously Occurring Cardiovascular Disease in Dogs. Amer. J. Public Health, 51 (1961):228.

Detweiler, D. K., Patterson, D. F., Luginbühl, H., Rhodes, W. H., Buchanan, J. W., Knight, D. H., and Hill, J. D.: Diseases of the Cardiovascular System. In *Canine Medicine*. Edited by E. J. Catcott. 1st Catcott ed. American Veterinary Publications, Inc., Santa Barbara, California (1968b):589.

Jones, T. C., and Zook, B. C.: Aging Changes in the Vascular System of Animals. Ann. N. Y. Acad. Sci., 127 (1965):671.

Kersten, U.: Klinische Untersuchungen am herzkranken Hund. Thesis, Hannover, Germany, 1968.

Kersten, U., v. Winterfeld, K., and Brass, W.: Statistische Erhebungen über Herzkrankheiten beim Hund. Kleintierpraxis 14 (1969):45.

Patterson, D. F.: Congenital Heart Disease in the Dog. Ann. N. Y. Acad. Sci., 127 (1965):541.

Patterson, D. F.: Epidemiologic and Genetic Studies of Congenital Heart Disease in the Dog. Circ. Res., 23 (1968):171.

Patterson, D. F., Detweiler, D. K., Hubben, K., and Botts, R. P.: Spontaneous Abnormal Cardiac Arrhythmias and Conduction Disturbances in the Dog; A Clinical and Pathological Study of 3000 Dogs. Amer. J. Vet. Res., 22 (1961):355.

Patterson, D. F., Hare, W. C. D., Shive, R. J., and Luginbühl, H. R.: Congenital Malformations of the Cardiovascular System Associated with Chromosomal Abnormalities (A Report of the Clinical, Pathologic, and Cytogenic Findings in 2 Dogs). Zbl. Veterinärmed., 13 (1966):669.

Pensinger, R. R.: Comparative Aspects of Mitral Valve Disease in Dogs. Ann. N. Y. Acad. Sci., 118 (1965):525.

Pensinger, R. R.: Chronic Congestive Heart Failure in Dogs — Clinical and Pathological Findings. Ann. N. Y. Acad. Sci., 147 (1968):330.

Taylor, D. H., and Sittnikow, K. L.: The Diagnosis of Canine Cardiac Disease. J. Small Anim. Pract., 9 (1968):589.

CHAPTER

13

ACQUIRED VALVULAR AND ENDOCARDIAL HEART DISEASE

Endocardial disease of inflammatory or degenerative origin may affect the valvular endocardium, the mural endocardium, or both. Valvular lesions usually result in detectable murmurs which are recognized during the physical examination, whereas mural endocardial lesions do not produce such obvious, clinically detectable signs. Diseases affecting only the mural endocardium are therefore diagnosed more frequently at necropsy than by clinical examination.

Acquired valvular heart disease is almost entirely due to chronic valvular fibrosis resulting in insufficiency (also called regurgitation or incompetence). Acquired valvular stenosis is extremely uncommon, although Tashjian and Mc-Coy (1960) have reported one case of acquired mitral valvular stenosis.

Mitral insufficiency resulting from chronic mitral (left atrioventricular) valvular fibrosis is the form of heart disease most frequently diagnosed in clinical practice. It is followed in frequency by chronic tricuspid (right atrioventricular) valvular fibrosis, which results in tricuspid insufficiency. The aortic (left semilunar) valve is only occasionally recognized as being diseased, and pulmonic (right semilunar) valve lesions almost never cause cardiac disease.

Valvular insufficiency is a clinical term which refers to functional incompetency of the atrioventricular or semilunar valve leaflets that results in regurgitation of blood from the ventricle into the atrium during ventricular systole, or from the great vessels into the ventricles during diastole. The causes of acquired valvular insufficiency include:

1. Chronic valvular fibrosis resulting in valvular incompetence (see pp. 322-361 and 371-376).
2. Severe ventricular dilatation with consequent dilation of the valve anulus

321

which results in valvular insufficiency. This may occur secondarily in congenital heart disease.

3. Ruptured chordae tendineae (see pp. 366-371).
4. Bacterial endocarditis (see pp. 378-381).
5. Papillary muscle dysfunction.
6. Ventricular muscle dysfunction (cardiomyopathy; see pp. 392-400).
7. Asynchronous ventricular contraction.
8. Atrial dysrhythmias.

CHRONIC MITRAL VALVULAR FIBROSIS (CMVF)

Chronic mitral valvular fibrosis resulting in mitral insufficiency is by far the most frequent cause of congestive heart failure in the dog. No single designation has been applied universally to the condition. It has been referred to as chronic valvular fibrosis, fibrotic valvular endocarditis, chronic valvular heart disease, mitral endocardiosis, leaky valve disease, nodular valvulitis, warty valve disease, proliferative fibrosis of the atrioventricular valves, vegetative valvular endocardiosis, fibrous endocarditis, and mitral insufficiency. The clinical features of chronic valvular fibrosis were first described in 1913, and according to Detweiler and Patterson (1965b), the pathologic lesions were first reviewed in 1925 and 1929.

INCIDENCE

In a clinical study of 4831 dogs (Detweiler et al., 1968), chronic valvular fibrosis was found clinically or at necropsy in 8.1 per cent of all dogs. In another study, 139 of 404 dogs (34 per cent) had chronic valvular fibrosis at necropsy (Jones and Zook, 1965): 228 of 550 dogs (42 per cent) had similar lesions at necropsy in a third study (Das and Tashjian, 1965). Stünzi (1962) found typical changes of chronic valvular fibrosis in 11 per cent of 789 dogs examined at necropsy. In all the studies reported, the incidence of chronic mitral valvular fibrosis increased with age.

Das and Tashjian (1965) found chronic mitral valvular fibrosis in 128 male dogs and 100 females in a series of 550 consecutive necropsies. In 343 dogs with valvular heart disease studied clinically by Kersten (1968), 180 had only mitral valvular disease; of these, 121 dogs (68 per cent) were male, and 59 (32 per cent) were female. Chronic mitral and tricuspid valvular fibrosis coexisted in 152 dogs. Detweiler and Patterson (1965b) observed specifically that male Cocker Spaniels are more prone to congestive heart failure than are females.

CLINICAL SIGNS

The symptomatology of chronic mitral valvular fibrosis producing mitral insufficiency is variable depending on the inciting factors and the phase of the disease process (see Table 13-1). Although our classification is arbitrary, it is helpful in making a prognosis and in determining a course of therapy. There is no sharp distinction between the phases, and the disease may develop insidiously and without apparent cause. The disease is progressive over a period of weeks, months, or years, and exacerbations and remissions are likely.

Chronic mitral insufficiency due to valvular fibrosis (*phase I/IV*) is often an incidental finding recognized during the routine clinical examination. It may be present for an indefinite period of time, without signs of cardiac decompensation.

As the disease progresses the heart and lungs become less compliant, and early signs of decompensation occur (*phase II/IV*). The most common sign in the early stages of the disease is a nocturnal, deeply resonant cough. The owner may report that the cough usually (but not always) begins in the early morning hours. The dog may retch at the end of a coughing spasm, producing a little white or blood-flecked phlegm. This retching, often misinterpreted by the owner as vomiting, may be the presenting complaint. In other cases, the presenting complaint may be that the dog "seems to have swallowed a bone which is now caught in the throat." Every effort should be made to rule out this situation, even if the veterinarian is certain that heart disease is present, since the owner may be sincerely convinced that a bone is present. The owner may have been unaware that heart disease occurs in dogs and would not expect such a diagnosis, especially if the dog's condition is otherwise good. Less frequently, the dog may be presented because of difficult breathing (*dyspnea*) or rapid breathing (*tachypnea*). Respiratory signs are often associated with the cardiac cough. The owner should be questioned about respiratory distress when a cough is the chief complaint. In many cases, the owner is so concerned about the cough that the presence of respiratory distress is overlooked.

As the disease progresses (*phase III/IV*), the cough becomes more frequent, occurring in paroxysms throughout the day. The cough may then be induced when the dog is excited, drinks water, or tugs on his leash. This hollow, rasping cough is suggestive of cardiac disease.

The progression of the disease process from phase II/IV to III/IV or IV/IV may not be seen by the veterinarian, since the owner often changes doctors because the cough was not "cured." The intensity and frequency of the cough and dyspnea continue to increase. If the dog is affected with *orthopnea*, an inability to breathe while lying down, the owner may report that the dog is restless at night.

Paroxysmal pulmonary edema is often reported as extreme restlessness at night. In such cases the owner brings the dog to the veterinarian, stating that only 30 minutes earlier he had feared for the dog's life because of intense breathing difficulties. Because the edema is paroxysmal in nature, the signs often subside before the dog is seen by the veterinarian.

When the heart can no longer compensate for the disease (*phase IV/IV*), gross pulmonary edema occurs and becomes progressively more severe.

Signs of right heart failure, such as hepatomegaly, ascites, subcutaneous edema, and peripheral venous engorgement, may develop as the increased pressures from the left heart and subsequently the lungs tax the right ventricle until it finally fails. Tricuspid valvular insufficiency (see pp. 371-376) often accompanies mitral insufficiency so that both ventricles fail simultaneously.

Syncope due to inadequate cardiac output is reported in some dogs with chronic mitral valvular fibrosis. It is most often associated with frequent atrial premature beats or paroxysmal atrial tachycardia (see p. 287). Since syncope occurs commonly with many conditions, a careful differential diagnosis is essential (see *Syncope*, p. 6).

Other signs of heart failure that result either directly from circulatory impairment or from other organ dysfunctions associated with heart disease include gastrointestinal disturbances, diminished appetite, vomiting, and diarrhea (Jaksch,

TABLE 13-1 CLINICAL AND RADIOGRAPHIC DESCRIPTION OF THE
PHASES OF CHRONIC MITRAL VALVULAR FIBROSIS*

PHASE	DESCRIPTION	CLINICAL SIGNS
I/IV	Compensated mitral valvular insufficiency	Murmur only; no signs of pulmonary or systemic disease related to mitral insufficiency; normal exercise tolerance
II/IV	Early phase of decompensating chronic mitral insufficiency, confined to left side (prodromal stage)	Occasional cough or respiratory embarrassment referable to mild degree of pulmonary congestion occurs after strenuous exertion; only left heart involved, and systemic signs are not present
III/IV	Cardiac dysfunction and decompensation; increased load on right ventricle and pulmonary hypertension may result in impending right ventricular disease	Signs of cough and pulmonary congestion present after exercise and at night; strain on right ventricle may produce signs of right heart failure
IV/IV	Congestive heart failure with left or left and right heart decompensation	Pulmonary edema, often with signs of severe right heart failure such as ascites, pleural effusion, and liver enlargement; signs develop in dogs at rest and are exaggerated by even minimal exercise

See opposite page for footnotes.

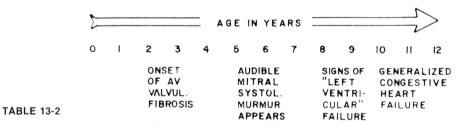

ACQUIRED HEART DISEASE AND CONGESTIVE HEART FAILURE

AGE IN YEARS

0   1   2   3   4   5   6   7   8   9   10   11   12

TABLE 13-2

ONSET OF AV VALVUL. FIBROSIS

AUDIBLE MITRAL SYSTOL. MURMUR APPEARS

SIGNS OF "LEFT VENTRICULAR" FAILURE

GENERALIZED CONGESTIVE HEART FAILURE

INTRAMURAL CORONARY ARTERIOSCLEROSIS, FOCAL MYOCARDIAL NECROSIS AND FIBROSIS

ATRIAL PREMATURE BEATS

ATRIAL FIBRILLATION

See legend on facing page.

TABLE 13-1   *Continued*

RADIOGRAPHIC SIGNS[†]	
Dorsoventral view	**Lateral view**
Slightly enlarged left auricle; left ventricle unremarkable	Slightly enlarged left atrium; left ventricle unremarkable
Left ventricular enlargement[‡] which may obscure enlargement of the left auricle; apex becomes rounded L/R <.05; L does not approximate R[§] $\dfrac{LH + RH}{LAT} > 2/3$	Left atrial enlargement eliminates distal bend of trachea; left ventricle enlarges; angle of trachea with thoracic spine decreases; caudal waist stretched; pulmonary veins approximate density of arteries and may be slightly dilated at junction with left atrium; lung field remains clear.
Left auricle may be visible again on left. border; left atrium tends to force the main stem bronchi apart; ventricular enlargement progresses to general cardiac enlargement L approximates R $\dfrac{LH + RH}{LAT} > 2/3$ [§]	Marked left atrial enlargement; craniocaudal diameter increases markedly due to right ventricular enlargement; intrapulmonary vascular structures blurred in hilar and middle zones of lung field, which appears hazy; intrapulmonary arteries and/or veins accentuated; occasional liver enlargement
Left auricle visible at left border; left atrium forces main stem bronchi apart; pulmonary congestion and pulmonary alveolar edema; occasionally pleural and pericardial effusion L approximates R[§] $\dfrac{LH + RH}{LAT} > 2/3$	Large to very large left atrium displacing left stem bronchus dorsally; moderate to extreme enlargement of cardiac silhouette; pulmonary alveolar edema (air-bronchograms, mottling); dense pulmonary arteries; occasionally large caudal vena cava; pleural and/or pericardial effusion; ascites; hepatomegaly

[*]The radiographic classification is based on that originally proposed by Hamlin (1968). The number of radiographic signs has been expanded and includes both lateral and dorsoventral views because we believe that the presence or absence of a single sign in one view, no matter how pronounced, may be deceiving. Radiographic signs compatible with pulmonary or systemic circulatory failure have also been included since they may be of help in proving the presence of heart failure. [†]See Figures 13-6 through 13-13, which illustrate the four phases. [‡]Before assessing enlargement, shifting of the cardiac apex must be considered. [§]See pp. 64-66. L = distance between left ventricular epicardium and left thoracic wall. R = distance between right ventricular epicardium and right thoracic wall. LH + RH = total maximum distance from left ventricular wall to right ventricular wall on dorsoventral radiograph. LAT = distance between left and right thoracic walls at level of maximum leftward and rightward deviation of the ventricles.

Table 13-2.   Schema of the time course and sequence of events as they may occur in a dog with acquired cardiovascular disease leading to congestive heart failure. Valvular fibrosis begins in the early years and slowly progresses, primarily affecting the atrioventricular valves, especially the mitral. Mitral insufficiency is likely to appear in the middle years and may be tolerated until late in life. Intramural coronary arteriosclerosis and focal myocardial necrosis become associated with the antecedent valvular changes during the later years and, when the effects of these multiple lesions are sufficiently severe, clinical signs of left-sided heart failure appear. Generalized congestive heart failure follows some months, or a year or two or even longer, after the onset of left-sided ventricular failure. A precipitating factor in the development of generalized heart failure may be the occurrence of atrial fibrillation, sometimes preceded by the appearance of atrial premature beats. However, generalized heart failure may occur without the prior or subsequent existence of these atrial arrhythmias. (Detweiler et al. Ann. N.Y. Acad. Sci. 147:318, 1968).

1966), as well as oliguria, anuria, or polyuria, weakness, lethargy, poor haircoat and hair loss, and generalized debility (cardiac cachexia; see p. 220).

CLINICAL COURSE

Atrioventricular valvular fibrosis begins early in life (2 to 3 years), and systolic murmurs are often audible by 5 to 7 years of age. Many dogs develop signs of left ventricular dysfunction (phase II/IV or III/IV) around 8 to 9 years of age, and generalized congestive heart failure (phase IV/IV) often occurs between 10 and 12 years of age (Table 13-2) (Detweiler et al., 1968). Although this is the usual course of chronic valvular heart disease in dogs, there are exceptions. Severe, terminal conditions have been recognized in dogs as young as five years old. In other dogs, clinical signs may not appear earlier than 12 or more years of age.

Chronic valvular fibrosis occurs in dogs of all breeds, but serious pathophysiological manifestations seem to be more frequent in the toy and medium-sized (up to 40 lb.) breeds. The reason for the prevalence of chronic mitral valvular fibrosis in the smaller breeds is not clear.

PHYSICAL EXAMINATION

Depending on the phase of the disease, the dog's general condition may vary from excellent to very weak, cachectic, and close to death.

Coughing and respiratory distress may be observed while the history is being obtained. However, many dogs stop coughing as soon as they enter the doctor's office, and failure to elicit a cough by tracheal palpation does not indicate that a cough is absent. Panting must be critically evaluated, since it is a frequent manifestation of excitement or anxiety in the dog.

The color of the mucous membranes is usually unremarkable, although an injected appearance with a muddy color is seen in the more advanced cases. Cyanosis is seen only in advanced cases where there is peripheral stasis of blood, or when the severity of the pulmonary edema interferes with gaseous exchange in the lung parenchyma (Jaksch, 1966).

Extension of the head and neck may improve ventilation if respiratory distress is present. In most cases the typical cardiac cough is readily elicited by tracheal palpation. Dental or periodontal disease is often present in older dogs. As a consequence, some believe that there is a cause-and-effect relationship between dental disease and chronic valvular fibrosis. However, statistical evidence has not yet been presented to confirm such a hypothesis.

On palpation of the thorax, a precordial thrill is felt when the intensity of the murmur is grade V/VI or VI/VI. The thrill is palpable over the point of maximal intensity at the caudoventral left sternal border and may radiate over the entire precordium in dogs with very intense murmurs. An apical thrust (left ventricular heave) at the ventral fourth to sixth left intercostal space is sometimes observed in dogs with advanced mitral insufficiency; however, it is obscured in obese dogs.

The abdomen is unremarkable unless right heart failure accompanies the mitral valve disease or unless concurrent disease processes are present in the abdomen. The abdominal muscles may feel hard and tense if the cardiac cough is severe. Ascites and hepatic or splenic engorgement are frequently associated with advanced right heart failure.

Subcutaneous edema is unusual even in the most advanced phases of heart failure (Jaksch, 1966). When subcutaneous edema due to heart disease is present, it is accompanied by ascites and abdominal enlargement due to right heart failure.

The palpable femoral pulse provides an important diagnostic clue. In normal dogs and in asymptomatic dogs with compensated mitral insufficiency (phase I/IV), the pulse is usually slow and strong. As the disease becomes more severe, the pulse becomes rapid and jerky. Other terms for a jerky pulse are water-hammer pulse and B-B shot pulse. A pulse deficit is detected when arrhythmias such as atrial fibrillation, atrial premature contractions, ventricular premature contractions, and paroxysmal tachycardia develop.

AUSCULTATION

The average heart rate in one group of dogs in congestive heart failure was 166 beats/min., compared with 144 beats/min. in a group of dogs not in heart failure (Wallace and Hamilton, 1962). The murmur may be a soft, early systolic murmur initially, but as the disease progresses it becomes more intense and holosystolic. An apical systolic murmur occurs with a loud, snapping first heart sound (Fig. 13-1). The second heart sound may be obscured by the intense murmur. A mixture of high- and low-frequency sounds characterizes this murmur, although occasionally a high-frequency, musical whoop or seagull-type sound may be heard instead of the holosystolic murmur (Fig. 13-2). The murmur is most intense at the left caudal sternal border. When it is severe, it radiates both cranially and dorsally on the left as well as to the right thorax.

The intensity of the first heart sound is increased initially in dogs with mitral valvular fibrosis (Fig. 13-1) (Gould, Ettinger, and Lyon, 1968), although it may

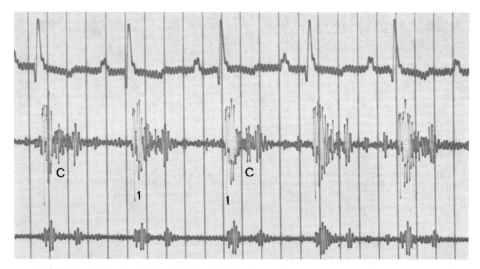

FIGURE 13-1 Lead II of the electrocardiogram and simultaneous wide-frequency (*middle*) and low-frequency (*bottom*) band phonocardiograms recorded over the left caudosternal border. The loud first heart sound (1), a holosystolic murmur, and a mid-systolic click (C) are most evident on the wide-band tracing.

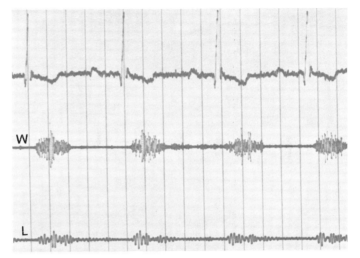

FIGURE 13-2 Lead II of the electrocardiogram and simultaneously recorded wide-frequency (W) and low-frequency (L) band phonocardiograms. The systolic murmur is diamond-shaped and was musical in quality—the so-called "systolic whoop." The low-frequency components are minimal, indicating that the higher frequency sounds predominate in this systolic murmur, which is occasionally associated with chronic mitral valvular fibrosis.

later be reduced in intensity. The intensity of the second heart sound may be increased over the pulmonic area if pulmonary hypertension develops. A low-frequency third and/or fourth heart sound caused by the rapid inflow of blood into the ventricle during diastole is usually audible in dogs in congestive heart failure (Fig. 13-3). When an intense holosystolic murmur obscures the second heart sound, the third heart sound is often mistaken for the second heart sound when it is auscultated at the cardiac apex. The presence of an audible third or fourth heart sound, or gallop rhythm, indicates that the dog is in congestive heart failure. When an intense murmur of mitral insufficiency radiates to the right thorax, it may be mistaken for the murmur of tricuspid insufficiency. However, mitral insufficiency and tricuspid insufficiency coexist so frequently that a presumptive diagnosis of combined mitral and tricuspid insufficiency is likely if a holosystolic murmur of mixed frequency is auscultated over both the mitral and tricuspid valve regions.

The intensity and rhythm of the heart sounds in mitral insufficiency are usually constant unless a cardiac arrhythmia is present. When a single premature atrial or ventricular contraction occurs, an early but weak first heart sound is auscultated. The intensity of the murmur is then diminished or absent, and the second heart sound may also be absent (Fig. 13-4). With paroxysmal tachycardia, the normal sinus rhythm is periodically disrupted by a burst of rapid beats which begins and ends abruptly. Murmurs are usually not heard during these paroxysms, perhaps because of the rapid heart rate and the incomplete ventricular filling. If atrial fibrillation becomes the dominant rhythm, the heart rate is rapid and irregular, and the intensity of the first heart sound is variable. The holosystolic murmur becomes variable in intensity or is absent, as may be the second heart sound (Fig. 13-5).

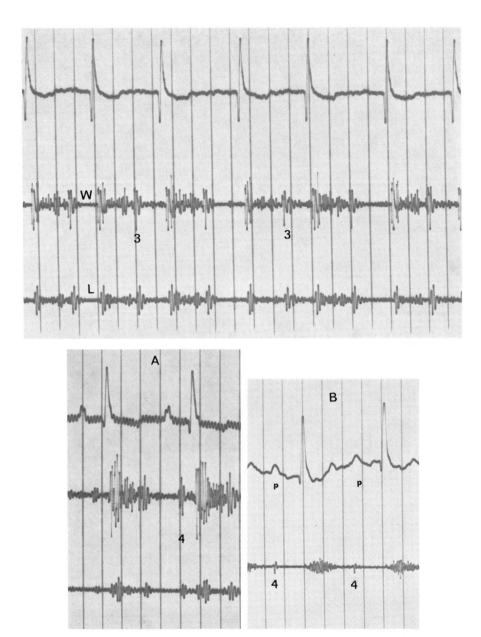

FIGURE 13-3   *Above*, Lead II of the electrocardiogram (at $1/2$ amplitude) and simultaneously recorded wide-frequency (W) and low-frequency (L) band phonocardiograms recorded over the left caudosternal border. In addition to the holosystolic murmur, a loud third heart sound (3), or gallop, is present on both the wide- and low-frequency bands. The gallop sound, associated with heart failure, is a low-frequency sound which may be misinterpreted as the second heart sound when a holosystolic murmur is present.

Below, In addition to a holosystolic murmur, a fourth heart sound is present in both of these tracings recorded from dogs in congestive heart failure. In tracing (*A*), the sound (4) occurs 0.08 sec. after the onset of the P wave, whereas it occurs simultaneously with the beginning of atrial electrical activity (p) in tracing (*B*).

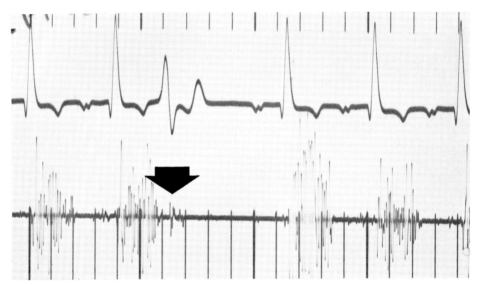

FIGURE 13-4 Premature contractions do not permit the ventricles to fill completely during diastole. The resultant contraction may then be ineffectual, and the intensities of both the first heart sound and the murmur are diminished (arrow). The second heart sound is often absent, since the ventricular contraction fails to generate enough pressure to open the valves initially. The negative P waves in the lead II electrocardiogram reflect an aberrant atrial rhythm produced by digitalis intoxication.

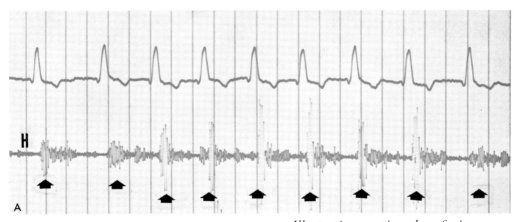

Illustration continued on facing page.

FIGURE 13-5 *A* and *B,* Atrial fibrillation is characterized by an irregular heart rate (variable R-R intervals), inconstant intensity of the first heart sound due to incomplete ventricular filling (arrow in *A;* [1] in *B*), and variation in the intensity of the murmur, all of which can be identified in these recordings. Lead II ECG in *A* and aVF (F) in *B*. Phonocardiograms recorded at high (H) and wide (W) band levels.

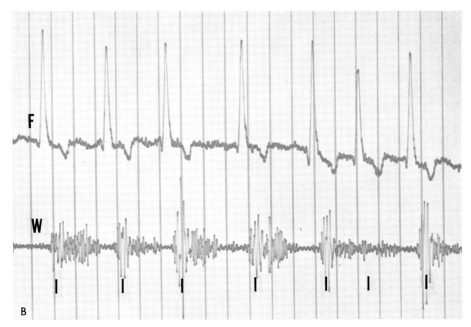

FIGURE 13–5   *Continued.*

RADIOGRAPHIC EXAMINATION

The radiographic appearance of chronic mitral valvular fibrosis varies according to the severity of the condition (Figs. 13-6 through 13-13). In both the lateral and the dorsoventral views, left atrial and left and right ventricular enlargement occurring with mitral insufficiency result in characteristic changes in the cardiac silhouette. It is not possible, however, to differentiate radiographically between mitral insufficiency resulting from chronic valvular fibrosis and mitral insufficiency due to other causes (see pp. 356-357). Mitral insufficiency is often detected radiographically when the dog is still fully compensated and when a systolic murmur is the only clinical sign of the disease (phase I/IV). The radiographic changes in the lung field are good indicators of impending left heart failure (see Chapter 3, pp. 88-90). Radiographic examination may also be used to obtain objective evidence of the effects of therapy (Figs. 13-14 and 13-15).

The lateral radiograph.   Left atrial enlargement is usually the earliest radiographic sign of mitral insufficiency; it is followed by left ventricular enlargement, which is more difficult to assess. The enlarged left atrium elevates the trachea, thus diminishing the angle between the trachea and the thoracic spine. It also eliminates the ventral bend in the distal extremity of the trachea. The enlarged left atrium occupies the dorsocaudal quadrant of the cardiac silhouette (see Fig. 13-16 *A* and *B*), and when it is markedly dilated it may extend as a wedge-shaped density into the diaphragmatic lung field. The wedge-shaped atrial extension represents the dilated portions of the pulmonary veins as they join the atrium. In the cranial hilar area, those dilated veins may appear as dense oval masses when seen on end; these tend to be mistaken for enlarged hilar nodes or tumor masses.

With marked atrial enlargement, the main stem bronchi become ventrodor-

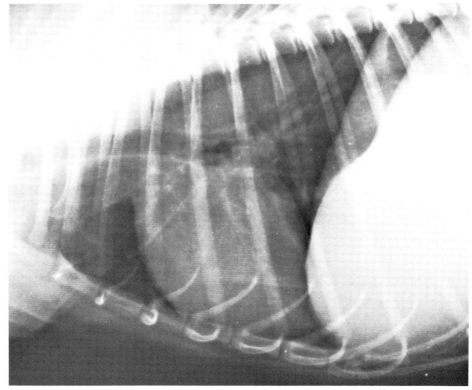

FIGURE 13-6 Lateral radiograph, 14 year old male Beagle with mitral insufficiency, phase I. The dog was examined because it had diarrhea. A grade III/VI holosystolic regurgitant murmur typical for mitral insufficiency was heard. The dog had no signs of cardiac disease, and the electrocardiogram was unremarkable. The heart size is nearly normal. The caudal waist of the cardiac silhouette is somewhat shallower than normal. The left atrium is slightly enlarged. Dogs with mitral insufficiency, phase I, are usually compensated and require no treatment.

sally compressed, and their normally superimposed lucent bands may be separated, thereby forming a V-shaped structure open caudally. In such cases, the left bronchus is displaced dorsally by the enlarged left atrium. The central portion of the left atrium can occasionally protrude dorsally between the two main stem bronchi. The left atrium forms an ill-defined oval mass occupying most of the dorsal half of the cardiac silhouette in extreme enlargement.

Dilatation of the mitral valve anulus as well as ventricular and atrial dilatation are responsible for the disappearance of the caudal cardiac waist and the straightening of the caudal cardiac border, which occasionally merges with the diaphragmatic silhouette. The disappearance of the cardiac waist makes it difficult to assess how much the enlarged ventricle contributes to the increase in the apicobasilar diameter of the heart. The craniocaudal diameter increases after the right ventricle begins to enlarge, and signs of left and right heart failure develop.

The dorsoventral radiograph. Protrusion of the enlarged left auricle over the left heart border is an early and characteristic finding in mitral insufficiency. As the disease progresses, left ventricular enlargement becomes visible as an increased rounding of the normally straight left cardiac border. The left ventricular

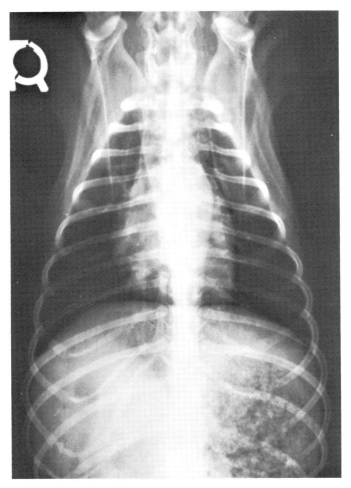

FIGURE 13-7   Dorsoventral radiograph, dog in Figure 13-6 (mitral insufficiency, phase I). The cardiac silhouette looks normal except for a small bulge in the cranial third of the left cardiac border, which represents the slightly enlarged left auricle.

border is displaced markedly to the left and caudally and gives the cardiac apex a rounder appearance than normal. The extended left ventricular border may obscure the protrusion of the left auricle temporarily unless it dilates simultaneously. A dense, often ill-defined mass within the caudal half of the cardiac silhouette represents the dilated central portion of the left atrium. Marked dilatation of its main portion forces the stem bronchi apart, changing their angle from acute to obtuse. If the lung field is clear, the caudal border of the left atrium appears as a double outline within the apical area.

Secondary right ventricular strain results in right ventricular enlargement and a farther rightward extension of the right cardiac border, thus increasing the transverse diameter of the cardiac silhouette.

The dilated pulmonary veins, indicating the backing up of blood caused by left ventricular failure, are often well outlined in the dorsoventral view. The engorged venous structures are easily distinguished from the pulmonary arteries by their confluence at the dilated left atrium.

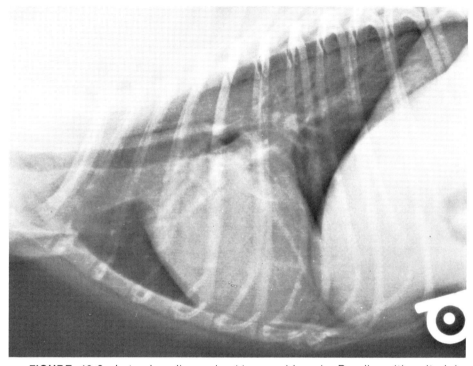

FIGURE 13-8 Lateral radiograph, 11-year-old male Poodle with mitral insufficiency, phase II. The dog had an occasional cardiac cough for three years. A holosystolic murmur of mitral insufficiency was heard, and the lung sounds were normal. The trachea is elevated, and the ventral bend in the distal trachea is absent. The apicobasilar distance is increased. The cranial waist has been preserved, but the caudal waist has become shallow. The craniocaudal diameter of the heart is slightly increased. The intrapulmonary vascular markings are accentuated. Veins and arteries are of similar density. The veins are slightly widened as they join the left atrium. The lung field has remained clear.

A classification of mitral insufficiency into four phases based on radiographic findings was proposed by Hamlin (1968) and is illustrated in Figures 13-6 through 13-13. He found that the radiographic findings and the prognosis obtained by such a classification correlated well. The clinical and radiographic findings in the four phases of mitral insufficiency are summarized in Table 13-1 (see pp. 324-325).

There is frequently a marked difference between the size and shape of the cardiac silhouette in the lateral and dorsoventral views. The increase in the apicobasilar distance is more obvious in the lateral radiographs of dogs with narrow, deep thoracic conformation than in those with a wide thorax. The apicobasilar elongation is less obvious in the lateral view in dogs with a wide, shallow thorax, but it may be pronounced in the dorsoventral radiograph, where it is often accompanied by extensive displacement of the apex of the heart to the left or, rarely, to the right.

Fluoroscopic examination can further demonstrate functional abnormalities such as arrhythmias or a weakly contracting heart. The morphologic changes are best evaluated on the routine radiograph.

(Text continues on page 344.)

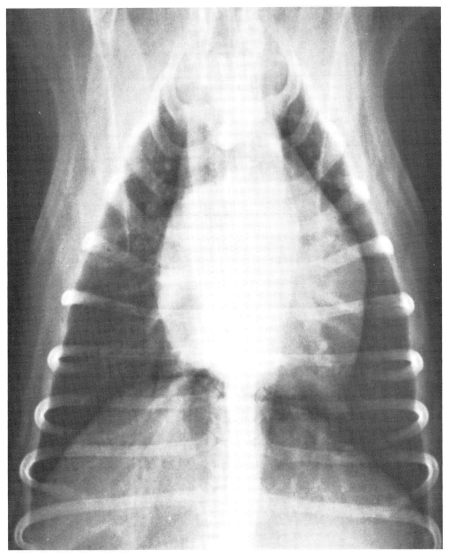

FIGURE 13-9 Dorsoventral radiograph, dog in Figure 13-8 (mitral insufficiency, phase II). The cardiac silhouette is rounded because the left ventricular border bulges, and the left cardiac border extends farther toward the thoracic wall than normal. The apex is wider than normal. The left ventricular enlargement impairs visualization of the dilated left auricle, which can only be seen as a small bulge protruding slightly over the left cardiac border.

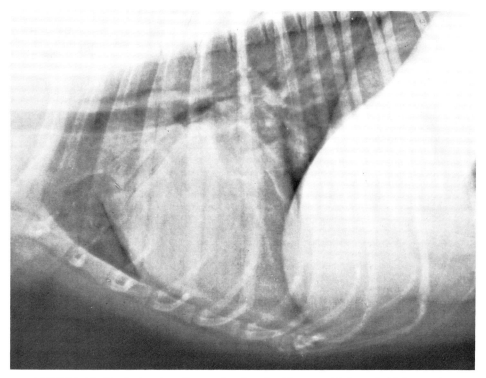

FIGURE 13-10 Lateral radiograph, dog in Figures 13-8 and 13-9, made one year later. Radiographically, the mitral insufficiency has progressed to phase III. The cardiac cough had become more frequent. Râles were not auscultated. In addition to the increased apicobasilar distance already visible in Figure 13-8, indicated by tracheal elevation, there is now a marked increase in the craniocaudal diameter of the heart. The increased diameter is due to further cranial extension of the right ventricular border and caudal extension of the left ventricular border, which now runs parallel with the ribs. The left atrium extends caudodorsally, and the caudal waist has now vanished completely. The cranial waist is less distinct than before. The caudal vena cava is denser than in Figure 13-8 and now appears dilated. The liver has enlarged and extends beyond the costal arch. The lung field is hazy, making it difficult to differentiate the intrapulmonary vascular markings. Mitral insufficiency, phase III, is characterized by interstitial pulmonary edema, which is also referred to as pulmonary congestion; this causes the increased fuzzy density of the lungs. This stress, in turn, precipitates right ventricular disease.

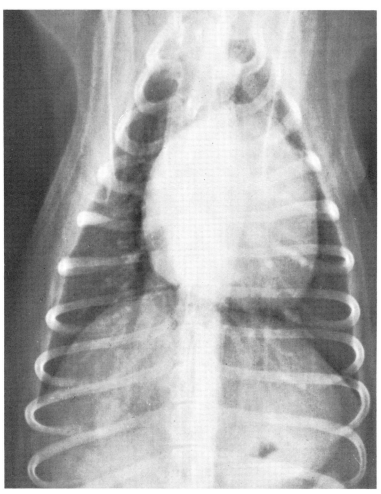

FIGURE 13-11 Dorsoventral radiograph, dog in Figures 13-8 to 13-10 (mitral insufficiency, phase III). The cardiac silhouette is larger than on the radiograph in Figure 13-9. The right ventricle is rounder and extends farther toward the right side than before. The left ventricular border is also rounder, and the bulging density of the left auricle protrudes beyond the left cardiac border. The apex is rounder than in Figure 13-9. There is a diffuse haziness of the lung field.

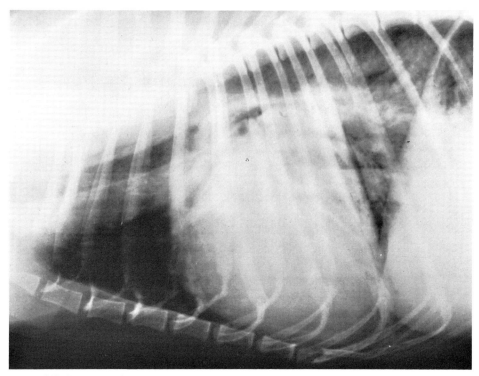

FIGURE 13-12 Left lateral radiograph, 10 year old female German Shepherd-mixed breed dog with mitral insufficiency, phase IV. The dog was examined because of respiratory distress and coughing of two weeks' duration. A loud holosystolic murmur, grade V/VI, and moist râles were auscultated. Treatment with digoxin and diuretics was initiated while the dog was hospitalized. There is extensive, generalized cardiac enlargement affecting all four cardiac chambers. The trachea is elevated and runs parallel with the spine. The left stem bronchus, which is dorsally displaced by the greatly dilated left atrium, is dorsoventrally compressed and is barely visible due to the greatly increased density of the hilar area. The cranial and caudal waists have disappeared. The right cardiac border remains in close contact with the sternum for a greater distance than normal; the cranial portion then curves rather steeply in a dorsal direction. The left cardiac border runs parallel with the ribs and joins the caudally bulging left atrium in a straight line. The caudal vena cava is denser than normal and is distended. Its slightly dorsal instead of ventral course is occasionally seen with right heart enlargement. There is a hazy and in some areas mottled, patchy density of the lung field, most pronounced in the hilar area, which obscures the vascular markings almost completely. The presence of a small amount of pleural effusion cannot be excluded because of the double outline visible in the apical lobar area. Notice that all the radiographic signs of mitral insufficiency, phase IV, are present: right and left heart enlargement with left heart failure, causing pulmonary alveolar edema; and right heart failure causing venous congestion of the systemic circulation.

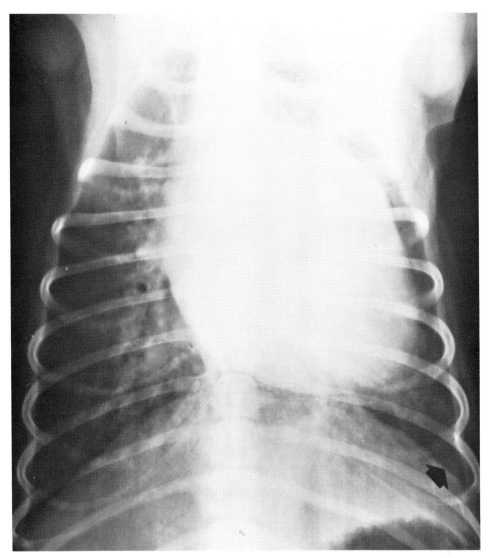

FIGURE 13-13   Dorsoventral radiograph, dog in Figure 13-12 (mitral insufficiency, phase IV). The cardiac silhouette is greatly enlarged, the outlines are blurred,
and the borders are more rounded than normal. The right and left ventricles are both
enlarged. The left ventricular enlargement has been accentuated by a shift of the
apex to the left side. The left auricular enlargement is obscured by the left ventricular
enlargement. The lung field is most dense in the hilar area, where it obscures the
details; this density gradually fades toward the periphery. The vascular markings are
indistinct and appear wider than normal. In the costophrenic angles the lung lobes
have retracted 1 to 2 mm. from the thoracic wall (arrow). The density between the
lucent lung lobe and the thoracic wall indicates a small amount of pleural effusion.

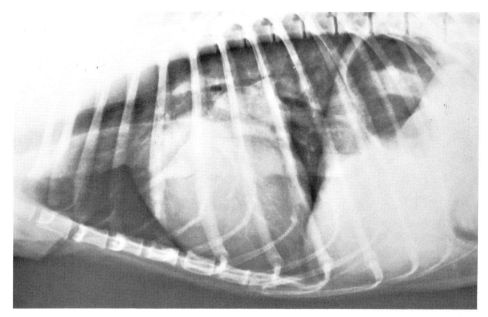

FIGURE 13-14   Left lateral radiograph, dog in Figures 13-12 and 13-13. Treatment of heart failure has resulted in regression of signs from those of phase IV to those of phase III. This radiograph was made three days after those in Figures 13-12 and 13-13. The cardiac silhouette is much better defined and its size has decreased markedly. The right cardiac border is in contact with the sternum for a shorter distance than on the previous radiograph (Fig. 13-12), and the dorsal curving of its cranial portion is less steep. The trachea forms a small angle with the thoracic spine, indicating a decrease in the apicobasilar distance. The left stem bronchus is much better visualized than before; however, it is still displaced dorsally. The left cardiac border regained a slight rounding, and the ventricle is separated from the atrium by a shallow waist. The left atrium remained greatly enlarged. The lung field is much more lucent than it was before treatment. The vascular markings are indistinctly outlined, but they can again be seen. The area of junction of the veins with the left atrium remains greatly distended. The caudal vena cava is still denser than normal. The radiographic signs of a possible pleural effusion have disappeared.

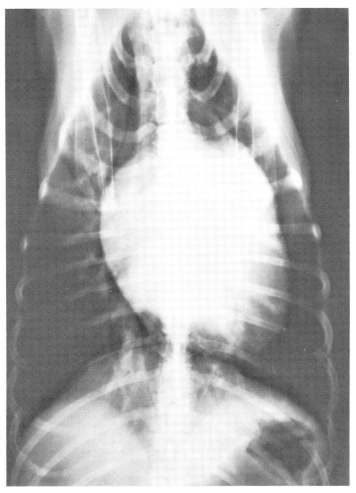

FIGURE 13-15   Dorsoventral radiograph, dog in Figures 13-12 to 13-14, made at the same time as Figure 13-14. The cardiac silhouette is better defined, smaller, and less rounded than on the previous radiograph (Fig. 13-13). The rounding of the right ventricular border has reduced considerably. The apex, which had been displaced to the left side, has returned toward the midline. The marked, persistent left ventricular enlargement can be evaluated by the proximity of the left cardiac border to the thoracic wall. The bulge of the left auricle is better visible now than on the previous radiograph, where it was obscured by the left ventricle. The lung field has become clear, and the costophrenic angles are sharp and lucent.

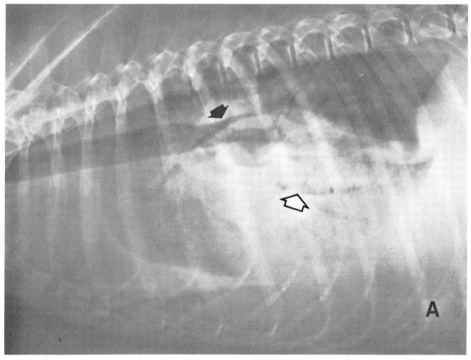

FIGURE 13-16 Left lateral plain radiograph (*A*) and selective left lateral ventricular angiocardiogram (*B*), 15 year old male dog of mixed breed in severe right and left congestive heart failure. The dog had previously been on digitalis therapy, but its condition had slowly deteriorated. The dog was dyspneic and weak and had an enlarging abdomen. In addition to the typical signs of mitral insufficiency and tricuspid insufficiency, atrial fibrillation was present on the electrocardiogram.

Radiograph (A) was made immediately before cardiac catheterization to show the radiographic signs of right and left heart failure: pleural and abdominal effusion; cardiac enlargement with elevation of the trachea and dorsal deviation of the left stem bronchus (black arrow), which is difficult to see because of the pleural effusion; and pulmonary edema, recognized despite the pleural effusion by the lucent, air-filled bronchi (air-bronchograms, clear arrow) in the infiltrated lung lobes.

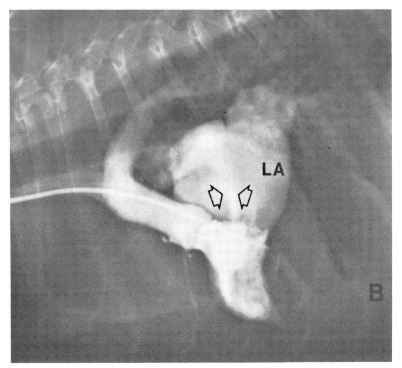

FIGURE 13–16   *(Continued)* *B,* Selective left ventricular angiocardiogram exposed 0.5 sec. after the beginning of the injection of Hypaque-M 75% (1 ml./kg. body weight). A large amount of contrast medium has flowed retrograde into the greatly dilated left atrium (LA). Between the two clear arrows is seen a denser band, which represents the jet of undiluted contrast medium forced backwards into the left atrium through the incompetent mitral valve. The left ventricle is in systole. A rough comparison of the amount of contrast medium ejected antegrade with the amount which has flowed retrograde through the incompetent mitral valve shows that probably less than half of the ventricular stroke volume has been ejected into the aorta.

ELECTROCARDIOGRAPHY

The electrocardiogram may yield little diagnostic information or may confirm the degree of cardiomegaly. All the arrhythmias described in Chapter 11 have been recognized in dogs with chronic mitral valvular fibrosis as well as other disease processes.

The electrocardiographic abnormalities other than arrhythmias associated with mitral insufficiency are basically accentuations of the normal electrocardiogram. The mean electrical axis in the frontal plane is usually within normal limits but may deviate to the left with gross left ventricular hypertrophy (Fig. 13-17). In such situations the axis is not likely to be less than 0°. Right-axis deviation develops occasionally when right ventricular hypertrophy accompanies chronic mitral and tricuspid valvular insufficiency (Fig. 13-18). Wallace and Hamilton (1962) reported that the mean electrical axis in the frontal plane in compensated dogs was 66°, and that it was 100° in dogs in congestive heart failure caused by chronic mitral valvular fibrosis. However, 15 of 17 dogs in the latter group had an axis under 100°, and the mean axis for the group was increased because two dogs had axes of 317° and 270°, respectively, which probably indicated conduction disturbances rather than right axis deviation.

The heart rate is often increased in dogs with serious chronic valvular fibrosis because compensatory tachycardia develops. The rhythm is usually sinus, but arrhythmias have been observed in as many as 53 per cent of dogs with mitral insufficiency that were in congestive heart failure (Wallace and Hamilton, 1962). Atrial and atrioventricular junctional premature contractions are often seen on the electrocardiogram (Fig. 13-19). Occurring often but less frequently than single premature contractions are paroxysmal atrial tachycardia, ventricular premature beats, and paroxysmal ventricular tachycardia (Fig. 13-20). Atrioventricular dissociation and ventricular tachycardia may occur in advanced and terminal mitral valve disease (Fig. 13-21). Atrial fibrillation is most often recognized late in the course of this disease and is always associated with combined right and left heart failure. It is seen most frequently, but not always, in male dogs (Fig. 13-22).

P mitrale (P wave > 0.04 sec.) is common in dogs with mitral valvular insufficiency because of left atrial enlargement (Fig. 13-23). Left ventricular hypertrophy is recognized on the electrocardiogram (Fig. 13-23) by prolongation of the QRS complex (> 0.05 sec. in small and medium-sized breeds or > 0.06 sec. in large breeds); increased amplitude of the QRS complex in leads II, III, and aVF (R wave > 2.5 to 3.0 mv.); left axis deviation in the frontal plane; and the presence of S-T repolarization changes (see pp. 134-143).

As mitral insufficiency progresses, pulmonary lesions develop and impair right heart function. Prolongation of the initial forces to the right (> 0.01 sec.) suggests right ventricular hypertrophy accompanying left ventricular hypertrophy. Other signs of right ventricular hypertrophy are the presence of an S wave in lead I and right axis deviation (see p. 143). When the right heart is stressed, right atrial strain is indicated by increased amplitude of the P wave or P pulmonale (P wave > 0.4 mv.).

(Text continues on page 351.)

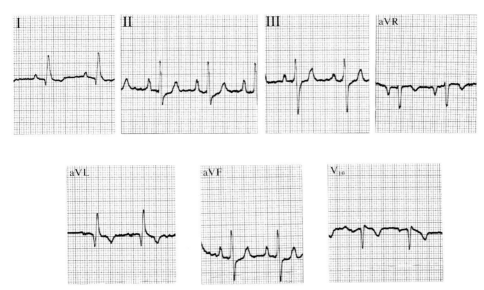

FIGURE 13-17 Electrocardiogram of a dog with advanced chronic mitral and tricuspid valvular fibrosis. The mean electrical axis in the frontal plane is 5°, which is consistent with left axis deviation; in addition, the maximum width of the QRS complexes is 0.06 sec. Both of these findings are compatible with left ventricular hypertrophy. Although it is neither a frequent nor a constant finding, left axis deviation may occur in dogs with left ventricular hypertrophy. P pulmonale is also present.

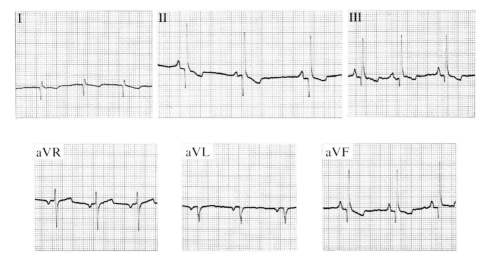

FIGURE 13-18 Right axis deviation. The mean electrical axis in the frontal plane in this dog with chronic mitral and tricuspid valvular fibrosis is 100°. Right axis deviation is not usually associated with acquired atrioventricular valvular insufficiency.

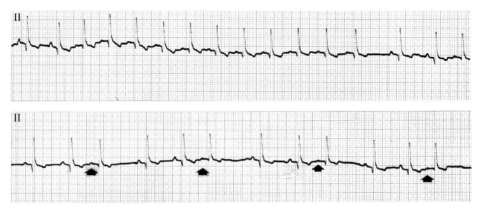

FIGURE 13-19 Supraventricular arrhythmias. The third beat in the top tracing, an atrial premature contraction, is the first beat of a run of paroxysmal atrial tachycardia during which the heart rate is 188 beats/minute. After the paroxysmal atrial tachycardia spontaneously ceases at the end of the top strip, a sinus rhythm is again present. In association with paroxysmal atrial tachycardia, the sinus rhythm is usually interrupted periodically by atrial premature contractions (arrows, bottom tracing). In these complexes, the P waves are abnormal and occur early and are similar to those occurring during the atrial tachycardia.

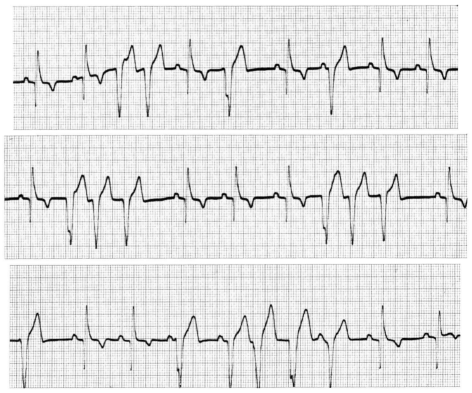

FIGURE 13-20 Chronic valvular heart disease is often associated with degenerative myocardial lesions which may stimulate ectopic ventricular foci. Ventricular premature contractions may occur singly, or in pairs, runs (3), or paroxysms (4 or more); all of these are demonstrated in these 3 tracings from a dog with advanced chronic mitral valvular fibrosis. P mitrale and left ventricular hypertrophy are also present. Lead II electrocardiogram.

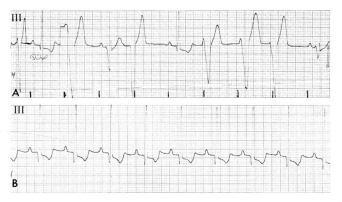

FIGURE 13-21   Ventricular tachycardia with capture and fusion. *A*, The atria and ventricles beat independently of each other in this arrhythmia. The black lines at the bottom of the tracing indicate the atrial rate. Wide, aberrant ventricular beats indicate the idioventricular rhythm (beats 1, 3, 5, 8, and 9). When the P wave arrives at the atrioventricular node when it is not refractory, the impulse captures the ventricle, resulting in a normal QRS complex called a "capture beat" (beats 2 and 6). When the P wave is conducted through the atrioventricular node and depolarizes the ventricle at the same time as does the idioventricular beat, a fusion beat with a configuration between that of the normal capture beat and the idioventricular beat results (beats 4, 7, and 10).

B, Following the administration of parenteral quinidine sulfate, a normal sinus rhythm resumes. If the idioventricular rate is greater than 100 beats/min., the rhythm is termed ventricular tachycardia. When it is less than 100 beats/min., the rhythm is referred to as atrioventricular dissociation.

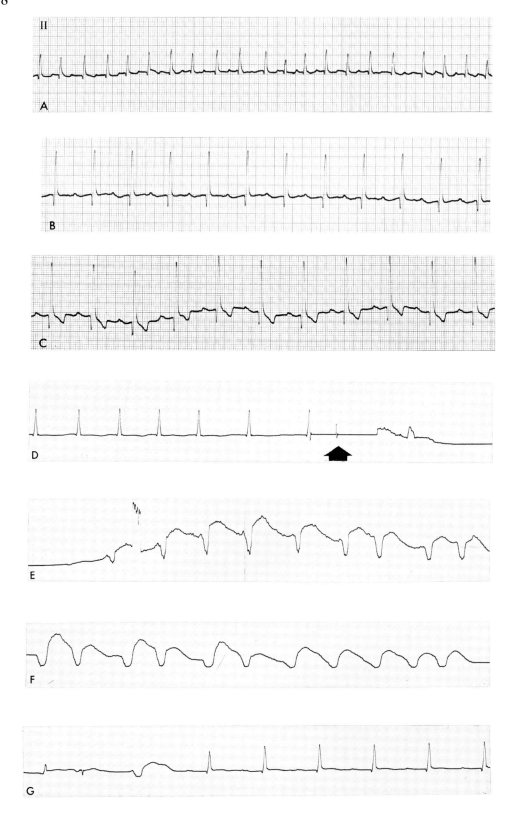

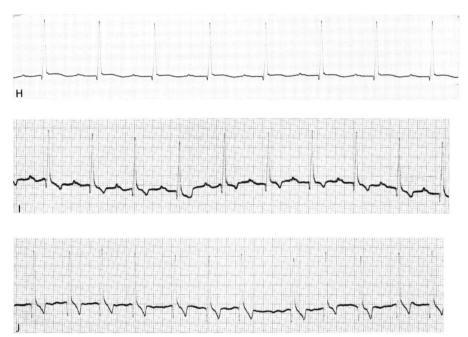

FIGURE 13-22   Lead II of the electrocardiogram, strips run at 50 mm./sec. *A*, The heart rate is 240 beats/minute. The rate is rapid and irregular, and the absence of P waves indicates atrial fibrillation. *B*, Tracing made immediately following successful direct current cardioversion. P waves and a sinus rhythm have been restored. A prolonged P-R interval is common following restoration of a sinus rhythm. *C*, Two months after cardioversion, the rhythm remains sinus. There is a pattern of P mitrale and left ventricular hypertrophy in this tracing. The dog was maintained on oral digoxin and quinidine.

D through *H*, Six months following cardioversion (*B*), the rhythm again reverted to atrial fibrillation (*D*). Cardioversion at 150 w./sec. (arrow) induced a brief ventricular tachycardia (*E, F,* and *G*), and a sinus rhythm was then restored (*G* and *H*). Notice again the prolonged P-R interval (*H*) immediately following conversion.

I, Four days following the second cardioversion, the rhythm remained sinus, and the dog was discharged on slightly higher dosages of digoxin and quinidine. *J*, Ten days after the second cardioversion, atrial fibrillation recurred. Further attempts at cardioversion were not considered, and the dog was maintained only on digoxin to maintain a slow ventricular rate.

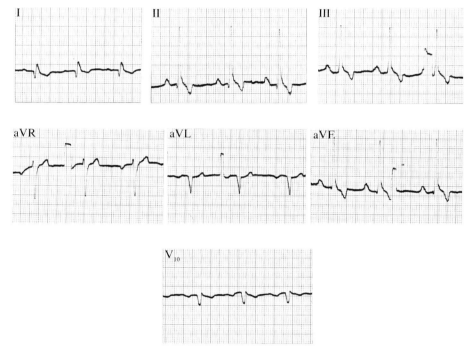

FIGURE 13-23 Representative electrocardiogram of a dog with advanced chronic mitral valvular fibrosis. Although the mean electrical axis in the frontal plane is normal (80°), the P wave is definitely prolonged, indicating left atrial enlargement. Prolongation of the QRS complexes, increased amplitude of the QRS complexes, and repolarization changes of the S-T segment are all consistent with advanced left ventricular hypertrophy. Because the QRS complexes are wider than 0.07 sec., left bundle branch block is also suggested; however, this is merely an intraventricular conduction delay due to the extreme left ventricular hypertrophy.

VECTORCARDIOGRAPHY

In the frontal plane, there is an increase in the initial forces to the right ($>$ 0.01 sec.), as well as an increase in the magnitude of the loop. In the horizontal plane, the terminal forces are directed leftward as usual but are prolonged terminally, especially in the dorsal direction (Fig. 13-24).

LABORATORY FINDINGS

In the absence of concurrent disease, the hematologic values are not markedly abnormal in dogs with chronic valvular fibrosis. The red blood cell count and packed cell volume may be slightly elevated. In dogs with mitral insufficiency, the blood volume in cc./kg. of body weight was 90 cc./kg. in dogs with mild disease, and increased to 120 cc./kg. in dogs with severe disease, as compared to 75 to 90 cc/kg. in normal dogs (Wallace, 1962). Detweiler and Patterson 1965b) reported a slight decrease in packed cell volume and hemoglobin levels, especially in dogs in right heart failure. The white blood cell count is normal unless an infection (often bronchopneumonia) develops, producing neutrophilia with a shift to the left. Blood glucose is not abnormal, but the blood urea nitrogen and serum glutamic pyruvic transaminase levels can both be moderately elevated (to 40 mg./ 100 ml. and 100 S. F. units, respectively) as a result of decreased renal blood flow and chronic hepatic congestion. Serum electrolytes are usually within normal limits. In dogs with heart failure, the average plasma protein concentration is 4.8 Gm. per cent, as compared to 6.5 to 7.0 Gm. per cent in normal dogs, according to Wallace (1962). This latter difference has not been a frequent finding in our clinic.

CARDIAC CATHETERIZATION

As the severity of mitral insufficiency increases, left atrial pressures increase. This is characterized by a large "V" wave and a prominent "Y" descent when left atrial pressures are recorded directly (Fig. 13-25) or when pressures are recorded from the pulmonary artery wedge position, which reflects left atrial pressure. Left ventricular pressures may remain normal, although the end diastolic pressure is greater than 10 mm. Hg (Figs. 13-25, 13-26) when heart failure results in a volume overload of the left ventricle. Right ventricular and pulmonary arterial systolic pressures increase in advanced mitral insufficiency. The right ventricular end diastolic pressure and the right atrial pressure remain normal unless right heart failure is present, in which case they too are elevated.

Wallace (1962) reported that the jugular venous pressure in dogs with mitral insufficiency was higher than that in normal dogs (0 to 20 mm. Hg, as compared to 0 to 6 mm. Hg). Systolic pulmonary arterial pressures were also elevated (35 to 55 mm. Hg as compared to 20 to 30 mm. Hg). No gross differences were observed in femoral artery pressures.

On indicator dilution curves, the peak dye concentration is delayed, indicating that the dye is not ejected from the ventricle as a bolus but instead gradually becomes diluted because of constant regurgitation from the ventricle into the atrium.

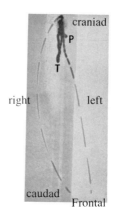

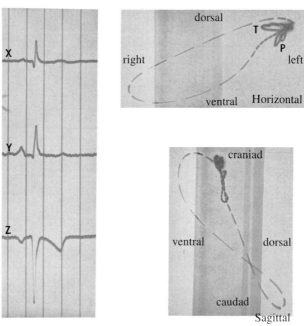

FIGURE 13-24 The vectorcardiogram recorded from a dog with chronic mitral valvular fibrosis demonstrates an accentuation of the normal loops. There is an increase in the initial rightward forces (frontal and horizontal loops); an increase in the overall length of the loops; and an increased area within the loops. The directions of the P and T loops are normal. The frontal loop was recorded at double amplitude.

The chamber enlargement, ventricular wall thickness, and degree of mitral regurgitation can be evaluated on selective left ventricular angiocardiograms (Fig. 13-16).

DIFFERENTIAL DIAGNOSIS

Congestive heart failure with pulmonary edema is often complicated by or incorrectly diagnosed as *pneumonia*. These conditions must be differentiated, since pulmonary infections are likely to complicate or occur concurrently with congestive heart failure.

Stertorous breathing in brachycephalic dogs or in dogs with respiratory conditions is often mistakenly identified as mitral and/or tricuspid insufficiency. This sound may mimic that of a murmur, thus falsely suggesting the presence of a cardiac abnormality. Respiratory sounds should be carefully differentiated from cardiac sounds, and their significance should be considered in view of the results of the overall examination.

Tricuspid insufficiency due to chronic tricuspid valvular fibrosis usually coexists with mitral insufficiency (see pp. 371-376), although it may occur alone or as the more prominent cardiac lesion. The murmur of tricuspid insufficiency is most intense at the third to fifth right intercostal space near the junction of the lower and middle thirds of the thorax. When the murmur is severe, it may radiate to the left thorax. The murmur of tricuspid insufficiency resembles that caused by chronic mitral valvular fibrosis, and it is often impossible to differentiate the two because the murmur of mitral insufficiency may radiate to the right thorax. Therefore, it is important to assess the signs of heart failure present — that is, right-sided failure, left-sided failure, or both — since the murmur of mitral insufficiency is more likely to be associated with left heart failure, tricuspid insufficiency with right heart failure, and mitral insufficiency and tricuspid insufficiency with biventricular heart failure.

Acute *rupture of the chordae tendineae* produces signs exactly like those seen with chronic mitral valvular fibrosis, phase IV/IV. The distinguishing sign in the differential diagnosis of these two conditions (which may also coexist) is the rapid onset (24 to 48 hours) of coughing, respiratory distress, and pulmonary edema in dogs with ruptured chordae tendineae (see pp. 366-371).

The systolic murmur characteristic of *anemic murmurs* and functional murmurs is short and high-pitched and is not holosystolic. There is usually little radiation, and the intensity varies from beat to beat. One should attempt to associate murmurs and cardiac enlargement with an organic condition unless the murmur is proved to be functional or unless anemia is present.

Cardiomyopathy resulting in mitral insufficiency (see Chapter 14) results in clinical signs similar to those that occur with chronic mitral valvular fibrosis. However, right heart failure is the most prominent feature of the former condition. In addition, dogs with idiopathic cardiomyopathy are usually young or middle-aged, and atrial fibrillation is the cardiac rhythm, whereas the cough dominates the clinical picture of chronic mitral valvular fibrosis.

A *congenital ventricular septal defect* produces a murmur similar to that of mitral insufficiency which is auscultated over the left caudal sternal border. However, the murmur of a ventricular septal defect extends to the right of the sternum,

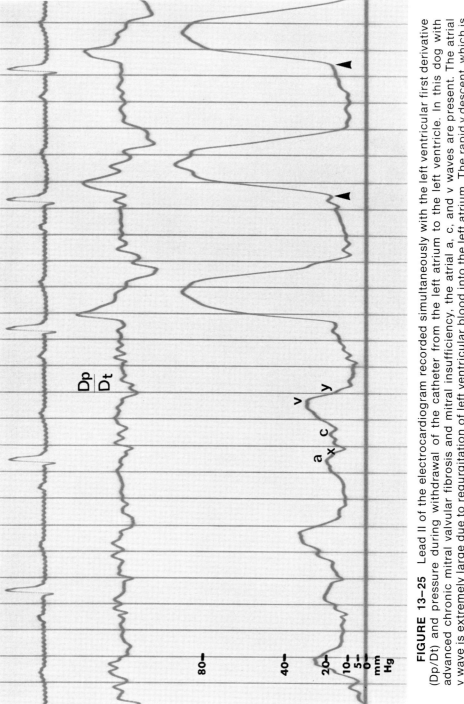

FIGURE 13-25   Lead II of the electrocardiogram recorded simultaneously with the left ventricular first derivative (Dp/Dt) and pressure during withdrawal of the catheter from the left atrium to the left ventricle. In this dog with advanced chronic mitral valvular fibrosis and mitral insufficiency, the atrial a, c, and v waves are present. The atrial v wave is extremely large due to regurgitation of left ventricular blood into the left atrium. The rapid y descent, which is a characteristic of mitral insufficiency, occurs as atrial blood flows rapidly into the left ventricle. The elevated left ventricular end-diastolic pressure (arrows) is a hemodynamic indication of the pressure of heart failure.

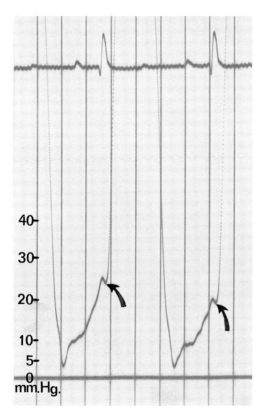

FIGURE 13-26 Elevated left ventricular end-diastolic pressure. When the pressure is recorded at an increased amplitude of mm. Hg per vertical mm., the end-diastolic pressure (arrows) is clearly recorded. Because small differences separate normal from abnormal end-diastolic pressures, it is preferable to use recordings such as this one when measuring the end-diastolic pressure. The left ventricular end-diastolic pressure in this tracing varies from 20 to 25 mm. Hg.

and a more prominent thrill is palpated along the right thoracic wall. Ventricular septal defects are first recognized in puppies, and heart failure usually develops early in life, when the defect is large (see Chapter 18). In comparison, chronic mitral valvular fibrosis usually develops after 5 years of age, and clinical signs occur even later. The electrocardiographic findings in ventricular septal defects may suggest right ventricular hypertrophy, rather than the left ventricular hypertrophy and left atrial dilatation that occur with mitral insufficiency.

The murmurs of *congenital aortic stenosis* and *pulmonic stenosis* are crescendo-decrescendo and more musical than that of mitral insufficiency. They are most intense over the aortic and pulmonic valves and radiate cranially on the thorax and to the right, as well as to the carotid arteries in dogs with aortic stenosis. These murmurs occur later in systole than does the murmur of mitral insufficiency and often do not obliterate the second heart sound. In dogs with aortic stenosis, the pulse is slow, small, and late-rising, rather than jerky, as it is in decompensating chronic mitral valvular fibrosis. Radiographically, an aortic bulge caused by poststenotic dilatation of the aortic arch is seen in dogs with aortic stenosis; this buldge is absent in dogs with chronic mitral valvular fibrosis. In dogs with pulmonic stenosis, bulging of the main pulmonary artery is the important differential diagnostic feature on radiographs.

RADIOGRAPHIC DIFFERENTIAL DIAGNOSIS

Although typical, the radiographic signs of chronic mitral valvular fibrosis are not pathognomonic for this disease. The various causes of mitral insufficiency cannot be differentiated radiographically. Furthermore, left atrial enlargement, left ventricular enlargement, and/or generalized enlargement of the cardiac silhouette as seen with secondary involvement of the right heart are also seen in a number of other disease conditions. An increased volume of blood flowing through the lungs and the left heart in left-to-right shunts, such as patent ductus arteriosus or large ventricular septal defect, or an increased total blood volume such as that secondary to severe chronic anemia, causes radiographic signs similar or identical to those of mitral insufficiency. Secondary generalized enlargement of the cardiac silhouette is also a sequela to heart failure from myocardial disease, pericarditis, or peritoneopericardial hernia, from which it can often be differentiated clinically, radiographically, or both.

Cardiac catheterization and angiocardiography provide one of the best means of obtaining detailed information about mitral insufficiency. This technique enables differentiation of hypertrophy from dilatation and is the method of choice for ruling out the presence of a congenital disease such as patent ductus ateriosus, aortic stenosis, or aortic insufficiency, which may secondarily initiate mitral insufficiency.

In most cases these conditions may be differentiated from mitral insufficiency resulting from chronic mitral valvular fibrosis by specific radiographic findings. Chronic anemia is associated with mild overcirculation and slight enlargement of the pulmonary artery segment, but no signs of venous congestion or pulmonary edema develop. Pericardial effusion results in a globular cardiac silhouette in both the lateral and the dorsoventral views. There is no prominent left atrium displacing the left stem bronchus dorsally. On the lateral view the left cardiac border is bowed caudally, in contrast to severe mitral insufficiency in which it is straight. Fluoroscopy may also be helpful in differentiating pericardial lesions (see Chapter 15). When the heart fails because of aortic stenosis, there is usually a dilated aortic arch. Shunting of blood from left to right, as occurs in patent ductus arteriosus, ventricular septal defect, and atrial septal defect, results in hypervascularity of the lung field. In addition, in a patent ductus arteriosus the cardiac silhouette is elongated owing to a widened aortic arch, and an aneurysmal bulge of the descending aorta, and an enlarged pulmonary artery segment are present. The generally enlarged cardiac silhouette seen in dogs with a peritoneopericardial diaphragmatic hernia is differentiated by the loculated gas pockets within the silhouette and the discontinuity of the diaphragmatic outline in one or both views.

PROGNOSIS

Most dogs with chronic mitral valvular fibrosis remain compensated and thus are asymptomatic throughout most of their lives (phase I/IV); if they develop congestive heart failure, it is usually late in life. When cardiac dysfunction occurs the condition progresses slowly, and therapy is often very helpful in retarding further circulatory disturbances in the early stages of the disease (phases II/IV and III/IV). Even as the disease progresses to congestive heart failure (phase IV/IV), therapeutic measures may often prove successful for a variable although short period of time—usually several months to a year.

THERAPY

Therapy is initiated according to the phase of the disease, and the treatment is usually symptomatic. Although therapeutic measures may improve circulatory function, the cause cannot be treated, and further pathology cannot be prevented from developing.

Asymptomatic dogs (Phase I/IV).   Neither therapy nor restriction of exercise is required. Sodium need not be restricted in the diet; however, food excessively high in sodium and poor quality protein should not be fed. Clinical examinations every 4 to 6 months are recommended when cardiac disease is evident. When clinical signs of heart failure are absent but the intensity of the systolic murmur increases, and when radiographic and/or electrocardiographic findings indicate progressing cardiac disease, the dog should be placed on a low sodium diet. Prophylactic digitalization is advised in those cases that are considered likely to progress to heart failure.

Dogs with early signs (Phase II/IV).   Initially, restriction of strenuous exercise and excitement, as well as of sodium and caloric intake, may relieve occasional episodes of dyspnea, cough, and fatigability. Before heart failure is obvious, dietary sodium restriction combined with administration of bronchodilators and occasional sedation may be extremely effective. Since the majority of cases do not progress beyond this point, the importance of such therapy should not be underestimated. In the authors' experience, bronchodilation is effectively accomplished with the drugs noted in Table 13-3, which are listed by generic name, preparation sizes available, trade names, and dosages used.

Dogs with advanced signs and heart failure (Phases III/IV and IV/IV). There is no substitute for the proper use of the cardiac glycosides when the heart is failing. Digoxin is the preferred drug for use in dogs in congestive heart failure (for dosage and routes of administration, see Chapter 7). Diuretic agents should be used in association with cardiac glycosides to control retention of sodium and water. Although they provide effective diuresis, diuretics should not be considered as a substitute or an alternative for digoxin in the treatment of congestive heart failure (see Chapter 9). In addition to therapy with digitalis and diuretics, sodium should be restricted as completely as possible. Some dogs will refuse to eat all low sodium diets. Rather than starve these animals, diuretic therapy may be used to help eliminate excessive quantities of salt used in the preparation of a palatable diet. Exercise should be restricted during the acute phases of congestive heart failure; hospitalization is often the only means of accomplishing this, since restriction at home may be difficult.

In addition to cardiac glycosides, diuretics, and salt restriction, bronchodilators may also be required to control the signs of coughing and dyspnea. Dihydrocodeinone (Hycodan), 2.5 mg. to 10 mg. two to four times daily, phenobarbital, or chloral hydrate may be utilized when all other agents are ineffective in relieving the cough. These agents are not substitutes for the proper cardiac therapy; instead, they should be used in addition to the previously mentioned drugs.

PATHOLOGIC FINDINGS

In chronic mitral valvular fibrosis, the mitral valve appears grossly thickened, with grayish-white nodules on the leaflet edges, and the leaflets are contracted to a variable degree depending on the stage of fibrosis (Das and Tashjian, 1965; Luginbühl and Detweiler, 1965) (Fig. 13-27). The commissures of the valve leaflets do not often fuse (Das and Tashjian, 1965). The chordae tendineae may be shortened or thickened (Luginbühl and Detweiler, 1965) but are rarely fused (Das and Tashjian, 1965). Detweiler et al. (1968) and Ettinger and Buergelt (1968; 1969) have noted that the chordae tendineae may be thin or ruptured. Das and Tashjian (1965) reported fibrosis at the attachment of the chordae tendineae to the papillary muscles. The mitral anulus is usually dilated in this condition.

In a series of 314 necropsies (Luginbühl and Detweiler, 1965), there was chronic fibrosis of the mitral valve in 193 dogs, of the tricuspid valve in 71 dogs, and of the aortic valve in 9 dogs; pulmonic valve lesions were not seen. Bretschneider (1962) reported that 83.3 per cent of 688 dogs with valvular endocarditis had chronic valvular fibrosis: the mitral valve was affected in 57.3 per cent; mitral and tricuspid valves in 26.6 per cent; tricuspid valve in only 7.5 per cent; the aortic valve in 2.1 per cent; the pulmonic valve in 0.4 per cent; and other combinations in 6.1 per cent.

Microscopically, the leaflets are thickened, with ". . . collagen and elastic fibrosis, edema, increased ground substance, and sometimes amyloid deposition and hemorrhage" (Detweiler et al., 1968). Luginbühl and Detweiler (1965) noted that these changes may involve the subendothelial valve layers and, in the more advanced cases, the fibrosa. Wagner (1968) recognized the earliest changes in the connective tissue ground substance, as a result of accumulation of water and stainable acid mucopolysaccharides.

TABLE   13-3   BRONCHODILATORS USED AT THE ANIMAL MEDICAL CENTER[*]

GENERIC NAME AND PREPARATION SIZE	TRADE NAME	DOSAGE
Aminophylline (theophylline with ethylenediamine) $1^{1}/_{2}$ gr. (100 mg.) tablets	–	$^{3}/_{4}$ to $1^{1}/_{2}$ gr., 2 to 4 times daily as needed
Theophylline elixir 80 mg./15 cc.	Elixophyllin Theolixir	0.2 cc/lb., 2 to 4 times daily as needed
Theophylline with glyceryl guaiacolate Capsule or 15 cc. = 100 mg. Theophylline + 90 mg. glyceral guaiacolate	Quibron	Capsules – 1 capsule 2 to 3 times daily Elixir – $^{1}/_{4}$ to 1 tbsp. 2 to 3 times daily
Theophylline with noscapine 100 mg. theophylline and 15 mg. noscapine per half-strength tablet	Theo-Nar	Half-strength tablets – $^{1}/_{2}$ to 1 tablet 2 to 3 times daily
Ethylpapaverine HCl and pentaerythritol tetranitrate 30 mg. ethylpapaverine plus 20 mg. pentaerythritol (tablet) or 50 mg. pentaerythritol (capsule)	Papavatral 20 (tablet) Papavatral LA (capsule)	$^{1}/_{2}$ to 1 tablet 2 to 3 times daily $^{1}/_{8}$ capsule twice daily
Aminophylline with ¼ or ½ grain phenobarbital	–	$^{1}/_{2}$ to 1 tablet 2 to 3 times daily

[*]There are many other single and combination bronchodilating products available as human or veterinary products which may be equally as effective as those commonly employed by the authors.

Chronic mitral valvular fibrosis is often accompanied by intramural coronary arteriosclerosis. This is most common in older dogs with chronic mitral valvular fibrosis and congestive heart failure, although it also occurs in younger dogs with congenital subaortic stenosis (Detweiler et al., 1968). In dogs with valvular fibrosis producing mitral insufficiency and coronary arteriosclerosis, myocardial fibrosis and necrosis develop, probably as a result of ischemia (Detweiler et al., 1968). This microscopic lesion has been referred to as microscopic intramural ventricular myocardial infarction (MIMI) (Detweiler, 1962; Hamlin, 1968).

In 1293 dogs necropsied, Hubben, Patterson, and Botts (1963) found 1.7 per cent to have telangiectases in the atrioventricular valves, but they stated that such a finding could not be related statistically to chronic valvular disease, age, sex, or breed.

Dilatation of the left atrium usually occurs first, followed by eccentric hypertrophy and dilatation of the left ventricle. Right ventricular enlargement is often observed as the insufficiency becomes more severe and as the strain placed on the right heart increases. As pulmonary hypertension and tricuspid insufficiency develop and the right ventricle enlarges, the right atrium may also dilate. Roughened fibrous plaques on the intimal surface of the left atrium are seen directly opposite the mitral valve orifice. Because these lesions are the result of forceful regurgitation of blood into the left atrium, they are called "jet" lesions.

As a result of the increasing severity of regurgitation, whereby atrial volume

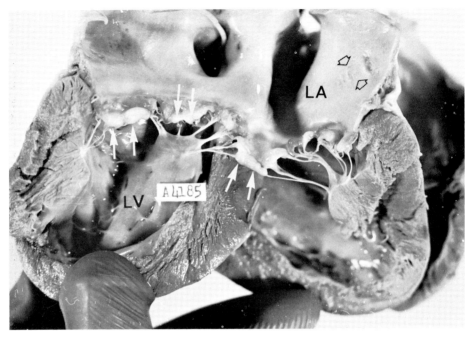

FIGURE 13-27 Postmortem specimen of opened left ventricle (LV) and left atrium (LA). The left ventricular wall is thickened, and the mitral valve leaflets are grossly thickened and contracted, with grayish-white nodules rolling in the free edges (white arrows). The valve leaflets are not fused, and the chordae tendineae appear normal. Jet lesions present on the left atrial wall (between clear arrows) result when the regurgitant streams of blood from the left ventricle continuously strike the atrial wall. (The authors thank Dr. S.-K. Liu, The Animal Medical Center, New York, N.Y., for taking this photograph.)

is increased, the left atrium gradually dilates to a tremendous size and becomes thickened. Splitting of the endocardium, progressing to left atrial tear, occasionally occurs (see pp. 361-366).

As the severity of mitral valvular insufficiency increases, circulatory failure develops, as well as extracardiac lesions. Clinically, the most significant of these lesions is pulmonary edema. The lung gradually loses its spongy texture and becomes hyperemic and congested. Grossly, it does not collapse, and it appears firm and red. The cut surface is wet, and varying amounts of frothy white or blood-tinged fluid can be expressed from the tissue.

ETIOLOGY

The etiology of chronic mitral valvular fibrosis is unknown, and numerous theories have evolved to explain its pathogenesis.

Stünzi (1962), Angrist (1964), Detweiler et al. (1968), and Wagner (1968) discuss the *possible* etiologic factors in chronic valvular disease of the dog. Some of the etiologic factors considered are:

1. Bacterial endocarditis which may have occurred earlier in life cannot be ruled out.

2. Viral valvulitis.

3. Autoimmune reaction or reaction to exogenous antigens. This possibility exists since valvular fibrinoid deposits along with myocardial necrosis and amyloid deposits in the vascular wall represent an altered immune state (Wagner, 1968).

4. Hemodynamic alterations.

5. Alterations of collagen tissue in age-related fashion (i.e., valve sclerosis and arteriosclerosis).

The possible relationship between rheumatic valvular disease in man and chronic valvular fibrosis in dogs has been discussed frequently but has been dismissed by Stünzi (1962) and by Detweiler et al. (1968) because of the difference in age prevalence and because Aschoff's nodules are not seen histologically in the dog. There is no evidence to suggest that chronic valvular fibrosis is initiated by bacterial endocarditis, since endocarditis would likely demonstrate intermediate microscopic stages of inflammation which have not been seen (Stünzi, 1962; Luginbühl and Detweiler, 1965).

Endocarditis as a separate disease entity occurs most often in the older dog (Lundh, 1964; Jones and Zook, 1965), as does chronic valvular fibrosis. However, the preferred location of the lesions in the two diseases differs. Chronic valvular fibrosis usually involves the mitral or mitral and tricuspid valves (Bretschneider, 1962; Luginbühl and Detweiler, 1965; Kersten, 1968), whereas bacterial or fibrinous endocarditis rarely affects the tricuspid valve (only 12 per cent of all cases of bacterial endocarditis according to Lundh, 1964). In comparison, the aortic valve, which is rarely affected with chronic valvular fibrosis, is often involved in bacterial endocarditis (34 per cent of all cases according to Lundh, 1964). This evidence further supports the hypothesis that chronic valvular fibrosis is not a likely sequela to bacterial valvular endocarditis.

ENDOCARDIAL RUPTURE AND LEFT ATRIAL SPLITTING

Endocardial splitting of the caudal left atrial wall, and occasionally the medial wall, has been reported as a pathologic condition by Stünzi (1962) and as a clinical syndrome by Buchanan and Kelly (1964). It is a complication of other cardiac conditions rather than a distinct disease entity.

In one study (Buchanan and Kelly, 1964), the disease affected the Dachshund and the Cocker Spaniel predominantly (13 of 22 dogs) and was seen mostly in male dogs (19 of 22 dogs). Hemopericardium was diagnosed clinically in five dogs and at necropsy in two others; all seven dogs so affected were male. The disease is usually a complication of chronic mitral valvular fibrosis, and death ensues quickly, usually within two hours when cardiac tamponade occurs.

The lesion begins as an incomplete rupture of the endocardium, upon which fibrin is deposited. The rupture then heals or develops into an extensive rupture producing hemopericardium (Luginbühl and Detweiler, 1965) (Fig. 13-28). Endocardial splitting of the interatrial septum resulting in acquired atrial septal defect has been reported in three dogs, and endocardial splitting with incomplete rupture has occurred secondary to patent ductus arteriosus (Buchanan and Kelly, 1964).

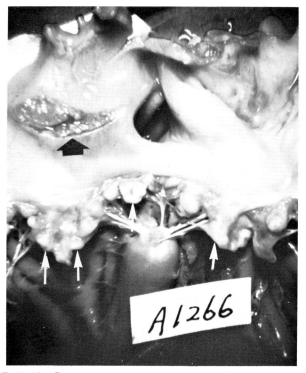

FIGURE 13-28 Postmortem specimen, dog with chronic mitral valvular fibrosis and left atrial tear. Rupture of the left atrial wall (black arrow) usually occurs at the site of a previous jet lesion. However, the rupture is usually in a horizontal plane approximately parallel to the valve anulus. Left atrial rupture is often a sequela to chronic mitral valvular fibrosis. The mitral valve leaflets in this specimen are severely fibrotic and shrunken (white arrows). From Gould, L., Ettinger, S., and Lyon, A.: Dis. Chest, 53 (1968): 545.

HISTORY

The history and physical examination of dogs with this lesion do not differ from those of the dog with chronic mitral valvular fibrosis (see pp. 322-329). In Buchanan and Kelly's study (1964), the dogs ranged in age from eight to 15 years, with an average age of 10.7 years.

AUSCULTATION

A holosystolic murmur of mixed frequency is heard over the mitral valve area and radiates dorsally, cranially, and to the right. The murmur is usually of sufficient intensity (grade V/VI to VI/VI) to produce a palpable precordial thrill. Arrhythmias suggesting supraventricular premature contractions or atrial fibrillation may be heard. In dogs which have not been treated for heart failure, a diastolic gallop rhythm is present. Buchanan and Kelly (1964) noted that heart sounds were not muffled in dogs with hemopericardium secondary to the left atrial tear. The authors have observed loud heart sounds and murmurs in all but one dog in which the complete left atrial rupture occurred within one hour of the original examination. In that dog, there was a noticeable decrease in the intensity of the murmur, with disappearance of the precordial thrill. At necropsy, 150 cc. of fresh blood was found in the pericardial sac. In this dog, the antemortem diagnosis was suggested by the sudden change in intensity of the murmur and by radiographs.

RADIOGRAPHIC EXAMINATION

The radiographic signs of endocardial splitting depend on the presence or absence of hemopericardium and have been described by Buchanan and Kelly (1964). If there is no hemopericardium, the radiographs are similar to those seen in phase IV/IV of mitral insufficiency (see pp. 338-339). Left atrial enlargement is usually extreme, indicated by a triangular extension of the cardiac silhouette into the diaphragmatic lobar area (Fig. 13-29 and 13-30). The left ventricular border remains straight in the lateral radiograph. The cardiac silhouette is usually dis-

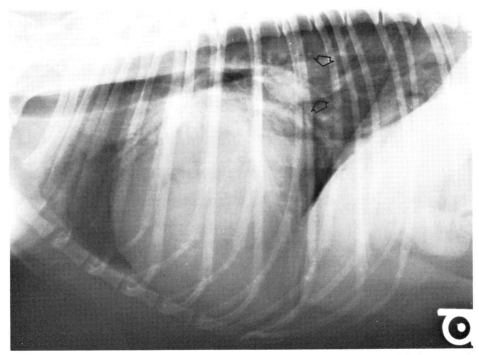

FIGURE 13-29 Left lateral radiograph of a 9 year old dog with hemoperi-cardium due to endocardial splitting and left atrial tear. The dog had had a deep cough for six weeks. A grade VI/VI murmur was auscultated at the left caudal sternal border. Immediately after radiographic examination the dog became cyanotic. The murmur diminished in intensity, and signs of acute heart failure developed. The dog succumbed despite intensive cardiac therapy. There is extreme enlargement of the cardiac silhouette in both cranial and caudal directions. The trachea runs parallel with the spine, and its distal extremity is elevated by the enlarged left atrium, which extends caudally into the lung field (clear arrows). The lung field is dense owing to the accentuated vascular structures, which have blurred outlines, and to a general-ized, hazy density indicating pulmonary congestion. The caudal vena cava is slightly widened and is denser than normal. Massive enlargement of the cardiac silhouette as seen in this case is compatible with pericardial effusion; however, the prominent left atrium and the presence of pulmonary congestion suggest left heart failure due to mitral insufficiency. Therefore, the two most likely diagnoses are left atrial tear or pericardial effusion due to chronic heart failure. At necropsy examination, 150 cc. of sanguineous fluid was found in the pericardial sac, and a massive clot was located at the apical area. Clots were also found on the epicardium of the left atrium. A tear 2.5 cm. in length which had apparently occurred within partially healed scar tissue was found in the left atrial wall.

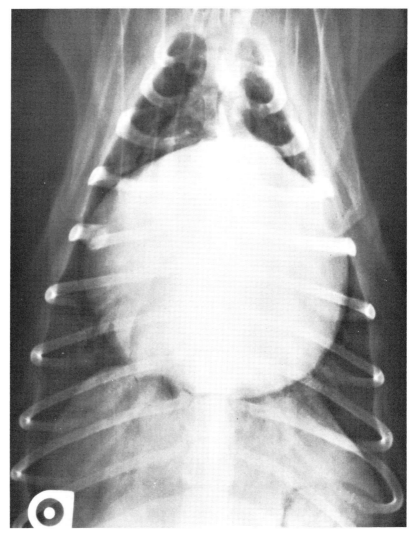

FIGURE 13-30   Dorsoventral radiograph, dog in Figure 13-29. The massively enlarged cardiac silhouette has a globular shape. Its surface is smooth, and all details within the shadow have been obliterated. A markedly enlarged, round cardiac silhouette in both lateral and dorsoventral views is a characteristic sign of peri-cardial effusion. The tentative diagnosis of left atrial tear cannot be made from the dorsoventral radiograph because the extreme enlargement of the cardiac silhouette obscures the enlarged left atrium.

similar in the lateral and dorsoventral views. If hemopericardium is present, the cardiac silhouette appears moderately to greatly enlarged and is evenly rounded in both views. With the exception of the enlarged left atrium, which can be seen only in the lateral radiograph, the radiographs are therefore similar to a moderately extensive pericardial effusion (see pp. 405-417). Since the left atrium cannot be seen on the dorsoventral radiograph, this view is not characteristic. Radiographic signs of left heart failure are usually present, but alveolar pulmonary edema seems to be unusual.

Because pericardial effusion may occur secondarily to congestive heart failure due to chronic mitral valvular fibrosis, differentiation of this condition from rupture of the left atrium may not be possible radiographically. Left atrial rupture can be expected when a dog with radiographic signs of phase IV/IV chronic mitral insufficiency suddenly develops a globular cardiac silhouette despite the administration of intensive therapy for heart failure (Harpster, 1969).

Extreme care in positioning the dog for radiographic examination is essential if left atrial rupture is suspected. An imminent tear may be provoked by forcing the dog to lie still in an uncomfortable position. The authors have seen three fatalities due to ruptured left atria during or shortly after radiographic examination.

ELECTROCARDIOGRAPHY

The electrocardiogram is the same as that seen with chronic mitral and tricuspid valvular fibrosis and insufficiency. The P wave is prolonged, and the QRS complex is likely to have features indicating left ventricular hypertrophy. Arrhythmias, especially atrial premature contractions, resulting from left atrial disease may be evident. Atrial fibrillation was recognized in two of 22 dogs with this condition (Buchanan and Kelly, 1964). A female Cocker Spaniel was observed by us with chronic mitral and tricuspid valvular fibrosis and left atrial rupture in which atrial premature contractions and a supraventricular rhythm occurred intermittently with paroxysmal atrial fibrillation (see Fig. 11-22).

CLINICAL PATHOLOGY

Pericardiocentesis of dogs with acute left atrial tear yields whole blood that clots. If the hemopericardium has been present for a period of time and no fresh hemorrhage has occurred, some clots form in the pericardial sac. The remainder of the blood is defibrinated and does not clot when removed (Harpster, 1969).

DIFFERENTIAL DIAGNOSIS

The differential diagnosis of endocardial splitting has been described by Buchanan and Kelly (1964). In chronic congestive heart failure due to mitral insufficiency, death is usually not sudden, and there is only minimal serous fluid collection in the pericardial sac.

After acute rupture of the chordae tendineae, the onset of signs is sudden, and a prior history of cough or dyspnea is absent. Pulmonary edema is the primary clinical sign. On radiographic examination, the cardiac silhouette is enlarged but not globular.

In pericardial effusion resulting from pericarditis or heart base tumors, the presenting signs of congestive heart failure, especially right-sided failure, have developed gradually. Coughing is noticeably absent. The heart sounds are muffled and often absent on auscultation. Wave amplitudes on the electrocardiogram are often diminished. Radiographically, the cardiac silhouette is large, globular, and homogeneous in appearance, and there is no marked left atrial enlargement (see Figs. 15-1 and 15-7). If a pneumopericardium is made after aspiration of pericardial fluid, a normal or only slightly enlarged cardiac silhouette is recognized within the air-filled pericardial sac. In addition, pericardial effusion is never extreme in left atrial tear, whereas it may be when other conditions produce pericardial effusion.

Peritoneopericardial hernia, a congenital defect that is usually seen in young dogs, is characterized by muffled heart sounds and diminished electrocardiographic amplitudes; these findings are similar to those in pericardial effusion. Radiographically, there is discontinuity of the diaphragmatic outline in the lateral and/or dorsoventral views, and loculated gas pockets are seen within the pericardial sac. An oral barium study demonstrating intestine within the cardiac silhouette should be used to prove the diagnosis (see Fig. 18-62). In some cases, physical examination confirms the presence of such a lesion when a hernia extending to the xiphoid is palpated cranial to the umbilicus.

ETIOLOGY

The etiology of rupture of the left atrial endocardium is unknown. However, dilatation of the left atrium in dogs with chronic mitral valvular disease and trauma to the caudal wall where the jet lesions most often occur must be considered as contributory factors. Neither the breed nor male predisposition to this condition has been explained.

TREATMENT

Because cardiac tamponade develops rapidly, it is unlikely that treatment of acute rupture of the left atrium with hemopericardium can be successful. Withdrawal of whole blood only improves function temporarily, since the hemorrhage will continue. If one can assume that the bleeding has stopped, withdrawal of pericardial fluid to reduce the hemopericardium will improve cardiac function and should therefore be attempted. If incomplete rupture is suspected, treatment of chronic mitral valvular fibrosis by intravenous digitalization and diuretics is suggested.

RUPTURE OF THE CHORDAE TENDINEAE

The chordae tendineae are fibrous collagen bands that extend from the papillary muscles to the edges of the atrioventricular valves. Their function is to prevent eversion of the valve leaflets into the atria during systole, since such eversion would result in valvular incompetence.

Rupture of the chordae tendineae may be classified as acute, subacute, or chronic, depending on the clinical syndrome produced (Ettinger and Buergelt, 1969). The acute syndrome is distinguishable clinically because of the sudden onset of acute congestive heart failure (Ettinger and Buergelt, 1968, 1969). The acute syndrome is usually caused by rupture of a first order chorda tendinea, which results in sudden, massive mitral insufficiency (Fig. 13-31). Dogs with this form of the syndrome die from massive pulmonary edema; large amounts of frothy, blood-tinged fluid pour from the oral and nasal cavities. In comparison, dogs with the subacute form of the disease have protracted chronic mitral valvular fibrosis and mitral insufficiency, as well as ruptured chordae tendineae

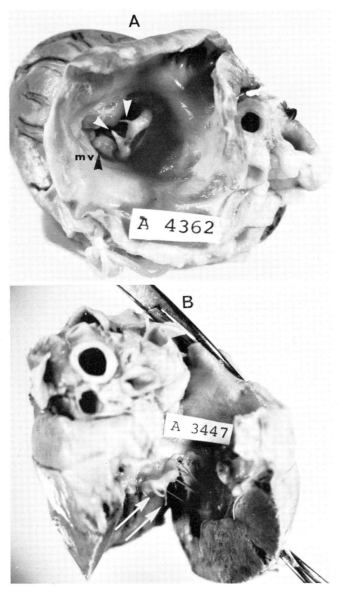

FIGURE 13-31   *A*, View of the mitral anulus from the left atrium. Two ruptured chordae tendineae (arrows) permit the septal leaflet to float toward the left atrium. There was also moderate (2+) mitral valvular fibrosis (MV). *B*, Two ruptured chordae tendineae (arrows) in a dog. The degree of mitral valvular insufficiency was recorded as moderate (2+) at necropsy. From Ettinger, S., and Buergelt, C.-D.: J.A.V.M.A., 155, (1969):535.

(Liu, Suter, and Ettinger, 1969). Dogs with chronic rupture of the chordae tendineae do not have symptomatic cardiac disease, and the condition is recognized only as an incidental necropsy finding. Since the subacute and chronic forms of the disease cannot be distinguished clinically from chronic mitral valvular fibrosis, the following discussion of the syndrome of rupture of the chordae tendineae is limited to the acute form only.

HISTORY AND PHYSICAL EXAMINATION

The dog is presented with extreme pulmonary edema, severe respiratory distress, cyanosis due to pulmonary embarrassment, and venous engorgement. A previous history of cardiac signs such as protracted dyspnea, orthopnea, or cough is remarkably absent. In 10 reported cases, the onset of clinical signs was 12 hours or less in six dogs, less than 24 hours in three dogs, and less than 48 hours in the tenth dog (Ettinger and Buergelt, 1969). If respiratory distress is severe, the dog may stand with its forelimbs abducted and its head and neck extended. The breeds in which this syndrome was recognized included six Poodles, two Dachshunds, one Cocker Spaniel, and one dog of mixed breed (Ettinger and Buergelt, 1969).

On physical examination, it is evident that the dog has been in good condition but is in obvious acute respiratory distress. A precordial thrill and a jerky pulse are recognized. A jugular pulse is especially obvious in dogs with short hair coats or in those which are clipped closely.

AUSCULTATION

A loud, harsh holosystolic murmur, grade V/VI to VI/VI, is loudest at the left caudal sternal border. The murmur usually radiates over the entire thorax and is occasionally so loud that it may be auscultated over most portions of the body. Because of the gross pulmonary edema, bubbling râles are heard even without the aid of a stethoscope, and the rapid heart rate, heart sounds, and murmurs may be difficult to distinguish from lung sounds. When the heart sounds are heard, there is a loud gallop rhythm due to the volume overload of the left atrium.

RADIOGRAPHIC EXAMINATION

Radiographic signs are similar to those seen in chronic mitral valve disease and left heart failure (Fig. 13-32 and 13-33). They are not indicative of the underlying cause. The alveolar pulmonary edema in the acute syndrome may be characterized by mottling and involvement of the peripheral lung field, which often remains free of such findings in slowly progressive heart failure of other origin. Because of the severity of the pulmonary distress associated with acutely ruptured chordae tendineae, radiography should be postponed until emergency treatment has taken effect. The clinician must decide whether the further stress placed upon the dog by radiographic examination is warranted. If radiographs are necessary to further evaluate the extent, origin, and progress of the respiratory lesions, the examination may be confined to a lateral radiograph only. Under no circumstances must the dog be positioned on its back. Of six dogs with ruptured chordae tendineae in which radiographs were made, gross pulmonary alveolar edema was recognized in four. Slight pulmonary congestion was present in one dog radiographed four days prior to sudden rupture. Slight left atrial enlargement was diagnosed in one dog, moderate enlargement in another, and severe enlargement in four (Ettinger and Buergelt, 1969).

ELECTROCARDIOGRAPHY

Electrocardiograms, like radiographs, are difficult to obtain from a patient in severe pulmonary distress. However, it is essential to have some basis on which to evaluate therapeutic effects, especially of cardiac glycosides. The dog should be restrained as little as possible and the leads attached in any position the dog assumes. Such an electrocardiographic tracing will indicate the cardiac rate and rhythm, and may suggest other abnormalities. In six dogs (Ettinger and Buergelt, 1969), the heart rate varied from 100 to 220 beats/minute. Sinus rhythm was present in four dogs, and one of these had first degree heart block. A ventricular rhythm and atrioventricular dissociation were present in the other two dogs. Left atrial dilatation was detected electrocardiographically in only one dog, in which there was prior evidence of chronic mitral valvular fibrosis and insufficiency.

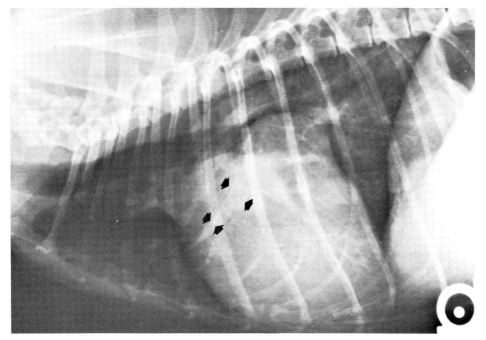

FIGURE 13-32 Lateral radiograph of a 15 year old dog examined because of a cough. A grade VI/VI murmur was auscultated at the left caudosternal border. The dog remained well for the next five days. Then pulmonary edema developed suddenly, and the dog died. At necropsy, chronic mitral and tricuspid valvular fibrosis and rupture of a chorda tendinea (first order) were found. On the radiograph, the trachea is only slightly elevated. The left stem bronchus is markedly displaced dorsally and is dorsoventrally compressed by the dilated left atrium. The caudal waist has almost disappeared, and there is left ventricular enlargement. The right heart is unremarkable. The lung field has remained clear. The hilar portions of the veins are dilated (arrows). The radiographic signs seen with imminent rupture of chordae tendineae are not diagnostic for this condition. Radiographs exposed after rupture has occurred indicate severe pulmonary congestion and alveolar edema.

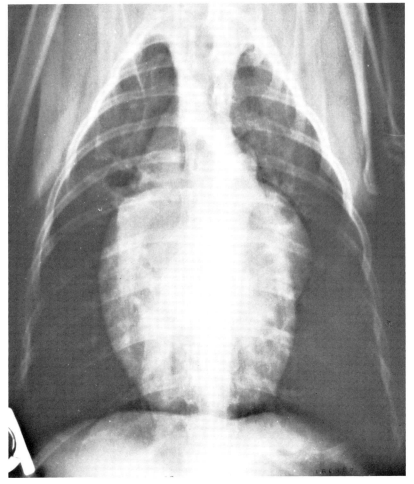

FIGURE 13-33 Dorsoventral radiograph, dog in Figure 13-32. The size of the cardiac silhouette is within normal limits for a dog of this age. The protrusion of the left auricle over the left cardiac border is the only radiographic sign indicating left heart disease.

Right atrial strain (P pulmonale) was present in three dogs, and five out of six had electrocardiographic evidence of left ventricular hypertrophy. The mean frontal plane electrical axis was normal, between 60° and 80°.

CARDIAC CATHETERIZATION

In dogs in which chordae tendineae from the septal leaflet of the mitral valve were experimentally transected (Haller and Morrow, 1955a, 1955b; Moscovitz et al., 1963), signs identical with those described in spontaneous rupture developed. On cardiac catheterization of these dogs, there was acute elevation of the left atrial "V" waves from 4 to 19.2 mm. Hg, followed by a precipitous "Y" descent of the left atrial pressure curve. These results demonstrate the severe mitral regurgitation that results from rupture of the chordae tendineae of the septal leaflet of the mitral valve. A major difference between such acute ruptures and chronic mitral valvular fibrosis and insufficiency is the sudden hemodynamic overload placed on the left atrium and pulmonary vascular bed. In chronic valvular disease, the left atrium has had time to compensate for increased pressure by dilatation and hypertrophy. In acute rupture of the chordae tendineae, the clinical syndrome is directly related to the inability of the left atrium to tolerate the burden of an acute hemodynamic overload.

DIFFERENTIAL DIAGNOSIS

Left atrial tear with cardiac tamponade may also be responsible for acute cardiac death. However, those dogs have a history of chronic valvular disease. In addition, sudden, massive hemorrhage into the pericardial sac may infrequently be accompanied terminally by muffling of the heart sounds and diminution of the electrocardiographic complexes.

Cardiac tamponade and acute pericarditis are rare and are accompanied by muffled heart sounds rather than by a loud, radiating systolic murmur. Radiographic examination is also helpful in the differential diagnosis of these conditions. Bronchopneumonia, heat prostration, and electric shock all may produce evidence of acute pulmonary edema. Elevated temperatures, rapid heart rates, and the lack of a loud cardiac murmur usually help to identify these conditions.

ETIOLOGY

The etiology of rupture of the chordae tendineae is unknown. Bacterial endocarditis, trauma, or other recognizable causes were absent in a study of 28 cases (Ettinger and Buergelt, 1969). The degree of chronic mitral valvular fibrosis was recorded in seven dogs with acute rupture of first order chordae tendineae. Two had only marginal fibrosis, and five had moderate fibrosis, but none had severe fibrotic lesions. It is not known whether chronic valvular disease modifies the course of the acute syndrome.

TREATMENT

Treatment of acute rupture of the chordae tendineae has been uniformly unsuccessful to date. Regardless of therapy, the signs advance rapidly, and death ensues because of pulmonary edema. The prognosis is very grave, but attempts at treatment should include intravenous digitalization and diuretic therapy, peripheral vasodilating agents and sedation (i.e., morphine), oxygen, rotating tourniquets, phlebotomy, and pulmonary defoaming agents.

CHRONIC TRICUSPID VALVULAR FIBROSIS

Chronic tricuspid valvular fibrosis is a disease entity that results in tricuspid valvular insufficiency in the same way that chronic mitral valvular fibrosis produces mitral insufficiency. Chronic tricuspid valvular fibrosis in the dog usually occurs in conjunction with chronic mitral valvular fibrosis but is also seen independently. Tricuspid insufficiency may also be associated with rupture of the chordae tendineae of the tricuspid valve (Ettinger and Buergelt, 1968), bacterial endocarditis, heartworm disease (Detweiler and Patterson, 1965a), and dilatation of the tricuspid valve anulus (e.g., functional tricuspid insufficiency), as well as with congenital lesions affecting the tricuspid valve. Functional tricuspid insufficiency due to right ventricular dilatation results from dilation of the anular ring so that the commissures of the leaflets of the tricuspid valve fail to coapt during right ventricular systole. In the presence of atrial fibrillation, tricuspid insufficiency and right heart failure become intensified.

The incidence of isolated tricuspid insufficiency in dogs is low. In 343 dogs with acquired valvular disease, only 11 had pure tricuspid insufficiency, but 152 had both mitral and tricuspid valvular fibrosis and insufficiency (Kersten, 1968). In another study, 7.5 per cent of 688 dogs with valvular endocarditis had tricuspid insufficiency, but 26.6 per cent had both mitral and tricuspid valvular fibrosis (Bretschneider, 1962). On necropsy studies, Das and Tashjian (1965) recognized combined mitral and tricuspid valvular fibrosis in almost 50 per cent of dogs with chronic valvular lesions.

HISTORY AND PHYSICAL EXAMINATION

The dog is usually presented with respiratory signs compatible with chronic mitral valvular fibrosis, since chronic tricuspid valvular fibrosis is usually associated with that condition. Whether the condition is isolated or combined with other diseases, the history includes progressive abdominal distention, anorexia, weight loss, diarrhea, and vomiting, all of which are due to congestion and edema of the liver, spleen, and gastrointestinal tract. Clinically, the signs of right heart failure predominate, although signs of left heart failure often occur simultaneously. Systolic jugular pulsations and venous engorgement of the superficial veins are evident. Hepatic enlargement due to venous congestion may produce signs of abdominal tenderness. Because of overfilling of the hepatic sinusoids, the jugular venous pressure increases when pressure is applied to the liver, thus demonstrating a positive *hepatojugular reflex*.

Peripheral edema does not result from right heart failure unless ascites is also present. Pleural and/or pericardial effusions develop in more advanced cases, as may icterus.

AUSCULTATION

A holosystolic murmur of mixed frequency similar to that of mitral insufficiency is auscultated at the right third to fifth intercostal space along the midthoracic wall. If the murmur is severe it may radiate to the left, and the condition becomes difficult to differentiate from combined mitral and tricuspid valvular insufficiency. When atrial fibrillation is present, the intensity of the murmur is variable, and the rhythm is irregular.

RADIOGRAPHIC EXAMINATION

Because tricuspid valvular fibrosis is rare as a separate lesion, typical radiographs demonstrating isolated tricuspid insufficiency are infrequent. On most radiographs, there is concurrent enlargement of the left heart even when clinical signs indicate that tricuspid valvular insufficiency is the predominant lesion. Right atrial enlargement as a radiographic sign of tricuspid insufficiency is more difficult to diagnose than is left atrial enlargement in early mitral insufficiency. As heart failure develops, the radiographic signs described below become more typical.

Because right atrial enlargement is difficult to assess unless it is marked in both the lateral and dorsoventral projections, it is essential to substantiate the suspicion by other radiographic signs such as dilatation of the caudal vena cava, widening of the cranial mediastinum, and signs of abdominal congestion.

On the lateral radiograph (Fig. 13-34), moderate to great right atrial enlargement is indicated by a slight dorsal deviation of the trachea cranial to the carina. The cranial mediastinal border extends farther ventrally than normal, and the caudal vena cava is denser and can be seen within the cardiac silhouette.

On the dorsoventral radiograph (Fig. 13-35), the right atrium can cause a craniolateral bulge in the cranial quadrant of the right cardiac silhouette, and the cranial vena cava may curve to the right before it joins the right atrium.

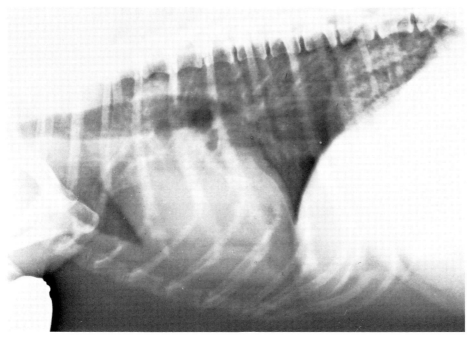

FIGURE 13-34 Left lateral radiograph, 14 year old dog with a history of recurrent diarrhea and enlarging abdomen. There were typical auscultatory signs of tricuspid insufficiency, and moderate liver enlargement was palpable. The trachea is elevated, but the slight ventral bend at the distal extremity has been preserved. The right cardiac border extends cranially to the third rib, and the cranial waist has disappeared. The right cardiac border runs parallel with the sternum to a greater extent than normal due to right ventricular enlargement. The left side of the heart is unremarkable. The caudal waist of the cardiac silhouette has been preserved. Dilatation of the caudal vena cava, often associated with right heart failure, is not present. The lung field has remained clear.

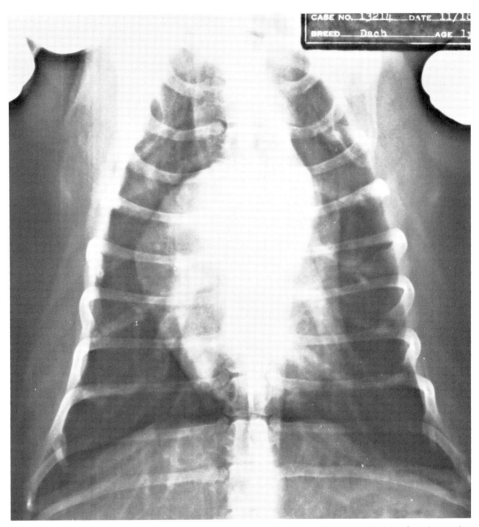

FIGURE 13-35 Dorsoventral radiograph, dog in Figure 13-34. A triangular protrusion of the cranial right cardiac border and farther extension of the right ventricular border to the right thoracic wall than normal indicate right atrial and right ventricular enlargement. The left heart is unremarkable. The lung field is clear.

Excessive enlargement of the right atrium has been reported in a dog with a rigid, anomalous tricuspid valve by Buchanan and Patterson (1965); the valve was both insufficient and stenotic. In a similar case seen by us (see Figure 18-35), a dog had pulmonic stenosis with secondary tricuspid insufficiency and heart failure which resulted in the right atrium being approximately the size of a normal heart.

Right ventricular enlargement is associated with chronic tricuspid valvular fibrosis and tricuspid insufficiency. In some dogs with right ventricular enlargement, the junction of the caudal vena cava with the cardiac silhouette appears elevated.

Pleural and pericardial effusion and congestion of the abdominal organs often follow the onset of right heart failure. Hepatomegaly and increased abdominal density due to ascites, with hazy outlines of the intestines and sometimes the abdominal wall, are common.

In numerous cases in which tricuspid insufficiency develops as a sequela to mitral insufficiency, the radiographic signs are those of a phase III/IV or IV/IV mitral insufficiency (see Table 13-1).

ELECTROCARDIOGRAPHY

P pulmonale and prolongation of the P-R interval occur as the right atrium enlarges. In the frontal plane, the mean electrical axis may be greater than 100°. It is not possible to diagnose tricuspid insufficiency electrocardiographically since signs of left ventricular hypertrophy often complicate and predominate on the electrocardiogram.

LABORATORY FINDINGS

Aspiration of ascitic fluid yields a thin, straw-colored transudate with a specific gravity under 1.018 and with small numbers of white and red blood cells. In long-standing cases, the fluid becomes blood-tinged, and the specific gravity increases. If a secondary infection is present, the number of white blood cells in the fluid is increased. In the presence of chronic passive liver congestion, liver enzyme levels are elevated. The serum glutamic pyruvic transaminase level is moderately elevated up to 240 Sigma Frankel units, and the alkaline phosphatase level has been recorded as high as 10 Bodansky units in dogs with isolated right heart failure. Retention of Bromsulphalein dye may be increased to 10 to 15 per cent after 30 minutes. Icterus and bilirubinemia are infrequent sequelae to tricuspid insufficiency.

DIFFERENTIAL DIAGNOSIS

Few conditions need be differentiated from tricuspid insufficiency. Mitral insufficiency with marked radiation of the murmur to the right thoracic wall represents a differential diagnostic problem (see pp. 322-361). If there are signs of biventricular failure, it is likely that both atrioventricular valves are affected. Ventricular septal defects result in a similar murmur and occasionally heart failure; however, severe congenital conditions are usually suspected in younger dogs, whereas chronic tricuspid valvular fibrosis is usually a problem in dogs over seven years of age. Heartworm disease may result in signs similar to those described for chronic tricuspid valvular fibrosis, such as right heart failure. Murmurs are usually but not always absent, and splitting of the second heart sound often develops with dirofilariasis. Microfilariae are absent in the peripheral blood in dogs with chronic tricuspid valvular fibrosis. The radiographic signs, especially the enlarged pulmonary arteries (see pp. 425-428), are usually adequate in suggesting heartworm disease.

Concurrent primary abdominal lesions such as neoplasia or hepatic dysfunction may also present problems in differential diagnosis because murmurs due to concurrent compensated atrioventricular valvular insufficiency can be auscultated. Such cases require a thorough medical examination. A pneumoperitoneum or an oral barium study may be helpful in demonstrating a primary abdominal lesion.

Whereas dogs with ascites due to tricuspid insufficiency often respond positively to diuretic therapy, exudates due to abdominal neoplasia are rarely eliminated by similar treatment. Neoplastic cells can be identified on cytologic examination of the ascitic fluid.

TREATMENT

Most dogs with chronic tricuspid valvular fibrosis respond to the classic measures applied in the treatment of congestive heart failure—i.e., digitalization, diuretics, and low sodium diets. If extreme abdominal distention and the resulting pressure on the diaphragm are responsible for respiratory embarrassment, aspiration of fluid is indicated. Fluid should be removed slowly to avoid a rapid fall in venous return to the heart and subsequent shock. Occasionally, large amounts of the fluid must be removed by aspiration before the dog responds satisfactorily to therapeutic measures.

AORTIC VALVULAR INSUFFICIENCY

Aortic valvular insufficiency (acquired or congenital) is recognized infrequently in dogs; when severe, it results in diastolic overloading of the left ventricle. The condition was diagnosed in 2 per cent of 688 dogs with all forms of valvular endocarditis by Bretschneider (1962). The etiology is uncertain except in dogs with bacterial endocarditis (Fisher, Ritchie, and Thomson, 1965) or congenital aortic stenosis, in which there is usually some degree of aortic valvular insufficiency (Carmichael et al., 1968). Trauma to an aortic valve leaflet, as may occur during cardiac catheterization or cardiac puncture, can produce aortic insufficiency. Buchanan (1965a) reported iatrogenic aortic insufficiency in dogs repeatedly subjected to cardiac puncture; he also reported a dog that had aortic insufficiency associated with a congenital ventricular septal defect. Aortic insufficiency has been recognized in a dog with a tetralogy of Fallot by us. The lesion has also been reported in a dog with aortic valvular bacterial endocarditis with rupture of the sinus of Valsalva into the pulmonary artery in which a continuous or machinery murmur was auscultated (Kleine, Bisgard, and Lewis, 1966).

HISTORY AND PHYSICAL EXAMINATION

Isolated aortic insufficiency may not be associated with any abnormal history until heart failure results in dullness, lethargy, and weight loss. A recurrent fever develops when the lesion results from bacterial endocarditis. As the severity of left ventricular hypertrophy increases, a prominent left ventricular heave may be observed and palpated over the cardiac apex. A jerky or waterhammer pulse which rises and falls sharply is characteristic in aortic insufficiency. In man, congestive heart failure occurs late in the course of the disease. Emboli originating from the endocardium may lodge in the brain, kidneys, and other organs, producing clinical signs of specific organ dysfunction and septicemia.

AUSCULTATION AND ELECTROCARDIOGRAPHY

A decrescendo diastolic murmur beginning with the second heart sound is auscultated over the aortic valve region. The murmur is a blowing sound of high frequency and low to moderate intensity (Fig. 13-36), and in the cases seen by the authors and by Fisher, Ritchie, and Thomson (1965), a mid- to late-systolic murmur was also present. When aortic insufficiency is associated with chronic mitral valvular fibrosis or congenital aortic stenosis, the intensity of the systolic murmur usually obscures the diastolic sounds; however, the diastolic murmur can be detected on the phonocardiogram. The electrocardiogram indicates left ventricular hypertrophy in advanced cases.

RADIOGRAPHIC EXAMINATION

Radiographs are not diagnostic in uncomplicated cases of aortic insufficiency. Isolated left ventricular enlargement resulting from the marked diastolic overload of the ventricle is difficult to assess unless left atrial enlargement occurs secondarily to ventricular or mitral anular ring dilatation. When aortic insufficiency occurs secondarily to congenital aortic stenosis, ventricular septal defect, tetralogy of Fallot, or acquired chronic mitral valvular fibrosis, radiographic signs attributable to the primary disease predominate.

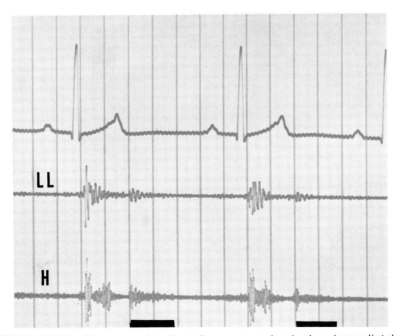

FIGURE 13-36 Decrescendo diastolic murmur beginning immediately after the second heart sound (black line). The murmur, due to aortic valvular insufficiency, occurred in a Great Dane after prolonged septicemia; a blood culture was positive for *beta* hemolytic *Streptococcus* sp. A systolic murmur was also present.

TREATMENT

Little is known about the treatment of acquired aortic insufficiency in the dog because the condition is encountered so infrequently. In one dog seen by the authors, beta-hemolytic streptococci (Lancefield group D) were isolated from a blood culture. This dog had signs of chronic lethargy and a persistent fever, but heart failure was absent. After treatment with antibiotics for four weeks, no bacteria were isolated from blood cultures. The diastolic murmur could not be auscultated two months later.

PULMONIC VALVULAR INSUFFICIENCY AND MITRAL STENOSIS

Pulmonic insufficiency is rare in dogs, but it may develop secondarily to dirofilariasis or patent ductus arteriosus with pulmonary hypertension (Detweiler and Patterson, 1965a). It has also been reported to occur after surgery for removal of heartworms, apparently as a result of trauma to the pulmonic valve leaflets (Hahn, 1962). Pulmonic insufficiency is identified on auscultation by a soft, blowing, decrescendo diastolic murmur of high frequency, and has been described by Hamlin et al. (1962) in a dog with iatrogenic pulmonic insufficiency following cardiac catheterization.

Mitral stenosis is rare in the dog. In one report, mitral stenosis, left atrial dilatation, and a left atrial mural thrombus were confirmed at necropsy in a 10 year old dog which had had atrial fibrillation with a grade III systolic murmur and a grade III rumbling diastolic murmur (Tashjian and McCoy, 1960). Detweiler (in Buchanan, 1965b) has also reported seeing this condition.

BACTERIAL ENDOCARDITIS

Endocarditis is a bacterial or nonbacterial inflammatory alteration of the endocardium and can be divided morphologically into mural or valvular endocarditis. Parietal or mural endocarditis involves the inner lining of the heart chambers (endocardium), particularly the left atrium. Deposition of calcium salts may follow necrosis of the subendocardial tissue and ulceration of the endocardium (Luginbühl and Detweiler, 1965). Mural endocarditis is usually a manifestation of other systemic diseases such as acute renal insufficiency or uremia (Jubb and Kennedy, 1963; Luginbühl and Detweiler, 1965), although mural endocarditis may also occur as an extension of a process originating from the valve leaflets. The inflammatory deposits in valvular endocarditis are referred to as vegetations or verrucae; verrucae are infrequently seen on the parietal or mural endocardium alone (Lundh, 1964). In a study of over 11,000 necropsies, Lundh (1964) reported an overall incidence of 0.58 per cent of spontaneous fibrinous endocarditis in the dog. The lesions were confined to the mitral valve in 34 of the 67 cases (54.8 per cent). In 46 (74.2 per cent), the mitral valve as well as one or more other valves was affected. Similarly, the aortic valve alone was involved in 12 of the 67 cases (19.4 per cent), but the aortic valve was affected in association with other valvular lesions in 21 (33.9 per cent) of the cases. Vegetations developed on the tricuspid valve in only four dogs (6.5 per cent), and there were lesions on the tricuspid valve and one or more other valves in eight dogs (12.9 per cent). The pulmonic valve was not affected in this study.

Comparison of various reports demonstrates the variable degree to which endocarditis is recognized at necropsy. Lundh (1964) reported an incidence of 0.58 per cent; Jones and Zook (1965) 5.8 per cent (58 of 991 necropsies); Shouse and Meier (1956) 6.6 per cent (40 of 600 necropsies); and in two earlier studies, by Schornagel in 1936 and Winquist in 1945, cited by Lundh (1964), the incidence was 0.74 per cent and 2.27 per cent, respectively. Such variable results suggest that the populations of dogs from which the necropsy material was obtained differed and/or that the criteria used to reach the diagnosis of endocarditis were variable.

HISTORY AND PHYSICAL EXAMINATION

The following discussion refers to both acute and chronic bacterial endocarditis. Dogs are presented with a nonspecific and nonpathognomonic history such as lethargy, weakness, anorexia, and chronic weight loss. There is usually evidence of a general lack of well-being. Shifting lameness and specific organ dysfunction may develop periodically if emboli lodge in the brain, muscles, lungs, kidney, gastrointestinal tract, or other organs. A chronic, recurrent fever may be reported by an astute owner or may be noticed if the veterinarian examines the dog repeatedly over an extended period for the nonspecific signs described above. Petechiae may be recognized in the eyes (Lillehei, Bobb, and Visscher, 1950). There are no apparent sex and breed predispositions, but endocarditis has been recognized most commonly at necropsy in older dogs (Lundh, 1964; Jones and Zook, 1965). Lundh (1964) noted a possible predilection of German Shepherds in the Stockholm region for this condition. A previous systemic disease, infection, or traumatic accident is occasionally reported by the owner.

Pallor, septicemia, lethargy, a systolic murmur, and sometimes evidence of a severe local infection such as dental abscess, pharyngitis, prostatitis, or anal sac abscess may be found on physical examination. Systemic infections such as bronchopneumonia or extension of local processes may also be related.

The spleen may be grossly enlarged on abdominal palpation. Embolization to the kidneys produces lumbar tenderness, hematuria, and proteinuria with evidence of leukocytes on microscopic examination of a urine specimen. Embolization can also be responsible for encephalitis and bronchopulmonary disease. In experimental dogs which developed bacterial endocarditis after arteriovenous fistulas were artificially induced, diagnosis was based upon the development of a fever, an elevated erythrocyte sedimentation rate, heart murmurs, petechiae in the eyes, recovery of organisms from the blood, and typical gross and microscopic necropsy findings (Lillehei, Bobb, and Visscher, 1950).

In the presence of chronic fever, signs of generalized septicemia, and a history that is compatible with endocarditis, hematologic studies such as a complete blood count and serial or daily blood cultures are indicated. Antibiotic therapy should be withheld temporarily, pending the results of the hematologic studies.

CARDIAC EXAMINATION

On auscultation of the heart, there may be a systolic or diastolic heart murmur. This murmur requires differentiation by physical and specialized examinations from murmurs caused by unrelated chronic valvular fibrosis, or, in the presence of pallor, an anemic murmur. The heart rate may be increased because of fever and/or anemia. On the electrocardiogram, disturbances of the cardiac rhythm are unusual in endocarditis, although Theran, Henry, and Thornton (1965) reported complete heart block with unifocal ventricular premature contractions in one dog with bacterial endocarditis. If the lesion continues to progress, active myocarditis with subsequent arrhythmias (ventricular premature contractions — single, paroxysmal, or continuous) is likely to develop. As the condition progresses, signs of generalized congestive heart failure may develop.

In one dog with bacterial endocarditis affecting the aortic valve, rupture of the sinus of Valsalva resulted in aortic insufficiency as well as shunting of blood from the aorta to the pulmonary artery, producing a continuous murmur. This condition, which required differentiation from a patent ductus arteriosus, was positively diagnosed by aortography (Kleine, Bisgard, and Lewis, 1966). Bacterial endocarditis associated with a ductus has been recognized by Buchanan (1968). Emboli from vegetative valvular endocarditis occluded the coronary arteries in two dogs (Nielsen and Nielsen, 1954). Because of the infrequency of this latter lesion, the clinical diagnosis of coronary occlusion is not warranted (see pp. 400-401). Supravalvular aortic medial necrosis was associated with bacterial endocarditis and myocarditis in one dog (Andrews and Kelly, 1970).

DIFFERENTIAL DIAGNOSIS

Because of the multiplicity of organ involvement, the diagnosis of bacterial endocarditis may be difficult. If the history and physical examination are compatible with those findings described above, and if a recurrent, chronic fever is present, the diagnosis of bacterial endocarditis should always be suspected, and serial blood cultures are indicated.

ETIOLOGY

According to Shouse and Meier (1956), Lundh (1964), and Luginbühl and Detweiler (1965), hemolytic and nonhemolytic streptococci, staphylococci, *Escherichia coli, Erysipelothrix rhusiopathiae,* and *Pseudomonas aeruginosa* have all been identified in dogs with bacterial endocarditis. Bone (1970) reported bacterial endocarditis caused by an L-form of *Pseudomonas aeruginosa. Streptococcus sp.* are apparently the most common cause. Lillehei, Bobb, and Visscher (1950) found that eight of 10 dogs developed bacterial endocarditis after arteriovenous fistulas producing a volume overload were created experimentally. The fistulas were large in the eight dogs that developed endocarditis and small in the other two, whose valves remained normal. The association of endocarditis with acute and subacute nephritis has been discussed by Stünzi (1962) and by Luginbühl and Detweiler (1965).

TREATMENT

When bacterial endocarditis is suspected, antibiotic treatment should be withheld temporarily so that serial blood cultures can be taken. If bacteria are isolated from the blood culture, antibiotic therapy should be instituted according to the results of sensitivity tests, and should be continued for at least three to four weeks. Blood cultures should be repeated during and after the completion of antibiotic therapy. One would expect blood cultures made during antibiotic therapy to be negative unless bacterial resistance has occurred. If circumstances do not allow therapy to be withheld until antibiotic sensitivity results are known, 1 to 2 million units of intramuscular procaine penicillin and 5 mg./lb. streptomycin may be administered twice daily (Detweiler and Patterson, 1966). Cardiac arrhythmias that develop when myocarditis becomes a complicating factor must be controlled with antiarrhythmic agents (see Chapter 8).

References

Andrews, E. J., and Kelly, D. F.: Naturally Occurring Aortic Medial Necrosis in a Dog. Amer. J. Vet. Res., 31 (1970):791.

Angrist, A.: Aging Heart Valves and a Unitary Pathological Hypothesis for Sclerosis. J. Geront., 19 (1964):135.

Bone, W. J.: L-Form of *Pseudomonas aeruginosa* the Etiologic Agent of Bacterial Endocarditis in a Dog. Vet. Med., 65 (1970):224.

Bretschneider, J.: Zur Pathologie und Pathogense der sog. Endocarditis Valvularis Chronica Fibrosa des Hundes. Inaug. Diss., Univ. Giessen, 1962.

Buchanan, J. W.: Selective Angiography and Angiocardiography in Dogs with Acquired Cardiovascular Disease. J. Amer. Vet. Radiol. Soc., 6 (1965a):5.

Buchanan, J. W.: Spontaneous Arrhythmias and Conduction Disturbances in Domestic Animals. Ann. N. Y. Acad. Sci., 127 (1965b):224.

Buchanan, J. W.: Patent Ductus Arteriosus and Persistent Right Aortic Arch Surgery in Dogs. J. Small Anim. Pract., 9 (1968):409.

Buchanan, J. W., and Kelly, A. M.: Endocardial Splitting of the Left Atrium in the Dog. J. Amer. Vet. Radiol. Soc., 5 (1964):28.

Buchanan, J. W., and Patterson, D. F.: Selective Angiography and Angiocardiography in Dogs with Congenital Cardiovascular Disease. J. Amer. Vet. Radiol. Soc., 6 (1965):21.

Carmichael, J. A., Liu, S.-K., Tashjian, R. J., Radford, G., and Lord, P.:A Case of Canine Aortic Stenosis and Aortic Valvular Insufficiency, with Particular Reference to Diagnostic Technique. J. Small Anim. Pract., 9 (1968):213.

Das, K. M., and Tashjian, R. J.: Chronic Mitral Valve Disease in the Dog. Vet Med., 60 (1965):1209.

Detweiler, D. K.: The Heart. In *Canine Medicine*. Edited by H. Hoskins, J. Lacroix, and K. Mayer. 2nd ed. American Veterinary Publications, Inc., Santa Barbara, California, 1962.

Detweiler, D. K., Luginbühl, H., Buchanan, J. W., and Patterson,D. F.: The Natural History of Acquired Cardiac Disability of the Dog. Ann. N. Y. Acad. Sci., 147 (1968): 318.

Detweiler, D. K., and Patterson, D. F.: Bacterial Endocarditis. In *Current Veterinary Therapy 1966-1967*. Edited by R. W. Kirk. W. B. Saunders, Philadelphia, 1966.

Detweiler, D. K., and Patterson, D. F.: A Phonograph Record of Heart Sounds and Murmurs of the Dog. Ann. N. Y. Acad. Sci., 127 (1965a):322.

Detweiler, D. K., and Patterson, D. F.: The Prevalence and Types of Cardiovascular Disease in Dogs. Ann. N. Y. Acad. Sci., 127 (1965b):481.

Ettinger, S., and Buergelt, C.-D.: Atrioventricular Dissociation (Incomplete) with Accrochage in a Dog with Ruptured Chordae Tendineae. Amer. J. Vet. Res., 29 (1968): 1499.

Ettinger, S., and Buergelt, C.-D.: Ruptured Chordae Tendineae in the dog. J. A. V. M. A., 155 (1969):535.

Fisher, E. W., Ritchie, D., and Thomson, A.: Aortic Incompetence in a Dog. Vet. Rec., 77 (1965):506.

Gould, L., Ettinger, S., and Lyon, A. F.: Intensity of the First Heart Sound and Arterial Pulse in Mitral Insufficiency. Dis. Chest, 53 (1968):545.

Hahn, A. W.: Auscultation of the Canine Heart. IV. Murmurs. Small Anim. Clin., 2 (1962): 13.

Haller, J., and Morrow, A.: Experimental Mitral Insufficiency. An Operative Method of Chronic Survival. Ann. Surg., 142 (1955a):37.

Haller, J., and Morrow, A.: Experimental Mitral Insufficiency. Surgery, 38 (1955b):518.

Hamlin, R. L.: Prognostic Value of Changes in the Cardiac Silhouette in Dogs with Mitral Insufficiency. J. A. V. M. A., 153 (1968):1436.

Hamlin, R. L., Smetzer, D. L., Smith, C. R., Crocker, H. D., and Marsland, W. P.: Iatrogenic Pulmonic Insufficiency in a Dog. J. A. V. M. A., 141 (1962):725.

Harpster, N. K.: Case Records of the Angell Memorial Animal Hospital (Left Atrial Tear). J. A. V. M. A., 154 (1969):413.

Hubben, K., Patterson, D. F., and Botts, R. P.: Telangiectasis in Canine Heart Valves. Zbl. Veterinärmed; 10 (1963):195.

Jaksch, W.: Kardiologische Probleme in der Kleintierpraxis V. Kleintierpraxis 11 (1966):19.

Jones, T. C., and Zook, B. C.: Aging Changes in the Vascular System of Animals. Ann. N. Y. Acad. Sci., 127 (1965):671.

Jubb, K. V. F., and Kennedy, P. C.: Pathology of Domestic Animals. 1st ed. Academic Press, New York, 1963.

Kersten, U.: Klinische Untersuchungen am herzkranken Hund. Thesis. Hannover, Germany, 1968.

Klein, L. J., Bisgard, G. E., and Lewis, R. E.: Rupture of the Aortic Sinus and Aortic Insufficiency in a Dog. J. A. V. M. A., 149 (1966):1050.

Lillehei, C. W., Bobb, J. R. R., and Visscher, M. B.: Occurrence of Endocarditis with Valvular Deformities in Dogs with Arteriovenous Fistulae. Proc. Soc. Exp. Biol. Med., 75 (1950):9.

Liu, S.-K., Suter, P. F., and Ettinger, S.: Pulmonary Alveolar Microlithiasis with Ruptured Chordae Tendineae in Mitral and Tricuspid Valves in a Dog. J. A. V. M. A., 155 (1969):1692.

Luginbühl, H., and Detweiler, D. L.: Cardiovascular Lesions in Dogs. Ann. N. Y. Acad. Sci., 127 (1965):517.

Lundh, T.: Fibrinous Endocarditis in Dogs. Acta Vet. Scand., 5 (1964):17.

Moscovitz, H., Donoso, E., Gelb, I., and Wilder, R.: An Atlas of Hemodynamics of the Cardiovascular System. Grune and Stratton, New York, 1963.

Nielsen, S. W., and Nielsen, L. B.: Coronary Embolism in Valvular Bacterial Endocarditis in Two Dogs. J. A. V. M. A., 125 (1954):376.

Shouse, C. L., and Meier, H.: Acute Vegetative Endocarditis in the Dog and Cat. J. A. V. M. A., 129 (1956):278.

Stünzi, H.: Zur Pathogenese der Endocarditis valvularis. Schweiz. Arch. Tierheilk., 104 (1962):135.

Tashjian, R. J., and McCoy, J. R.: Acquired Mitral Stenosis Resulting in Left Atrial Dilatation with Thrombosis. A Case Report. Cornell Vet., 50 (1960):485.

Theran, P., Henry, W. B., and Thornton, G. W.: Case Records of the Angell Memorial Animal Hospital (Bacterial Endocarditis). J. A. V. M. A., 146 (1965):54.

Wagner, B.: Myocardial Disease in Man and Dog, Some Properties. Ann. N. Y. Acad. Sci., 147 (1968):354.

Wallace, C. R.: Cardiac Catheterization to Aid in Diagnosis of Cardiovascular Disease. Small Anim. Clin., 2 (1962):332.

Wallace, C. R., and Hamilton, W. F.: Study of Spontaneous Congestive Heart Failure in the Dog. Circ. Res., 11 (1962):301.

CHAPTER

14

ACQUIRED DISEASES OF THE MYOCARDIUM

The classification of pathologic conditions of the myocardium has resulted in a multiplicity of terms and confusion in their definitions (Friedberg, 1966; Mc-Guire, 1969; Witham and Hurst, 1970). In the following chapter, myocardial diseases have been subdivided into three distinguishable groups which are widely accepted in human cardiology and are properly adaptable to the needs of canine cardiology.

1. *Cardiomyopathies of known origin (myocarditis and myocardial degeneration).* Refers specifically to states in which there is satisfactory evidence of inflammation or degeneration of the myocardium.

2. *Idiopathic cardiomyopathy.* Refers to myocardial diseases of unknown etiology. The outstanding features are cardiac dilatation and congestive heart failure. Atrial fibrillation seems to be a constant feature in the dog, and embolization may develop.

3. *Ischemic myocardial disease.* Massive myocardial infarction resulting in ischemia due to occlusion of major coronary vessels is unusual in the dog. Alterations in the major coronary artery circulation are also not the cause of progressive changes that develop in the hearts of older dogs (Pensinger, 1968). However, microinfarction of the intramural myocardium and intramural coronary arteriosclerosis have been associated with chronic mitral valvular fibrosis (Detweiler, 1962), congenital subaortic stenosis (Flickinger and Patterson, 1967), and angiopathies in older dogs (Dahme and Reif, 1964; Luginbühl and Detweiler, 1965).

Neoplastic disease, both primary and metastatic, is discussed in another section (see pp. 471-473) because the lesions are rarely limited to the myocardium; instead, they usually invade several portions of the cardiovascular system.

Myocardial degeneration was thought to be less common in carnivorous than in herbivorous animals (Jubb and Kennedy, 1963). However, an increasing number of myocardial diseases have been reported in dogs by several authors (Jones and Zook, 1965; Detweiler et al., 1968a; Kersten, 1968; Taylor and Sittnikow, 1968; Ettinger, Bolton, and Lord, 1970).

The criteria by which myocardial disease has been recognized have varied among authors. In studies in which myocardial abnormalities were reported frequently, the diagnosis was often based only on the presence of abnormal electrocardiographic findings such as ectopic beats, conduction disturbances, and repolarization or ischemic changes in the S-T segment, and/or on radiographic evidence of cardiomegaly. On the basis of signs noted on physical, electrocardiographic, and radiographic examinations, Detweiler et al. (1968a) reported an overall frequency of chronic myocardial disease in 3.4 per cent of 4831 cases screened for cardiovascular disease in Philadelphia, Pennsylvania. In this study, the incidence increased with age from 0.7 per cent in dogs under one year of age to 14.9 per cent in dogs over 13 years old.

Kersten (1968) reported myocardial disease in 356 dogs, or approximately 2.5 per cent of all dogs examined at the veterinary college in Hannover, Germany. Of 754 dogs classified as having cardiac abnormalities, 47.8 per cent were classified as having myocardial disease; however, this figure does not include those dogs which had both valvular heart disease and myocardial damage. In Kersten's study, myocardial disease was recognized in dogs ranging in age from one to over 13 years, the incidence increasing markedly with age. No sex predisposition could be determined, but the incidence of myocardial disease was higher in certain breeds—the Boxer, Spitz, German Shorthaired Pointer, and Saint Bernard—than could have been anticipated from the clinic population of these breeds.

Taylor and Sittnikow (1968) reported that of 4126 dogs treated at the College of Veterinary Medicine in Helsinki, Finland, myocardial disease was recognized in 67 of 112 dogs with acquired cardiac conditions; it usually occurred in dogs over six years old. In 14 dogs, myocardial disease was associated with valvular disease. The authors related the high incidence of myocardial disease to the fact that a large number of dogs had myocardial disease secondary to clinical conditions such as pyometra and uremia.

Of 5852 clinical patients at the medical clinic of the veterinary college in Munich, Germany, myocardial lesions were demonstrated in 32 dogs at necropsy. In only 25 were there clinical signs compatible with myocarditis (Bohn, 1967).

Jones and Zook (1965) reported myocardial lesions of all forms in 77 dogs (7.8 per cent) from a total of 991 necropsy examinations in Boston, Massachusetts. In that study, there was no correlation between the incidence of myocardial lesions and age.

Detweiler et al. (1968b) noted that inflammatory myocardial changes from all causes were diagnosed in about 10 per cent of the hearts studied at necropsy examination in Philadelphia, Pennsylvania. Of 30 dogs with myocarditis, only two were considered to have myocardial disease of primary origin. In the remaining 28 cases, myocardial disease was secondary to infectious disease, neoplasia, or toxemia resulting from metabolic disturbances. They further noted that focal rather than diffuse microscopic myocardial lesions are more common at necropsy. Even when lesions were present microscopically, clinical myocarditis might not have been evident.

Some studies have considered only the presence of electrocardiographic abnormalities as the basis for the clinical diagnosis of myocardial disease, whereas others restrict the diagnosis to those cases in which there is a specific inflammatory, degenerative, or ischemic lesion recognized at necropsy. The authors diagnose clinical myocardial disease when the history, physical examination, and cardiac examination, especially the electrocardiogram, are compatible with the findings presented below.

CARDIOMYOPATHIES (MYOCARDITIS AND DEGENERATIVE MYOCARDIAL DISEASE)

Myocarditis denotes inflammation of the myocardium. Active myocardial inflammatory changes, as well as chronic myocardial degeneration, may be associated with most of the common viral, bacterial, mycotic, and protozoan diseases known to affect dogs (Lannek, 1949; Luginbühl and Detweiler, 1965; Detweiler et al., 1968b). There is also a known relationship between the presence of chronic valvular fibrosis and myocarditis. Other conditions known to be associated with cardiomyopathy include hyperthyroidism, hypothyroidism, anemia, malnutrition, electrolyte imbalances, parasitic infections, uremia, and pancreatitis. Toxemias and poisonings, neoplasia, intestinal foreign bodies, pyometra-endometritis, diabetes mellitus, pleuritis, pericarditis, and pericardial effusion may also be related to cardiomyopathy.

HISTORY AND PHYSICAL EXAMINATION

Diseases of the myocardium are often associated with such nonspecific clinical signs as prolonged fever, weakness, fatigue, physical inactivity, anorexia, coughing, and dyspnea. As the disease process advances, signs of congestive heart failure may develop. Dogs with myocarditis may be presented in a state of collapse or near-collapse, and are extremely weak. Myocarditis may often be unrecognized because the signs of the primary condition, such as pneumonia, gastroenteritis, or poisoning, predominate, and a further cardiac examination is not performed.

Older dogs should be evaluated routinely for signs referable to myocarditis when chronic diseases, uremia, pyometra, or neoplasia produce nonspecific signs of weakness. When chronic mitral valvular fibrosis is complicated by myocarditis, the interpretation of signs indicating myocardial disease is easier if serial electrocardiograms are recorded.

CARDIAC EXAMINATION

Findings on auscultation may vary depending on the etiology and progression of the disease. Heart murmurs are likely to be absent unless valvular, congenital, or anemic heart disease accompanies myocarditis. The intensity of the heart sounds is decreased when the force of myocardial contraction diminishes. If an irregular rhythm and heart sounds of variable intensity are present, an electrocardiogram should be recorded to determine the site of origin and the significance of the arrhythmia. If the right atrium contracts against closed atrioventricular valves, there is a retrograde pulse in the jugular vein (canon "a" waves). Bradycardia or tachycardia may occur (Bohn, 1967). Tachycardia and a gallop rhythm denote congestive heart failure and occur late in the disease process. A pulse deficit and/or irregularity of the pulse strength are also associated with cardiac arrhythmias. If circulatory failure develops and persists, extracardiac signs of heart failure such as pulmonary congestion and edema, hepatomegaly, pleural effusion, and edema may be present (Bohn, 1967). In our experience, heart failure develops rapidly, and death is likely to occur without signs of chronic congestive heart failure.

ELECTROCARDIOGRAPHY

All types of arrhythmias, such as ventricular premature contractions, atrioventricular dissociation, paroxysmal or persistent supraventricular tachycardia, heart block, and atrial or ventricular flutter or fibrillation, are associated with myocarditis. Aberrant (wide and irregular) QRS complexes, nonspecific changes of the S-T segment such as depression, elevation, or general deformity, and alteration of the T wave may also be seen. The amplitudes of all waves of the electrocardiogram may be diminished (Lannek, 1949; Gratzl, 1963; Detweiler et al., 1968b). It is incorrect to specifically correlate all electrocardiographic changes with myocarditis. However, any cardiac arrhythmia which arises from a premature ectopic focus should be associated with increased myocardial irritability.

RADIOGRAPHIC EXAMINATION

The radiographic findings are not characteristic and do not assist in making a specific diagnosis of myocardial disease. However, cardiomegaly and extracardiac signs of heart failure may suggest myocarditis (Figs. 14-1 and 14-2). Cardiac enlargement involving the right or left ventricle, or both, has been found in 50 to 70 per cent of all cases (Bohn, 1967; Kersten, 1968; Taylor and Sittnikow, 1968). Left atrial enlargement is present when myocardial disease accompanies chronic mitral valvular disease.

Extracardiac signs such as pulmonary congestion and pulmonary alveolar edema may be seen if the left ventricle fails. If right ventricular function is disturbed, dilation of the caudal and cranial venae cavae, hepatomegaly, pleural effusion, pericardial effusion, and ascites may occur. However, generalized enlargement of the cardiac silhouette and a globular shape are often the only radiographic signs indicating cardiac disease. Therefore, it may be difficult to differentiate this condition from cardiomegaly associated with pericardial effusion. Contrast studies of the heart would be useful in differentiating these conditions.

LABORATORY FINDINGS

Although myocardial disease cannot be identified specifically by clinical laboratory analyses, positive findings may indicate a primary disease responsible for a secondary myocarditis. Leukocytosis and increased red blood cell sedimentation rates are present in most conditions associated with myocarditis. Occasionally, a positive blood culture is obtained when there is generalized septicemia.

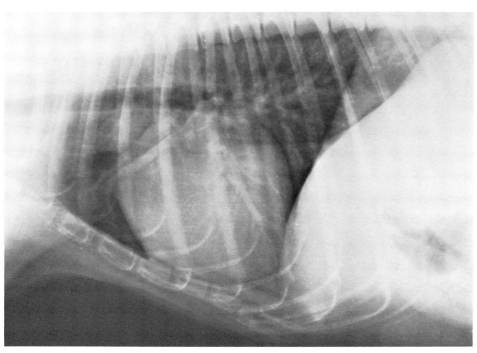

FIGURE 14-1 Left lateral radiograph, 6 year old female Irish Terrier which was examined because an arrhythmia was auscultated prior to induction of anesthesia for an elective ovariohysterectomy. Ventricular premature contractions were diagnosed on the electrocardiogram. Since the physical examination and laboratory tests suggested no specific cause for the condition, idiopathic myocarditis was diagnosed.

The craniocaudal diameter of the cardiac silhouette is increased, and the silhouette is rounder than normal; therefore, the heart appears enlarged. The trachea is not elevated. The cranial and caudal waists have both been preserved. The left atrium is not enlarged; however, the pulmonary vasculature appears denser than normal, and the outlines are blurred by a diffuse haziness of the lung field. The caudal vena cava is denser than normal and can be followed within the cardiac silhouette.

The radiograph indicates slight right and left ventricular enlargement, with no enlargement of the left atrium. The hazy lung field would be compatible with pulmonary congestion due to mitral insufficiency if the left atrium were enlarged. The possibility of a primary pulmonary condition causing the haziness cannot be excluded radiographically. In the absence of clinical signs referable to such a condition, pulmonary congestion due to some degree of left heart failure can be assumed. The radiographic signs of left heart failure, although not in themselves diagnostic, substantiate the clinical diagnosis of myocarditis.

The serum glutamic oxaloacetic transaminase (SGOT) and serum glutamic pyruvic transaminase (SGPT) are greater than 60 S. F. units when myocardial necrosis is present. Although elevations of the transaminase values do not assist in the prognosis, absence of such elevations may assist in making the differential diagnosis (Crawley and Swenson, 1963). According to Crawley and Swenson (1963), the serum lactic dehydrogenase (LDH) is not an effective test to determine the presence of myocardial necrosis in the dog; even when there are 10-fold elevations of serum lactic dehydrogenase in dogs with cardiac disease, the values may still be within the normal range for this enzyme.

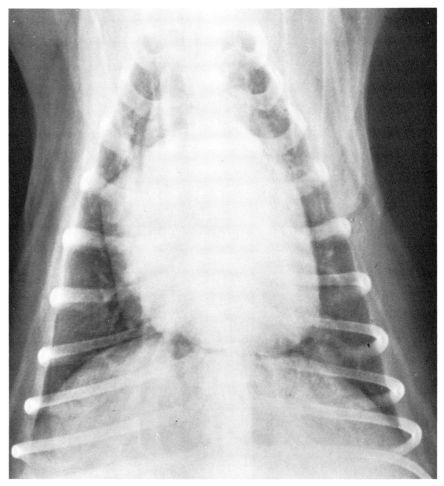

FIGURE 14-2   Dorsoventral radiograph, dog in Figure 14-1. The cranial portion of the right cardiac border extends farther to the right side than normal, suggesting mild right ventricular enlargement. The left cardiac border is slightly rounded. The slight, generalized cardiac enlargement seen on the lateral radiograph is thus confirmed on the dorsoventral view. The haziness of the lung field is less pronounced than on the lateral radiograph.

DIFFERENTIAL DIAGNOSIS

Since the causes of myocardial disease are so numerous, they are difficult if not impossible to differentiate accurately. It is important to determine whether the myocardial lesion is primary or secondary. Since the initial signs may be nonspecific, the clinician must explore the history in detail to determine the possible inciting factor. A thorough medical examination is necessary to determine whether there are noncardiac medical problems which are responsible for secondary cardiac manifestations. Angiocardiography may be of value in determining the size of the cardiac chambers as well as in demonstrating or excluding valvular heart disease.

TREATMENT

In addition to cardiac therapy for treatment of myocarditis, treatment of the inciting factors must be as complete and specific as possible. The form and route of administration of cardiac therapy varies, depending on the inciting cause as well as on the severity of the condition.

When cardiac output is diminished because of chronic cardiac disease, such as mitral valvular fibrosis, ectopic impulses are often abolished or reduced in frequency by digitalization, since this drug increases the cardiac output and improves coronary arterial and myocardial perfusion (Fig. 14-3). If a persistent ventricular tachycardia is present, digitalis therapy is usually contraindicated. If there is doubt as to the need for digitalization, small doses of a rapid-acting agent such as ouabain may be administered intravenously every 30 minutes, utilizing continuous electrocardiographic monitoring. *If the ectopic impulses increase in frequency, or if more advanced arrhythmias develop during digitalization, cardiac glycoside therapy must be discontinued immediately.* Because ouabain is metabolized rapidly, arrhythmias induced by it are quickly resolved. Antiarrhythmic therapy should be instituted immediately if serious arrhythmias occur (see below). If the number of ectopic impulses diminishes after the patient has been digitalized, maintenance therapy with digitalis should be instituted.

Intravenous antiarrhythmic agents are indicated for the dog presented in collapse with a weak pulse, irregular heart rate, and electrocardiographic signs of atrioventricular dissociation or ventricular tachycardia (Fig. 14-4). Lidocaine without epinephrine (see pp. 245-246) is administered by slow intravenous infusion until the arrhythmia diminishes or disappears entirely. Then a slow intravenous drip or intermittent intravenous therapy with lidocaine is continued at a rate adequate to control the arrhythmia. Since an excessive amount of lidocaine can induce convulsive seizures, the drug should be used cautiously. If convulsions occur, the infusion is discontinued, and the seizures usually cease within 30 to

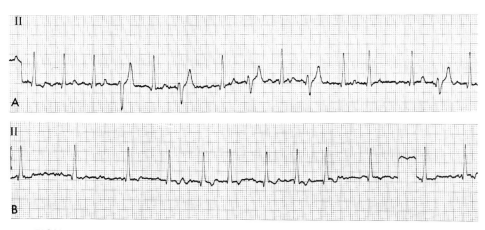

FIGURE 14-3 Atrial fibrillation with ventricular premature contractions. *A*, Atrial fibrillation with multiple unifocal ventricular premature contractions. In this case, the presence of ventricular premature contractions was thought to be the result of diminished cardiac output and congestive heart failure rather than a focal area of inflammation. When cardiac output improved after digitalization, the electrocardiogram was devoid of ventricular premature contractions and showed only atrial fibrillation (B).

120 seconds. However, the clinician should be prepared to insert an endotracheal tube and administer a short-acting barbiturate if the convulsions persist. Procainamide may be preferred by some to lidocaine for intravenous infusion in the treatment of acute arrhythmias.

While the arrhythmia is being converted medically with lidocaine, a calculated dose of quinidine (see pp. 239-242) should be administered either orally or intramuscularly. Quinidine is effective via either route in approximately 30 minutes. Intravenous lidocaine is used cautiously until an adequate blood level of quinidine has been obtained. If procainamide (see pp. 242-244) is preferred to quinidine, it may be given intravenously, intramuscularly, or orally. Because its effect is more rapid than that of quinidine, lidocaine therapy can be omitted. Although procainamide acts more rapidly than quinidine, its effects also dissipate more rapidly, requiring that it be administered every four to six hours.

Single or occasional multiple ventricular premature contractions do not require the same intensive therapy as does ventricular tachycardia. Most occasional ventricular premature contractions are suppressed with oral antiarrhythmic agents such as quinidine or procainamide. When high doses of one drug have been unsuccessful in controlling the frequency of ventricular premature contractions, or if the toxic reactions from the high dose required have been too severe, a combination of two antiarrhythmic agents at lower doses has been used successfully by the authors (Fig. 14-5).

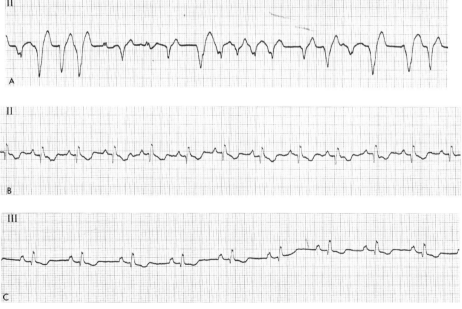

FIGURE 14-4   Ventricular tachycardia due to myocarditis. A, The electrocardiogram demonstrates a persistent ventricular tachycardia which developed in a dog presented for collapse which had an irregular and rapid heart rate on auscultation. A blood culture from this dog was positive for Streptococcus sp. B, The electrocardiogram shows the normal sinus rhythm that was restored shortly after intravenous infusion of lidocaine. C, Electrocardiogram recorded two days after restoration of the normal rhythm. The dog was maintained on an oral quinidine preparation and was treated with antibiotics for four weeks, according to the results of antibiotic sensitivity tests on the positive blood culture.

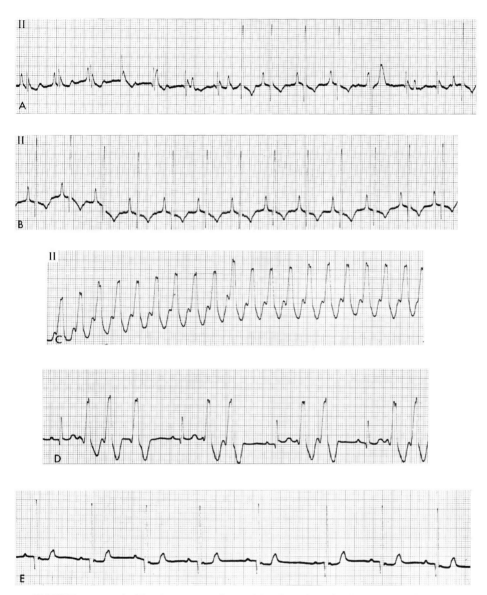

FIGURE 14-5 *A,* Tracing from dog with chronic mitral valvular fibrosis and congestive heart failure. The rhythm is that of atrioventricular dissociation; four capture beats with normal-appearing P-QRS-T complexes are in the middle of the strip. Although a sinus rhythm was restored with either oral quinidine or procainamide alone, the dog developed signs of intoxication after each agent was administered. By combining lower doses of both, a sinus rhythm was maintained (*B*) without signs of intoxication.

C, Tracing of ventricular tachycardia from dog with idiopathic myocarditis presented because of a syncopal episode and acute collapse. Following oral quinidine therapy, occasional beats originating from the sinoatrial node were conducted; even at toxic levels, ventricular premature contractions still persisted (*D*) which could not be abolished with quinidine or procainamide alone. Using a combination of quinidine and procainamide, a normal sinus rhythm (*E*) was maintained until all drug therapy was discontinued after 60 days.

IDIOPATHIC CARDIOMYOPATHY (PRIMARY MYOCARDIAL DISEASE; MYOCARDIOPATHY)

The large breeds of dogs such as the Boxer, Bouvier des Flandres, Doberman Pinscher, English Bulldog, German Shepherd, Great Dane, Irish Setter, Irish Wolfhound, Newfoundland, and St. Bernard develop an idiopathic cardiomyopathy. It is characterized by biventricular cardiac dilatation with dilation of the atrioventricular anular rings which leads to mitral and tricuspid valvular incompetence and massive atrial dilatation. Atrial fibrillation appears to be the predominant rhythm when the condition is clinically recognizable. Congestive heart failure is progressive, with clinical signs of right heart failure usually occurring first and signs of left heart failure developing subsequently or simultaneously. The condition differs from chronic valvular fibrosis in that the atrioventricular valves are normal or nearly normal in size, contour, and thickness, and are usually free of fibrotic nodules. Whereas atrial fibrillation develops late in the course of chronic mitral valvular fibrosis, and then only infrequently, in idiopathic cardiomyopathy it is associated with the onset of clinical signs and may even develop before clinical signs are present (Fig. 14-6) (Ettinger, Bolton, and Lord, 1970).

HISTORY AND PHYSICAL EXAMINATION

The dogs, usually between two and seven years of age, are presented in varying degrees of right and left heart failure. Weight loss and general debility are the most striking signs. When right heart failure is severe, ascites is associated with the condition. In most cases, the dog is reported to have been normal until weight loss and lethargy developed. From that time the progression of the disease is usually rapid, with ascites and other clinical signs developing often over a period of two to four weeks. Clinical signs of left heart failure occur occasionally during the early stages of the disease although respiratory distress and coughing are frequently present in the history. Although the condition has been recognized in more male than female dogs it is not apparent whether there is a specific sex predisposition for this disease.

Clinical signs other than weight loss and weakness include dyspnea, coughing (in some but not all cases), anorexia, and abdominal distention. Jugular venous distention and engorgement of subcutaneous veins are evident. An irregular apical

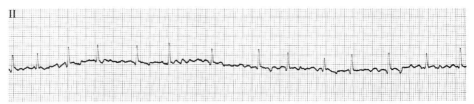

FIGURE 14-6 Lead II of the electrocardiogram recorded from a 2 year old male Irish Wolfhound with idiopathic cardiomyopathy. The rhythm is that of atrial fibrillation, and the ventricular rate varies from 140 to 160 beats/minute. The dog was not on glycoside therapy when this tracing was recorded, and signs of heart failure other than moderate weight loss had not yet developed.

cardiac beat and left ventricular heave are often obvious, especially in cachectic dogs. The rapid, irregular heart rate is palpated best over the point of maximal intensity at the left caudal sternal border. The pulse is also irregular and varies in rate, rhythm, and strength. The distended abdomen is filled with a straw-colored to lightly blood-tinged ascitic fluid, the specific gravity of which varies with the content of protein and red blood cells.

AUSCULTATION

An irregular tachycardia is the most prominent feature on auscultation. In the decompensated dog, the heart rate is greater than 180 beats/min. and is frequently as high as 240 to 280 beats/min. When the heart is auscultated simultaneously with palpation of the femoral arteries, a marked pulse deficit is apparent. The intensity of the first heart sound varies from beat to beat, and the second heart sound may be absent (Fig. 14-7). A diastolic gallop sound may be so loud as to be confused with the first heart sound, making proper identification of the heart sounds difficult. At the left caudal sternal border, a short systolic, musical murmur of low to moderate intensity (grade I/VI to III/VI), or no murmur at all, may be auscultated. Because of the variations in ventricular filling in the presence of atrial fibrillation, if a murmur is present it is often variable in both intensity and duration. In some cases, coarse, bubbling pulmonary râles reflect the advanced

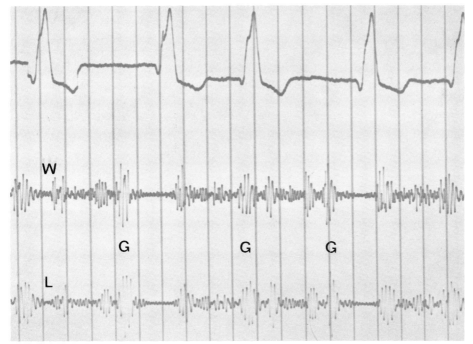

FIGURE 14-7 Atrial fibrillation and idiopathic cardiomyopathy. Lead II of the electrocardiogram recorded simultaneously with wide-frequency (W) and low-frequency (L) band phonocardiograms. Notice the variable intensities of the first and second heart sounds. The diastolic gallop sound (G) is so loud and consistent that it could easily be mistaken for the first heart sound on auscultation.

degree of pulmonary congestion and the presence of pulmonary alveolar edema. Bronchial tones are frequently transmitted throughout the thoracic cavity.

ELECTROCARDIOGRAPHY

The irregular tachycardia is evident on the electrocardiogram. However, when the rate becomes very rapid, the irregularity may be less obvious due to the shorter R-R intervals associated with the tachycardia. In atrial fibrillation, "f" waves replace the normal sinus P waves (see pp. 292-299). Although the configuration of the QRS complex is nearly normal, its duration is increased to 0.06 sec. and often 0.07 sec., consistent with left ventricular hypertrophy and occasionally with left bundle branch block. The QRS complex is sometimes aberrantly conducted and appears abnormal.

The presence of single or multiple ventricular premature contractions is not uncommon, especially late in the disease. These may result from myocardial degeneration or from ischemic myocarditis due to a deficient coronary circulation or perhaps microinfarctions. The vectorcardiogram demonstrates large, prolonged QRS loops with correspondingly large T loops (Fig. 14-8).

RADIOGRAPHIC EXAMINATION

The cardiac silhouette is moderately to greatly enlarged and has all the features common to advanced chronic mitral valvular disease with secondary right heart failure (see pp. 338-339) (Figs. 14-9 and 14-10). Marked venous distention is often seen, and the veins are two to three times wider than in normal dogs and taper rapidly in the peripheral lung field. The intrapulmonary veins appear larger and denser than the pulmonary arteries. Although the pulmonary parenchyma appears hazy, the engorged veins remain clearly visible. The outlines of the vascular structures are irregular and blurred, and alveolar edema may be confined to the hilar region. With pulmonary congestion and pulmonary edema developing in dogs which have chronic mitral valvular disease, the veins are usually not as prominent as they are in dogs with idiopathic cardiomyopathy.

CARDIAC CATHETERIZATION

The hemodynamic data obtained during cardiac catheterization do not differ appreciably from those obtained from dogs with mitral insufficiency due to chronic mitral valvular fibrosis (see pp. 354-355). The atrial pressures are elevated, and the left atrial pressure exceeds the right atrial pressure. Atrial a, c, and v waves, which occur when a sinus rhythm is present, are replaced in atrial fibrillation by a single, large atrial v wave. Although we have found that the ventricular systolic pressures are normal in dogs with idiopathic cardiomyopathy, the left ventricular and right ventricular end diastolic pressures have been elevated in dogs considered to be clinically in heart failure. These pressures fell after ouabain was administered intravenously during cardiac catheterization. Angiocardiography demonstrates the degree of dilatation of the mitral anulus and the severity of mitral regurgitation by late filling of the aorta and dilution of the contrast medium, which oscillates backwards and forwards several times between the left ventricle and atrium before being ejected into the aorta.

Text continues on page 398.

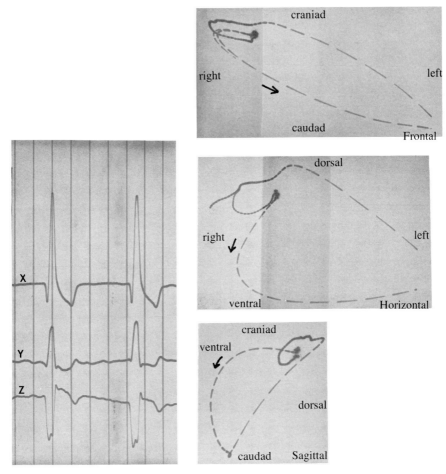

FIGURE 14-8 Vectorcardiogram of a dog with idiopathic cardiomyopathy. Atrial fibrillation is indicated on the scalar leads by the lack of a P wave and on the vectorcardiogram by the lack of a P loop. Notice the accentuated vectorcardiogram in all three planes, indicative of cardiac enlargement. Electrocardiographic S-T depression is demonstrated on the vectorcardiogram when the loops fail to close. The direction and shape of the three loops are accentuations of normal, indicating cardiac enlargement.

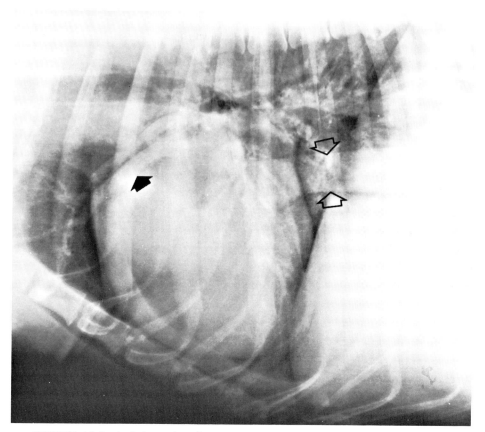

FIGURE 14-9 Left lateral radiograph of a 2½ year old female Great Dane with a history of debilitation, lethargy, and weight loss for one month. The heart rate was rapid and irregular, with heart sounds of variable intensity; atrial fibrillation was recognized on the electrocardiogram. Severe dyspnea and ascites were present. Radiographically, the cardiac silhouette is greatly enlarged. The cranial and caudal waists have disappeared. Both ventricles are enlarged. The left atrium bulges caudo-dorsally into the diaphragmatic lung field. The apical lobar veins (black arrow) are dilated and denser than normal. Enlarged vascular densities, congestion, and ensuing pulmonary alveolar edema make the diaphragmatic lung field appear denser than normal. The vascular structures are not well outlined. The caudal vena cava (clear arrows) is markedly enlarged and can be followed within the cardiac silhouette. Except for the extreme enlargement of the pulmonary arteries and veins, the radiographic appearance resembles that of mitral insufficiency with right and left heart failure in small breeds.

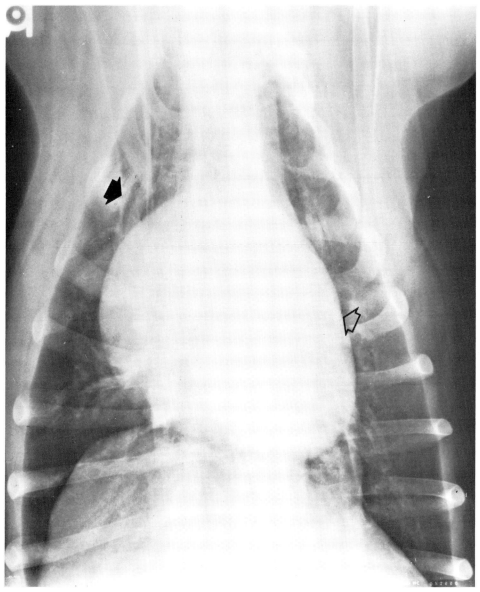

FIGURE 14-10 Dorsoventral radiograph, dog in Figure 14-9. The cardiac silhouette is enlarged. The right ventricular border bulges, and the apex and left ventricular border are rounded. A slight bulge (clear arrow) represents the dilated left auricle. The bulge is small because the rest of the auricle is obscured by the large left ventricle. The lung field is hazy. The large apical lobar vein and artery are well visualized (black arrow). Because the veins are larger than the arteries and since there is no vascular distortion, severe heartworm disease, which can cause dilatation of the pulmonary arteries, can be excluded in making the differential diagnosis.

DIFFERENTIAL DIAGNOSIS

Since signs of right heart failure predominate initially, specific cardiac diseases which affect primarily the right ventricle, such as chronic tricuspid valvular fibrosis, dirofilariasis, pericardial effusion, and some congenital heart diseases, must be differentiated from idiopathic cardiomyopathy. Chronic tricuspid valvular fibrosis is usually concurrent with chronic mitral valvular fibrosis, and both are associated with a loud, holosystolic, regurgitant murmur which is absent in dogs with idiopathic cardiomyopathy. Chronic tricuspid valvular fibrosis is also associated with a protracted history, in comparison to that of idiopathic cardiomyopathy, which develops rapidly and is associated with atrial fibrillation. In heartworm disease, microfilariae are often present in the peripheral blood, right axis deviation is often seen on the electrocardiogram, and specific radiographic findings such as a prominent pulmonary artery segment and large, distorted pulmonary arteries that may end abruptly in the peripheral lung field are present (see Chapter 16). In moderate to advanced heartworm disease, splitting of the second heart sound is often prominent over the pulmonic valve. Pericardial effusion is usually suggested if there are muffled heart sounds on auscultation and if a large, globular cardiac silhouette is seen on radiographic examination. Congenital cardiac lesions are differentiated on the basis of the electrocardiogram, absence of typical cardiac murmurs, and radiographic findings that are typical for the specific congenital heart defect.

Congenital mitral insufficiency as described by Hamlin, Smetzer, and Smith (1965) is not initially associated with atrial fibrillation and right heart failure. In dogs with idiopathic cardiomyopathy seen by us, there was no history of systolic murmurs prior to the onset of clinical signs, nor were signs of heart failure ever present previously. In addition, the condition usually occurs in middle-aged dogs, whereas congenital mitral insufficiency has been seen in dogs under one year of age.

Since there are a number of other medical problems which can result in cachexia and ascites (such as abdominal neoplasia, hypoproteinemia, and hepatic cirrhosis), a complete medical examination with clinical laboratory tests is recommended for dogs suspected of having idiopathic cardiomyopathy.

TREATMENT

Dogs presented with idiopathic cardiomyopathy are usually in moderately advanced to severe congestive heart failure. Digitalization should be undertaken immediately to reduce the cardiac rate and improve myocardial contractility. The dosage and route of administration of digitalis vary with the severity of the signs of heart failure (see Chapter 7). If a ventricular arrhythmia is present, a trial dose of ouabain with continuous electrocardiographic monitoring is indicated to determine the dog's response. If the arrhythmia persists or is aggravated, cardiac glycoside therapy must be discontinued and antiarrhythmic therapy instituted. If the arrhythmia is reduced, glycoside therapy may then be resumed.

In dogs with severe ascites, diuretic therapy may not prove successful initially. In such cases, paracentesis of the bulk of the abdominal fluid is indicated. Following paracentesis, however, the same diuretic therapy is often effective in controlling further fluid accumulation.

After the dog has been digitalized and congestive heart failure is under con-

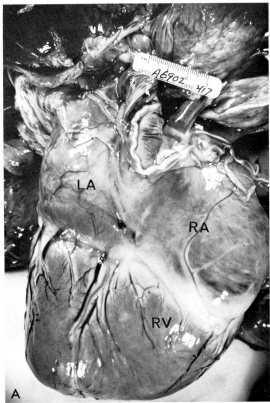

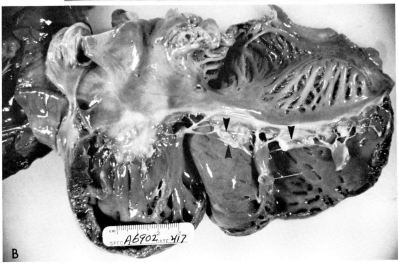

FIGURE 14-11 Postmortem specimen, dog with idiopathic cardiomyopathy. *A,* Generalized cardiomegaly with severe left atrial (LA) and right atrial (RA) dilatation. The right ventricle (RV) is extremely enlarged; this is responsible for the rounding of the cardiac apex. The marked enlargement of the atria and ventricles results in dilatation of the atrioventricular valve ring and subsequent atrioventricular valvular insufficiency.

B, Opened right ventricle. The right ventricular wall is thin and extremely dilated. The chordae tendineae extending from the papillary muscles to the valve leaflets (arrows) are normal. The valve leaflets are normal for a middle-aged dog; they are translucent and without significant fibrotic changes (see Fig. 13-27 for comparison). (The authors are grateful to Dr. S.-K. Liu, The Animal Medical Center, New York, N. Y., for taking these photographs.)

399

trol, medical or electrical conversion of the rhythm to normal should be considered. Twenty-four hours prior to direct current cardioversion, quinidine sulfate is begun (see Chapter 8) and digitalis therapy is withheld. If medical therapy alone is successful in restoring a normal sinus rhythm (see Fig. 11-23), digitalis therapy is reinstituted immediately. If direct current cardioversion is necessary (see Fig. 11-24), digitalis therapy is begun after the procedure regardless of the success or failure of conversion. Maintenance levels of quinidine should also be administered if conversion to a sinus rhythm occurs during either medical therapy or direct current shock.

PROGNOSIS

Long-term survival of dogs with idiopathic cardiomyopathy is not likely. In our experience, survival for more than six to 12 months is unusual after the signs of atrial fibrillation and congestive heart failure have appeared.

PATHOLOGY

Extensive pathologic descriptions of this condition have not been presented. Grossly, the heart is generally enlarged, and there is dilatation of all chambers. In addition, the atrioventricular anular rings are both dilated, producing mitral and tricuspid valvular incompetence. The mitral and tricuspid valve leaflets are normal for middle-aged dogs, demonstrating only a moderate degree of thickening and/or fibrosis. Fibrotic nodules typical of chronic mitral valvular fibrosis and chronic tricuspid valvular fibrosis are absent (Fig. 14-11).

Left atrial ball thrombi occasionally develop late in the disease and may be responsible for embolic phenomena resulting in concurrent organ disease.

Sections of the right and left ventricular myocardium may reveal small focal regions of fibrosis; however, these are neither extensive nor consistent, and they do not always help to differentiate dogs with this disease from normal dogs.

Microscopic examination of the ventricular myocardium does not reveal lesions which could be considered pathognomonic for idiopathic cardiomyopathy.

ISCHEMIC MYOCARDIAL DISEASE (MYOCARDIAL INFARCTION; CORONARY EMBOLISM; HEART ATTACK)

Coronary embolism with myocardial infarction is rarely diagnosed in the dog either clinically or at necropsy. The origin of the coronary emboli that have been described is associated with neoplastic tissue from the lungs (Luginbühl and Detweiler, 1965), bacterial endocarditis (Nielsen and Nielsen, 1954), and generalized septicemia (Sandersleben, 1961). It is important to realize that gross myocardial infarction is uncommon and that a diagnosis of myocardial infarction is usually made only at necropsy; even then, histologic verification is usually necessary. Of 314 dogs examined at necropsy for cardiac abnormalities, only six had myocardial infarction; the infarctions were visible macroscopically in two dogs, and in the other four the infarctions were recognized on histopathologic examination (Luginbühl and Detweiler, 1965).

Myocardial infarctions, which occur frequently in human beings (the so-called "heart attack"), do not have a true counterpart in dogs, and such a diagnosis should be considered only in the most unusual circumstances. There are no specific signs for this condition which would lead the clinician to make the diagnosis. However, focal areas of intramural myocardial necrosis and the sequelae thereof, such as myocardial fibrosis, are relatively common in the left ventricle of dogs. Microscopic intramural ventricular myocardial infarctions and the associated lesion of coronary arteriosclerosis have been reviewed by Detweiler et al. (1968a). The lesions occur almost exclusively in the left ventricular wall, especially in older dogs with chronic mitral valvular fibrosis and mitral insufficiency or in young dogs with congenital subaortic stenosis (Flickinger and Patterson, 1967). Intramural arteriosclerosis and subsequent left ventricular ischemia may contribute to the frequency of heart failure in older dogs. Hamlin (1968) has also emphasized the importance of microscopic intramural myocardial infarction (MIMI) in valvular heart disease in the dog.

The marked anatomic, physiologic, and pathologic differences between the coronary artery circulations of dog and man, and the significance of these differences have been summarized by Pensinger (1968).

References

Bohn, F. K.: Vergleich klinischer elektrokardiographischer und pathologisch-anatomischer Befunde bei lokalisierten und generalisierten Myokarderkrankungen beim Hund. Zbl. Veterinärmed. [A], 14 (1967):416.

Crawley, G. J., and Swenson, M. J.: Blood Serum Enzymes as Diagnostic Aids in Canine Heart Disease. Amer. J. Vet. Res., 24 (1963):1271.

Dahme, E., and Reif, E.: Weitere Untersuchungen zur Pathomorphologie des Kranzarteriensystems beim Hund. Berlin. Münchn. Tierärztl. Wschr., 73 (1964):181.

Detweiler, D. K.: Wesen und Häufigkeit von Herzkrankheiten bei Hunden. Zbl. Veterinärmed., 9 (1962):317.

Detweiler, D. K., Luginbühl, H., Buchanan, J. W., and Patterson, D. F.: The Natural History of Acquired Cardiac Disability of the Dog. Ann. N. Y. Acad. Sci., 147 (1968a): 318.

Detweiler, D. K., Patterson, D. F., Luginbühl, H., Rhodes, W. H., Buchanan, J. W., Knight, D. H., and Hill, J. D.: Diseases of the Cardiovascular System. In Canine Medicine. Edited by E. J. Catcott. 1st Catcott ed. American Veterinary Publications, Inc., Santa Barbara, California (1968b):589.

Ettinger, S., Bolton, G. R. and Lord, P. F.: Idiopathic Cardiomyopathy in the Dog. (Abs.) J. A. V. M. A., 156 (1970):1225.

Flickinger, G. L., and Patterson, D. F.: Coronary Lesions Associated with Subaortic Stenosis in the Dog. J. Path. Bact., 93 (1967):133.

Friedberg, C. K.: Diseases of the Heart. W. B. Saunders, Philadelphia, 3rd ed. 1966.

Gratzel, E.: Das Elektrokardiogramm bei der Myocarditis des Hundes. Proc. 17th Ann. World Vet. Congress, (1963):1073.

Hamlin, R. L.: Prognostic Value of Changes in the Cardiac Silhouette in Dogs with Mitral Insufficiency. J. A. V. M. A., 153 (1968):1436.

Hamlin, R. L., Smetzer, D. L., and Smith, C. R.: Congenital Mitral Insufficiency in the Dog. J. A. V. M. A., 146 (1965):1088.

Jones, T. C., and Zook, B. C.: Aging Changes in the Vascular System of Animals. Ann. N. Y. Acad. Sci., 127 (1965):671.

Jubb, K. V. F., and Kennedy, P. C.: Pathology of Domestic Animals. Academic Press, New York, 1963.

Kersten, U.: Klinische Untersuchungen am herzkranken Hund. Thesis. Hannover, Germany, 1968.

Lannek, N.: A Clinical and Experimental Study on the Electrocardiogram in Dogs. Thesis. Stockholm, Sweden, 1949.

Luginbühl, H., and Detweiler, D. K.: Cardiovascular Lesions in Dogs. Ann. N. Y. Acad. Sci., 127 (1965):517.

McGuire, J.: The Cardiomyopathies (Primary Myocardial Disease, Myocardiosis, Idiopathic Cardiac Hypertrophy, Myocardiopathy, Cardiopathy, Idiopathic Cardiomyopathy). Seminars Roentgenol., 4 (1969):299.

Nielsen, S. W., and Nielsen, L. B.: Coronary Embolism in Valvular Bacterial Endocarditis in Two Dogs. J. A. V. M. A., 125 (1954):376.

Pensinger, R. R.: Chronic Congestive Heart Failure in Dogs—Clinical and Pathological Findings. Ann. N. Y. Acad. Sci., 147 (1968):330.

Sandersleben, J. V.: Der Infarkt und Seine Bedeutung beim Haustier. Deutsch. Tierärztl. Wschr., 68 (1961):590.

Taylor, D. H., and Sittnikow, K. L.: The Diagnosis of Canine Cardiac Disease. J. Small Anim. Pract., 9 (1968):589.

Witham, A. C., and Hurst, J. W.: Myocardial Disease: Introduction and Classification. In *The Heart—Arteries and Veins*. Edited by J. W. Hurst and R. B. Logue. McGraw-Hill Book Company, New York, 2nd ed., 1970.

15

DISEASES OF
THE PERICARDIUM

Most acquired diseases involving the pericardium result in an accumulation of fluid within the pericardial sac. The effusion can be inflammatory or noninflammatory, and occurs secondarily to a variety of cardiac and systemic diseases, as well as to pathologic processes involving the immediate surroundings of the heart such as the pleura or the mediastinum. Although pericardial effusions and inflammations of the pericardium occur infrequently when compared to the overall incidence of heart disease, they comprise an important group of diseases which may be responsible for signs of heart failure. In 314 dogs in which heart disease was diagnosed at necropsy, 46 had pericardial disease as follows: hemopericardium, 11; hydropericardium, 10; fibrinous or uremic pericarditis, 12; metastatic tumors, 4; subacute pericarditis, 3; acute pericarditis, 1; adhesions, 2; hemorrhage, 1; fibrosis, 1; and absence of the pericardium, 1 (Detweiler, 1962).

It is convenient for diagnostic and differential diagnostic purposes to classify the effusions on the basis of their being bloody, transudate, or exudate (Table 15-1). Hemopericardium can result from cardiac neoplasia, heart base tumors, metastatic cardiac tumors, or rupture of a coronary vessel or other portion of the heart due to other pathology or trauma.

Clear or straw-colored pericardial transudates result from congestive heart failure, hypoproteinemia, and peritoneopericardial hernias. Serous pericardial effusions are the most frequently encountered type of pericardial effusion (Gratzl, 1965).

Pericardial exudates from pericarditis are variable in appearance depending on the etiologic agent at cause. Benign or idiopathic pericardial effusion is characterized by a serosanguineous, port wine–colored, nonclotting, sterile fluid. Bacterial and viral agents, toxemias, and extension of pleural inflammations to the pericardium (Jubb and Kennedy, 1963) may result in exudative pericardial effusions.

PERICARDITIS AND PERICARDIAL EFFUSION

Pericarditis refers to an inflammation of the fibrous and serous layers that surround the heart. In the dog, pericarditis is usually effusive rather than constrictive. Because the diseases of the pericardium, regardless of their etiology, have common features, they are discussed together. The types of effusions, etiology, and characteristic features are summarized in Table 15-1.

TABLE 15-1 DIFFERENTIAL DIAGNOSIS OF PERICARDIAL EFFUSION

TYPE OF PERICARDIAL EFFUSION	ETIOLOGY	CHARACTERISTIC FEATURES
Blood	1. Heart base tumors	Usually brachycephalic breeds over 8 years old, blood usually nonclotting.
	2. Other neoplasia (metastatic)	
	3. Left atrial rupture	Usually occurs in male dogs of smaller breeds, over 8 years old.
	4. Physical trauma	
	5. Iatrogenic trauma	Due to cardiac puncture or cardiac catheterization.
Transudate	1. Congestive heart failure	Effusion not commonly recognized by physical or radiographic examination.
	2. Hypoproteinemia	
	3. Secondary to peritoneoperi-cardial diaphragmatic hernia	
Exudate (Pericarditis)	1. Benign idiopathic pericardial effusion	Fluid serosanguineous; port wine color, nonclotting, and sterile (Luginbühl and Detweiler, 1965).
	2. Infectious pericarditis	Serous exudate in distemper and leptospirosis; sanguinous exudate in tuberculosis (Labie, 1962); or in conjunction with pleuritis and coccidioidomycosis.

HISTORY AND PHYSICAL EXAMINATION

Since pericarditis is usually secondary to another disease, the history varies depending on the signs of the primary condition—i.e., trauma, chronic heart disease, systemic infections, or neoplasia. If the pericardial fluid does not interfere with venous return or impair cardiac function, clinical signs will be absent. As the disease progresses, signs such as dyspnea, generalized debilitation, and abdominal distention are noticed. If the condition is of infectious origin, chronic fever may be present.

The signs noticed on physical examination vary with the amount of fluid trapped within the pericardial sac and the rapidity with which it collects. As the effusion becomes extensive, peripheral venous pressure rises owing to impairment of venous return to the heart. This increase in venous pressure is recognized by peripheral venous distention and a prominent jugular pulse. Elevation of central venous pressure leads to an elevated caudal vena caval pressure which is then responsible for hepatomegaly, ascites, and eventually generalized peripheral edema. Cardiac tamponade results when the tension of the trapped pericardial fluid compresses the heart and prevents proper cardiac filling. The restriction in cardiac filling results in diminished arterial blood pressure, which is indicated by a rapid, weak peripheral pulse and by blanching of the mucous membranes. As pericardial effusion progresses toward a terminal state, effusions develop in the pleural cavity.

It is more likely for a dog to sustain a large effusion when it develops slowly, because the pericardium stretches, and the circulatory system can then adapt gradually to the abnormal hemodynamic situation. When the effusion develops rapidly, as in left atrial rupture (see pp. 361-366), death due to tamponade may be sudden, even when relatively small amounts of fluid are present.

The triad of increased venous pressures, decreased peripheral arterial pressure, and muffled heart sounds (see next paragraph) is highly suggestive of pericardial effusion.

AUSCULTATION

Characteristically, heart sounds are muffled or of diminished intensity when a significant amount of fluid has collected within the pericardial sac. However, if only a small amount of pericardial fluid is present, as is common in hydro-pericardium secondary to congestive heart failure, the intensity of the heart sounds is not diminished significantly. The muffled heart sounds of advanced pericardial effusion remain unchanged even when the dog's position is varied in an attempt to bring the heart closer to the thoracic wall. The heart rate increases as the effusion becomes more extensive, and the stroke volume decreases as less blood is returned to the heart per unit of time.

Pericardial hemorrhage resulting from endocardial splitting and rupture of the left atrial wall (see pp. 361-366) usually cannot be detected by auscultation unless cardiac tamponade is produced. Even in cases of left atrial tear, the holo-systolic murmur of mitral and tricuspid valvular insufficiency is more likely to be auscultated than are muffled heart sounds.

ELECTROCARDIOGRAPHY

Electrocardiography is usually of little value in the differential diagnosis of pericardial effusion. Electrocardiographic complexes of low amplitude and changes in the S–T segment may occur, but they are not specific for pericardial effusion. In some instances, the electrocardiogram is normal even in severe peri-cardial effusion, and no changes are recorded even after large amounts of the pericardial fluid are withdrawn.

RADIOGRAPHIC EXAMINATION

The radiographic signs of pericardial effusion have been described by Rhodes, Patterson, and Detweiler (1963), Buchanan and Kelly (1964), and Carlson (1967). The reliability of the radiographic signs depends on the amount of fluid that has accumulated in the pericardial sac. Small amounts of pericardial fluid are difficult to differentiate from cardiac enlargement and are therefore not diagnosed. In comparison, large amounts of fluid always produce significant radiographic changes, but the size of the cardiac silhouette on the radiograph does not neces-sarily indicate the amount of fluid present within the pericardial sac. The heart may be of normal size, the enlargement being entirely due to the accumulated fluid; or only small amounts of fluid may be present if pericardial effusion and cardiac enlargement are concurrent. The radiographic appearance is similar in both cases.

It may be difficult to evaluate pericardial effusion if massive pleural effusion obscures the cardiac silhouette (Figs. 15-1 and 15-2). In such cases the thoracic fluid should be removed before exposing further radiographs. A standing lateral radiograph is often beneficial when pleural effusions are present (Fig. 15-3).

Massive pericardial effusion is usually characterized by a greatly enlarged, globular cardiac silhouette in both the lateral and dorsoventral projections (Figs. 15-7 and 15-8). The high density of the silhouette prevents recognition of structures such as the caudal vena cava within the silhouette. The borders of the silhouette are markedly even, and all protrusions such as the right auricle, the left atrial bulge, and the apical rounding are absent. However, the cardiac silhouette may be flattened wherever it touches the thoracic wall. The hilar area is displaced dorsally, but the structures remain visible except in those cases where effusion is secondary to heart base tumors or endocardial splitting and rupture of the left atrium. The lung field is often not affected, since pulmonary hypertension does not develop in the presence of restricted cardiac filling (see Fig. 15-1). The diaphragm may be indented by the cardiac silhouette, but its outline is uninterrupted.

In the lateral radiograph, the left cardiac border, which remains relatively straight even in massive cardiac enlargement, becomes rounded. The caudal vena cava is dilated, and the cranial mediastinum extends farther ventrally than normal. These signs are frequently combined with ascites, hepatomegaly, splenomegaly, and/or blurring of the details in the abdomen. In the dorsoventral radiograph, the mediastinum appears wider than normal.

Radiographs are seldom helpful in determining the etiology of the effusion, since inflammatory and noninflammatory fluids cannot be differentiated. However, tumors of the mediastinum and the heart base (Figs. 15-9 and 15-10) or splitting of the endocardium with a ruptured left atrium can often be suggested or ruled out. Radiographs also assist in evaluating the effects of therapy (Figs. 15-4. 15-5, and 15-6).

Fluoroscopy can further assist in diagnosing pericardial effusion. The normal pulsations of the ventral portions of the silhouette are absent or weakened, and undulation of the border is seen instead. This is so because fluid tends to collect in these areas (Mellins, Kottmeier, and Kiely, 1959). The pulsations at the hilar area appear nearly normal and therefore contrast with the lack of motion of the rest of the cardiac silhouette. Soulen, Lapayowker, and Cortes (1958) demonstrated that gravity has no significant effect on the fluid distribution; that is, the heart neither floats nor sinks in the fluid.

DIFFERENTIAL DIAGNOSIS

The triad of clinical signs of increased central venous pressure, heart sounds that are muffled or of decreased intensity, and decreased arterial blood pressure as indicated by weak pulse and blanching of the mucous membranes is definitely suggestive of pericardial effusion and cardiac tamponade. Heart sounds of decreased intensity are also heard in obese dogs, in dogs with emphysema, pleural effusion, thoracic masses, diaphragmatic or peritoneopericardial diaphragmatic

Text continues page 417.

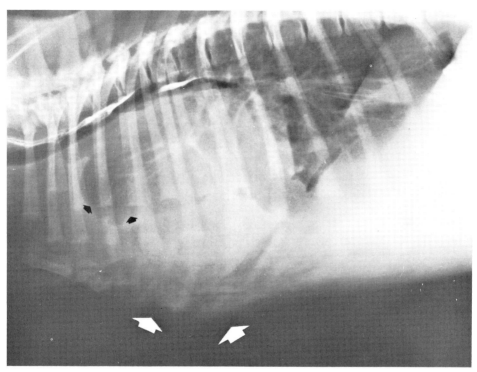

FIGURE 15-1 Left lateral radiograph, 4 month old male Great Pyrenees with pleural and pericardial effusion. An esophagram was done with barium to outline the mediastinal and hilar structures. The dog had been debilitated for two weeks and then developed dyspnea suddenly. No heart sounds could be heard. The pulse was thready and weak, and a jugular pulse was noticed. The mucous membranes were blanched. Ascites and pleural and pericardial effusion were diagnosed on the initial radiographs, and medical treatment was initiated. This radiograph was exposed after two days of treatment. The thorax is denser than normal, and there is lack of contrast among the different structures in the cranial and ventral portions due to accumulation of fluid in the pleural space. The lobes of the lungs are retracted and are visible as darker areas within the fluid (black arrows). Although the cardiac silhouette is not entirely visible, it appears markedly enlarged. The trachea is displaced dorsally and appears squeezed between the enlarged cardiac silhouette and the spine. The ventral bend of the distal extremity of the trachea is straightened, but no dorsal bulge of the left atrium is visible. Neither displacement nor obstruction of the esophagus is seen on the esophagram. The caudal border of the cardiac silhouette is rounder than normal and extends far caudally. The caudal vena cava, which is barely visible, appears engorged. The lung field is unremarkable. Because of the pleural effusion, it is difficult to recognize the pericardial effusion. Upon reexamination of the radiograph, it was noticed that from the third sternebral body caudally, the sternebrae were not distinctly outlined; instead, their densities merged with the surrounding soft tissue structures. In addition, there was a slight ventral protrusion of the soft tissue in this area (white arrows). This finding, and the discovery of a cyst-like hemorrhagic structure in the pericardial sac at the time of exploratory surgery, led to the diagnosis of pleural and pericardial effusion, probably of traumatic origin.

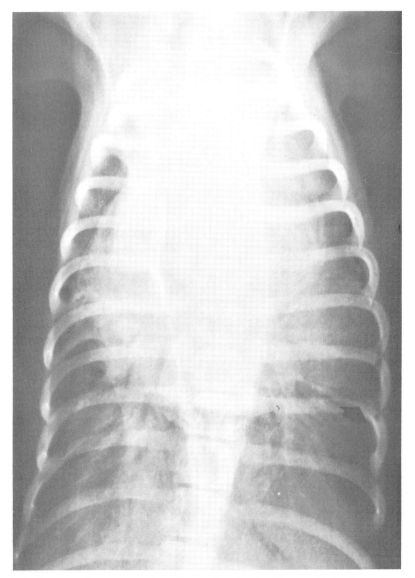

FIGURE 15-2 Dorsoventral radiograph, dog in Figure 15-1. The pleural fluid makes identification of structures even more difficult here than on the lateral radiograph. The cardiac silhouette, which appears blurred because of the effusion, is globular. The cranial mediastinum is much wider than normal. The appearance of fluid-filled interlobar spaces (arrow) helps to make the diagnosis of pleural effusion in this type of radiograph.

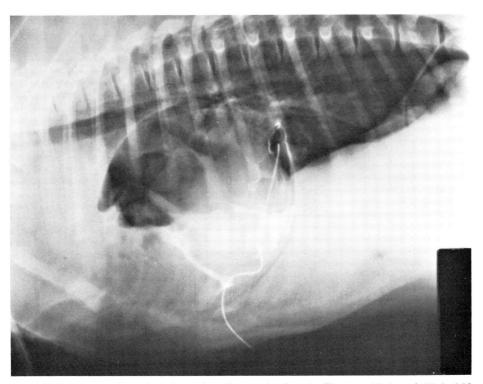

FIGURE 15-3   Standing lateral radiograph, dog in Figures 15-1 and 15-2. 350 ml. of fluid was withdrawn by pericardiocentesis and was replaced by 150 ml. of room air. To outline the nonopaque catheter, 1 ml. of Hypaque 50% was injected immediately before the radiograph was exposed. The cranial thorax has a ground-glass-like appearance. The injected air dilated the dorsal half of the pericardial sac, and the pericardium is seen as a linear structure approximately 1 to 1.5 mm. in diameter. However, there is no continuous horizontal fluid level in the pericardium, as might have been expected with an uncomplicated pericardial effusion. Instead, there are several dense structures suggesting the presence of masses such as fibrinous clots in the pericardium. This assumption was even more likely because it was impossible to withdraw more fluid despite both rotation of the dog to make the fluid shift to the deepest point and repeated changes in the position of the catheter. The craniocaudal diameter of the cardiac silhouette appears normal. In the hilar area, slight left atrial enlargement is indicated.

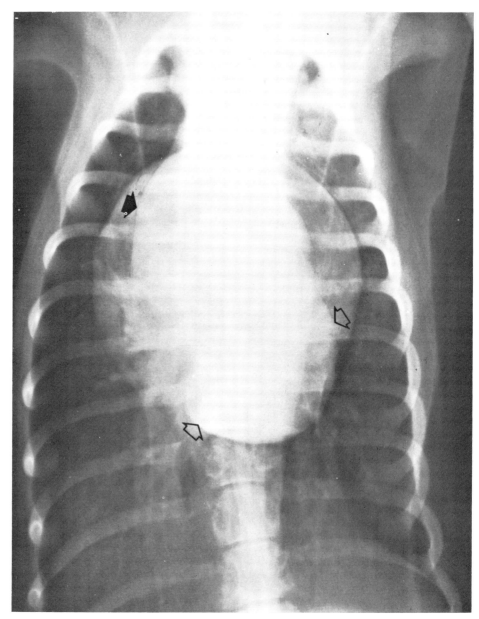

FIGURE 15-4 Dorsoventral radiograph, dog in Figures 15-1 through 15-3, made one day after the pneumopericardium shown in Figure 15-3. Some air remains in the pericardial sac, but additional fluid has accumulated, as indicated by the diminished contrast between the cardiac silhouette and the surrounding pericardial space. A well-delineated density on the right side (black arrow) represents the cranial vena cava and left atrium. The outline of the cardiac silhouette is indistinct. The cardiac apex and a dense mass are superimposed (clear arrows). This mass corresponds to the cyst-like fluid-filled structure which was found at the time of surgery. The mass was located at the apex within the pericardium, which was attached to the sternum.

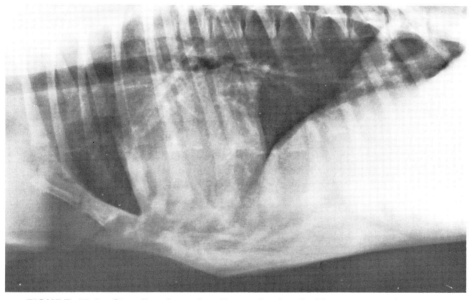

FIGURE 15-5 Standing lateral radiograph, dog in Figures 15-1 through 15-4, made one month postoperatively. The dog had regained its normal activity. The cardiac silhouette is slightly enlarged and appears to adhere to the sternum and to the ventral diaphragm. The left atrium is enlarged. The diaphragm extends farther cranially than normal and therefore appears more inclined. In addition, the separation between the cardiac silhouette and the diaphragm is ill-defined. The bulge in the subcutis of the ventral thorax has almost completely disappeared.

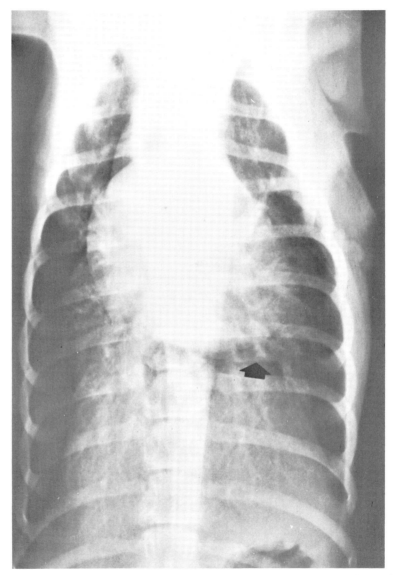

FIGURE 15-6 Dorsoventral radiograph, dog in Figures 15-1 through 15-5, made one month postoperatively. The cardiac silhouette is of nearly normal size. There is a double shadow (arrow) surrounding the apex, which is connected to the diaphragm by a thickened cardiophrenic ligament. This density is a remnant of the surgical procedure. The diaphragm has an elliptical appearance; therefore, the costophrenic angles are deeper and more acute than normal. Merging of the outline of the diaphragm with the caudal cardiac border is less obvious than in the lateral view.

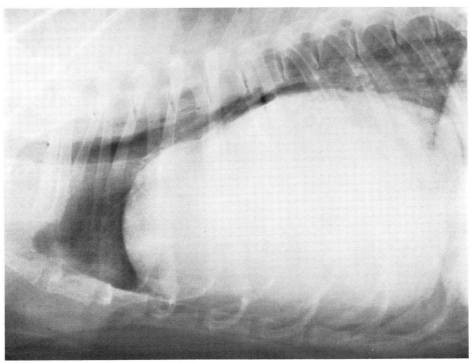

FIGURE 15-7   Lateral radiograph, 14½ year old female Poodle with a history of dyspnea and wheezing. The heart sounds were muffled, the pulse was rapid and weak, and harsh lung sounds were heard. The abdomen was not enlarged. The huge cardiac silhouette fills most of the thoracic cavity. It is dorsoventrally compressed, and the cranial and caudal borders are globular. The structures of the hilar area appear compressed; however, there is no sign of left atrial enlargement. The density of the silhouette is homogeneous, and an ill-defined border demarcates the cardiac silhouette from the diaphragm. The diaphragmatic lobes of the lung are dense. The extreme extension of the caudal border of the cardiac silhouette and the absence of a left atrial bulge rule out extreme cardiac enlargement as is occasionally seen with severe heart failure. At necropsy, diffuse infiltration of the pericardial sac by mesothelioma was seen.

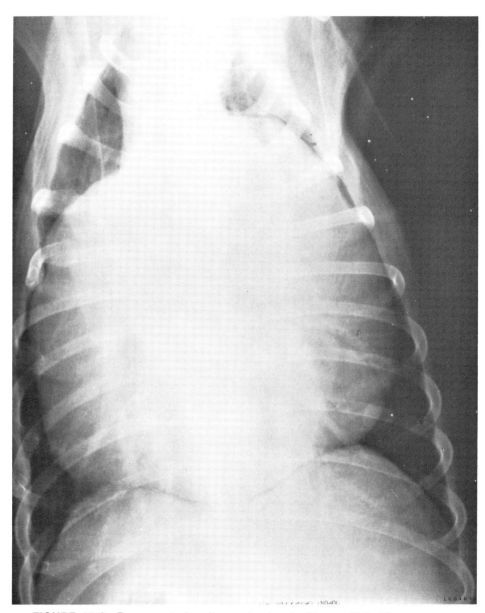

FIGURE 15-8 Dorsoventral radiograph, dog in Figure 15-7. The extreme enlargement of the cardiac silhouette is also obvious in this projection. The silhouette flattens where it touches the thoracic wall, and some indentation is also seen where it meets the diaphragm. There is no defect in the diaphragm. A globular cardiac silhouette in both the lateral and dorsoventral views is diagnostic for pericardial effusion.

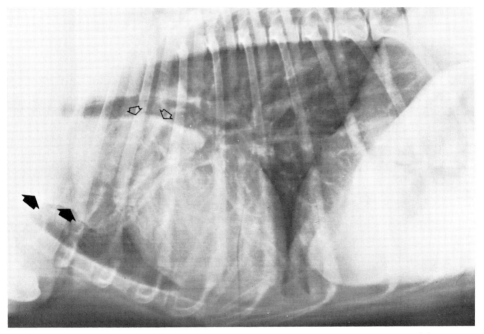

FIGURE 15-9 Left lateral radiograph, 8 year old male Boxer examined because of a cough which did not respond to therapy. The cardiac silhouette is slightly enlarged on the right side. There is a dense mass in the cranial mediastinum. The ventral outline of the mediastinum is scalloped (black arrows) and extends ventrally to within approximately 1.5 cm. of the sternum. The trachea is slightly displaced dorsally, and the dorsal border of the mass is superimposed on the lucency of the trachea (clear arrows). The caudal vena cava joins the caudal border of the heart at a higher point than normal, which sometimes indicates right atrial and right ventricular enlargement. A heart base tumor was diagnosed clinically and proved on postmortem examination.

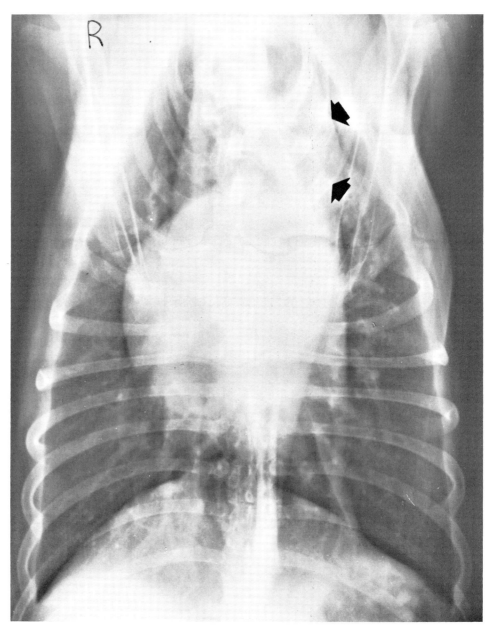

FIGURE 15-10 Dorsoventral radiograph, dog in Figure 15-9. The right ventricular enlargement is more obvious in this view than it was in the lateral (Fig. 15-9). The left side of the heart is unremarkable. The aortic arch is wider and extends farther to the left side than normal. A round density approximately 4 cm. in diameter is located cranial and to the left of the aortic arch. It extends to about the first rib. Heart base tumors often impinge on the cranial vena cava. An angiogram made after injection of contrast medium into the jugular vein is sometimes helpful in doubtful cases to outline indirectly the impingement of the tumor mass on the cranial vena cava if it does not protrude beyond the borders of the mediastinum, as it does in this case.

TABLE 15-2 RADIOGRAPHIC DIFFERENTIAL DIAGNOSIS OF PERICARDIAL EFFUSIONS

DISEASE	TYPICAL RADIOGRAPHIC SIGNS WHICH MAY ASSIST IN MAKING A DIAGNOSIS
General cardiac enlargement and heart failure due to acquired or congenital disease	Often marked difference in shape of cardiac silhouette in lateral and dorsoventral radiographs. The silhouette is not as smooth and evenly rounded as it is in pericardial effusion. The enlarged left atrium is always seen bulging dorsocaudally. The caudal cardiac border in the lateral radiograph remains straight or may even be convex as it joins the enlarged left atrium. If fluoroscopy is done, the pulsations, although weaker than normal, are the same in the hilar area and at the left and right cardiac borders.
Endocardial splitting with left atrial rupture	Because of the hemopericardium, the shape of the cardiac silhouette is identical to that seen with every other type of effusion; however, the greatly enlarged left atrium, which can always be seen in the lateral radiograph in this condition, helps to identify the etiology.
Heart base tumors and metastatic neoplasia	Some pericardial effusion is almost invariably present. It is very important to scrutinize the hilar area and the cranial mediastinum for round or oval densities which may displace the trachea dorsally or to the right. The aortic arch may also be displaced. An esophagram may be helpful to show displacement of the esophagus in the precordial mediastinum or at the base of the heart. Venous angiography can be used to indicate vascular displacement or obstruction by a tumor mass. The tumor may be outlined in the arterial phase.
Massive right atrial enlargement secondary to severe tricuspid insufficiency	The right atrium may enlarge to such an extent that a globular cardiac silhouette, most obvious on the right side, is produced.
Peritoneopericardial diaphragmatic hernia	Small gas pockets trapped in the intestinal loops are often present within the cardiac silhouette. There is discontinuity of the diaphragmatic outline in the lateral and/or dorsoventral radiograph. Abnormal positioning of liver and stomach is often present. Oral barium administration serves to prove the diagnosis.

hernia, and in dogs in which myocardial contractility and cardiac output are diminished. Although most of these conditions can be differentiated clinically, radiographic examination with or without contrast medium can be of great value in differentiating some lesions (Table 15-2).

Several methods have been proposed to secure the radiographic differential diagnosis of pericardial effusion. After removal of the pericardial fluid, part of its volume is replaced with air (Patterson and Botts, 1961; Buchanan, 1965). Radiographs are then made in the lateral recumbent, dorsoventral, and standing lateral positions (horizontal beam to see fluid level) (Figs. 15-3 and 15-4). The size of the heart can then be properly evaluated.

Positive or negative (CO_2) contrast material injected via the jugular or cephalic vein can be used to outline the right atrial and right ventricular chambers and thus to differentiate cardiac enlargement from pericardial effusion. Displacement or compression of the cranial vena cava by tumors can be visualized using angiocardiography (Patterson and Botts, 1961; Buchanan, 1965).

TREATMENT

When fluid collects within the pericardial sac and cardiac function is restricted, it is imperative that the fluid be removed. The methods used for removing pericardial fluids vary with the underlying cause of the effusion. Re-accumulation of fluid is avoided by medical treatment of the underlying cause or by surgical intervention to remove the cause or to produce a pericardial window. When valvular insufficiency results in severe congestive heart failure, pericardial fluid may collect. This fluid can usually be eliminated if cardiac therapy for the underlying disease process, including digitalization, diuretics, cage rest, and a low sodium diet, is effective in controlling the heart failure.

Aspiration of a small amount of pericardial fluid to determine its character is necessary before specific therapeutic measures can be taken. Aspiration also has a beneficial therapeutic effect on cardiac function. Removal of the pericardial effusion is a simple and safe technique. It is usually best performed with the dog in right lateral recumbency. The skin over the left fourth to sixth intercostal spaces near the costochondral arch is antiseptically prepared and locally anesthetized. The intercostal space to be penetrated for pericardial puncture is determined by digital localization of the cardiac apical beat if possible.

An 18- or 20-gauge needle attached directly to a syringe is adequate for removing samples of fluid for inspection. However, we prefer the following method: A 16-gauge needle combined with a polyethylene catheter (Venocath) is attached to a three-way stopcock and a 30-cc. syringe. A rubber tube is attached to the stopcock so that after fluid is withdrawn into the syringe it may be evacuated by opening the stopcock to the rubber tubing. After the pericardial sac has been penetrated, the syringe and stopcock are temporarily removed, and the polyethylene catheter is introduced through the needle. The needle is then removed and secured safely outside the thoracic wall. The external end of the polyethylene catheter is then attached to the 3-way stopcock and syringe. This method gives the operator more maneuverability. Removal of the needle diminishes the likelihood of cardiac trauma (especially in restless dogs). The catheter, well placed in the pericardial sac, is not likely to slip out of the sac if the dog moves suddenly. Disadvantages of this technique are that the internal diameter of the catheter is small, making fluid withdrawal more time-consuming, and that when the catheter is sharply bent or a vacuum is produced, its lumen will collapse.

For pericardial puncture, the needle is passed through the skin and intercostal space at an angle slightly less than perpendicular to the thoracic wall, pointing medially and somewhat dorsally. As it strikes the pericardial surface, a scratchy feeling is transmitted through the needle. The pericardial sac is penetrated using a short thrust; penetration is usually recognized by a sudden decrease in resistance. If the needle penetrates too far and touches the epicardium or enters the heart, a short burst of ectopic beats results which can usually be recognized by the aberrant motion of the needle or by direct electrocardiographic visualization. The barrel of the syringe may be forced open by the excessive intrapericardial pressure, but this pressure would be greater if the needle had penetrated the left ventricle.

Initially, only a small amount of pericardial fluid is withdrawn, and sterile aliquots are prepared for bacteriologic culture, cytologic analysis, and clinical laboratory tests, including determination of clotting ability. The types of fluid that may be removed from the sac are listed in Table 15-1. If a sanguineous fluid which clots completely is withdrawn, further attempts at aspiration should be discontinued immediately. Sanguineous fluid that does not clot suggests the presence of defibrinated blood, which is usually associated with heart base tumors or pericardial metastatic neoplasia.

If the nature of the fluid is not immediately apparent, a venous blood sample should be compared with the aspirated fluid; if the effusion is whole blood, it should clot as quickly as the venous blood. If the pericardial fluid is whole blood, laboratory examination of the pericardial and venous samples should demonstrate similar hematologic qualities. In benign pericardial effusion, the fluid is a port wine color, and little if any will clot. If the fluid is nonclotting, withdrawal should be continued at a slow but steady rate, to avoid shock, and as much fluid as possible should be removed.

If a polyethylene catheter has been introduced, the dog may be rotated to shift the fluid to the dependent regions in an effort to remove all the fluid. A second pericardial tap from the right thoracic wall is occasionally indicated to remove additional fluid. After the fluid has been removed, a pneumopericardium may be made by injecting a volume of carbon dioxide, nitrogen, or air equal to about half the volume of fluid removed. Radiographs of a dog with an induced pneumopericardium are made with the dog in different positions, including a standing lateral position (Fig. 15-3 and 15-4). The pneumopericardium outlines the heart and pericardial sac, and effectively demonstrates the quantity of fluid remaining in the pericardial sac. A radiolucent catheter may be filled with contrast medium to show its location within the pericardial sac (Fig. 15-3).

When nonsanguineous, sterile pericardial fluid re-accumulates rapidly after several attempts at removal, additional attempts at pericardiocentesis are rarely helpful. Surgical intervention may then be recommended for diagnostic purposes and to create a pericardial window. A pericardial window permits the fluid to drain into the pleural space, where it is reabsorbed or may be removed more easily. In addition, the recurrent signs of pericardial effusion and tamponade are thus avoided while specific therapy is being given. Nonsanguineous effusion with pericarditis due to a pericardial cyst was surgically corrected after numerous pericardiocentesis procedures were ineffective in controlling recurrent pericardial effusion (Marion et al., 1970).

Specific antibiotic therapy should be instituted if a definite organism is isolated in cultures made from the pericardial fluid.

PROGNOSIS

Benign pericardial effusion has been treated successfully by Detweiler et al. (1968), but the condition tends to recur (Price and Mullen, 1966).

Sanguineous effusions are not always fatal. In some cases they may stop spontaneously, and in other cases surgical exploration is indicated. One case induced during cardiac catheterization was successfully repaired surgically after the rents in the myocardium were sutured (Buchanan and Pyle, 1966). Pericardial hemorrhage due to primary or secondary neoplasia is usually terminal.

PERICARDIAL TRAUMA AND RUPTURE

Traumatic rupture of the pericardium has been reported (Kohler, 1958; Teuscher, 1958; Pallaske, 1959). These cases have only been recognized at necropsy. The dogs died suddenly after showing signs of circulatory collapse. Rupture of the right ventricle occurred in one of the cases (Pallaske, 1959), and left ventricular incarceration developed in another (Teuscher, 1958).

Other diseases such as chronic mitral valvular fibrosis, congenital heart disease with right-to-left shunts, and idiopathic pulmonary hypertension may result in right ventricular hypertrophy and pulmonary hypertension. However, the term cor pulmonale is used only when right ventricular hypertrophy occurs secondarily to primary pulmonary vascular or parenchymal disease.

HEARTWORM DISEASE (DIROFILARIA IMMITIS)

Adult heartworms *(Dirofilaria immitis)* lodge in the right atrium, right ventricle, right ventricular outflow tract, pulmonary arteries, and venae cavae, and occasionally in other organs. The major effect of heartworms in the body is obstruction of the pulmonary vascular bed, resulting in pulmonary hypertension with subsequent right heart failure. Heartworms are also responsible for serious circulatory and parenchymal damage within the liver and for the "liver failure syndrome," recognized in regions where the disease is enzootic (Jackson, von Lichtenberg, and Otto, 1962; von Lichtenberg, Jackson, and Otto, 1962; R. F. Jackson, 1969c).

Dirofilariasis is most common in the Atlantic and Gulf Coast regions of the United States (Thrasher, Ash, and Little, 1963; Thrasher and Clanton, 1968; Thrasher et al., 1968), but the disease is also recognized in other parts of the United States (Augustine, 1938; Mann and Fratta, 1952; Otto and Bauman, 1959; Wallenstein and Tibola, 1960; Rothstein et al., 1961; Groves and Koutz, 1964; Lillis, 1964; Hirth, Huizinga, and Nielsen, 1966; Marquardt and Fabian, 1966; McGreevy et al., 1970). It has been diagnosed in many parts of the world, particularly in the tropics, subtropics, and north and south temperate zones (Otto, 1969).

The microfilariae of the nonpathogenic *Dipetalonema reconditum* must be differentiated from those of *D. immitis.* Epidemiologic studies made before the two parasites were differentiated by Newton and Wright (1956) cannot be considered valid.

In a general study of dogs in the state of Georgia, Thrasher and Clanton (1968) found the microfilariae of *D. immitis* in 19.6 per cent of all dogs examined and those of *D. reconditum* in 4.7 per cent of all dogs. In a similar study of dogs in Atlanta, Georgia, Thrasher et al. (1968) compared the frequency of *D. immitis* and *D. reconditum* in privately owned dogs with that in dogs from a pound. Of 273 privately owned dogs, 5.4 per cent had microfilariae of *D. immitis* and 14.6 per cent had microfilariae of *D. reconditum.* Microfilariae of both *D. reconditum* and *D. immitis* were present in 0.7 per cent of the 273 dogs. In comparison, when 40 dogs from the pound were examined, 12.5 per cent had microfilariae of *D. immitis* and 37.5 per cent had those of *D. reconditum.* Mixed infection with both *D. reconditum* and *D. immitis* was found in 7.5 per cent of the 40 dogs. From the same study, it was determined that the incidence of *D. immitis* is higher in yard dogs than in house dogs, or in dogs that are both house and yard dogs. There was no sex predisposition for *D. immitis;* however, a 3:1 male:female ratio was determined in dogs with microfilariae of *D. reconditum.* It was also determined that the length of hair of the dogs is unrelated to the frequency of *D. immitis* infection.

The incidence of *D. immitis* and *D. reconditum* infections is lower in dogs in the Eastern, Northeastern, and Midwestern (Zydeck, Chodkowski, & Bennett,

1970) United States than in the Southern United States. Dirofilariasis is often recognized in dogs that have lived in the South or in dogs living near lakes, ponds, or the seashore, where mosquitos, the intermediate host for the parasite, are common.

HISTORY AND PHYSICAL EXAMINATION

The history and findings on physical examination vary with the chronicity and severity of the infection. We thus differentiate between asymptomatic infections and clinically apparent disease, which can occur in an acute form (the liver failure syndrome) or in a more chronic form, with cardiac and pulmonary signs.

In most dogs with heartworm disease, blood tests (direct smear or modified Knott technique), electrocardiography, and radiography help to provide definitive diagnostic data. If microfilariae are not present and the diagnosis remains doubtful, cardiac catheterization and angiocardiography may help to provide a definitive diagnosis.

Chronic infection.   In asymptomatic dogs, microfilariae found on a blood smear may be the only suggestion of heartworm disease. The asymptomatic form can become symptomatic at any time as pathologic changes continue to develop. As the condition progresses, loss of stamina and body weight as well as general listlessness, vomiting, exertional fatigue, poor haircoat, and dehydration develop. In other cases, a persistent soft cough may be the first sign recognized (Thrasher, 1965). As the condition becomes further advanced, a hacking cough is present, and the dog tires rapidly. Apparently in an attempt to alleviate respiratory distress, the forelimbs are often held in abduction. Although interstitial dehydration occurs, ascitic fluid is retained as right heart failure leads to hepatic congestion. Syncope and convulsions (Henderson, 1967; Patton and Garner, 1970) and anemia, as well as advanced congestive heart failure, may be present in dogs with advanced heartworm disease.

Acute vena caval or liver failure syndrome (Jackson, von Lichtenberg, and Otto, 1962).   Dogs developing the acute vena caval syndrome usually have had no previous clinical signs other than perhaps a cough. Although the acute vena caval syndrome can occur at any age, dogs affected are usually between 3 and 5 years of age (R. F. Jackson, 1969c). The condition usually begins from 12 to 24 hours before the dog is presented to the veterinarian for weakness, collapse, anorexia, and discolored urine (hemoglobinuria). At the time of examination, rapid respiration and a cough are noticed, as is a forceful heartbeat, although murmurs are usually absent. Ascites does not develop in the acute condition, and many dogs are reported to be anemic. As its name infers, the syndrome occurs acutely, and death due to hepatic and renal failure ensues within 12 to 72 hours from the time of initial examination. The severity of clinical signs can be directly related to the number of adult worms in the venae cavae at necropsy. However, severe signs sometimes occur in dogs with relatively few worms.

CARDIAC EXAMINATION

Examination of the asymptomatic patient is usually unrevealing; auscultation of the heart and lungs and the electrocardiogram are within normal limits. For this reason, blood should be collected routinely for examination for microfilariae in endemic regions (see pp. 429-430). As cardiac disability becomes moderately advanced, pulmonary artery pressures become increased so that closure of the pulmonic valve is delayed slightly. This produces a split second heart sound that is best heard over the pulmonic valve region (Fig. 16-1). Splitting of the second heart sound may not be heard with each beat, and it is more obvious during inspiration than expiration because of an increased volume of blood in the right ventricle during this phase of respiration, further delaying valve closure. At this stage of the disease the electrocardiogram may be normal, or moderate right axis deviation and P pulmonale may be present.

When pulmonary hypertension becomes advanced and signs of heart disease are obvious, splitting of the second heart sound is usually constant, and right axis deviation in the frontal plane of the electrocardiogram is usually obvious (Fig. 16-2). An $S_I S_{II} S_{III}$ pattern may develop during the moderately severe and advanced stages of heartworm disease because of hypertrophy of the right ventricle. A deep S wave in lead $CV_6 LU$ is present in most dogs with moderately severe and advanced heartworm disease when right ventricular hypertrophy is present.

Systolic murmurs are not usually a feature of heartworm disease, although Yarns and Tashjian (1967) reported that systolic murmurs are more common in dogs with heartworm disease than in normal dogs. Detweiler and Patterson (1965) reported that pulmonic insufficiency occasionally develops in heartworm disease, producing a diastolic murmur audible over the pulmonic valve region. In one study (Yarns and Tashjian, 1967), the phonocardiogram of heartworm-infected dogs demonstrated a prolonged interval from the onset of the Q wave on the electrocardiogram to the second heart sound when the two were recorded simultaneously. In the same study, electrocardiograms indicated a tendency for clockwise rotation of the mean electrical axis in the frontal plane and counterclockwise rotation of the horizontal axis. Atrial and ventricular premature contractions occasionally occur in dogs with heartworms. Atrial fibrillation is infrequently associated with heartworm disease.

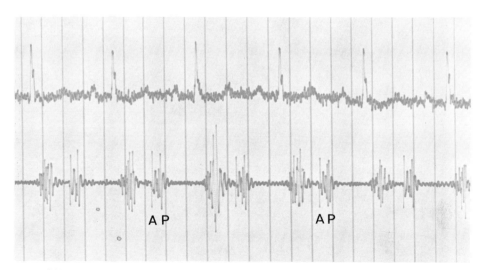

FIGURE 16-1 Lead II of the electrocardiogram recorded simultaneously with phonocardiogram from dog with moderately advanced dirofilariasis. Wide splitting of the second heart sound, 0.04 sec. between the aortic (A) and pulmonic (P) components, is due to delayed closure of the pulmonic valve.

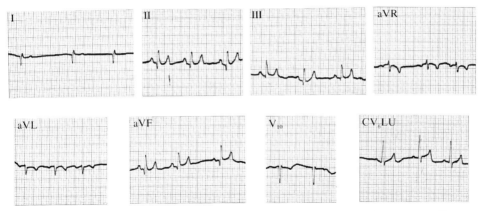

FIGURE 16-2 Right axis deviation. Dog with symptomatic heartworm disease presented for fatigue, dyspnea, and a chronic cough. The mean electrical axis in the frontal plane is 110°, suggesting moderate right ventricular hypertrophy. The depth of the S wave in lead CV$_6$LU (0.2 to 0.3 mv.) is not helpful in this case in proving the presence of right ventricular hypertrophy. Following arsenical therapy the signs regressed, and the dog was able to participate in normal physical activity without tiring.

The vectorcardiogram will vary depending on the degree of right ventricular hypertrophy. Early in the disease and when the infection is not severe, the vectorcardiogram is normal. As the degree of right ventricular hypertrophy progresses, there is an increase in the initial rightward forces in the frontal and horizontal planes. In some advanced cases, the forces are oriented almost entirely to the right, mimicking the vectorcardiogram of significant pulmonic stenosis.

RADIOGRAPHIC EXAMINATION

Thoracic radiographs are valuable in differentiating dirofilariasis from other heart diseases and in determining the severity of the cardiac, pulmonary, and vascular changes. The radiographic signs depend on the duration and severity of the disease, but the findings may not always correspond with the severity of the clinical signs. The radiographic findings in dogs with dirofilariasis have been described repeatedly and were summarized by W. F. Jackson (1969a). The cardiac and pulmonary changes have been demonstrated in detail, using angiocardiographic techniques (Tashjian et al., 1970).

Little diagnostic information is obtained from radiographs of asymptomatic dogs harboring only a small to moderate number of heartworms, or from those of young dogs even when a large number of worms are present. Dogs with acute vena caval occlusion may also have few changes in the heart and lungs because the rapid development of the disease has left no time for compensatory cardiac and pulmonary changes. However, in some cases the caudal vena cava appears enlarged.

The most serious radiographic changes are seen in adult dogs with large numbers of worms in the pulmonary arteries causing severe vascular thickening (Figs. 16-3 and 16-4). The radiographic signs of cor pulmonale and the secondary changes of the pulmonary arteries are the most severe in dogs with chronic heartworm disease and migration of large numbers of worms into the pulmonary vascular bed (W. F. Jackson, 1969a).

When pulmonary signs are severe, they are pathognomonic for dirofilariasis, even in those cases in which blood tests for microfilariae are negative. There are increased, sometimes patchy densities disseminated over the lung field which could be mistaken for pulmonary infiltrates or even disseminated tumor masses. However, when analyzed closely the densities can be differentiated into those of vascular origin and those due to pulmonary embolism. The pulmonary arteries in the hilar and middle zones of the lungs are three to four times their normal diameter and appear as bandlike structures adjacent to the lucent bronchi. When the surrounding parenchyma is infiltrated, the arterial borders appear hazy, incorrectly suggesting that the densities are infiltrates rather than arterial structures. As pulmonary pressures increase, the pulmonary arteries frequently become distorted and are sometimes displaced. Abrupt ending or "pruning" of the arteries is a characteristic finding in dirofilariasis (Figs. 16-3 and 16-4). If the veins and arteries are carefully distinguished according to location and origin (see page 62), it will be noticed that the diameter of the veins remains essentially normal in this disease, whereas on the dorsoventral radiograph the diameter of the pulmonary arteries is more than 60 per cent of the diameter of a rib, the normal limit recognized by W. F. Jackson (1969a).

The abrupt ending of some arteries as they reach the peripheral zone of the lung represents arterial occlusion by worm embolization; this is sometimes followed by incomplete infarction and later by scarring of the affected portions of the lung lobes. Complete infarction is rare in the dog. Pulmonary emboli result in round, irregular, semi-dense infiltrates with hazy borders. According to W. F. Jackson (1969a), regression of these densities can be followed over subsequent radiographs. Local areas of atelectasis, which appear as ill-defined opacities that are less dense than areas of infarction, are seen with arterial obstruction (Tashjian et al., 1970). Pulmonary fibrosis appears as nodular or linear interstitial densities (Fig. 16-3).

On the lateral radiograph, right ventricular enlargement is slight to moderate and is seldom as severe as that seen with secondary right heart failure in valvular diseases. The enlarged conus arteriosus and the dilation of the pulmonary artery displace the right cardiac border cranially and make the cranial waist disappear. The craniocaudal diameter of the cardiac silhouette is increased, but the apicobasilar distance does not increase as much as it does in left heart failure. Although the trachea may be elevated slightly, the ventral bend of the distal trachea is usually preserved; it may even be accentuated when there is right atrial enlargement. The left atrium and ventricle are usually unremarkable. When right heart failure ensues, the caudal vena cava and the precordial mediastinum appear dense and enlarged.

On the dorsoventral radiograph (Fig. 16-4), the right cardiac border is rounder and bulges farther toward the right thoracic wall than normal. The shape of the heart in dirofilariasis has been referred to as a mirror image of a capital "D" (W. F. Jackson, 1969a). The pulmonary artery segment may be markedly enlarged (Fig. 16-4), appearing as a semicircular protrusion at approximately 1 to 2 o'clock on the cardiac silhouette. The apex frequently shifts toward the left thoracic wall because of right ventricular hypertrophy; this must not be falsely diagnosed as left ventricular enlargement.

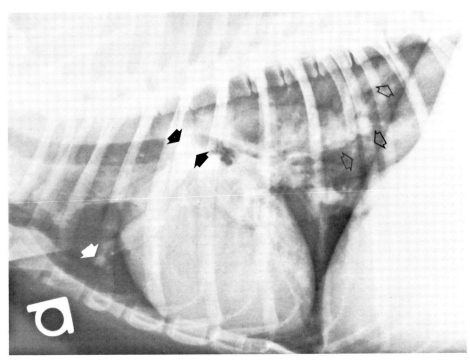

FIGURE 16-3 Left lateral radiograph, 6 year old female dog of mixed breed with severe pulmonary vascular changes due to heartworm disease. The dog was examined because of listlessness, inappetence, and weight loss for two weeks. Polydipsia and weakness had appeared in the last few days. At the time of clinical examination the dog was afebrile, and respiration seemed normal. Hematuria was found on urinalysis. On the radiograph, the right cardiac border is rounder than normal; it runs more parallel to and is in closer contact with the sternum than normal. The dorsal portion of the cranial border extends far cranially, and the cranial waist is accentuated. The area of the left atrium is unremarkable, and the ventral bend at the distal extremity of the trachea is therefore preserved. The left heart is unremarkable. The caudal vena cava is denser and wider than normal. Several band-like densities are seen in the lung field. In the apical lobar area these densities can be identified as a greatly distended left apical lobar artery (black arrows) and a distended, peripherally pruned right apical lobar artery (white arrow). In the diaphragmatic lung field the greatly distended right and left pulmonary arteries are difficult to distinguish from each other and from their markedly dilated and distorted branches. Several less dense, rounded opacities with indistinct borders are seen peripherally in the diaphragmatic lung field (clear arrows). They represent infarcts or atelectatic areas due to embolization. Other than these densities the lung field is clear, and the veins are unaffected. The radiographic findings were confirmed when a thoracotomy was done. A large number of adult heartworms was removed from the main pulmonary artery and its branches. It is notable that microfilariae were not detected in the peripheral blood (wet film examination and modified Knott concentration method).

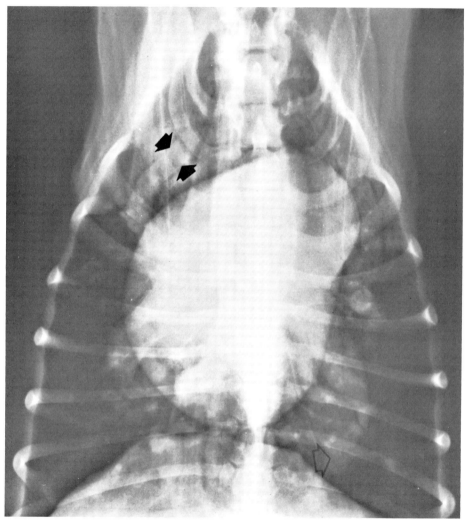

FIGURE 16-4   Dorsoventral radiograph, dog in Figure 16-3. The right ventricular enlargement seen in the lateral radiograph is also seen in this view. In addition, there is extreme distention of the pulmonary artery segment between 12 and 3 o'clock due to an accumulation of adult heartworms in the conus arteriosus and the main pulmonary artery. The right apical lobar artery is distended (black arrows). The left diaphragmatic lobar artery tapers abruptly. Medial to this artery a less dense opacity (clear arrow) is seen, representing an infarct or an atelectatic lung area.

LABORATORY FINDINGS

The two major difficulties encountered when examining blood for micro-filariae are the periodicity of *D. immitis* in the blood stream and the differentiation of *D. immitis* from the nonpathogenic *D. reconditum*. Otto (1969) reported that there may be up to 50 times more microfilariae of *D. immitis* in the bloodstream in the early evening and night than during other hours of the day. He concluded that there is probably a concentration of microfilariae in the spleen. If heartworms are suspected and if microfilariae are not found, it is thus advisable to withdraw and examine blood samples in the late afternoon and evening. In a study of dogs in which adult heartworms are found, R. F. Jackson (1969a) reported that 8 per cent did not have microfilariae when blood concentration tests were performed.

First, to determine if microfilariae are present in the blood, a wet film prep-aration should be examined microscopically under low magnification. Using the wet film preparation, *D. immitis* and *D. reconditum* can be differentiated accord-ing to the motion specific for each type. Microfilariae of *D. immitis* coil and un-coil rapidly but do not have a significant degree of forward movement, whereas microfilariae of *D. reconditum* have a snake-like motion and move in and out of the field rapidly.

The most reliable method for identifying microfilariae in the blood is the modified Knott technique, introduced by Newton and Wright (1956), for the concentration of microfilariae in a blood sample. In this technique, 1 ml. of blood is added to 10 ml. of 2 per cent formalin solution. The solution of blood and formalin is then centrifuged for 5 to 8 minutes at 1000 to 1500 rpm. The super-natant is poured off, and the sediment is mixed with an equal volume of aqueous 1:1000 methylene blue stain. A drop of the stained sediment is then examined microscopically for microfilariae. The microfilariae are differentiated as indicated in Table 16-1. Another method reported by Wylie (1970) that effectively demon-strates microfilariae, utilizes lysis of the blood (in a solution of 5 ml. triton ×100 and 8 Gm. Na_2CO_3 in 1000 ml. water). The lysed solution is forced through a 25 mm. filter pad which is then examined for microfilariae under a microscope after staining with methylene blue.

Other methods utilizing stains for the differentiation of microfilariae have been reported by Rothstein and Brown (1960), who used acridine orange to stain the microfilariae and were then able to use their movement as a distinguishing

TABLE 16-1 MICROSCOPIC CHARACTERISTICS OF *DIROFILARIA IMMITIS* AND *DIPETALONEMA RECONDITUM**

CHARACTERISTICS SPECIFIC FOR MICROFILARIAE	D. IMMITIS	D. RECONDITUM
Number present	Few to many	Few
Size	*Bigger* 6.1 to 7.2 μ by 286 to 340 μ	4.7 to 5.8 μ by 258 to 292 μ
Anterior end	Tapered sides	Parallel sides
Tail end	Straight	Button-hooked

*Revised from Lindsey, J. R.: J.A.V.M.A., 146 (1965): 1106.

factor, and by Sawyer, Rubin, and Jackson (1965), who reported that a fresh blood smear stained with 1:50 1 per cent brilliant cresol blue reveals the cephalic hook on *Dipetalonema sp.*

Bilirubinuria and bilirubinemia may be present in dogs with chronic heartworm disease, and both are regularly associated with the acute vena caval obstruction syndrome. The serum glutamic pyruvic transaminase level is elevated when liver damage and liver necrosis occur. Bromsulphalein dye (BSP) is retained when hepatic circulation is decreased or when there is a decrease in the amount of functional hepatic tissue owing to heartworm disease. Dogs with advanced heartworm disease frequently have elevated blood urea nitrogen and creatinine levels because of altered renal function. Leukocytosis, due to secondary bronchopneumonia and systemic infections, and eosinophilia, indicating an allergic reaction to the adult heartworms, are not uncommon. Significant increases in total serum protein and in the globulin fraction have been reported in dogs with heartworm disease (Snyder, Liu, and Tashjian, 1967). The total protein was 6.18 Gm./100 cc., compared to 5.71 Gm./100 cc. in normal dogs; as determined by electrophoresis, the globulin fraction in dirofilariasis was 4.19 Gm./100 cc., compared to 3.08 Gm./100 cc. in normal dogs; and because of the increase in the *gamma* globulin fraction, the albumin:globulin (A:G) ratio was 0.53, compared to 0.98 in normal dogs. Although they are statistically significant, the blood protein changes are unlikely to assist the clinician, since the reported values overlap with the normal ranges for dogs. Wallace and Hamilton (1962) reported a total blood protein level of 6.0 Gm./100 cc.; the protein contents of thoracic effusate and ascitic fluid measured 2.4 Gm./100 cc. and 3.8 Gm./100 cc., respectively, in dogs with advanced heartworm disease.

The statistical analysis of numerous clinical pathologic tests, as well as serology, in a group of experimentally infected dogs did not reveal significantly different data than did the same studies in noninfected dogs (Tulloch et al., 1970).

CARDIAC CATHETERIZATION

In a study of 34 dogs infected with heartworms but not in congestive heart failure, Yarns and Tashjian (1967) reported a moderate increase in the main pulmonary artery pressure and the right ventricular systolic pressure as compared with control dogs. Wallace and Hamilton (1962) found that the pressures in dogs with heartworm disease varied with the severity of the infection. Those dogs not in failure had considerably lower pressures in the jugular vein, right atrium, right ventricle, main pulmonary artery, and pulmonary wedge positions than did dogs in heart failure due to heartworm disease. A summary of the results of cardiac catheterization pressure studies from two different reports is presented in Table 16-2.

Yarns and Tashjian (1967) noted that the cardiac output and cardiac index did not differ between normal dogs and those with heartworm disease but not in failure. In another study, Wallace (1962) reported an increase in the diastolic heart volume (20 to 60 cc./kg., compared to 15 to 20 cc./kg. in normal dogs). The total blood volume of dogs with heartworm disease was 90 to 125 cc./kg., compared to 75 to 90 cc./kg. in normal dogs. The heart rate was only increased in severe cases in which heart failure had developed. Femoral artery, left ventricular, and aortic pressures were not significantly different between heartworm-infected dogs and normal dogs (Wallace and Hamilton, 1962; Yarns and Tashjian, 1967).

TABLE 16-2   RIGHT HEART PRESSURE IN DOGS WITH HEARTWORM DISEASE

CATHETER POSITION	AVERAGE PRESSURES (mm. Hg)		
	Dogs in Failure	Dogs not in Failure	Normal Dogs*
Right atrium	11.5†	2.5†	3 to 4
Right ventricle	90†	42† 31‡	15 to 40
Main pulmonary artery (systole)	—	28‡	15 to 30
Pulmonary artery wedge	14†	8† 15‡	10

*From Table 5-3, p. 186.
†Wallace, C. R., and Hamilton, W. F., Circ. Res., 11 (1962): 301.
‡Yarns, D. A., and Tashjian, R. J.: Amer. J. Vet. Res., 28 (1967): 1461.

The circulation time from the cephalic vein to the third eyelid or oral mucosa is increased in heartworm disease. W. F. Jackson (1962) reported that when 10 per cent sodium fluorescein is injected into the cephalic vein (1 ml. per 30 lb. of body weight in the normal dog), it reaches the third eyelid or oral mucosa in less than 12 seconds. If fluorescence of the injected dye, as recognized by the Wood's lamp, occurs more than 15 sec. after the injection, an increased circulation time such as occurs in dogs with heartworm disease is indicated. In the experiments of Yarns and Tashjian (1967), the circulation time from the right ventricle to the left ventricle, as determined from angiocardiograms, averaged 3.3 sec. in normal dogs and 4.5 sec. in heartworm-infected dogs.

ANGIOCARDIOGRAPHY

Angiocardiographic findings in heartworm-infected dogs have been reported by Hobson (1959), Hahn (1960), and Tashjian et al. (1970). Liu, Yarns, and Tashjian (1969) published data on postmortem pulmonary angiograms of dogs which have previously been examined by antemortem angiocardiography. Using angiocardiography, detailed visualization of the secondary changes in the right heart and in the pulmonary arteries and their smaller branches is obtained (Fig. 16-5 and 16-6). In addition, the adult heartworms can be recognized as filling defects in the right heart and pulmonary arteries (Tashjian et al., 1970). The characteristic filling defects are fine, linear lucencies 1 to 2 mm. in diameter which are parallel to the long axes of the arterial walls and are sourrounded by contrast material (Hahn, 1960; Tashjian et al., 1970). Hahn (1960) referred to these changes, which he found in all of 14 severely infected dogs, as "streaking . . . or reticulation." The presence of linear lucencies in the pulmonary arteries is diagnostic for the presence of adult heartworms. However, adult worms are not always outlined, especially if only a few worms are present or if there is excessive dilatation of the pulmonary arteries.

When making the diagnosis of heartworm disease, the indirect signs such as the vascular changes referred to below are more consistently reliable than is visualization of the worms. On the basis of angiocardiographic findings, however, the severity of the vascular changes can be estimated. As the vascular changes progress, there is increasing dilatation of the pulmonary arteries in the hilar and

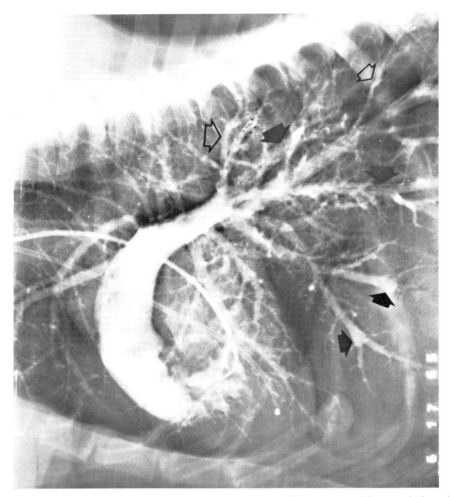

FIGURE 16-5 Right lateral selective angiocardiogram, middle-aged female Great Dane with moderately severe heartworm infection. The changes in the peripheral pulmonary arteries are visualized by injection of contrast medium into the right ventricle. The distention of the arteries is not as obvious as it was in the dog in Figures 16-3 and 16-4. Filling defects caused by adult heartworms lodging in the diaphragmatic lobar arteries are recognized as fine linear lucencies (white arrows) 1 to 1.5 mm. in diameter which are parallel with the long axis of the arterial walls. Some of the smaller arterial branches are distorted. Dilatation and pruning of the peripheral arteries due to vascular occlusion caused by emboli or by fibrocellular intimal proliferation are also seen (black arrows). (Courtesy of Drs. S.–K. Liu and D. A. Yarns, The Animal Medical Center, New York, N. Y.)

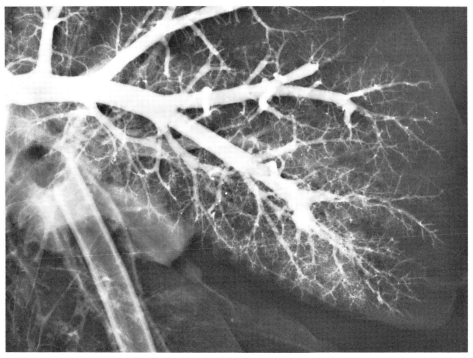

FIGURE 16-6 Detail from a postmortem pulmonary arteriogram, dog in Figure 16-5. The details of the changes in the smaller arterial branches, which are difficult to recognize in a routine antemortem angiocardiogram, are best outlined by this type of study. The abrupt pruning or truncation of the pulmonary arteries as they reach the peripheral zone of the lungs is obvious. The smaller branches are irregular in diameter and sometimes distorted and/or pruned. (Courtesy of Drs. S.–K. Liu and D. A. Yarns, The Animal Medical Center, New York, N. Y.)

middle zones of the lungs, accompanied by distortion of these arteries. Slight alterations in the pattern of arterial arborization develop in mild cases and progress to truncation and loss of normal tapering and arborization of the pulmonary arteries in more severe cases (Fig. 16-6).

Pruning or loss of the normal tapering of the arteries is a result of vascular occlusion, either by embolism of the worms or fibrocellular intimal proliferation, or villous projections (Liu, Yarns, and Tashjian, 1969). Arterial changes are usually most marked in the diaphragmatic lobes. The margins of the peripheral vessels become serrated or scalloped, presumably because of intimal proliferation. Opacification of the pulmonary vasculature is prolonged in severely infected dogs, and pooling of contrast medium in the greatly dilated arteries has been seen by us in a heartworm-infected dog in heart failure. In severe cases, the bronchial arteries enlarge to provide the necessary blood supply to the lung parenchyma distal to sites of obstruction of the pulmonary arteries (Liu, 1969).

Early in the disease, the changes in the right heart are unremarkable. In moderate to severe cases, dilatation and hypertrophy of the right ventricle are seen, and the main pulmonary artery dilates, forming the cranial border of the cardiac silhouette. If tricuspid insufficiency occurs, there is marked regurgitation of contrast medium into the enlarged right atrium and the caudal vena cava, and radiographic signs of right heart failure may be seen. Dilatation of the right coronary artery as a result of the right ventricular hypertrophy has also been described (Tashjian et al., 1970).

DIFFERENTIAL DIAGNOSIS OF HEARTWORM DISEASE

Thoracic radiographs are essential for the evaluation of secondary changes in the heart and lungs in dirofilariasis. These changes must be clearly differentiated from similar changes produced by other heart diseases. The major radiographic differential diagnostic features of heartworm disease are presented in Table 16-3.

TABLE 16-3 RADIOGRAPHIC FEATURES UTILIZED IN THE DIFFERENTIAL DIAGNOSIS OF HEARTWORM DISEASE

CONDITION	HEART	LUNG FIELD
Congestive right and left heart failure due to mitral insufficiency	Obvious left atrial enlargement; loss of distal bend of trachea; loss of caudal waist; right and left ventricular enlargement; usually no protrusion of pulmonary artery segment	Arteries not as dilated as in severe heartworm disease; coalescing, patchy densities due to pulmonary edema (see p. 90); air bronchograms and air alveolograms located primarily around hilus
Pulmonic stenosis	Cardiac silhouette the same as in heartworm disease; often very prominent poststenotic dilatation of main pulmonary artery	Field remains clear; pulmonary arteries immediately distal to the poststenotic dilatation are normal in size; no signs of pulmonary emboli
Cor pulmonale other than that due to heartworm disease	Cardiac silhouette similar to that in heartworm disease	Arteries denser and often more curved in dorsoventral view than in normal dog, but no significant arterial enlargement; sometimes signs of pulmonary disease such as bronchiectasis or fibrosis are visible
Tumor metastases to the lung	Little or no right heart enlargement; no prominent pulmonary artery segment	Tumors rounded and have distinct or indistinct outlines but never coalesce; masses persist or increase in size in subsequent radiographs; dilated arteries seen end on may mimic tumors; a second radiograph made in a different projection will reveal the true nature of the density

Because heartworm disease is not usually associated with murmurs, it can be differentiated from most other heart diseases by their typical murmurs. In addition, the radiographic and electrocardiographic findings are markedly different from those findings associated with heartworm disease.

Lethargy, weakness, and/or dyspnea resulting from noncardiac conditions such as chronic adrenal cortical hypofunction, chronic anemia, and functional hypoglycemia must occasionally be differentiated from similar signs due to heartworm disease.

THERAPY

When heartworm infection has been diagnosed, either by identification of the microfilariae of *D. immitis* or by cardiac and radiographic examinations, medical therapy or surgical removal of the parasites is recommended. Chemotherapy and surgery are occasionally used together. Chemotherapy may be inadvisable only in older patients in which laboratory data indicate concurrent organ dysfunction, thereby increasing the danger of medical therapy.

The subject of chemotherapy versus surgical therapy has been controversial for many years. Over the past 10 years, therapeutic agents have become available which can be used without exceeding a 1 to 5 per cent mortality rate. Practical surgical procedures for the removal of heartworms have been developed. However, since surgical mortality is often as high as 30 to 40 per cent, surgery is recommended only for the treatment of poor risk cases in which chemotherapy is inadvisable.

Surgical therapy for adult heartworms. W. F. Jackson (1969b) reviewed the three basic surgical methods for removal of heartworms:

1. Arteriotomy of the right and left pulmonary arteries affords poor access to the worms in the right ventricle, right atrium, and venae cavae (Weipers and Lawson, 1965)

2. Right ventriculotomy (Essex, 1950; Rubin and Brooks, 1964) below the pulmonary artery through an opening kept tight by a purse-string suture is unsatisfactory in that worms in the right atrium, venae cavae, and terminal left pulmonary artery cannot be removed (Kurokawa et al., 1954; Jackson, Knowles, and Wallace, 1962).

3. Pulmonary arteriotomy after temporary occlusion of the venae cavae is the most reliable technique, but it is difficult to probe the right atrium and the venae cavae from this incision (Johnson, 1951; Roenigk, 1958; Pollard, Ashby, and Derrick, 1959; Wilcox, 1960; Abadie et al. 1970).

W. F. Jackson (1969b) concluded that surgery is rarely recommended and cannot be endorsed generally for the treatment of heartworm disease.

Chemotherapy for adult worms.   Medical therapy to kill the adult heartworms is recommended in almost every case – in asymptomatic dogs as well as those with clinical signs. Prior to chemotherapy the dog's condition must be evaluated to determine whether he can withstand adverse reactions that may result from embolization of the parasites as well as toxic reactions due to chemotherapy and/or the breakdown products of the worms. If heart failure, gross hepatic dysfunction, uremia, or signs of severe respiratory disease are present, treatment of adult heartworms should be withheld until these organs are functioning more effectively. Adequate hepatic and renal function is especially important, since storage and excretion of arsenic, the main ingredient of the filaricides, is accomplished by these organs. An exception is the acute vena caval syndrome, in which therapy must be instituted immediately regardless of complicating conditions (Henderson, 1967).

Therapy prior to treatment with filaricides could include alleviation of anemia; rehydration of the patient with isotonic fluids; the use of lipotrophic agents such as methionine, choline, and inositol (Lufa); administration of B complex vitamins to anorectic dogs; and the oral or parenteral administration of vitamin C to prevent hepatotoxic reactions (R. F. Jackson, 1969b). In addition, therapy with digitalis and diuretics is required if heart failure is present, and antibiotics are indicated when respiratory tract infections are present. During and following filaricide therapy, cage rest for one to two weeks, followed by marked restriction of exercise for two more weeks, is recommended to avoid complications resulting from pulmonary embolization of the dead worms.

After successful chemotherapy has destroyed the adult worms, the dog's condition usually returns to normal in six months to one year. However, it should be emphasized that pulmonary, hepatic, and renal complications may persist following massive infection and therapy. Although many dogs are capable of entirely normal activity, some never regain exercise tolerance.

A 1 per cent solution of thiacetarsamide sodium (Caparsolate) is recommended for chemotherapy of adult heartworms. Thiacetarsamide is a trivalent arsenic compound that concentrates in the worm in higher levels than it does in the tissues of the host. Although a number of dosage regimens have been used in the past, the method recommended by the American Veterinary Medical Association's Panel on Heartworms (1969) is 0.1 ml. of 1 per cent solution of thiacetarsamide per pound of body weight administered intravenously twice daily for two days. When the drug is administered in this manner, there is a sudden discharge of microfilariae from the female, followed by slow death of both male and female worms over a period of several weeks.

Pulmonary embarassment with coughing and occasional anaphylactic reactions may occur during therapy. Antibiotics, antihistamines, and corticosteroids have been used to prevent such reactions, although there is no evidence to support or deny the rationale of such therapy. Because thiacetarsamide is a tissue irritant, perivascular injection may result in tissue edema and sloughing, and extreme caution must be exercised to prevent perivenous injection. Proper needle placement before and after infusion of the arsenical may be ascertained by flushing the needle thoroughly with saline or water. The injection site must also be closely observed during intravenous administration. Should perivenous injection occur, the region should be infiltrated immediately with a solution of a vasodilator, such as phentolamine (Regitine), and sterile water, or with water alone. Henderson (1967) noted an adverse host reaction following filaricide therapy one to two weeks after treatment, with signs such as depression, anorexia, cough, and dyspnea.

When severe complications develop during chemotherapy, arsenical injections should be discontinued. Such complications include jaundice, uremia, and persistent vomiting, all of which are signs of arsenic poisoning. Intravenous fluid therapy, preferably with balanced electrolytes, should be instituted until dehydration is overcome, but care must be taken to avoid fluid or sodium overloading. Sudden spiking of the body temperature, another sign indicating complications resulting from chemotherapy, is likely to be related to pulmonary embolism. Temporary incoordination with head tilting and loss of vision may occur as a reaction to arsenic filaricides.

Dogs with the acute vena caval syndrome require intensive and immediate therapy. In addition to thiacetarsamide, these dogs may require peritoneal dialysis, intravenous fluid therapy, and red blood cells if anemia due to hemoglobinuria is present.

Chemotherapy for microfilariae. Treatment instituted to destroy adult heartworms does not eliminate microfilariae present in the blood. Six weeks following the treatment for the adult worms, the circulating microfilariae should be destroyed to prevent their transmission and subsequent progression to adult worms. Veterinary microfilaricides available include dithiazanine iodide (Dizan), diethylcarbamazine (Caricide), fenthion (Talodex), and stibophen (Fuadin). Only dithiazanine iodide and diethylcarbamazine are used commonly to destroy the microfilariae. Fenthion is an organic phosphate recently introduced to the profession, and clinical studies of the drug other than those made by the manufacturer are not yet available.

Dithiazanine iodide is a cyanine dye that is also used for the treatment of intestinal nematodes in the dog. The product does not affect the adult heartworms. It is used initially at a daily oral dose of 2 to 3 mg./lb. body weight for three days. The blood is then reexamined for microfilariae, and if microfilariae are still present the dosage is increased to 5 mg./lb. body weight daily until the blood is free of microfilariae, usually in two to three days. A characteristic malodorous, blue-stained diarrhea develops during the course of therapy. Chapman and Smith (1961) reported that dithiazanine iodide was successful in killing microfilariae when administered in a single dose of 25 mg./lb. They also noted that diarrhea can be prevented if a light meal is fed before the drug is administered.

Diethylcarbamazine, a substituted piperazine, is administered orally as a microfilaricide at 10 to 20 mg./lb. three times daily for three weeks. Fenthion, an injectable organic phosphate, is recommended by the manufacturer as a micro-filaricide, using 7 mg./lb. body weight subcutaneously every two weeks until the microfilariae are no longer present on the blood smear. (Lambert et al., 1970).

Products commonly used for treating parasites in dogs, such as dichlorvos (Task), should not be administered to dogs that harbor adult heartworms, since these products may be responsible for migration of the heartworms from the right ventricle to the pulmonary artery and lungs, resulting in massive pulmonary embolization and sudden death.

When microfilariae are found in puppies (under three to four months old), their presence is probably a result of transplacental transmission. In such cases, treatment for adult heartworms is not necessary, and microfilaricides can be used safely (R. F. Jackson, 1969a).

PREVENTION OF HEARTWORM DISEASE

Various prophylactic regimens have been advocated to prevent heartworm disease in enzootic areas. Thiacetarsamide sodium (Caparsolate) may be given once or twice annually to kill adult worms at the dosage schedule given above; then diethylcarbamazine (Caracide) is administered beginning 1 to 2 months before the mosquito season and continuing throughout the season. One of the recommended prophylactic dosages of diethylcarbamazine is 1.5 mg./lb. given once daily (American Veterinary Medical Association, 1969). In an experiment in which a continuous dosage of diethylcarbamazine was administered (3.1 mg./kg.), Kume, Ohishi, and Kobayashi (1967) found that the number of developing larvae decreased from 33 per cent in control dogs to 0.6 per cent in dogs given the microfilaricide, and at 5.5 mg./kg. daily, larval development was prevented entirely. Tulloch, et al. (1970) found that 5.0 mg./kg. of diethylcarbamazine given daily prevented the development of infective larvae when injected subcutaneously. Warne, Tipton, and Furusho (1969) found that 5.5 mg./kg. of diethylcarbamazine 6 to 7 days per week, from the beginning of the mosquito season until 30 days after the season ended, was an effective method of preventing the development of most microfilariae. Fowler et al. (1970) demonstrated the equal efficacy of diethylcarbamazine (3.3 mg. per kg. per day orally) and fenthion (2.2 to 4.6 mg. per kg. per day or 13.2 mg. per kg. every two weeks subcutaneously) in preventing the development of microfilaria into adult worms.

LIFE CYCLE OF D. IMMITIS

After hatching from ova in the uterus of the adult ovoviviparous female heart-worm, the microfilariae pass into the blood stream of the dog. When the adult heartworm dies (natural or drug-induced), the microfilariae may survive in the blood stream for as long as two to three years. Several mosquito species in the United States, *Culex pipiens, Anopheles freeborni, A. quadrimaculatus, Aedes vexans,* and some of the salt marsh mosquitoes, act as intermediate hosts for *D. immitis* (Otto, 1969). The mosquitoes feed around the muzzle, eyes, and pelvic region of the dog (Otto, 1969). The mosquito bites the host, and by sucking the blood ingests the microfilariae, which then travel to the mosquito's malpighian tubules, develop into first-stage larvae, and molt to the second and third stages. After approximately 2 weeks (Otto, 1969), the third stage microfilariae are ready to be transmitted back to the primary host, the dog, by another mosquito bite. After reintroduction into the dog, the larvae live in subcutaneous, intramuscular, adipose, and subserosal venous tissues. The larvae live subcutaneously for the first 80 days, after which they invade the venous system (Orihel, 1961). Young adult worms may be recovered from the heart in 67 to 80 days after infection (Orihel, 1961). Six to seven months after infection, heartworms are capable of releasing microfilariae into the blood stream. Otto (1969) reported that some adult worms may live and produce microfilariae for as long as five years.

Adult heartworms measure from 1.0 to 2.0 mm. in diameter. The mature adult male worms are from 150 to 180 mm. long, and the females are from 250 to 300 mm. long (Otto and Bauman, 1959). The anterior end of both male and female worms is rounded and has six papillae and a small mouth. The posterior end of the male worm is coiled spirally, with several pairs of caudal papillae; it is straight in the female (Jackson and Wallace, 1966).

Microfilariae and heartworms have also been found in the timber wolf, coyote, red fox, gray fox, dingo, and domestic cat (Otto, 1969). Pulmonary "coin" lesions due to dirofilariasis have been reported as a rare finding in man in the United States (Faust, 1962; Beaver and Orihel, 1965; Beskin, Colvin, and Beaver, 1966).

The intermediate host for *D. reconditum,* a parasite of the subcutaneous tissues, is the flea rather than the mosquito. The microfilariae are injected into the subcutaneous tissue by a flea bite, and the larvae may then be found in the blood stream. *Dipetalonema reconditum* does not produce cardiovascular lesions.

PATHOLOGIC CHANGES IN HEARTWORM DISEASE

The pathologic changes in heartworm disease have been well described. They vary with the severity of the infection, individual susceptibility, and the duration and form of the disease. The severity of the disease is not always related to the number of adult worms found in their preferred sites, the right heart, especially the right ventricular outflow tract, and the pulmonary arteries. Macroscopically, dilatation and hypertrophy of the right ventricle occur. The main pulmonary arteries are dilated and distorted, and their walls are thickened.

Occasionally, adult worms have been found in the bronchioles (Turk, Gaafar, and Lynd, 1956), in the eyes and in an interdigital cyst (Schnelle and Jones, 1945), in the brain (Tajuchi, Takehara, and Uriu, 1959; Patton and Garner, 1970), in the femoral arteries (Horne, 1967), and in the peritoneal cavity (Abbott, 1961;

Tulloch, *et al.*, 1970). Liu, Das, and Tashjian (1966) described a dog in which 166 worms were found in the left and right ventricles, left and right atria, cranial and caudal venae cavae, aorta, pulmonary artery, left and right external and internal iliac arteries, left and right femoral arteries, left and right popliteal arteries, and testicular arteries. Villose intimal proliferation, endarteritis, and granulomatous lesions were seen in the involved arteries.

The following microscopic lesions have been reported in dogs with heart-worm disease: villose endarteritis of the large pulmonary arteries, medial hyperplasia of the smooth musculature of the pulmonary arteries, pulmonary thrombosis, hemorrhagic infarction in the lung, hepatic congestion and degeneration, and fibrosis and hyalinization of Bowman's capsules in the kidneys (Hennigar and Ferguson, 1957; Adcock, 1961; Hirth, Huizinga, and Nielsen, 1966). The pulmonary vascular changes and pulmonary collateral circulation in dirofilariasis have been summarized by Liu, Yarns, and Tashjian (1969), and by Liu et al. (1969). A postmortem pulmonary arteriogram demonstrating dilatation, obstruction, and pruning of the pulmonary lobar arteries and their branches is shown in Figures 16-5 and 16-6 (pp. 432-433).

Cutaneous lesions such as erythema and patchy alopecia, especially on the forelimbs and thorax, have been considered to be due to the larvae of *D. immitis*. However, it has not been proved that these lesions are a direct result of such a parasitic infection (Muller and Kirk, 1969).

Jackson, von Lichtenberg, and Otto (1962), von Lichtenberg, Jackson, and Otto (1962), and R. F. Jackson (1969c) have reviewed the acute vena caval syndrome that develops when adult worms obstruct the caudal vena cava. Worms are usually also present in the right atrium, right ventricle, pulmonary artery, and pulmonary arterioles. The signs of the acute vena caval syndrome in dogs result from concurrent cardiac and hepatic failure caused by nodular necrosis of the liver and biliary stasis. Heartworms not obstructing the vena cava may be found in dogs that do not have the clinical vena caval syndrome. At necropsy, dogs with the acute vena caval syndrome have a larger number of heartworms than do asymptomatic dogs, and they usually have twice the number of heartworms found in dogs with chronic heartworm disease (R. F. Jackson, 1969c). Therefore, it is suggested that heavy, acute infection with maturation of a large number of worms over a relatively short period of time is responsible for the dramatic clinical condition (Sawyer and Weinstein, 1963).

COLLAPSED TRACHEA

The syndrome of collapsed trachea is characterized by dorsoventral flattening of the trachea and is responsible for clinical signs of respiratory distress and a chronic, "honking" cough. Cardiac enlargement and pulmonary emphysema may develop simultaneously. Collapsed trachea is included in this chapter because it produces clinical signs of cor pulmonale. According to O'Brien, Buchanan, and Kelly (1966), the macroscopic changes are accompanied by squamous metaplasia of the tracheal epithelium.

The syndrome is most often recognized in dogs of the toy and miniature breeds, usually but not always between the ages of three and eight years. Reports by Schiller, Helper, and Small (1964) and Zook and Hathaway (1966) indicate that it may occasionally be congenital.

HISTORY AND PHYSICAL EXAMINATION

The dog is presented to the veterinarian because of a chronic, honking cough. The owner often reports that the cough is most severe during the day, especially when the dog is excited or after it drinks water. It may also occur whenever the dog pulls on its leash, thereby bringing the collar tightly against the trachea and stimulating the cough. Severe respiratory distress and cyanosis can develop, making the condition a true emergency which may be temporarily relieved by hospitalizing the dog in a quiet section of the hospital, away from noisy distractions and the anxious owner.

When the history is reviewed, it is often evident that a mild cough has been present for a long time, sometimes since the dog was a puppy. The dog may have been treated previously for cardiac and respiratory diseases or for almost any condition that can affect the head, neck, and thoracic region and be associated with a cough. Although it has been suggested that the condition usually occurs in obese dogs (O'Brien, Buchanan, and Kelly, 1966), the authors have recognized the condition frequently in dogs of normal weight and in thin dogs. Excessive weight, however, aggravates the respiratory difficulties associated with collapsed trachea.

When the dog is examined, it may seem normal, or it may be in various degrees of respiratory distress which are occasionally severe enough to produce cyanosis. In the latter instance a complete physical examination is difficult to perform and may aggravate the dog's anxiety and respiratory difficulty. Abdominal breathing occurs with severe respiratory distress and cyanosis, and hypoxia may result in syncope. If the dog is not in respiratory distress, palpation of the trachea can be performed safely. Palpation cranial to the thoracic inlet suggests dorso-ventral flattening of the trachea, and the edges of the cartilaginous rings are palpable. Such palpation of the trachea usually elicits the honking cough pathognomonic for collapsed trachea.

On auscultation of the thorax, dry, coarse, rattling râles (rhonchi) are heard which may be described in some cases as sonorous or of low frequency. The râles are heard throughout respiration and often obscure the heart sounds. If the dog is calm enough so that the heart sounds can be auscultated, murmurs are usually absent; however, because chronic mitral valvular fibrosis may also be present, a systolic murmur may be heard. Accentuation of the pulmonic component of the second heart sound may give the heart sounds a snapping quality.

Electrocardiography is not diagnostic for collapsed trachea, although P pulmonale and a rapid heart rate are common. Right axis deviation suggesting right ventricular hypertrophy has not occurred in cases seen by the authors.

RADIOGRAPHIC EXAMINATION

The radiographic signs and difficulties encountered in diagnosing collapsed trachea have been described by O'Brien, Buchanan, and Kelly (1966). Since radiography can yield both false positive and false negative results, accurate positioning of the dog is important. O'Brien, Buchanan, and Kelly (1966) advise taking radiographs with the dog's head extended and the neck slightly bent dorsally. Artifacts are common when the head is bent ventrally during the exposure.

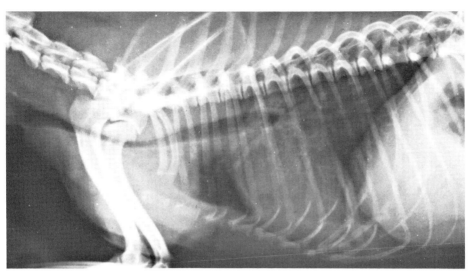

FIGURE 16-7 Left lateral radiograph, 8 year old, male Yorkshire Terrier examined because of a honking cough and expiratory wheezing. Collapse of the trachea was palpable at the thoracic inlet. There is fusiform narrowing of the distal portion of the cervical trachea. The caudal intrathoracic portion of the trachea is of normal width and runs parallel with the spine. The cardiac silhouette is normal in size. The caudal waist is flattened. The caudal vena cava appears slightly wider than normal, and the liver is enlarged. The lung field is denser than normal, and the vascular markings are blurred.

In typical cases (Figs. 16-7 to 16-9), a gradual dorsoventral narrowing of the tracheal lumen beginning at about the midcervical region is seen in the lateral radiograph. As a result, the tracheal lumen is nearly occluded at the thoracic inlet and becomes wider again in the thoracic cavity. The outlines of the tracheal border are often serrated or scalloped, at times appearing hazy. Widening of the trachea is seen in dorsoventral radiographs exposed with adequate penetration. Collapse of the intrathoracic portion of the trachea is not as common as collapse at the thoracic inlet. A collapse in the lateral direction has been seen in one dog after central chondrotomy, and in another it occurred spontaneously.

Because of the elasticity of the membranous portion and the tracheal cartilages, the lumen of the trachea varies in diameter during respiration. The diameters of the cervical and intrathoracic tracheal segments respond to respiration in opposite ways. During inspiration, the cervical trachea tends to become narrower, and the thoracic trachea widens because of the decreased pressure in the thoracic cavity, especially when the resistance in the upper respiratory passages is increased. During expiration, the cervical segment dilates and the intrathoracic segment narrows. This is accentuated if expiratory resistance is increased by holding the muzzle and the nares closed. When the muscle and fibroelastic transverse membrane are elongated, the cartilages flare and offer no resistance to ventrodorsal deformity. The luminal changes at inspiration and expiration become accentuated and are noticed as variable width of the tracheal lumen on the radiograph.

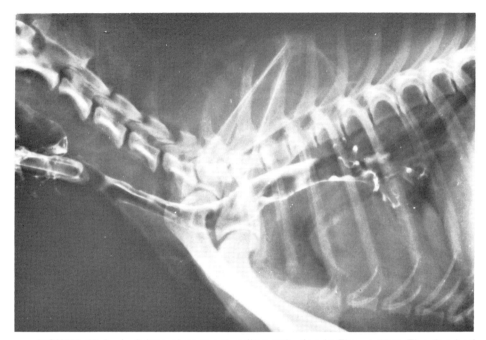

FIGURE 16-8 Left lateral contrast radiograph, dog in Figure 16-7. The dog had been anesthetized and intubated. A thin rubber catheter was passed through the tracheal catheter, and 1 ml. of oily Dionosil was injected into the distal cervical trachea. The dog was then rotated and tilted first head down and then head up to allow the oily contrast medium to disperse evenly. Immediately afterward, radiographs were exposed at the beginning of inspiration. The endotracheal tube is visible at the larynx. The contrast medium outlines the fusiform narrowing beginning at the fourth cervical vertebra and extending distally to about the seventh cervical vertebra. The intrathoracic portion of the trachea is of normal width before it bifurcates into the lobar branches.

The radiographic diagnosis of tracheal collapse is delicate, and one must not be surprised if repeated radiographs reveal a varying degree of narrowing of the tracheal lumen. Falsely positive and falsely negative results are common. Tracheal collapse is falsely suggested when soft tissue shadows or the esophagus is directly superimposed on the lucent tracheal lumen. Such false indications of a collapsed trachea occur often, especially in obese dogs. Furthermore, the reader should be aware of the fact that the trachea of many older dogs tends to become dorsoventrally deformed, even in clinically normal dogs.

Falsely positive radiographs also result from lateral displacement and rotation of the trachea. In such cases, the trachea lies ventral and to the right of the esophagus, with the fibroelastic membrane adjacent to the esophagus. On both lateral and dorsoventral radiographs, this gives the impression that the trachea is narrowed, as shown in Figures 16-10 and 16-11.

Falsely negative results have been observed when the trachea was only moderately narrowed at the thoracic inlet, and the collapse was found at necropsy to be at the carina. In other cases, false negative findings were the result of edema and inflammatory swelling of the tracheal mucosa, as well as of the presence of viscous mucous material within the trachea which obscured the tracheal lumen.

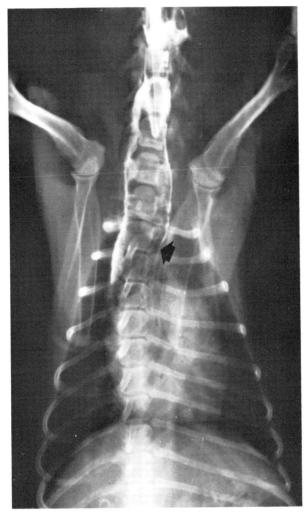

FIGURE 16-9 Ventrodorsal contrast radiograph, dog in Figures 16-7 and 16-8. The exposure was made following the lateral radiograph in Figure 16-8 to demonstrate the transverse widening of the trachea. This widening is associated with the dorsoventral collapse due to lengthening of the fibroelastic dorsal membrane, which is often difficult to see on the plain radiograph. The widening begins at the fourth cervical vertebra and extends for a short distance into the thorax. The lumen then narrows slightly (arrow). Notice that in older dogs of the small breeds the trachea almost always appears wider in the dorsoventral than in the lateral view.

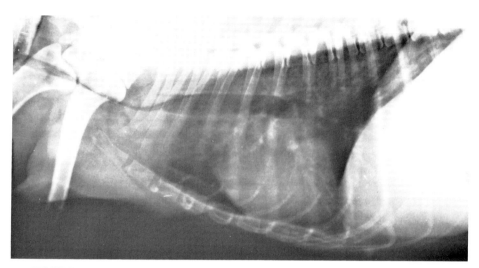

FIGURE 16-10   Lateral radiograph, 14½-year-old female dog of mixed breed which developed a deep cough within three weeks after orthopedic surgery had been performed. The air-filled structure of the trachea seems to be drastically narrowed from the distal cervical area to immediately caudal to the first rib. The remaining intrathoracic trachea is unremarkable. The right heart is slightly larger than normal. The bronchial markings are accentuated and at times appear blurred. The apparent narrowing of the tracheal lumen is aggravated by an overlying soft tissue mass (see Fig. 16-11).

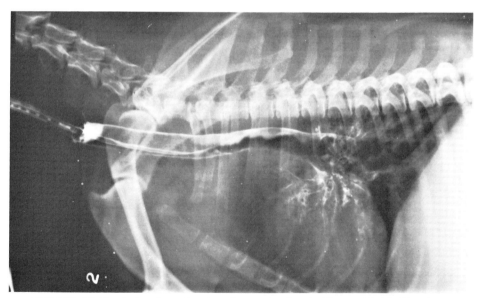

FIGURE 16-11   Lateral contrast radiograph, dog in Figure 16-10. The dog was anesthetized with a short-acting barbiturate and intubated. 2.5 ml. of oily Dionosil was injected into the distal cervical portion of the trachea. The dog was rotated and tilted first head down and then head up so that the contrast medium would disperse evenly. Then the radiograph was exposed during inspiration while the peripheral resistance was slightly increased by partial occlusion of the endotracheal tube. The trachea no longer looks collapsed. A pendulous, double line is visible in the tracheal lumen between the dorsal and ventral outlines. This somewhat puzzling appearance

Legend continues on opposite page.

SPECIAL EXAMINATIONS

When the clinical condition is unresponsive to symptomatic medical therapy, specialized procedures may be necessary to confirm the diagnosis and to assist in the proper selection of future therapy. Bronchoscopy performed under a short-acting anesthetic is helpful in demonstrating dorsoventral narrowing of the trachea and in eliminating other tracheal conditions such as foreign bodies or collapse of the larynx. Bronchoscopy also provides the opportunity to obtain samples of the bronchial secretions for laboratory tests. The lumen of the collapsed trachea appears as a flattened ellipse. The dorsal fibroelastic membrane is stretched and may become pendulous (O'Brien, Buchanan, and Kelly, 1966). A thick, purulent or mucoid material present throughout the entire trachea is often apparent during the bronchoscopic examination. The bronchi appear normal distal to the bifurcation or carina. Dorsoventral flattening of the trachea not palpable during the clinical examination may be recognized while the dog is under anesthesia, but even then, in obese dogs with a short, fat neck, the trachea is often not distinctly palpable.

In order to obtain a specimen of the tracheal exudate for analysis, a sterile swab secured within a polyethylene tube is passed through the bronchoscope immediately after a small amount of sterile fluid is injected through the bronchoscope. The swab is then extended beyond the outer polyethylene sheath, rotated to secure an adequate sample of tracheal exudate, and then withdrawn into the outer sheath of the tube. The swab is then removed and submitted for bacteriologic examination and culture.

Contrast studies such as esophagrams and tracheograms have been used to clarify the diagnosis in doubtful cases. O'Brien, Buchanan, and Kelly (1966) reported that soft tissue superimpositions mimicking tracheal collapse in two dogs could be distinguished by an esophageal contrast study and tracheal intubation.

We have injected contrast medium directly into the trachea by inserting an 18-gauge needle between the third and fourth tracheal rings (Figs. 16-8 and 16-11). The dogs were lightly sedated, and, with the heads bent dorsally, 1 to 2 ml. of 2 per cent lidocaine was injected to obtain local anesthesia of the tracheal mucosa and to prevent coughing. After several minutes, 1 to 1.5 ml. of propyliodone (Dionosil Oily) was injected slowly into the tracheal lumen, and the dogs were then rotated around their long axes to obtain even dispersion of the contrast

---

can be explained by a slight rotation of the trachea around its long axis and around the soft tissue shadow of the esophagus, which is located to the left and slightly dorsal to the trachea and depresses the left tracheal border. The most dorsal outline represents the right border of the trachea. The bottom outline represents the ventral border of the trachea. The double outline extending into the trachea represents both the left tracheal border being depressed by the overlying esophagus and the outline of the elongated, somewhat pendulous dorsal membrane of the trachea. In the ventrodorsal view (not shown), the trachea was displaced to the right side but was not widened. In another radiograph (not shown) made with elevated tracheal pressure, there was no ballooning of the dorsal tracheal membrane at the thoracic inlet. The oblique position of the trachea and the overlying esophagus can make tracheal collapse appear more serious than it really is.

medium. Radiographs in the lateral, dorsoventral, and oblique projections were made immediately because the contrast medium was rapidly expectorated.

Tracheal insufflation of tantalum dust, a contrast agent for bronchography, provides a satisfactory method for visualizing the mucosal surface of the trachea on radiographs.

DIFFERENTIAL DIAGNOSIS

Respiratory signs similar to those of collapsed trachea have been reported by Leonard (1956, 1957, 1960) in dogs with collapse of the larynx, eversion of the lateral ventricles of the larynx, stenotic nares, and elongation of the soft palate. These conditions are usually differentiated during the physical examination, during examination under anesthesia, and by radiographs of the trachea.

Chronic mitral and tricuspid valvular disease, with its typical history, clinical signs, and holosystolic murmur, can be confused with and may often coexist with the syndrome of collapsed trachea.

The differentiation of chronic bronchitis or tracheitis from collapsed trachea is difficult, mainly because a dog with a chronic cough due to collapsed trachea also develops an inflammation of the mucous linings of the bronchi and trachea. When the condition has been of short duration or if the dog has recently been kenneled, a presumptive diagnosis of tracheobronchitis is warranted. If the cough persists after prolonged antitussive therapy, further evaluation may be required to make the differential diagnosis. The loud honking cough is usually very suggestive of a collapsed trachea.

THERAPY

For most dogs with collapsed trachea, bronchodilating preparations, alone or in combination with other bronchodilators, expectorants, and sedatives, usually relieve the acute clinical signs (see Table 13-3, p. 359). For more excitable dogs or those that do not respond to this treatment, other bronchodilator-sedative combinations (such as Elixir of Isuprel and Quadrinal) may prove effective. Corticosteroid therapy may provide temporary relief but should not be continued indefinitely. Antitussive preparations such as dihydrocodeinone (Hycodan) and other narcotics may be required to control the cough. However, they often result in generalized depression and may not relieve coughing except in hypnotic doses.

The use of steam vaporizers is especially helpful in some dogs in which viscid tracheal secretions collect within the tracheal lumen. In some dogs, isoproterenol (Isuprel) nebulizers are effective when two to three short bursts are sprayed into the dog's mouth. However, not all dogs will tolerate the use of a nebulizer, and if the dog becomes too excited, this form of therapy is not recommended.

When palliative therapy is no longer successful, or if the diagnosis is uncertain, bronchoscopy should be performed in order to examine the pharynx and larynx as well as to obtain a culture of the tracheal secretion. After bacteriologic analysis, proper antibiotic therapy should be instituted in addition to the use of bronchodilators and expectorants. Long-term antibiotic therapy (14 to 21 days) and the judicious use of corticosteroids to reduce tracheal inflammation may be indicated.

Digitalis and diuretics are indicated when heart failure occurs. In some cases where all other drugs fail to provide relief, dramatic results have occurred after the dog has been digitalized.

To date, surgical therapy has not proved fully effective. In most cases, surgical techniques such as ventral chondrotomy and the use of artificial tubes to support the trachea (Schiller, Helper, and Small, 1964) have not been shown to relieve the collapsed trachea syndrome consistently.

COR PULMONALE DUE TO PRIMARY LUNG DISEASE

HISTORY AND PHYSICAL EXAMINATION

The history is likely to include signs related to chronic respiratory disease, such as labored and difficult breathing, rapid breathing, wheezing, or a chronic cough. These signs are most often recognized in dogs past middle age and are usually accentuated in obese dogs. It is noteworthy that only a very small number of pulmonary parenchymal diseases result in cor pulmonale in dogs.

When inadequate total ventilation or alveolar hypoventilation results from chronic respiratory disease, the thorax becomes barrel-shaped as the rib cage expands to increase total pulmonary volume. As the pulmonary elasticity is decreased, diminished thoracic movement furthers inadequate gaseous exchange. The dog then begins to utilize the abdominal muscles, resulting in abdominal pumping to provide further assistance in moving air into and out of the lungs. The forelimbs may also be held in abduction to increase the size of the thoracic cavity, and the head and neck are extended to further improve ventilation. During periods of acute respiratory distress, hypoxemia, which causes pulmonary vasoconstriction and acidosis, may result in cyanosis and syncope.

Auscultation of the heart and lungs is an important part of the examination of the dog with cor pulmonale. Inspiratory and expiratory lung sounds should be auscultated, and then, with respiratory sounds eliminated as completely as possible, the heart sounds are evaluated. The lung sounds usually suggest the presence of inspiratory or expiratory râles. The abnormal respiratory sounds or râles vary with the amount of fluid secretion present in the alveoli, bronchioles, bronchi, and trachea. Obstructive bronchial disease may be responsible for sibilant or whistling râles, whereas alveolar disease or destruction may be suggested by crackling râles at the end of inspiration. A low-frequency expiratory sound referred to as an "expiratory grunt" may result when dogs with emphysema attempt to force air out of the lungs. An increased inspiratory effort with sibilant râles may be recognized in advanced stages of generalized pulmonary fibrosis.

The heart sounds are normal as long as the pulmonary arterial pressure remains normal or only slightly elevated. If moderate pulmonary hypertension develops, the intensity of the pulmonic component of the second heart sound is increased, resulting in a heart sound that is described as snapping in quality. As pulmonary hypertension becomes more severe, outflow of blood from the right ventricle is delayed; closure of the pulmonic valve may then be delayed momentarily, and splitting of the second heart sound develops (see Chapter 2).

ELECTROCARDIOGRAPHY

Little or no specific information relative to cor pulmonale is obtained from the electrocardiogram. However, P pulmonale, best recognized in leads II, III, and aVF, and an atrial repolarization (T_a) wave may develop. Very rarely, the degree of pulmonary hypertension becomes severe, and right axis deviation may occur as right ventricular hypertrophy develops. Arrhythmias are unusual with cor pulmonale.

RADIOGRAPHIC EXAMINATION

The radiographic diagnosis of cor pulmonale secondary to primary lung disease is often based on the exclusion of other conditions capable of producing similar signs (see Table 16-4).

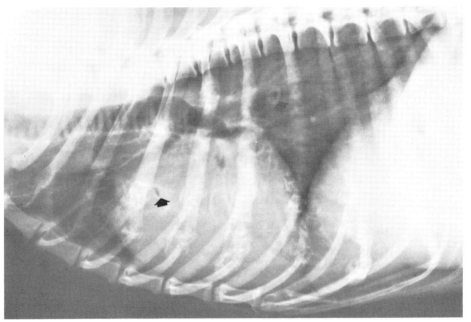

FIGURE 16-12 Lateral radiograph, 12 year old male Dachshund with chronic cough due to bronchitis and secondary heart disease referred to as cor pulmonale. Murmurs were auscultated over both the tricuspid and mitral valve areas. Dry râles could occasionally be heard over the lung field. P mitrale and P pulmonale, a tall, wide QRS complex, and deep T waves were seen on the electrocardiogram. Right and left ventricular hypertrophy was diagnosed. On the radiograph, the right cardiac border is in close contact with the sternum and then extends cranially into the third intercostal space. The craniocaudal diameter of the heart is increased; however, the portion representing the right ventricle markedly surpasses that representing the left ventricle. The trachea, with marked calcification of its rings, runs parallel with the spine except for its caudal extremity, which has the normal ventral bend, indicating that left atrial enlargement is not significant. The left ventricle is of nearly normal size. There is an increased linear density of the lung field due to thickening and calcification of the bronchial walls. In some areas saccular widenings (arrow) are present, suggesting bronchiectasis; at this time these structures are not filled with exudates and therefore appear lucent. The calcification of the tracheal rings and the bronchial walls is not pathologic *per se*; it is seen frequently in old dogs of the so-called chondrodystrophoid breeds such as Dachshunds and Beagles. The vascular markings are small and are not well visualized.

On the lateral radiograph, right ventricular enlargement is seen without significant left atrial or left ventricular enlargement (Fig. 16-12).

On the dorsoventral radiograph (Fig. 16-13), a small notch may be seen at the point where the enlarged right ventricle joins the interventricular septum. The left ventricle is normal in size, but shifting of the apex may mimic left ventricular enlargement. The pulmonary artery segment may also be slightly enlarged.

Positive radiographic signs in the lung field are essential if a diagnosis of cor pulmonale is to be considered. In severe pulmonary fibrosis, well delineated,

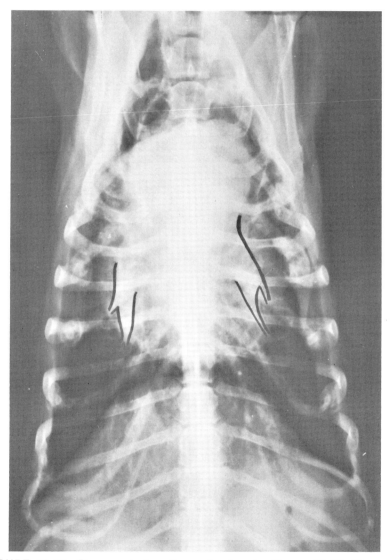

FIGURE 16-13 Dorsoventral radiograph, dog in Figure 16-12. The rounded right and left ventricular borders indicate mild, generalized cardiac enlargement. The apex appears wider than normal. The enlargement of the left ventricle as it appears on this radiograph may have been accentuated by a shift of the apex to the left side. The pulmonary artery segment is dense but does not extend beyond the left cardiac border. The linear markings in the lung field are not as prominent as in the lateral radiograph. Black lines have been used to indicate the rapid thinning of the pulmonary arteries.

linear densities, small nodules, or an irregular, honeycombed pattern prevails. However, in older dogs, mild signs of fibrosis are normal, and thickening of the bronchial walls or dilatation of the lumina producing bronchiectasis is seen occasionally. Groups of emphysematous alveoli, sometimes interspersed with fibrotic areas so that the lung field is hyperlucent, is another radiographic feature occasionally seen in cor pulmonale. Chronic inflammatory changes are recognized as ill-defined interstitial densities which are less dense than alveolar infiltrates; these densities remain unchanged over long periods of time and do not coalesce.

In pulmonary hypertension, the arteries in the central lung field appear denser than normal but are not dilated significantly. Their outlines are not as discrete as in the normal lung, and in the dorsoventral radiograph an accentuated curving of the cranial direction may be noticed. The branching of the pulmonary arteries is normal, but the arteries taper more rapidly in the periphery, and knot-like thickenings are occasionally seen at their bifurcations (see pp. 86-88).

DIFFERENTIAL DIAGNOSIS

Noncardiac conditions producing signs similar to those recognized with cor pulmonale include heat stroke, hyperexcitable or neurogenic dyspnea, and bronchial asthma. In addition, pulmonary disease secondary to cardiac disease also requires differentiation.

1. Heat prostration may cause severe respiratory embarassment. It is often recognized when hot weather is associated with the acute onset of signs, although it may also occur at other times. A rectal temperature greater than 106° F. and the typical appearance of a dog in severe respiratory distress, presented with tachypnea and a dripping, wet tongue extending far out of the open mouth, suggest heat prostration. Since similar physical findings develop acutely in eclampsia, such a possibility must be excluded.

2. Hyperexcitable or neurogenic dyspnea may develop with signs of tachypnea after only brief excitement. Dyspnea of this nature may be difficult to differentiate from primary pulmonary disease; however, it usually does not respond to parenteral bronchodilators unless such therapy is accompanied by sedation. Inherently excitable dogs with chronic lung disease are prone to frequent episodes of neurogenic dyspnea.

3. Bronchial asthma (also referred to as mucinous degeneration of the bronchial epithelium [Jubb and Kennedy, 1963; Schiefer, 1968]) is thought to be of allergic origin. In the presence of respiratory signs outlined above, the absence of signs suggesting other disease, and the rapid therapeutic response to corticosteroids or bronchodilators, it is likely that an asthmatic condition is present. Since bronchial asthma can lead to bronchiectasis, emphysema and pulmonary arterial hypertension as sequelae to asthma should not be excluded. In asthmatic states, the cause of the allergy should be eliminated if possible.

4. Cardiac dyspnea resulting from mitral insufficiency or heartworm disease must be differentiated from cor pulmonale. Congenital cardiac diseases which stress the right heart (patent ductus arteriosus, ventricular septal defect, atrial septal defect, tetralogy of Fallot) are usually distinguishable by their characteristic murmurs as well as by electrocardiographic and radiographic findings.

Since the clinical features do not always suggest the diagnosis, radiography can provide additional help. In Table 16-4, a number of conditions which produce signs similar to those of cor pulmonale are listed and their radiographic features are presented.

TABLE 16-4 RADIOGRAPHIC DIFFERENTIAL DIAGNOSIS OF COR PULMONALE

CONDITION	RADIOGRAPHIC SIGNS
Acquired diseases	
Dirofilariasis	Right ventricular enlargement, prominent pulmonary artery segment; dilated, distorted, pruned, or truncated pulmonary arteries with abnormal branching; occasional patchy densities due to infarction or atelectasis usually located in diaphragmatic lobes; unremarkable pulmonary veins and left heart
Pneumonia	Little or no cardiac enlargement; typical alveolar infiltrates with air bronchograms, air alveolograms, and confluence of densities (see p. 90), or interstitial infiltrates with hypervascularity of the lung field in the early phases of the disease
Bronchitis and bronchial asthma	Little or no cardiac enlargement; cor pulmonale may develop as disease progresses; lung field may be unremarkable in acute conditions; in subacute conditions, an increase of hazy linear densities of bronchial origin is noticeable; in long-standing cases, cylindrical or saccular widenings of the bronchi can develop (bronchiectasis) with interspersed emphysematous areas in the lung field
Tumors (primary or secondary)	Right ventricular enlargement mild if present; interstitial densities have well-defined or indistinct outlines and do not tend to coalesce; a miliary pattern can occur and linear densities develop with lymphatic metastases of the tumor
Heat prostration	No significant cardiac enlargement; pulmonary congestion and edema may develop
Cardiomyopathy	Varying degrees of cardiac enlargement occur; occasionally signs of pulmonary congestion or edema develop
Mitral valvular insufficiency	Left atrial and left ventricular enlargement are often accompanied by right ventricular enlargement; pulmonary venous congestion or alveolar edema develop progressively, as does dilatation of the pulmonary veins
Congenital heart diseases	
Pulmonic stenosis	Right ventricular enlargement only, with pulmonary artery segment enlargement due to poststenotic dilatation; lung field, pulmonary arteries, and pulmonary veins remain normal
Diseases with right-to-left shunts (patent ductus arteriosus, ventricular septal defect, atrial septal defect)	Left atrial and ventricular enlargement are followed by right ventricular enlargement as pulmonary hypertension develops. Hypervascularized lung field and signs of secondary pulmonary congestion or pulmonary edema (see p. 90) are seen
Tetralogy of Fallot and complicated pulmonic stenosis	Right ventricular enlargement occurs to varying degrees; lucent, hypovascularized lung field (see p. 85) is also present

TREATMENT

Obesity and poor physical condition are not beneficial to any dog, least of all one with chronic lung disease. It is important to stress the need to reduce excessive weight and to help improve body condition by frequent light exercise. The control of bronchopulmonary infection with antibiotics is essential, and long-term antibiotic therapy may be indicated for dogs with chronic pulmonary infections.

Bronchodilating agents such as those listed in Table 13-3 (p. 359) often provide symptomatic relief from the signs of chronic respiratory disease. To control the signs of pulmonary dysfunction, products such as Elixir of Isuprel, Quadrinal, or other bronchodilating agents combined with an expectorant and a sedative are indicated if heart failure is absent. Antihistamines may relieve chronic respiratory signs caused by fluid accumulation in the posterior nasopharynx. If the expectorants in the oral medications are not effective, good results may be achieved with vaporized water. Wetting agents (such as Alevaire, Tergemist, or Mucomyst) may be added to the water if it is to be nebulized, but their advantages have not been clearly demonstrated, and nebulization is not well accepted by most dogs.

Corticosteroids are useful for treating bronchospasm or improving alveolar capillary diffusion (Neal, Nair, and Hecht, 1968). Although suppression of the cough with narcotic antitussives is desirable to prevent further weakening and destruction of the alveolar and bronchial structures, respiratory depression must be avoided. Cough suppression should not be so intense that it impairs the elimination of bronchial secretions. Nevertheless, suppression of excessive nonproductive coughing is a primary objective of treatment for cor pulmonale.

Oxygen therapy is necessary for severely dyspneic, hypoxemic, and cyanotic dogs. Carbon dioxide narcosis resulting in failure to stimulate the respiratory centers of the central nervous system is avoided by the utilization of continuous low-flow rates of oxygen rather than a complete oxygen atmosphere.

If congestive heart failure develops, specific cardiac therapy is indicated. However, one should recognize the limitations of the cardiac glycosides if the primary etiology of the pulmonary dysfunction cannot be treated.

References

Abadie, S. H., Black, E., Dupuy, H. J., and Gonzalez, R.: A Procedure for the Surgical Removal of *Dirofilaria immitis.* J.A.V.M.A., 156 (1970): 884.

Abbott, P. K.: *Dirofilaria immitis* in the Peritoneal Cavity. Aust. Vet. J., 37 (1961): 467.

Adcock, J. L.: Pulmonary Arterial Lesions in Canine Dirofilariasis. Amer. J. Vet. Res., 22 (1961): 655.

American Veterinary Medical Association: Recommendations of the Symposium Panel: Treatment and Prevention of Heartworm Disease in Dogs. J.A.V.M.A., 154 (1969): 397.

Augustine, D. L.: Observations on the Occurrence of Heartworms, *Dirofilaria immitis,* in New England Dogs. Amer. J. Hyg., 28 (1938): 390.

Beaver, P. C., and Orihel, T. C.: Human Infection with Filariae of Animals in the United States. Amer. J. Trop. Med., 14 (1965): 1010.

Beskin, C. A., Colvin, S. H., and Beaver, P. C.: Pulmonary Dirofilariasis. J.A.M.A., 198 (1966): 665.

Brill, I. C.: Cor Pulmonale: A Semantic Consideration, with Brief Notes on Diagnosis and Treatment. Dis. Chest, 33 (1958): 658.

Chapman, N. F., and Smith, A. W.: Effects of Dithiazinine Iodide on *Dirofilaria immitis* in Dogs. J.A.V.M.A., 138 (1961): 605.

Detweiler, D. K., and Patterson, D. F.: A Phonograph Record of Heart Sounds and Murmurs of the Dog. Ann. N.Y. Acad. Sci., 127 (1965): 322.

Essex, H. E.: Certain Operative Procedures on the Mammalian Heart. Vet. Med., 45 (1950): 85.

Faust, E. C.: Human Infection with Dirofilaria. Bull. W. H. O., 27 (1962): 642.

Fowler, J. L., Warne, R. J., Furusho, Y., and Sugiyama, H.: Testing Fenthion, Dichlorvos, and Diethylcarbamazine for Prophylactic Effects Against the Developing Stages of *Dirofilaria immitis.* Amer. J. Vet. Res., 31 (1970); 903.

Groves, H. F., and Koutz, F. R.: Survey of Microfilariae in Ohio Dogs. J.A.V.M.A., 144 (1964): 600.

Hahn, A. W.: Angiocardiography in Canine Dirofilariasis. II. Utilization of a Rapid Film Changing Technique. J.A.V.M.A., 136 (1960): 355.

Henderson, J. W.: Diagnosis, Treatment, and Preventive Therapy for Heartworms. J.A.V.M.A., 151 (1967): 1737.

Hennigar, G. R., and Ferguson, R. W.: Pulmonary Vascular Sclerosis as a Result of *Dirofilaria immitis* Infection in Dogs. J.A.V.M.A., 131 (1957): 336.

Hirth, R. S., Huizinga, H. W., and Nielsen, S. W.: Dirofilariasis in Connecticut Dogs. J.A.V.M.A., 148 (1966): 1508.

Hobson, H. P.: Angiocardiography in Canine Dirofilariasis. I. Preliminary Studies. J.A.V.M.A., 135 (1959): 537.

Horne, R. D.: Recent Advances in Canine Dirofilariasis. 12th Gaines Vet. Symp., St. Louis, Missouri, 1967, p. 17.

Jackson, R. F.: Diagnosis of Heartworm Disease by Examination of the Blood. J.A.V.M.A., 154 (1969a): 374.

Jackson, R. F.: Treatment of Heartworm-Infected Dogs with Chemical Agents. J.A.V.M.A., 154 (1969b): 390.

Jackson, R. F.: The Venae Cavae or Liver Failure Syndrome of Heartworm Disease. J.A.V.M.A., 154 (1969c): 384.

Jackson, R. F., von Lichtenberg, F., and Otto, G. F.: Occurrence of Adult Heartworms in the Venae Cavae of Dogs. J.A.V.M.A., 141 (1962): 117.

Jackson, W. F.: Circulation Time in Heartworm Disease. Small Anim. Clin., 2 (1962): 336.

Jackson, W. F.: Radiographic Examination of the Heartworm-Infected Patient. J.A.V.M.A., 154 (1969a): 380.

Jackson, W. F.: Surgical Treatment of Heartworm Disease. J.A.V.M.A., 154 (1969b): 383.

Jackson, W. F., Knowles, J. O., and Wallace, C. R.: Heartworm Surgery Simplified. Small Anim. Clin., 2 (1962): 342.

Jackson, W. F., and Wallace, C. R.: Canine Dirofilariasis. In *Current Veterinary Therapy 1966-1967*. Edited by R. W. Kirk. W. B. Saunders Co., Philadelphia, 1966, p. 108.

Johnson, L. E.: The Surgical Removal of *Dirofilaria immitis*. Proc. Ohio State University Annual Conference, Columbus, Ohio, 1951.

Jubb, K. V. F., and Kennedy, P. C.: Pathology of Domestic Animals. Academic Press, New York, Vol. 1, 1963.

Kume, S., Ohishi, I., and Kobayashi, S.: Prophylactic Therapy Against the Developing Stages of *Dirofilaria immitis:* Supplemental Studies. Amer. J. Vet. Res., 28 (1967): 975.

Kurokawa, K., Odaira, S., Hideyuki, H., Moriwaki, H., Yeshizaki, S., and Sakimoto, Y.: Surgical Treatment of Canine Cardiofilariasis. Bull. Nippon Vet. Zootech. Coll., 3 (1954): 67.

Lambert, G., Merritt, F. R., Fuller, D. A., and McWilliams, P. F.: Evaluation of a New Microfilaricide in Dogs. Vet. Med., 65 (1970):676.

Leonard, H. C.: Collapse of the Larynx and Adjacent Structures in the Dog. J.A.V.M.A., 137 (1960): 360.

Leonard, H. C.: Eversion of the Lateral Ventricles of the Larynx in Dogs — Five Cases. J.A.V.M.A., 131 (1957): 83.

Leonard, H. C.: Surgical Relief for Stenotic Nares in a Dog. J.A.V.M.A., 128 (1956): 530.

Lillis, W. G.: *Dirofilaria immitis* in Dogs and Cats from South Central New Jersey. J. Parasit., 50 (1964): 802.

Lindsey, J. R.: Identification of Canine Microfilariae. J.A.V.M.A., 146 (1965): 1106.

Liu, S. –K.: Pulmonary Vascular Changes in Canine Dirofilariasis. Proc. 4th Int. Conf., World Ass. for the Advancement of Vet. Parasit. In press, 1970.

Liu, S. –K., Das, K. M., and Tashjian, R. J.: Adult *Dirofilaria immitis* in the Arterial System of a Dog. J.A.V.M.A., 148 (1966): 1501.

Liu, S. –K., Yarns, D. A., Carmichael, J. A., and Tashjian, R. J.: Pulmonary Collateral Circulation in Canine Dirofilariasis. Amer. J. Vet. Res., 30 (1969): 1723.

Liu, S. –K., Yarns, D. A., and Tashjian, R. J.: Postmortem Pulmonary Arteriography in Canine Dirofilariasis. Amer. J. Vet. Res., 30 (1969): 319.

Mann, P. H., and Fratta, I.: The Incidence of Coccidia, Heartworm, and Intestinal Helminths in Dogs and Cats in Northern New Jersey. J. Parasit., 38 (1952): 496.

Marquardt, W. C., and Fabian, W. E.: The Distribution in Illinois of Filariids of Dogs. J. Parasit., 52 (1966): 318.

McGreevy, P. B., Conrad, R. D., Bulgin, M. S., and Stitzel, K. A.: Canine Filariasis in Northern California. Amer. J. Vet. Res., 31 (1970):1325.

Muller, G. H., and Kirk, R. W.: Small Animal Dermatology. W. B. Saunders Co., Philadelphia, 1969.

Neal, R. W., Nair, K. G., and Hecht, H. H.: A Pathophysiological Classification of Cor Pulmonale: With General Remarks on Therapy. Mod. Conc. Cardiovasc. Dis., 37 (1968): 107.

Newton, W. L., and Wright, W. H.: The Occurrence of a Dog Filariid Other than *Dirofilaria immitis* in the United States. J. Parasit., 52 (1956): 311.

Newton, W. L., and Wright, W. H.: A Reevaluation of the Canine Filariasis Problem in the United States. Vet. Med., 52 (1957): 75.

O'Brien, J. A., Buchanan, J. W., and Kelly, D. F.: Tracheal Collapse in the Dog. J. Amer. Vet. Radiol. Soc., 7 (1966): 12.

Orihel, T. C.: Morphology of the Larval Stages of *Dirofilaria immitis* in the Dog. J. Parasit., 47 (1961): 251.

Otto, G. F.: Geographical Distribution, Vectors, and Life Cycle of *Dirofilaria immitis*. J.A.V.M.A., 154 (1969): 370.

Otto, G. F., and Bauman, P. M.: Canine Filariasis. Vet. Med., 54 (1959): 87.

Patton, C. S., and Garner, F. M.: Cerebral Infarction Caused by Heartworms *(Dirofilaria immitis)* in a Dog. J.A.V.M.A., 156 (1970): 600.

Pollard, H. S., Ashby, R., and Derrick, J. R.: Surgical Removal of Heartworms by Open Cardiotomy Using Total Venous Occlusion. Texas Rep. Biol. Med., 17 (1959): 603.

Roenigk, W. J.: Surgical Removal of Canine Heartworms by Pulmonary Arteriotomy. J.A.V.M.A., 133 (1958): 581.

Rothstein, N., and Brown, M. L.: Vital Staining and Differentiation of Microfilariae. Amer. J. Vet. Res., 21 (1960): 1090.

Rothstein, N., Kinnaman, K. E., Brown, M. L., and Carithers, R. W.: Canine Microfilariasis in Eastern United States. J. Parasit., 47 (1961): 661.

Rubin, E. F., and Brooks, F. T.: The Midsternal Approach for Removal of Heartworms by Ventriculotomy. J.A.V.M.A., 144 (1964): 237.

Sawyer, T. K., and Weinstein, P. P.: Experimentally Induced Canine Dirofilariasis. J.A.V.M.A., 143 (1963): 975.

Sawyer, T. K., Rubin, E. F., and Jackson, R. F.: The Cephalic Hook in Microfilariae of *Dipetalonema reconditum* in the Differentiation of Canine Filariasis. Proc. Helminth Soc. Washington, 32 (1965): 15.

Schiefer, B.: Zur Frage des Asthma bronchiale bei Hunden. Die Kleintierpraxis, 13 (1968): 109.

Schiller, A. G., Helper, L. C., and Small, E.: Treatment of Tracheal Collapse in the Dog. J.A.V.M.A., 145 (1964): 669.

Schnelle, G. B., and Jones, T. C.: *Dirofilaria immitis* in the Eye and in an Interdigital Cyst. J.A.V.M.A., 107 (1945): 14.

Snyder, J. W., Liu, S. –K., and Tashjian, R. J.: Blood Chemical and Cellular Changes in Canine Dirofilariasis. Amer. J. Vet. Res., 28 (1967): 1705.

Tajuchi, M., Takehara, B., and Uriu, I.: A Case Report on a Dog with Advanced *Dirofilaria immitis* in the Lateral Ventricles of Its Brain. J. Jap. Vet. Med. Ass., 12 (1959): 430.

Tashjian, R. J., Liu, S. –K., Yarns, D. A., Das, K. M., and Stein, H. L.: Angiocardiography in Canine Heartworm Disease. Amer. J. Vet. Res., 31 (1970): 415.

Thrasher, J. P.: Canine Dirofilariasis. Scope, 1 (1965): 2.

Thrasher, J. P., Ash, L. R., and Little, M. D.: Filarial Infections of Dogs in New Orleans. J.A.V.M.A., 143 (1963): 605.

Thrasher, J. P., and Clanton, J. R., Jr.: Epizootiologic Observations of Canine Filariasis in Georgia. J.A.V.M.A., 152 (1968): 1517.

Thrasher, J. P., Gould, K. G., Lynch, M. J., and Harris, C. C.: Filarial Infections of Dogs in Atlanta, Georgia. J.A.V.M.A., 153 (1968): 1059.

Tulloch, G. S., Pacheco, G., Casey, H. W., Bills, W. E., Davis, I., and Anderson, R.: Prepatent Clinical, Pathologic, and Serologic Changes in Dogs Infected with *Dirofilaria immitis* and Treated with Diethylcarbamazine. Amer. J. Vet. Res., 31 (1970): 437.

Turk, R. D., Gaafar, S. M., and Lynd, F. T.: A Note on the Occurrence of the Nematodes *Dirofilaria immitis* and *Ancylostoma braziliense* in Unusual Locations. J.A.V.M.A., 129 (1956): 425.

von Lichtenberg, F., Jackson, R. F., and Otto, G. F.: Hepatic Lesions in Dogs with Dirofilariasis. J.A.V.M.A., 141 (1962): 121.

Wallace, C. R.: Cardiac Catheterization to Aid in Diagnosis of Cardiovascular Disease. Small Anim. Clin., 2 (1962): 332.

Wallace, C. R., and Hamilton, W. F.: Study of Spontaneous Congestive Heart Failure in the Dog. Circ. Res., 11 (1962): 301.

Wallenstein, W. L., and Tibola, B. J.: Survey of Canine Filariasis. J.A.V.M.A., 137 (1960): 712.

Warne, R. J., Tipton, V. J., and Furusho, Y.: Canine Heartworm Disease in Japan: Screening of Selected Drugs against *Dirofilaria immitis* in vivo. Amer. J. Vet. Res., 30 (1969): 27.

Weipers, W. L., and Lawson, D. D.: Heart and Great Vessels. In *Canine Surgery*. 1st Archibald ed. Edited by J. Archibald. American Veterinary Publications, Inc., Santa Barbara, California. 1965:421.

White, P. D.: Heart Disease. The Macmillan Company, New York, 1st ed., 1931.

Wilcox, H. S.: Pulmonary Arteriotomy for Removal of *Dirofilaria immitis* in the Dog. J.A.V.M.A., 136 (1960): 328.

Wylie, J. P.: Detection of Microfilariae by a Filter Technique. J.A.V.M.A., 156 (1970): 1403.

Yarns, D. A., and Tashjian, R. J.: Cardiopulmonary Values in Normal and Heartworm-Infected Dogs. Amer. J. Vet. Res., 28 (1967): 1461.

Zook, B. C., and Hathaway, J. E.: Tracheal Stenosis and Congenital Cardiac Anomalies in a Dog. J.A.V.M.A., 149 (1966): 298.

Zydeck, F. A., Chodkowski, I., and Bennett, R. R.: Incidence of Microfilariasis in Dogs in Detroit, Michigan. J.A.V.M.A., 156 (1970): 890.

17

MISCELLANEOUS CONDITIONS AFFECTING THE CARDIOVASCULAR SYSTEM

ARTERIOVENOUS FISTULAS

An arteriovenous fistula is a pathologic direct communication between an artery and a vein resulting in formation of an aneurysmal sac and elimination of the capillary bed. Arteriovenous fistulas may be acquired or congenital. The diagnosis of an arteriovenous fistula is made when a continuous machinery-like murmur is heard over the area of the aneurysmal sac. The murmur, accentuated in systole, is accompanied by a palpable continuous thrill which disappears when pressure is applied proximal to the fistula.

A large arteriovenous shunt located centrally can shunt 20 to 50 per cent of the cardiac output directly to the venous system, eliminating passage through a capillary bed. This results in increased venous return, increased right atrial pressure, and a compensatory increase in heart rate and cardiac output. The circulatory dynamics of large arteriovenous fistulas such as patent ductus arteriosus impose a strain on the heart due to high cardiac output and predispose the dog to congestive heart failure.

When pressure is applied proximal to or over the aneurysmal sac of the arteriovenous fistula, the arteriovenous shunt is abolished, and the increased venous return to the heart diminishes, resulting in reduction of the heart rate. Applied clinically, this simple diagnostic test is called the *Branham test*. In small arteriovenous fistulas located far from the heart, this test, requiring occlusion of the arteriovenous shunt, may not prove positive since the venous return is not

456

appreciably reduced. The increase in venous pressure is responsible for formation of the aneurysmal sac and for venous engorgement distal to the fistula. The aneurysm pulsates prominently over the fistula.

When the arteriovenous fistula is large, the heart enlarges in response to the increased venous return and volume overload. Small peripheral arteriovenous fistulas do not result in significant cardiac enlargement, and radiography is not beneficial in making the diagnosis. A-V fistulas are reported to occur in many areas of the body in man (Holman, 1968; Gomes, 1970). In the dog, A-V fistulas other than patent ductus arteriosus have been reported in the orbit resulting in exophthalmos (Rubin and Patterson, 1965), in the cervical region (Wallace and Hamilton, 1962), and on the forelimb (Buchanan, 1965; Ettinger et al., 1968).

There is a soft tissue swelling or aneurysmal sac in the area of the arteriovenous fistula, over which a continuous bruit can be palpated. When a stethoscope is placed over the aneurysmal sac, a continuous or machinery murmur with systolic accentuation is heard. When surgical correction of peripheral arteriovenous fistulas is contemplated, angiography by direct arterial puncture and injection of 50% Hypaque can demonstrate the precise anatomic location of the fistula.

Treatment of arteriovenous fistulas by surgical excision or arterial ligation is essential to prevent heart failure, local pain, destruction of bone, or ulceration of skin. Following correction, the cardiac output is decreased, and the heart usually returns to normal size (Ettinger et al., 1968).

SUDDEN DEATH IN DOBERMAN PINSCHERS

The entity of sudden death in Doberman Pinschers (James and Drake, 1968) occurs in dogs which have had no previous history of cardiac disease. The syndrome occurred in 11 dogs between three days and 10 years of age, and male and female dogs were affected equally. At necropsy, there was neither cardiac dilatation nor hypertrophy, and the coronary arteries and ventricular myocardium appeared grossly normal. Microscopically, there were areas in the region of the bundle of His which had been replaced by fat, but inflammatory cells were not seen. The lumina of the small coronary arteries were narrow, and medial degeneration and endothelial proliferation were seen in these arteries. Focal degeneration of the bundle of His was accompanied by formation of cartilage and bone in the adjacent central fibrous body. This degeneration is thought to result from chronic ischemia and metabolic competition with cartilage and newly formed bone for the decreased blood supply. The condition described by James and Drake (1968) may be heritable.

ARTERIAL HYPERTENSION

An average femoral artery pressure greater than 145 mm. Hg has been defined as spontaneous hypertension (Katz, Skom, and Wakerlin, 1957). However, clearly recognizable clinical signs resulting from arterial hypertension are unusual. The diagnosis of arterial hypertension in a dog should be withheld unless there is confirmed evidence of elevated arterial pressures, as demonstrated by direct arterial blood pressure measurements. Detweiler et al. (1968) reviewed the pathogenesis and occurrence of both spontaneous and experimental hypertension in the dog.

Pheochromocytomas (epinephrine-secreting adrenal tumors) associated with adrenal hypertensive lesions were found at necropsy in seven dogs (Howard and Nielsen, 1965a). All had histologic evidence of hypertension, such as arteriolar medial hyperplasia and sclerosis in the lungs, spleen, and kidney, as well as fibrosis of Bowman's capsule. In these dogs clinical signs that are compatible with hypertension were lethargy, weakness, and periods of respiratory distress with pulmonary edema, as well as periods of incoordination. The severity of the clinical signs varied depending on the size and character of the tumor mass. Arterial pressure measurements and electrocardiograms were not available for any of the dogs affected.

Although pheochromocytomas have also been reported in dogs by other investigators (Mulligan, 1949; Smith and Jones, 1957; Moulton, 1961; Jubb and Kennedy, 1963; Meier, 1963), the incidence of the condition is low. There seems to be a specific breed predisposition to pheochromocytomas in the Boxer, according to Howard and Nielsen (1965b).

Left ventricular hypertrophy and histologic findings compatible with hypertension have also been found repeatedly in dogs with chronic interstitial nephritis (Dahme, 1957; Pirie, Mackey, and Fisher, 1965). Arterial pressures in non-uremic dogs were not significantly elevated, although uremic dogs had pressures 20 mm. Hg above the normal range (Spörri and Leemann, 1961). Bloom (1954) demonstrated that of nine dogs with arterial hypertension, six had no renal disease and three had chronic pyelonephritis. In contrast, Anderson and Fisher (1968) were able to demonstrate hypertension in some dogs with acute and sub-acute nephritis and in almost all dogs with chronic nephritis. They concluded that a positive relationship existed between renal disease and hypertension.

ANEURYSM OF THE HEART AND GREAT VESSELS

Aneurysmal dilatation of a portion of the heart or a great vessel has been reported in two dogs, although neither dog had clinical signs which would have suggested the antemortem diagnosis. During a routine experimental thoracotomy in an otherwise normal young dog, Danhof (1960) found a small aneurysmal dilatation of the right ventricle. Dilatation of the wall of the aorta with subsequent aneurysm can be produced by migration of *Spirocerca lupi* larvae, according to Bailey (1963). The larvae invade and destroy the elastic fibers of the thoracic aorta, leaving small scars or aneurysms. Radiographs of a 13-year-old dog of mixed breed with aortic aneurysm of undetermined origin which had signs such as right hindlimb paralysis and pain suggesting embolism in the iliac artery are shown in Figures 17-1 and 17-2.

AORTIC AND ARTERIAL EMBOLISM

Thrombo-embolic occlusions (obstructions) of the distal aorta and the bifurcation of the iliac arteries are relatively common in the cat (Holzworth, Simpson, and Wind, 1955; Buchanan, Baker, and Hill, 1966) but are rare in the

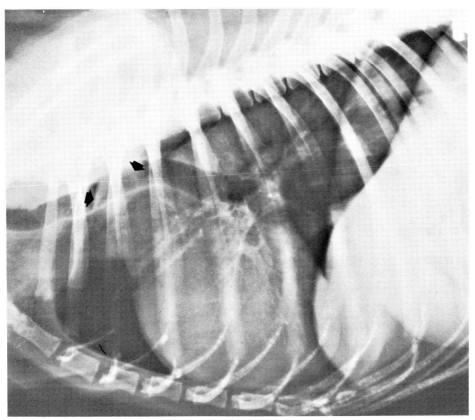

FIGURE 17-1   Left lateral radiograph, 13½ year old male dog of mixed breed with aortic aneurysm and embolization to the right iliac artery. The dog has signs of pain, knuckling over, and paresis of the right hindlimb. This limb was cold, and there was no femoral pulse. The tentative diagnosis was a saddle thrombus. An extreme dorsal deviation of the trachea at the third intercostal space and a mass (arrows) in the area of the aortic arch or the precardial mediastinum, which was responsible for the displacement, are the most prominent radiographic features. At the level of the third rib the mass and the trachea are superimposed. The aortic arch is not directly visible. As the aorta emerges from the hilar shadow, a marked widening becomes apparent; however, within a short distance the diameter of the descending aorta becomes normal. The right ventricle appears rounded and slightly larger than normal. The lung field is clear. The radiographic appearance is similar to that of a heartbase or mediastinal tumor with the exception that signs of pericardial effusion are not present. The marked dilatation of the aortic arch is characteristic of an aneurysm. This must be differentiated from poststenotic dilatation as occurs with aortic stenosis.

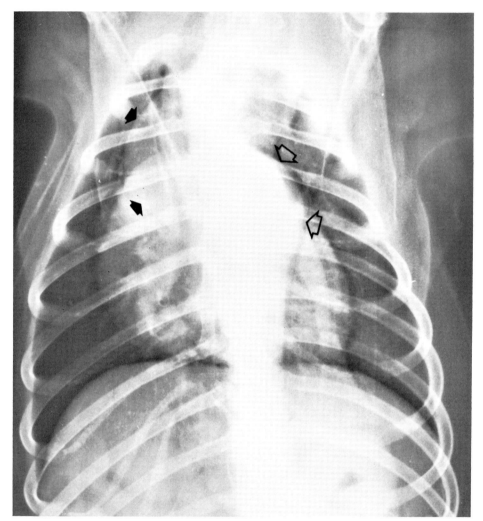

FIGURE 17-2 Dorsoventral radiograph, dog in Figure 17-1. The trachea deviates to the right side in the precardial mediastinum. A mediastinal mass (black arrows) protrudes markedly to the right. The left border of the mediastinum also extends slightly farther to the left side than normal. The right cardiac border appears markedly rounded, indicating right heart enlargement. The left ventricle is unremarkable. The descending portion of the aortic arch is much wider than normal and extends beyond the left cranial cardiac border (clear arrows), simulating an enlarged pulmonary artery segment. The pulmonary artery segment is, however, unremarkable. The left pulmonary artery is well delineated. Marked enlargement of the aortic arch in an old dog can occur due to displacement or aneurysm of the aorta. In a young dog, aortic stenosis and patent ductus arteriosus would have to be considered in making the differential diagnosis.

dog. The etiology of most spontaneous cases of aortic or arterial embolism in the dog is related to mural or valvular endocarditis in the left heart. Emboli have been found in the terminal aorta (Shouse and Meier, 1956; Nims, 1962; Ishmael and Udall, 1966; Axelson, Secord, and Weber, 1968), in the iliac and/or femoral artery (Shouse and Meier, 1956; Denholm, 1963; Kraft and Kraft, 1965; Baxter, 1967), and in a brachial artery (Shouse and Meier, 1956).

The clinical signs are usually acute onset of pain in the hindlimbs and paresis or paralysis in one or both hindlimbs. On physical examination, the affected limbs are cold and the muscles are swollen and tender. The cardinal sign is absence of the femoral pulse. The tail and bladder may be paralyzed. Depending on the extent of the embolic occlusions, the location of the emboli, and the development of collateral circulation, the dog's condition may deteriorate rapidly, as shock develops, or the dog may improve progressively, as in a case reported by Kraft and Kraft (1965). Infarction of abdominal organs such as the kidney, spleen, or gastrointestinal tract may complicate the disease process. Because vegetative valvular bacterial endocarditis is often reported in dogs with this condition (Shouse and Meier, 1956; Ishmael and Udall, 1966; Baxter, 1967), a systolic murmur may be auscultated if the atrioventricular valves have been made incompetent. The emboli in the dog described in Figures 17-1 and 17-2 apparently originated from an aortic aneurysm. Electrocardiographic findings in dogs with this condition have not been described.

If diagnostic studies are needed to demonstrate the area of occlusion caused by the embolism prior to surgery, aortography should be performed. The contrast medium may be injected into the left ventricle, by the method described by Imhoff and Tashjian (1961), or into the descending aorta through a catheter advanced retrograde from the common carotid artery.

If the condition is recognized early, embolectomy may be indicated (Denholm, 1963). However, if bacterial endocarditis is present, as it is in most cases, successful treatment is often precluded since new emboli to the arteries, brain, kidneys, spleen, and gastrointestinal tract are likely to develop. If medical therapy is to be successful, blood cultures should be made and long-term therapy instituted according to antibiotic sensitivity testing. The value of anticoagulants, analgesics, fibrinolytic enzymes, arterial dilating agents, and cage rest for this condition is not known at this time.

Venous thrombosis and embolism are not major problems in the dog except in certain neoplastic diseases and dirofilariasis (see Chapter 16).

SIMULTANEOUS SYNCHRONOUS CONTRACTION OF THE HEART AND DIAPHRAGM

Forceful, rhythmic abdominal and diaphragmatic contractions synchronous with the heart beat characterize this condition (Wyssman, 1940; Detweiler, 1955; Grauwiler, 1959; Smith, 1965; Ettinger, Suter, and Gould, 1969, Bohn and Patterson, 1970). The history usually includes persistent vomiting for several days, such as occurs with uremia, leptospirosis, intestinal foreign body, or gastroenteritis. Occasionally the condition occurs in dogs without any history of disease or following a traumatic accident (Bohn and Patterson, 1970). The forceful contractions at the left side of the costal arch may lead to the false impression that the heart has been displaced into this area. The electrocardiogram is usually normal, although changes in the S-T segment and T wave could develop. If the electrocardiogram and the movements produced by the abdominal pulsations are recorded simultaneously, the relationship of the diaphragmatic contraction to each cardiac cycle is shown (Fig. 17-3). The condition can be differentiated from a pulsating abdominal aneurysm and from abnormally forceful cardiac contractions by employing fluoroscopy. In some cases, the abnormal contractions are limited to the left hemidiaphragm.

In this condition, the phrenic nerve is stimulated by each cardiac contraction; the phrenic nerve, in turn, stimulates the diaphragm to contract either unilaterally or bilaterally in synchrony with the heart. It is theorized that hyperirritability of the phrenic nerve is caused by alkalosis or hypocalcemia induced by prolonged vomiting. Although blood gas analyses have not been reported from dogs with this syndrome, gross electrolyte disturbances such as hypocalcemia (4.3 mEq/L.)

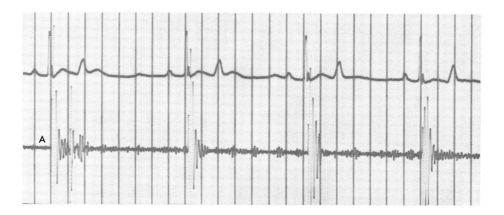

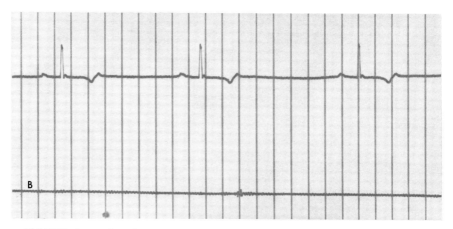

FIGURE 17-3 Lead II of the electrocardiogram recorded simultaneously with sounds produced by the synchronous simultaneous excursion of the thoracic wall and diaphragm with each heart beat (A). Two hours following the administration of intravenous phenobarbital, the movements of the thoracic wall were diminished, and when the electrocardiogram and sound recordings were made again, using the same recording device at the same amplitude, pulsations of the thoracic wall were not demonstrable (B).

and hypochloremia (104 mEq/L.) were present in one case seen by the authors. The electrolyte levels in this case were actually lower than they seemed because the dog was grossly dehydrated, as proved by an elevated total protein of 8 Gm./100 ml. When adjusted to a normal state of hydration, the calcium and chloride levels would be even lower.

Detweiler (1955) reported that the intravenous administration of Ringer's solution was effective in treating this condition in one dog, and Ettinger, Suter, and Gould (1969) reported that 0.5 gr. sodium phenobarbital administered intravenously reduced the force of the contractions almost immediately; all contractions had subsided within 8 hours. In another case treated by the authors in which prolonged vomiting was probably due to uremia (BUN, 154 mg./100 ml.; creatinine, 8.4 mg./100 ml.), phenobarbital (0.5 gr.) reduced the intensity of the contractions almost immediately and abolished them within 8 hours. Combined therapy with phenobarbital, Ringer's solution, and supplemental calcium is probably indicated in most cases.

SECONDARY CARDIAC DISEASE IN RESPONSE TO EXTRACARDIAC DISEASE

UREMIA

Clinical cardiac signs are usually absent until late in the course of uremia. Then, prolongation of the Q-T interval and peaked, narrow T waves of high amplitude are seen on the electrocardiogram as a result of hypocalcemia and hyperkalemia (Fig. 17-4). Terminally, hyperkalemia is responsible for slowing of atrial conduction and for diminished response of the heart to electrical stimulation. Simultaneous indirect and direct measurements of arterial pressure in dogs with chronic interstitial nephritis made by Spörri and Leemann (1961) demonstrated that arterial blood pressures did not increase if the blood urea nitrogen was normal. In uremic dogs, the diastolic blood pressures became elevated by approximately 20 mm. Hg; the systolic pressures were normal but decreased one to four days prior to death. Anderson and Fisher (1968) reported the existence of hypertension in dogs which were uremic.

Angiopathies were found regularly by Dahme (1955, 1957) and by Pirie,

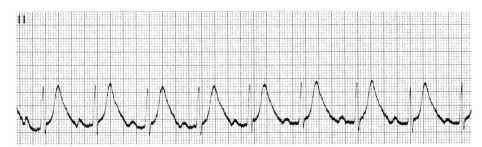

FIGURE 17-4   Hyperkalemic T waves. Tall, peaked T waves occur in terminal uremic states when the serum potassium, creatinine, and blood urea nitrogen levels are markedly elevated. This tracing was recorded from a dog with a blood urea nitrogen level of 120 mg./100 ml. Necropsy proved the clinical impression of chronic interstitial nephritis and terminal uremia.

Mackey, and Fisher (1965) when renal disease was present. Because left ventricular hypertrophy frequently coexisted with chronic interstitial nephritis, Nieberle and Cohrs (1952) interpreted left ventricular hypertrophy as a sign of arterial hypertension. However, Spörri and Leemann (1961) caution against such a simplified conclusion because secondary factors such as anemia, which often occurs with chronic interstitial nephritis, may be responsible for the left ventricular hypertrophy. Endocardial and pericardial lesions which develop secondarily to uremia are discussed in Chapters 13 and 15.

HYPERTHYROIDISM

Cardiac disease secondary to hyperthyroidism is unusual in the dog. Iatrogenic cardiac effects due to overtreatment with thyroid tablets are occasionally recognized. The only spontaneous clinical abnormality recognized in a dog with both chronic mitral valvular fibrosis and a functional thyroid adenocarcinoma was

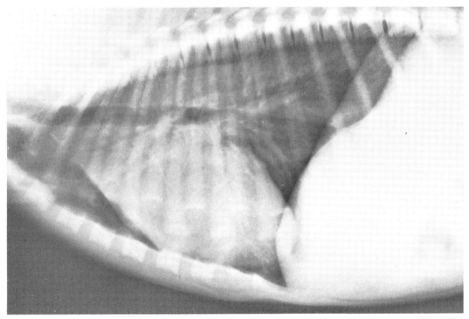

FIGURE 17-5   Lateral radiograph, 10 week old male Saluki with severe anemia due to bone marrow depression caused by uremia. At necropsy, severe bilateral fibrosis of the kidneys was seen. A loud anemic murmur had been heard on auscultation. The heart is larger than normal due to elongation of the long axis. The inclination of the apicobasilar line is markedly increased, and the right heart and the aortic arch extend into the second intercostal space. There is slight enlargement of the left atrium. When compared with the enlarged right ventricle, the left ventricle appears normal in size. The lung field is slightly denser than normal for a dog of this age, and the vascular markings in the diaphragmatic lobes are accentuated. In a dog of this age the prominent aortic arch and the increased apicobasilar diameter would usually indicate congenital heart diseases such as patent ductus arteriosus, ventricular septal defect, or aortic stenosis. The tentative diagnosis of congenital heart disease was proved incorrect at necropsy. At necropsy the aortic arch was very wide, and there was marked right and left ventricular hypertrophy, but no congenital lesion could be found. The radiographic and gross pathologic changes can be explained as an adaptation of the juvenile heart to the stress of severe anemia.

an increased heart rate (Reed et al., 1963). After removal of the mass from the neck, the heart rate returned to normal. In man, the heart rate is often increased in hyperthyroidism. A waterhammer pulse, visible arterial pulsations in the neck, and occasionally atrial fibrillation also occur in man.

SEVERE CHRONIC ANEMIA

In severe chronic anemia, a rapid circulation time and increased cardiac output are mediated by tachycardia, peripheral vasodilation, decreased vascular resistance, and a rapid ejection rate. The sum of these physiologic alterations has been referred to as a hyperkinetic state by Duke and Abelman (1969). The hemodynamic alterations that occur with anemia resemble those that develop in other

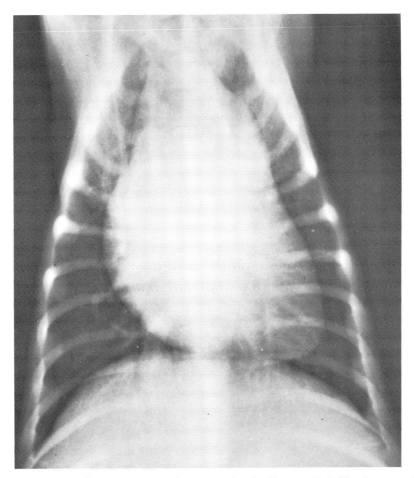

FIGURE 17-6 Dorsoventral radiograph, dog in Figure 17-5. The increased size of the cardiac silhouette is even more obvious in this view than in the lateral radiograph. Both the long diameter and the transverse diameter of the heart have increased. The right cardiac border is rounder than normal. Left ventricular enlargement is indicated by the rounded apex and the proximity of the left cardiac border to the thoracic wall. The prominent aortic arch, which extends into the cranial mediastinum and to the left side, could indicate aneurysmal enlargement as is seen with patent ductus arteriosus, or it could indicate a poststenotic dilatation as in aortic stenosis.

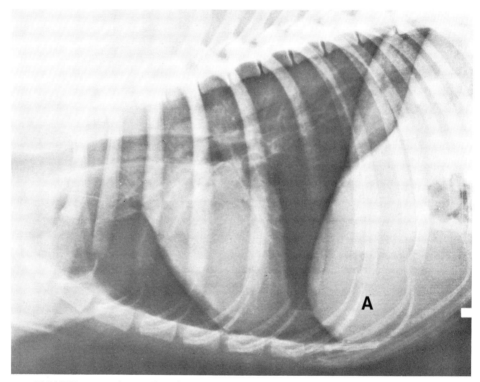

FIGURE 17-7 Lateral radiographs, 1 year old female German Shepherd dog. The dog had been hit by a car and was in acute hemorrhagic shock due to splenic rupture when the first radiograph (A) was made. The dog was given massive transfusions of whole blood and lactated Ringer's solution, and four hours later, after she had improved markedly, and the central venous pressure had returned to a low normal value, the second radiograph (B) was made.

A, the cardiac silhouette looks triangular and is smaller than normal. The decrease in size is mainly due to a diminished craniocaudal diameter. The cranial and caudal waists have become shallower than normal. The left cardiac border is straight, and the apex is narrower than normal. The lung field is lucent, and the intrapulmonary vascular markings are barely visible. The caudal vena cava and the thoracic aorta are small.

(Illustration continues on opposite page.)

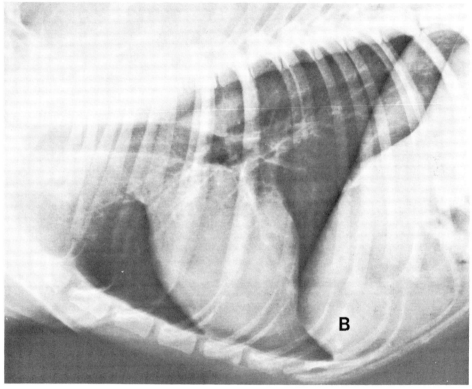

B, the heart is markedly larger than on the previous radiograph. The cranial and caudal waists are present, and a fusiform widening of the heart is seen before it narrows at the apex. The apex is wider than in *A.* The intrapulmonary vascular markings are denser than before but are still smaller than normal. The caudal vena cava is slightly larger and denser than before, and the aorta looks normal. The difference in cardiac size between the two radiographs is considered significant. The change in size owing to systole and diastole is not considerable. Although changes in cardiac size from systole to diastole may have influenced somewhat the dramatic change in radiographic appearance in the present case, these changes cannot be entirely responsible for the difference in cardiac size observed in these two radiographs.

high cardiac output states such as arteriovenous fistulas (see pp. 456-457, ac- quired and Ch. 18, congenital), hyperthyroidism (see above), and sepsis (Hermreck and Thal, 1969). Functional heart murmurs are often heard when the hemoglobin level falls below 6 Gm./100 ml. of blood. The short, high-frequency, early sys- tolic murmur is usually loudest over the mitral or pulmonic valve area and is thought to result either from increased flow across the pulmonic valve or from dilatation of the mitral valve anulus with subsequent mitral insufficiency following cardiac enlargement. Detweiler and Patterson (1965) have reported the occurrence of anemic diastolic murmurs as well as systolic murmurs. Radiographic indications of chronic severe anemia are cardiac enlargement and occasionally signs of pul- monary hypervascularity (Fig. 17-5 and 17-6). These signs are not observed in acute anemia due to acute blood loss. When acute blood loss results in shock, the heart size is diminished and a hypovascular lung field prevails (Fig. 17-7*A* and 17-7*B*). Detweiler et al. (1968) reported nonspecific electrocardiographic ab- normalities such as alteration of the QRS complex, S-T segment, and T wave in anemic states.

POLYCYTHEMIA VERA

In a case of polycythemia vera reported by Carb (1969), the electrocardio- gram suggested left ventricular hypertrophy, but this could not be positively cor- related with polycythemia vera. Necropsy findings were not available since the dog responded to therapy. It was suggested that left ventricular hypertrophy could have resulted from the chronic burden placed on the heart by the necessity of pumping more viscid blood.

ADRENAL CORTICAL HYPERFUNCTION (CUSHING'S SYNDROME)

Hyperfunction of the adrenal cortex is associated with clinical findings of bilateral alopecia, polydipsia, and polyuria. Laboratory findings include slight hyperglycemia, lymphopenia, eosinopenia, hypercholesterolemia, increased excretion of urinary 17-ketogenic steroids, and hypokalemia (Siegel et al., 1967). Although cardiac signs are not prominent with hyperfunction of the adrenal cortex, hypokalemia may be associated with prolongation of the Q-T interval on the electrocardiogram (Fig. 17-8). In one dog with an adrenocortical carcinoma, the heart rate was approximately 100 beats/min., and the Q-T interval was con- sidered prolonged at 0.24 sec.; the blood potassium level, between 2.4 and 2.6 mEq./L., was low (Siegel et al., 1967).

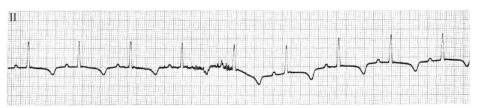

FIGURE 17-8 Q-T prolongation due to hypokalemia. Severe depression of serum potassium levels results initially in prolongation of the Q-T interval. This dog had a serum potassium of 2.5 mg./100 ml. The electrocardiographic tracing demon- strates a prolonged Q-T interval (0.32 sec.).

ADRENAL CORTICAL HYPOFUNCTION (ADDISON'S DISEASE)

The clinical signs of adrenocortical insufficiency (Addison's disease) are those of profound asthenia, ataxia, and chronic gastrointestinal crises such as emesis and diarrhea (Siegel, Schryver, and Fidler, 1967). Hypotension is characteristically another feature of this syndrome and may be responsible for syncopal attacks. Marshak, Webster, and Skelly (1960) reported one case in which the mean systolic blood pressure was 80 mm. Hg during an addisonian crisis. The diagnosis of this condition is based on typical clinical signs and on the laboratory findings of hyponatremia, hyperkalemia, eosinophilia, decreased urinary excretion of adrenocortical steroids, and diminished blood cortisol levels. Hyponatremia has not been a consistent finding in some of the cases seen by us. Reduced adrenal glucocorticoid production may result in hypoglycemia, whereas the

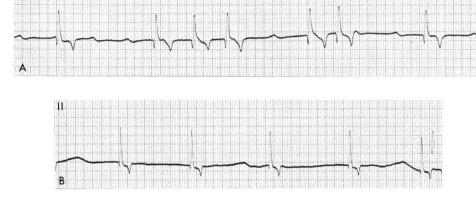

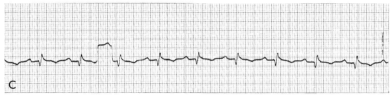

FIGURE 17-9 Adrenal cortical hypofunction. A, Hyperkalemia (potassium = 8.4 mEq./l.) is responsible for this advanced form of second degree atrioventricular block, which appears similar to complete heart block except for the slightly greater ventricular rate. The dog was presented because of acute collapse with a history of asthenia and chronic gastrointestinal disturbances, suggesting an acute addisonian crisis. An electrocardiogram was recorded when a slow, irregular heart rate was auscultated during physical examination. The P waves occur regularly at a rate of 150/minute. The ventricular rate is irregular and slow, 64 beats/minute, when counted for an entire minute. The irregular ventricular rate suggests a high degree of vagal influence on the supraventricular pacemaker (area of atrioventricular junctional tissue or bundle of His) stimulating the ventricles. The tracing was made at double amplitude, 20 mm. = 1 mv.

B, Prior to the intravenous infusion of hydrocortisone and glucose in saline (blood sugar = 12 mg./100 cc.; serum sodium = 139 mEq./l.), an electrocardiogram was again recorded. P waves are now entirely absent, and sinoatrial arrest has developed with complete heart block. The ventricular rate is 33 beats/minute. This tracing was made at paper speed of 25 mm./sec. and double amplitude.

C, Following the intravenous infusions, the dog's clinical response was dramatic, and the cardiac rhythm returned to normal. Blood cortisol levels were zero prior to the administration of prednisone and fluorohydrocortisone.

insufficient production of aldosterone, the mineralocorticoid fraction produced by the adrenal cortex, accounts for the decreased blood sodium and increased blood potassium levels. Hyperkalemia is also caused by diminished glomerular filtration and acidosis.

The cardiovascular examination is usually nonspecific. The cardiac silhouette may be abnormally small for the patient's size (see Fig. 3-22).

Radiographic examination of some dogs with Addison's disease may demonstrate a striking reduction in cardiac size, but this is not always consistent. When microcardia is present, the craniocaudal diameter is markedly decreased, and the apex appears narrower than normal. The heart's nearly triangular appearance is best seen in the lateral radiograph. The appearance of the lung field, more lucent than normal, might have resulted from reduced filling of the intrapulmonary vasculature, indicating diminished perfusion and/or overinflation of the lung.

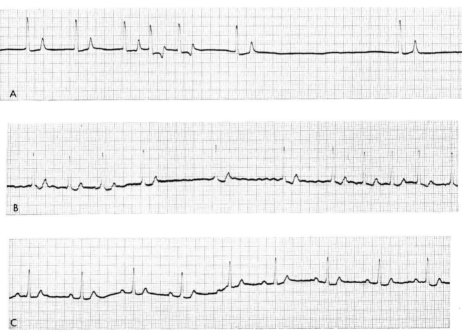

FIGURE 17-10 Adrenal cortical hypofunction. *A,* Sinoatrial arrest and an atrioventricular junctional rhythm (demonstrating marked vagal effects) resulted in a variable heart rate in a dog presented because of syncopal seizures and generalized asthenia. Based on the history and on blood serum chemistries (sodium = 136 mEq./l.; potassium = 9.1 mEq./l.; blood urea nitrogen = 180 mg./100 ml.; and creatinine = 5.4 mg./100 ml.), an acute addisonian crisis was diagnosed. The sinoatrial arrest and tall, peaked T waves were considered to be the result of hyperkalemia. A rapid clinical recovery occurred following the administration of intravenous hydrocortisone and intramuscular desoxycorticosterone acetate. Although the ventricular rate increased as the addisonian crisis became less intense, atrial fibrillation was the dominant cardiac rhythm (middle). There were no signs of underlying heart disease, as determined by auscultation and radiographic examination of the thorax. Because the ventricular rate began to increase spontaneously above 160 beats/minute, direct current cardioversion was employed to restore a normal rhythm (bottom). Following cardioversion the dog was maintained on oral quinidine for one month, in addition to daily therapy with fluorohydrocortisone and prednisone. Lead II electrocardiograms.

After initiation of therapy with corticosteroids, the radiographic signs are reversed.

Hyperkalemia produces peaked T waves of high amplitude as well as prolongation of the Q-T interval on the electrocardiogram. Prolongation of the P-R interval and QRS complex, complete atrioventricular block, and sinoatrial arrest develop progressively as the electrolyte imbalance increases. Complete atrioventricular block was reported in one dog (Marshak, Webster, and Skelly, 1960). In a number of dogs examined by the authors, complete heart block and/or sinoatrial arrest was diagnosed when the dogs were hospitalized during an acute episode of adrenocortical hypofunction (Figs. 17-9 and 17-10). Following therapy with intravenous hydrocortisone, glucose, and fluids, dogs that recover demonstrate a normal electrocardiogram as the electrolyte imbalance is relieved. In one dog that recovered, atrial fibrillation rather than a normal sinus rhythm developed; this required electrical cardioversion.

Long-term therapy of chronic adrenocortical hypofunction requires the administration of a mineralocorticoid such as 9-alpha-fluorohydrocortisone (Florinef) and a glucocortocoid such as cortisone.

CARDIAC NEOPLASIA

Primary and metastatic cardiac tumors are not common in dogs (Loppnow, 1961; Detweiler, 1962; Dobberstein and Tamaschke, 1962). Tumors are recognized primarily in the pericardium, myocardium, and atria. When aortic body tumors are included in the broad category of cardiac neoplasia because of their location at the base of the heart, the incidence of tumors rises sharply. In a series of 314 necropsies of dogs with cardiac disease, 17 (5.5 per cent) had some form of cardiac neoplasia (Detweiler, 1962).

Luginbühl and Detweiler (1965) reviewed the primary cardiac tumors previously reported, as well as those recognized in their laboratory. They listed the following primary cardiac tumors: hemangioendothelioma, mixed cell sarcoma, spindle cell sarcoma, round cell sarcoma, lymphangioendothelioma, hemangioma, fibroma, rhabdomyoma, chondroma, fibromyxoma, myxoma, and teratoma.

Metastatic tumors known to involve the heart include hemangiosarcoma, melanosarcoma, fibrosarcoma, chondrosarcoma, osteosarcoma, leiomyofibrosarcoma, adenocarcinoma, reticulum cell sarcoma, and lymphosarcoma (Loppnow, 1961; Sandersleben, 1961; Dobberstein and Tamaschke, 1962; Colby and Collins, 1965; Palumbo, 1967; Stünzi and Mann, 1970).

The history and clinical signs referable to cardiac neoplasia vary depending on the site and the extent of the tumor. Myocardial neoplasia is likely to produce signs similar to myocarditis (pp. 385-391). In such cases, clinical signs alone do not usually enable recognition of either primary or metastatic tumors from other causes of myocarditis, and the diagnosis is usually made at necropsy.

Primary or metastatic tumors involving the pericardium are likely to cause serosanguineous pericardial effusion (see Chapter 15).

Tumors occupying space within the heart are usually hemangioendotheliomas; these have a predilection for the right atrium (Luginbühl and Detweiler, 1965; Geib, 1967; Gilmore in Kleine, 1968; Harpster, 1969; Stünzi and Mann, 1970). Signs of right heart failure are likely to occur, and a murmur will be heard if the valves are made insufficient or stenotic by the mass (Buchanan, 1965). Metastasis to the lungs and respiratory signs which are not likely to respond to cardiac therapy usually occur. Pleural effusion may also be present. In most cases, diagnosis is difficult. However, if cytology of the pericardial effusate is positive for neoplastic cells, there would be evidence of cardiac neoplasia. Angiocardiography may demonstrate a filling defect of the right atrium and/or ventricle because of primary or metastatic neoplastic involvement (Patterson, 1961; Buchanan, 1965). Electrocardiography is likely to demonstrate atrial arrhythmias and conduction disturbances (complete heart block, paroxysmal atrial tachycardia, atrial premature beats) when tumors invade the atria (Patterson in Brodey and Prier, 1962).

A recent report describes primary hemangiosarcoma of the right atrium, observed most often in German Shepherds.

AORTIC BODY TUMORS (HEART BASE TUMORS)

Aortic body tumors, or chemodectomas, arise from chemoreceptor tissue in the region of the heart base. Aberrant thyroid and parathyroid tissue and malignant lymphoma and other neoplasias may also be found in some heart base tumors (Nilsson, 1955; Kast, 1958; Moulton, 1961). The neoplasia grows within the pericardial sac, usually in the periadventitial tissue between the aorta and the pulmonary artery, at the base of the heart (Nilsson, 1955; Johnson, 1968). Others arise between the pulmonary artery and the left atrial appendage or between the aorta and the right atrial appendage (Luginbühl and Detweiler, 1965). Heart base tumors often invade the adventitia of the great vessels and atrial myocardium.

Boston Terriers, Boxers, and English Bulldogs have a definite predisposition to aortic body tumors (Luginbühl and Detweiler, 1965). The Boston Terrier and the Boxer were affected in 25 of 33, 8 of 12, 13 of 13, 46 of 56, and 15 of 20 cases (Nilsson, 1955; Jubb and Kennedy, 1957; Howard and Nielsen, 1965; Luginbühl and Detweiler, 1965; and Johnson, 1968, respectively). These authors have observed that male dogs are affected most frequently. In addition, aortic body tumors usually occur in dogs over eight years old, the age ranges reported being four to 16 years (Luginbühl and Detweiler, 1965) and six to 15 years (Johnson, 1968).

The neoplasm is a slow-growing tumor which is often recognized as an incidental finding at necropsy (Kurtz and Finco, 1969). It may metastasize to the lungs and mediastinal lymph nodes (Nilsson, 1956; Brodey and Prier, 1962; Jubb and Kennedy, 1963; Johnson, 1968). When the neoplasm invades the pericardium, sanguinous pericardial effusion results, and clinical signs of congestive heart failure such as subcutaneous edema and ascites may develop. Edema of the head, neck, and forelimbs may occur if pressure is placed directly on the cranial vena cava near the mass. Johnson (1968) reported 20 dogs with aortic body tumors, of which 15 were in congestive heart failure. The clinical signs most frequently associated with the symptomatic state are cough, dyspnea, weight loss and emaciation, cyanosis, and vomiting (Bloom, 1943; Nilsson, 1955; Moulton, 1961; Brodey and Prier, 1962; Johnson, 1968).

If the dog is in congestive heart failure due to pericardial effusion, the heart sounds are muffled or inaudible. Radiography of the thorax often indicates pericardial effusion (see pp. 405-406 and Figs. 15-9 and 15-10). In many cases, a mass may be seen in the region of the aortic arch, and it may occasionally displace the trachea, the esophagus, or both. Complexes of diminished amplitude may be seen on the electrocardiogram (Fig. 17-11). Although pericardiocentesis may provide temporary relief of the clinical signs, the fluid recurs, and heart failure reappears

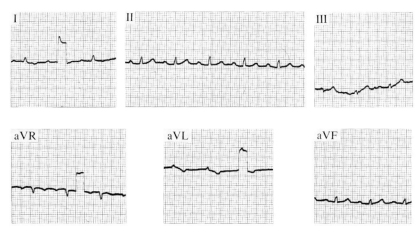

FIGURE 17-11   Electrocardiographic complexes of decreased amplitude occurring in all leads as a result of massive pericardial effusion. The amplitude of the QRS complexes never reaches 0.7 mv., the minimum amplitude considered for the electrocardiographic diagnosis of decreased amplitude. This dog had pericardial effusion secondary to a granulomatous tubercular mass involving the left atrium and pericardium.

over a variable period of time. Surgical excision of the tumors does not afford a very good prognosis, since they are not usually recognized until their size and degree of infiltration are too far advanced. Prior to that time, they do not cause clinical signs.

Angiocardiography may demonstrate the tumor either indirectly, because the cranial vena cava is displaced, or directly, by opacifying the mass with contrast medium entering through vessels branching from the arch of the aorta (Patterson, 1961).

Johnson (1968) reported testicular interstitial cell tumors in eight Boston Terriers and Boxer dogs in 223 necropsies performed on these breeds between 1949 and 1966. Of the eight dogs, six (five Boxers and one Boston Terrier) also had concurrent aortic body tumors. He suggested a relationship between aortic body tumors and testicular interstitial cell tumors in these two breeds.

CAROTID BODY TUMORS

Carotid body tumors arise from chemoreceptor tissue at the bifurcation of the carotid artery and are usually closer to the external carotid artery (Hubben, Patterson, and Detweiler, 1960). Of nine cases reported (Jubb and Kennedy, 1957; Scotti, 1958; Hubben, Patterson, and Detweiler, 1960; Kurtz and Finco, 1969), five Boxton Terriers, three Boxers, and one Cocker Spaniel were affected. Seven of the nine dogs were male, and all but one were over eight years of age. Most significantly, five of the nine also had an aortic body tumor.

Clinically, carotid body tumors are suggested when a mass develops in the angle of the mandible in brachycephalic dogs. Complete heart block, supraventricular trachycardia, and atrial premature contractions have been associated with this condition (Hubben, Patterson, and Detweiler, 1960). Because of the frequent association of this tumor with aortic body tumors, the dog should be carefully evaluated for the presence of combined tumors.

References

Arteriovenous Fistulas

Buchanan, J. W.: Selective Angiography and Angiocardiography in Dogs with Acquired Cardiovascular Disease. J. Amer. Vet. Radiol. Soc., 6 (1965):5.

Ettinger, S., Campbell, L., Suter, P. F., DeAngelis, M., and Butler, H. C.: Peripheral Arteriovenous Fistula in a Dog. J. A. V. M. A., 153 (1968):1055.

Gomes, M. R.: Arteriovenous fistulas: A review and ten year experience at the Mayo Clinic. Mayo Clin. Proc., 45 (1970):81.

Holman, E.: Abnormal Arteriovenus Communications. Charles C Thomas, Springfield, 1968.

Rubin, L., and Patterson, D. F.: Arteriovenous Fistula of the Orbit in a Dog. Cornell Vet., 55 (1965):471.

Wallace, C. R., and Hamilton, W. F.: Study of Spontaneous Congestive Heart Failure in the Dog. Circ. Res., 11 (1962):301.

Sudden Death in Doberman Pinschers

James, T. N., and Drake, E. H.: Sudden Death in Doberman Pinschers. Ann. Intern. Med., 68 (1968):821.

Arterial Hypertension

Anderson, L. J., and Fisher, E. W.: The Blood Pressure in Canine Interstitial Nephritis. Res. Vet. Sci., 9 (1968):304.

Bloom, F.: Pathology of the Dog and Cat. American Veterinary Publications, Inc., Santa Barbara, California, 1954.

Dahme, E.: Ueber die Beurteilung der Angiopathien bei chronisch sklerosierenden Nierenerkrankungen des Hundes. Arch. Exp. Veterinärmed., 11 (1957):611.

Detweiler, D. K., Patterson, D. F., Luginbühl, H., Rhodes, W. H., Buchanan, J. W., Knight, D. H., and Hill, J. D.: Diseases of the Cardiovascular System. In *Canine Medicine*. Edited by E. J. Catcott. 1st Catcott ed. American Veterinary Publications, Inc., Santa Barbara, California, 1968, p. 589.

Howard, E. B., and Nielsen, S. W.: Pheochromocytomas Associated with Hypertensive Lesions in Dogs. J. A. V. M. A., 147 (1965a):245.

Howard, E. B., and Nielsen, S. W.: Neoplasia of the Boxer Dog. J. A. V. M. A., 147 (1965b):1121.

Jubb, K. V. F., and Kennedy, P. C.: Pathology of Domestic Animals. Academic Press, New York, 1963.

Katz, J. I., Skom, J. H., and Wakerlin, G. E.: Pathogenesis of Spontaneous and Pyelonephritic Hypertension in the Dog. Circ. Res., 13 (1957):29.

Meier, H.: Etiologic Considerations of Spontaneous Tumors in Animals with Special Reference to the Endocrine System. Ann. N. Y. Acad. Sci., 108 (1963):881.

Moulton, J. E.: Tumors in Domestic Animals. University of California Press, Berkeley, California, 1961.

Mulligan, R. M.: Neoplasms of the Dog. Williams and Wilkins Co., Baltimore, 1949.

Pirie, H. M., Mackey, L. J., and Fisher, E. W.: The Relationship between Renal Disease and Arterial Lesions in the Dog. Ann. N. Y. Acad. Sci., 127 (1965):861.

Smith, H. A., and Jones, T. C.: Veterinary Pathology. Lea & Febiger, Philadelphia, 1957.

Spörri, H., and Leemann, W.: Das Verhalten des Blutdruckes bei Hunden mit chronischinterstitieller Nephritis. Zbl. Veterinärmed., 8 (1961):523.

Aneurysm of the Heart and Great Vessels

Bailey, W. S.: Epizootiology of Cancer in Animals. Ann. N. Y. Acad. Sci., 108 (1963):890.

Danhof, I. E.: Right Ventricular Aneurysm. J. A. V. M. A., 137, (1960):465.

Aortic and Arterial Embolism

Axelson, R. D., Secord, A. C., and Weber, L. G.: Aortic Embolism in a Dog—A Case Report. Anim. Hosp., 4 (1968):183.

Baxter, J. S.: Embolism of the Femoral Artery. Vet. Rec., 81 (1967):569.

Buchanan, J. W., Baker, G. J., and Hill, J. D.: Aortic Embolism in Cats: Prevalence, Surgical Treatment, and Electrocardiography. Vet. Rec., 79 (1966):496.

Denholm, T. C.: Thrombosis of the Femoral Artery in a Dog. Vet. Rec., 75 (1963):970.

Holzworth, J., Simpson, R., and Wind, A.: Aortic Thrombosis with Posterior Paralysis in the Cat. Cornell Vet., 45 (1955):468.

Imhoff, R. K., and Tashjian, R. J.: Diagnosis of Aortic Embolism by Aortography. J. A. V. M. A., 139 (1961):203.

Ishmael, J., and Udall, N. D.: A Case of Aortic Thrombosis in the Dog. Vet. Rec., 79 (1966):570.

Kraft, C. G., and Kraft, A. M.: Thromboembolic Occlusion of the Iliac Arteries in a Dog. J. A. V. M. A., 147 (1965):944.

Nims, R.: Embolectomy in the Dog. J. A. V. M. A., 140 (1962):668.

Shouse, C. L., and Meier, H.: Acute Vegetative Endocarditis in the Dog and Cat. J. A. V. M. A., 129 (1956):278.

Simultaneous Synchronous Contraction of the Heart and Diaphragm

Bohn, F. K., and Patterson, D. F.: Long Standing Unilateral Contraction of the Diaphragm with the Heart Beat. J. A. V. M. A., 156 (1970):1411.

Detweiler, D. K.: Contraction of the Diaphragm Synchronous with the Heartbeat in Dogs. J. A. V. M. A., 126 (1955):445.

Ettinger, S., Suter, P. F., and Gould, L.: Synchronous Myocardial and Diaphragmatic Contractions in a Dog. J.A.M.A., 208 (1969):2475.

Grauwiler, J.: Ueber einen Fall von herzsynchronen Zwerchfellskontraktionen beim Hund. Berlin. München. Tierärztl. Wschr., 72 (1959):383.

Smith, L. K.: Contraction of the Diaphragm Synchronous with the Heartbeat in a Dog. J. A. V. M. A., 146 (1965):611.

Wyssman, E.: Über Zwerchfellkrämpfe bei unseren Haustieren. Schweiz. Arch. Tierheilk, 82 (1940):175.

Secondary Cardiac Disease in Response to Extracardiac Disease

Anderson, L. J., and Fisher, E. W.: The Blood Pressure in Canine Interstitial Nephritis. Res. Vet. Sci., 9 (1968):304.

Carb, A. V.: Polycythemia Vera in a Dog. J. A. V. M. A., 154 (1969):289.

Dahme, E.: Morphologische Studien zur formalen Genese der Schrumpfniere des Hundes: chronische-interstitielle Nephritis. Mh. Tierheilk., 7 (1955):17.

Dahme, E.: Ueber die Beurteilung der Angiopathien bei chronisch sklerosierenden Nierenerkrankungen des Hundes. Arch. Exp. Veterinärmed., 11 (1957):611.

Detweiler, D. K., and Patterson, D. F.: A Phonograph Record of Heart Sounds and Murmurs of the Dog. Ann. N. Y. Acad. Sci., 127 (1965):322.

Detweiler, D. K., Patterson, D. F., Luginbühl, H., Rhodes, W. H., Buchanan, J. W., Knight, D. H., and Hill, J. D.: Diseases of the Cardiovascular System. In *Canine Medicine*. Edited by E. J. Catcott. 1st Catcott ed. American Veterinary Publications, Inc., Santa Barbara, California, 1968, p. 589.

Duke, M., and Abelman, W. H.: The Hemodynamic Response to Chronic Anemia. Circulation, 39 (1969):503.

Hermreck, A. S., and Thal, A. P.: Mechanisms for the High Circulatory Requirements in Sepsis and Shock. Surgery, 170 (1969):677.

Marshak, R. R., Webster, G. D., and Skelly, J. F.: Observations on a Case of Primary Adrenocortical Insufficiency in a Dog. J. A. V. M. A., 136 (1960):274.

Nieberle, K., and Cohrs, P.: Lehrbuch der speziellen pathologischen Anatomie der Haustiere. 3rd ed. Gustav Fischer, Jena, Germany, 1952.

Pirie, H. M., Mackey, L. J., and Fisher, E. W.: The Relationship between Renal Disease and Arterial Lesions in the Dog. Ann. N. Y. Acad. Sci., 127 (1965):861.

Reed, C. F., Pensinger, R. R., Ferrigan, L. W., and Parkes, L.: Functioning Adenocarcinoma in a Dog with Mitral Insufficiency. J. Amer. Vet. Radiol. Soc., 4 (1963):36.

Siegel, E. T., O'Brien, J. B., Pyle, L., and Schryver, H. F.: Functional Adrenocortical Carcinoma in a Dog. J. A. V. M. A., 150 (1967):760.

Siegel, E. T., Schryver, H. F., and Fidler, I.: Clinico-Pathologic Conference (Adrenocortical Atrophy). J. A. V. M. A., 150 (1967):423.

Spörri, H., and Leemann, W.: Das Verhalten des Blutdruckes bei Hunden mit chronisch-interstitieller Nephritis. Zbl. Veterinärmed., 8 (1961):523.

Cardiac Neoplasia

Bloom, F.: Structure and Histogenesis of Tumors of the Aortic Bodies in Dogs. Arch. Path., 36 (1943):1.

Brodey, R. S., and Prier, J. E.: Clinico-Pathologic Conference (Malignant Aortic Body Tumor with Pulmonary Metastasis). J. A. V. M. A., 141 (1962):739.

Buchanan, J. W.: Selective Angiography and Angiocardiography in Dogs with Acquired Cardiovascular Disease. J. Amer. Vet. Rad. Soc., 6 (1965):5.

Colby, E. D., and Collins, W. G.: Reticulum-Cell Sarcoma with Cardiac Involvement. Vet. Med., 60 (1965):1021.

Detweiler, D. K.: Wesen und Häufigkeit von Herzkrankheiten bei Hunden. Zbl. Veterinärmed., 9 (1962):317.

Dobberstein, J., and Tamaschke, C.: Die Blastome des Herzens. In *Joest's Handbuch der speziellen pathologischen Anatomie der Haustiere*. Edited by J. Dobberstein, G. Pallaske, and J. Stünzi. Paul Parey, Berlin, Germany, 3rd ed, Vol. 2, 1962, p. 167.

Geib, W.: Primary Angiomatous Tumors of the Heart and Great Vessels: A report of two cases in the dog. Cor. Vet., 57 (1967):292.

Harpster, N. K.: Case Records of the Angell Memorial Animal Hospital (Left Atrial Tear). J. A. V. M. A., 154 (1969):413.

Howard, E. B., and Nielsen, S. W.: Neoplasia in the Boxer Dog. Amer. J. Vet. Res., 26 (1965):1121.

Hubben, K., Patterson, D. F., and Detweiler, D. K.: Carotid Body Tumor in the Dog. J. A. V. M. A., 137 (1960):411.

Johnson, K. H.: Aortic Body Tumors in the Dog. J. A. V. M. A., 152 (1968):154.

Jubb, K. V. F., and Kennedy, P. C.: Pathology of Domestic Animals. 1st ed. Academic Press, New York, 1963.

Jubb, K. V. F., and Kennedy, P. C.: Tumors of the Nonchromaffin Paraganglia in Dogs. Cancer, 10 (1957):89.

Kast, A.: Herzbasistumoren beim Hund. Zbl. Veterinärmed., 5 (1958):459.

Kleine, L. J.: Case Records of the Angell Memorial Animal Hospital (Hemangioendothelioma of the Heart). J. A. V. M. A., 153 (1968):325.

Kleine, L. J., Zook, B. C., and Munson, T. O.: Primary Cardiac Hemangiosarcomas in Dogs. J. A. V. M. A., 157 (1970):326.

Kurtz, H. J., and Finco, D. R.: Carotid Body and Aortic Body Tumors in a Dog — A Case Report. Amer. J. Vet. Res., 30 (1969):1247.

Lieberman, L. L.: Malignant Hemangio-Endothelioma of the Canine Heart. J. A. V. M. A., 126 (1955):296.

Loppnow, H.: Zur Kasuistik primärer Herztumoren beim Hund (zwei Fälle von Hämangiom am rechten Herzohr). Berlin. München. Tierärztl. Wschr., 74 (1961):214.

Luginbühl, H., and Detweiler, D. K.: Cardiovascular Lesions in Dogs. Ann. N. Y. Acad. Sci., 127 (1965):517.

Moulton, J. E.: Tumors in Domestic Animals. 1st ed. University of California Press, Berkeley, California, 1961.

Nilsson, A.: A Case of Metastatic Tumor of the Glomus Aorticus in a Dog. Nord. Vet.-Med., 8 (1956):875.

Nilsson, T.: Heart-Base Tumors in the Dog. Acta Path. Microbiol. Scand., 37 (1955):385.

Palumbo, N. E.: Canine Cardiac Disease Due to Metastatic Carcinoma. J. A. V. M. A., 150 (1967):396.

Patterson, D. F.: Angiocardiography. J. Amer. Vet. Radiol. Soc., 1 (1961):26.

Riser, W. H., and Bailey, L. K.: Heart Base Tumor in a Dog. North Amer. Vet., 30 (1949):388.

Roberts, S. R.: Myxoma of the Heart in a Dog. J. A. V. M. A., 134 (1959):185.

Sandersleben, J. von: Die Leukosen und Retikulose beim Hund. Arch. Exp. Veterinärmed., 15 (1961):620, 687.

Scotti, T. M.: The Carotid Body Tumor in Dogs. J. A. V. M. A., 132 (1958):413.

Stünzi, H., and Mann, M.: Pathologisch-anatomische Befunde beim Hämopericard des Hundes. Schweiz. Arch. Tierheilk. 112 (1970):233.

CHAPTER
18

CONGENITAL HEART DISEASE

A discussion of the incidence and method of classification of congenital heart diseases may be found in Chapter 12 (pp. 318-319). We believe that the recognition of congenital heart disease in the dog is important for the following reasons:

1. It is important to recognize congenital heart disease when a recently purchased dog is presented to the veterinarian for physical examination and vaccination. If an abnormality is found, the veterinarian should discuss with the owner the advantages of returning the dog, especially since the prospect of a normal lifespan may be poor.

2. If the owner decides to keep the dog, it should be explained that cardiac therapy may be necessary later in the dog's life. However, medical therapy and restriction of exercise and sodium intake are not indicated until the dog shows signs of heart failure.

3. Surgical correction of certain congenital defects is feasible. The advisability of a surgical procedure should be discussed with the owner after the prognosis, expense, and mortality rate for the procedure are reviewed.

4. Congenital cardiac defects may occasionally be associated with other congenital lesions. Therefore, an additional effort should be made to rule out the likelihood of concurrent congenital anomalies.

PATENT DUCTUS ARTERIOSUS

The ductus arteriosus arises from the left sixth aortic arch and is a short arterial connection which functions in fetal life to circumvent pulmonary circulation and thus carry blood from the pulmonary artery to the distal portion of the   477 aortic arch and systemic circulation. When it remains patent beyond the first days of postnatal life, it is a congenital cardiac lesion and is referred to as a patent ductus arteriosus (PDA).

In the fetus, pulmonary circulation is minimal because of high pulmonary resistance, and blood is oxygenated in the placental vessels rather than in the nonfunctional fetal lungs. Immediately after birth and inflation of the lungs, the pressure in the right heart and the pulmonary arteries diminishes while the systemic pressure rises surpassing right ventricular pressure. Normally, closure of the ductus arteriosus occurs during the first weeks after birth, probably in response to changes in blood oxygen saturation (Buchanan, 1968). A nonpatent fibrous cord known as the ligamentum arteriosum persists after closure of the ductus arteriosus as a result of intimal proliferation, smooth muscle degeneration, and fibrosis (Buchanan, 1968).

If the ductus remains patent after birth, the rising pressure in the aorta and the left ventricle, which surpasses that in the right heart, reverses the direction of blood flow from the aorta into the pulmonary artery and occasionally into the right

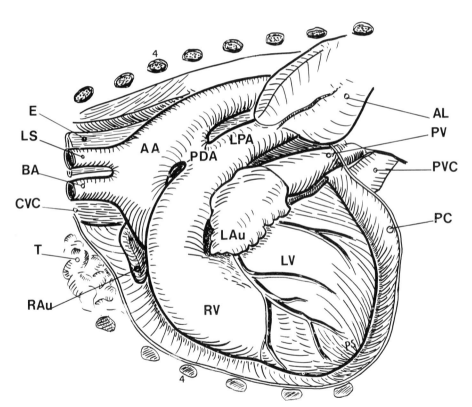

FIGURE 18-1 Drawing of the heart and great vessels from a 4 month old German Shepherd dog with a patent ductus arteriosus, viewed from the left side. The pericardium has been opened to show the details more clearly. (E) esophagus; (LS) left subclavian artery; (BA) brachiocephalic artery; (CVC) cranial vena cava; (T) thymus; (RAu) right auricle; (AA) aortic arch; (PDA) patent ductus arteriosus connecting the descending aorta with the left pulmonary artery (LPA); (RV) right ventricle; (LV) left ventricle; (AL) left apical lobe of the lung; (PV) pulmonary vein entering the left atrium; (PVC) caudal vena cava; (PC) pericardial sac; (4) transection of the fourth rib.

ventricle (Fig. 18-1). The shunting occurs in both systole and diastole, thereby decreasing the amount of blood reaching the systemic circulation. In order to maintain adequate systemic circulation for normal life function, the total blood volume increases, and the left ventricle is thus forced to increase output above normal levels.

Since oxygenated blood from the aorta is shunted into the pulmonary artery, which normally transports venous blood, the condition is referred to as an arterio-venous fistula. Patent ductus arteriosus is the most common form of arteriovenous fistula in dogs (see p. 456). Patent ductus arteriosus was recognized by a number of investigators prior to 1960 (Brooks, 1912; Hare and Orr, 1931; Cordy and Ribelin, 1950; Detweiler, 1952; Spörri and Scheitlin, 1952; Walters and Bramer, 1952; von Sandersleben, 1953; Dolowy et al., 1957; Saunders, 1957; Schmutzer, Marable, and Maloney, 1958; Pallaske, 1959). Since the 1960's, the condition has been frequently recognized and corrected surgically. Frese (1961) reported a patent ductus arteriosus that coexisted with a persistent right aortic arch. The size of the lumen of the ductus was, however, relatively small, and clinical signs were absent. Hare and Orr (1931) reported patent ductus arteriosus in a dog with ventricular septal defect. Patterson (1965) reported the occurrence of the following malformations in association with a patent ductus arteriosus: patent foramen ovale, pulmonic stenosis, tetralogy of Fallot, and persistent right aortic arch (see Figs. 18-19 and 18-20).

Purebred dogs such as the Poodle, Collie, and Pomeranian are most often affected, according to Patterson and Detweiler (1967), and Patterson (1968), and we have often observed the condition in German Shepherds as well.

HISTORY AND CARDIAC EXAMINATION

Dogs with this lesion may develop signs of severe heart failure in the first few weeks or months of life. Nine of 15 puppies with patent ductus arteriosus died between 2 and 6 weeks of age in a study by Patterson (1968). When this period has passed, many dogs with patent ductus arteriosus remain asymptomatic for variable lengths of time, and the condition is then usually recognized on routine physical examination. Then clinical signs develop after the dog reaches maturity, often between the ages of 8 months and 3 years. Older dogs with a patent ductus arteriosus (5 and 6 years old) without clinical signs have been described by Pierau et al. (1964) and by Schmidt, Hohaus, and Röder (1967). Frequently, a previously normal-appearing, well-nourished dog is presented to the veterinarian because of fatigue, lack of stamina, dyspnea, exertional dyspnea, hindlimb weakness, weight loss, and abdominal swelling. Coughing after excitement or exercise as well as fainting or seizures have been seen clinically by Buchanan (1968) and by the authors. Unrelated diseases such as tonsillitis, leptospirosis, or pneumonia place an additional burden on the heart and may be responsible for decompensation (Spörri and Scheitlin, 1952; Pallaske, 1959).

The color of the mucous membranes is usually normal. However, when pulmonary hypertension develops it results in a gradual reversal of the shunt of blood from right to left (pulmonary artery to aorta), instead of from left to right (aorta to pulmonary artery), and unoxygenated blood is shunted into the systemic circulation. Cyanosis may then develop. Because the unoxygenated blood enters the aorta distal to the aortic arch, blood supply to the head and neck is normal, and the mucous membranes are not cyanotic. However, the remainder of the body may appear blue because the blood perfusing these areas is not fully saturated with oxygen. Such advanced pulmonary hypertension with reversed shunting of blood is unusual; it occurred in only four of 61 dogs with patent ductus arteriosus reported by Detweiler and Patterson (1965) and in three of 53 dogs reported by Buchanan (1968).

Palpation of the thorax usually but not always reveals the characteristic continuous thrill over the cranial left thorax. The abdomen is unremarkable unless ascites and abdominal distention develop secondarily to right heart failure. There is a characteristic waterhammer pulse (also termed "B-B shot" or jerky pulse) in the femoral arteries which has rapid rates of rise and decline due to the wide pulse pressure in the aorta. The wide aortic pulse results from low diastolic aortic pressure, since the blood flows continuously from the aorta into the pulmonary artery and right ventricle.

AUSCULTATION

The continuous or machinery-like murmur, pathognomonic for arteriovenous fistulas, is heard over the aortic-pulmonic valve region. The murmur, continuous throughout systole and diastole, is accentuated during late systole and early diastole (Fig. 18-2), and the systolic component of the murmur may radiate

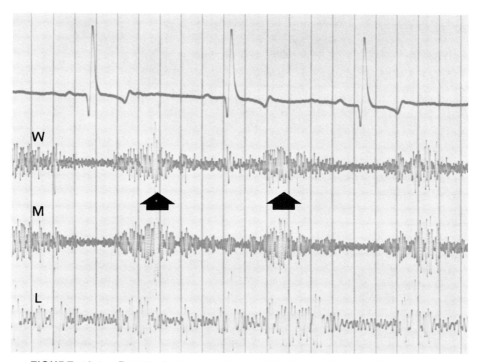

FIGURE 18-2 Patent ductus arteriosus. Machinery-like continuous murmur. The simultaneously recorded lead II electrocardiogram and the wide-band (W), medium-band (M), and low-band (L) phonocardiograms demonstrate a continuous murmur through systole and diastole. The murmur is most intense, however, during late systole and early diastole (arrows). Lead II Electrocardiogram.

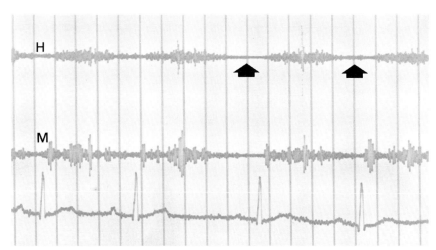

FIGURE 18-3 Patent ductus arteriosus. High-frequency (H) and medium-frequency (M) bands of the phonocardiogram recorded simultaneously with lead II of the electrocardiogram. When the heart rate is slow, the systolic-diastolic murmur of a patent ductus arteriosus may be diminished or may disappear in late diastole (arrows). As a result, the murmur is not as distinctive of a patent ductus arteriosus as is the continuous murmur shown in Figure 18-2.

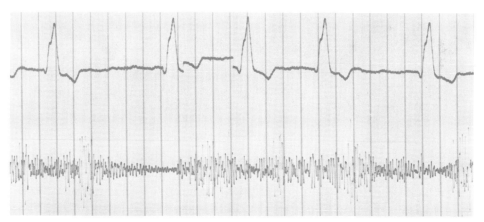

FIGURE 18-4 Patent ductus arteriosus with atrial fibrillation. Wide-band phonocardiogram and lead II of the electrocardiogram recorded simultaneously. The typical waxing and waning, continuous murmur does not occur during atrial fibrillation. When the R-R interval is prolonged, the murmur is diminished in intensity, as is seen between the first and second beats; when the R-R interval is shorter, the murmur is louder and does not diminish. A standardization impulse is present in the baseline of the electrocardiogram between the second and third QRS complexes.

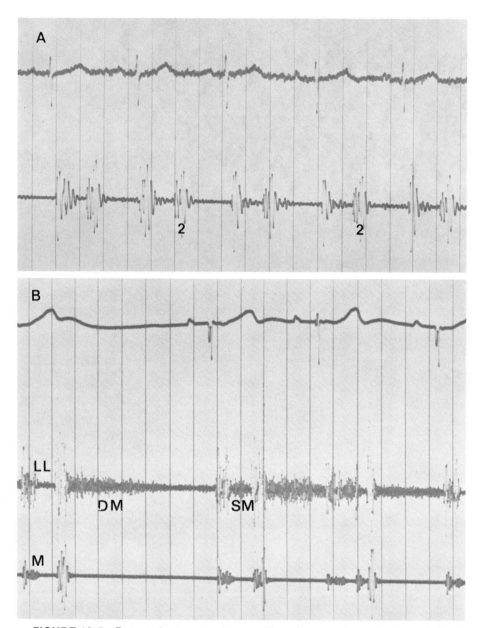

FIGURE 18-5 Patent ductus arteriosus with pulmonary hypertension. *A,* Lead I of the electrocardiogram recorded simultaneously with a wide-band phonocardiogram. Because of the similarity of left and right heart pressures in the presence of severe pulmonary hypertension, shunting of blood is minimal, and neither a systolic nor a diastolic murmur could be auscultated. Splitting of the second heart sound due to pulmonary hypertension is present (2). *B,* When a log-log channel (LL) phonocardiogram is recorded, the high-frequency sounds are accentuated. Now a diastolic murmur (DM) beginning after the second heart sound and a short systolic murmur (SM) are recognizable because of turbulence resulting from shunting of blood through the ductus from left to right. The medium-frequency band (M) records only a short systolic murmur. In this case, cardiac murmurs were not recognizable clinically with a stethoscope.

to the cervical vessels. The machinery murmur is auscultated over the cranial left precordium but may be confined to a very narrow area over the aortic and pulmonic region. Occasionally, the murmur may be auscultated *only* cranial and just dorsal to the manubrium sterni, and this area should therefore be auscultated if a patent ductus arteriosus is suspected. Infrequently, the murmur radiates widely over the thorax. Although the systolic murmur of mitral insufficiency, a result of mitral valvular incompetence following anular dilatation (Buchanan and Patterson, 1965), may be auscultated over the remaining valve regions, in some cases only the classic machinery murmur is heard over the left cranial thorax. In the young dog, the murmur of the patent ductus arteriosus may not be recognized unless all valve areas are auscultated carefully. With very slow and irregular heart rates, the diastolic murmur may not blend immediately into the systolic murmur, so that the sound is not continuous, giving the false impression of another lesion (Fig. 18-3). Similarly, when atrial fibrillation occurs, the typical waxing and waning of the machinery murmur may not be heard because of the irregular rate (Detweiler, 1957) (Fig. 18-4).

If pulmonary hypertension develops, only a systolic murmur occurs since the left-to-right shunt is limited to the systolic phase (Fig. 18-5). When pulmonary hypertension is severe and a right-to-left shunt occurs, there may be no murmur, and splitting of the second heart sound may be recognized (Brodey and Prier, 1962; Detweiler and Patterson, 1965). If the patent ductus is small, the murmur may be absent (Patterson, 1968). Pierau et al. (1964) reported that there was no murmur in a German Shepherd with a patent ductus arteriosus shunting from left to right. The dog was asymptomatic, and the diameter of the ductus was 1 cm. The authors hypothesized that the aneurysmal widening of the ductus itself could have caused the disappearance of the murmur.

In a series of puppies with patent ductus arteriosus, the murmur was first heard on the fifth to fourteenth day of life, and then only during systole; the machinery murmur developed by the end of the third week of life (Patterson, 1968). In another dog in which the patent ductus was corrected surgically at 4 weeks of age, the continuous murmur developed between the fourth and eighth days of life (Buchanan, Soma, and Patterson, 1967).

ELECTROCARDIOGRAPHY

The electrocardiogram characteristically demonstrates deep Q waves, tall R waves, and large negative T waves in leads II, III, and aVF. These findings are consistent with the diastolic overload syndrome that occurs in dogs with patent ductus arteriosus (Fig. 18-6). The amplitude of the R wave is greater than 30 mm. in lead II. Although the R wave is often large in young dogs (see p. 135), an amplitude over 30 mm. is highly suggestive of patent ductus arteriosus. Changes of the S-T segment are seen in most leads. Although the cardiac rhythm is usually normal, atrial fibrillation (see Fig. 18-3) may develop (Detweiler, 1957), and ectopic ventricular arrhythmias may occur in association with congestive heart failure.

The vectorcardiogram demonstrates normally directed but accentuated forces — i.e., left, caudal, and ventral. There is often prolongation of the initial forces to the right (Fig. 18-7).

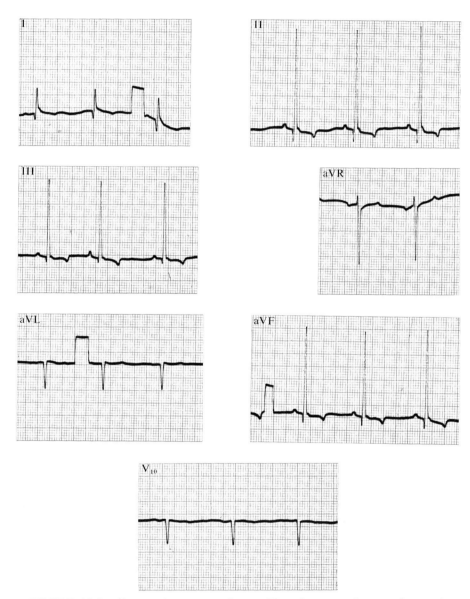

FIGURE 18-6   Patent ductus arteriosus. The electrocardiogram in most un-complicated cases of patent ductus arteriosus is typical for the disease. The mean electrical axis in the frontal plane is normal. The P and T waves and the QRS complexes are properly oriented, but the amplitude of the R wave in leads II and aVF, and occasionally lead III, is greater than 30 mm. Frequently, deep Q and T waves occur as well. In advanced cases (not demonstrated), there may be an increased depolarization time of both the atria and the ventricles, indicated by wide P waves and QRS complexes.

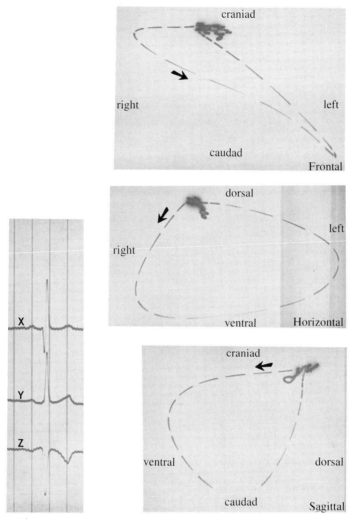

FIGURE 18-7   The vectorcardiogram associated with patent ductus arteriosus indicates an increase in the initial rightward forces (> 0.01 sec.) owing to hypertrophy of the interventricular septum. Also, there is an increase in the amplitude of all forces, indicated by increases in both size of the loops and area within the loops. The P and T loops, which are not clearly demonstrated in this tracing, are normally directed.

RADIOGRAPHIC EXAMINATION

The radiographic signs in most dogs with patent ductus arteriosus are characteristic unless the dog is in severe heart failure. The signs vary greatly, depending on the severity of the shunt and the duration of the condition. The radiographic appearance of the thorax in dogs with patent ductus arteriosus has been described in detail (Hamlin, 1960, 1968; Detweiler, 1962; Buchanan, 1968).

In the *lateral radiograph* (Fig. 18-8), marked enlargement of the cardiac silhouette and elevation of the trachea are usually present owing to an increase in the apicobasilar diameter of the heart. The left atrium is enlarged to varying degrees, depending on the severity of the shunt of blood, the duration of the disease, the degree of secondary mitral insufficiency produced by dilatation of the mitral anulus, and the degree of failure present. The left ventricular enlargement is often more difficult to see. The degree of enlargement depends on the same factors as mentioned for atrial enlargement. The right ventricle is enlarged in most dogs with patent ductus arteriosus. In characteristic cases, the widened aortic arch bulges cranially and thus eliminates the cranial waist of the heart. In radiographs which have been exposed with enough penetration, the enlarged aortic arch can be seen in the precardial mediastinum. The diameter of the apical lobar arteries and veins is increased due to the increased pulmonary circulation in left-to-right shunts, and their diameters exceed the smallest diameter of the dorsal third of the fourth rib (Buchanan, 1968). Overcirculation is also indicated by the increased density of the lung field. In some cases a number of small, straight, parallel, band-like densities representing dilated arteries and veins can be seen in the diaphragmatic lobar area.

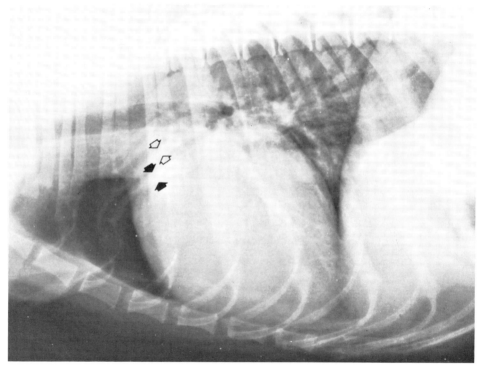

FIGURE 18-8 Left lateral radiograph, 4 year old female Springer Spaniel which had a continuous, machinery-like murmur typical of a patent ductus arteriosus. The dog had been asymptomatic but had recently developed mild signs of ensuing right and left heart failure. The dog was successfully operated on for an uncomplicated patent ductus arteriosus. Mild, generalized cardiac enlargement is indicated by elevation of the trachea and an increase in the craniocaudal diameter of the cardiac silhouette. The ventral bend at the distal extremity of the trachea has been eliminated, and there is slight left atrial enlargement. The cranial waist of the cardiac silhouette has disappeared. The caudal waist is still present. The caudal vena cava is slightly denser than normal. There was slight liver enlargement on abdominal radiographs (not shown). The lung field is less lucent than normal, and there is some blurring of the slightly dilated pulmonary arteries and veins. The right apical lobar vein (dark arrows) and the right apical lobar artery (clear arrows) are indicated. Their diameters do not exceed the diameter of the proximal third of the fourth rib.

The *dorsoventral radiograph* usually demonstrates more typical radiographic signs of patent ductus arteriosus than does the lateral projection. The cardiac silhouette is elongated, owing in part to the wide cranial bulging of the aortic arch. The right cardiac border is rounder than normal, and there are three bulging densities on the left cardiac border (Fig. 18-9). When all three bulging densities are present, they are pathognomonic for patent ductus arteriosus. The first bulge

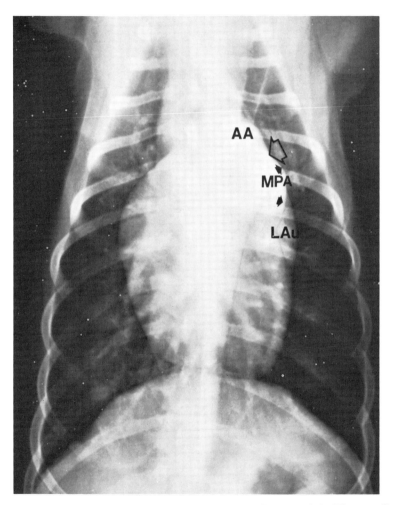

FIGURE 18-9 Dorsoventral radiograph, dog in Figure 18-8. The cardiac silhouette is elongated, and the aortic arch (AA) extends far cranially, with an aneurysmal widening to the left side (clear arrow). Caudal to the aortic bulge, a second bulge (small black arrows) represents the pulmonary artery segment (MPA) of the cardiac silhouette, which is within normal limits. Caudal to the pulmonary artery segment, a third, flat bulge indicates enlargement of the left auricle (LAu). This triad of bulges is diagnostic for patent ductus arteriosus. The left ventricular border is nearly normal. The slight bulge of the right ventricular border indicates mild right ventricular enlargement. The prominent pulmonary arteries are not as well defined as in the lateral radiograph (Fig. 18-8).

is caused by an aneurysmal widening of the descending portion of the aortic arch where the ductus arises. It is seen in most radiographs which have been exposed with sufficient penetration. The pulmonary artery segment, slightly wider than normal, is the second bulge. The third bulge results from the protrusion of the left auricle beyond the left cardiac border. It is located caudal to the pulmonary artery segment. The left ventricular border is frequently rounder than normal. The apex of the heart is widened, and dilated intrapulmonary arteries and veins are visualized on the dorsoventral view.

Radiographs made after surgical correction of patent ductus arteriosus demonstrate the reversibility of most of these signs. The cardiac silhouette begins to diminish in size within days. The left atrium becomes smaller immediately after surgery but usually remains slightly larger than normal. The signs of pulmonary overcirculation disappear immediately. The widened aortic arch persists but eventually diminishes somewhat in size.

In dogs with patent ductus arteriosus which are in heart failure, the generalized cardiac enlargement becomes so prominent that the details described above are often no longer discernible. Pulmonary congestion and alveolar edema further obscure the details, making it difficult to differentiate the condition from mitral insufficiency and heart failure, or from other congenital heart diseases and secondary

TABLE 18-1   ROENTGEN ANALYSIS OF COMMON CONGENITAL HEART DISEASES

APPEARANCE OF LUNG FIELD AND MUCOUS MEMBRANES	MALFORMATION	APPROXIMATE FREQUENCY*	CARDIAC SILHOUETTE
Overcirculation or hypervascularity and no cyanosis; left-to-right shunting of blood	Patent ductus arteriosus	30%	Elongated cardiac silhouette; enlarged aortic arch; aneurysmal widening of the aortic arch; enlarged pulmonary artery segment
	Uncomplicated ventricular septal defect	7%	Enlarged right ventricle, left atrium, and pulmonary artery segment
	Uncomplicated atrial septal defect	4%	Enlarged right atrium, left atrium, and right ventricle
Unremarkable vascular markings and no cyanosis; no shunting of blood; congestion may develop secondary to heart failure	Pulmonic stenosis	21%	Enlarged right ventricle and pulmonary artery segment; normal left heart
	Aortic stenosis	15%	Prominent aortic arch; occasionally, left ventricular and left atrial enlargement occurring secondarily
	Persistent right aortic arch or other vascular ring anomalies	8%	Cardiac silhouette unremarkable; esophageal dilatation and secondary aspiration pneumonia
	Persistent left cranial vena cava	5%	None, unless complicated anomaly
	Mitral insufficiency	3%	Enlarged left atrium and left ventricle; secondarily, enlargement of right ventricle and pulmonary congestion
Undercirculation or hypovascularity and cyanosis (see also Table 18-2)	Tetralogy of Fallot	4%	Enlarged right ventricle; variable pulmonary artery segment, usually small
	Atrial septal defect with tricuspid stenosis	—	Enlarged right atrium and possibly left atrium

Data from Patterson, D. F.: Circ. Res., 23 ,1968.; 171. Used by permission.

TABLE 18-2   ROENTGEN DIAGNOSIS OF CONGENITAL HEART DISEASE (UNCOMMON ALTERNATIVES TO CONGENITAL DISEASES INCLUDED IN TABLE 18-1)*

APPEARANCE OF LUNG FIELD AND MUCOUS MEMBRANES	MALFORMATION
Pulmonary vasculature increased and cyanosis present	Truncus arteriosus
	Pulmonary vein anomaly (draining into the right side of the heart)
	Aortic atresia or hypoplasia with ventricular septal defect
	Pulmonary vasculature obstruction secondary to intracardiac or extracardiac shunts: Eisenmenger complex with atrial septal defect, ventricular septal defect, or patent ductus arteriosus. The hallmark in these cases is centrally increased pulmonary vasculature and peripherally diminished pulmonary vasculature.
Decreased pulmonary vasculture and cyanosis	Pulmonic stenosis with: atrial septal defect (trilogy of Fallot); tetralogy of Fallot with atrial septal defect (pentalogy of Fallot); ventricular septal defect; single ventricle
	Tricuspid anomalies combined with: atrial septal defect or pulmonic stenosis, or both (Ebstein's anomaly)
	Severe pulmonic stenosis
Unremarkable pulmonary vasculture and no cyanosis; failure, congestion, and/or cyanosis may develop secondarily	Fibroelastosis (globular heart)
	Anomalies of the coronary arteries
Increased pulmonary vasculature and no cyanosis	Aorticopulmonary window
	Partial pulmonary vein anomaly
	Fibroelastosis (venous congestion)
	Pulmonary vasculature obstruction secondary to intracardiac or extracardiac shunts: Eisenmenger complex with atrial septal defect, ventricular septal defect, or patent ductus arteriosus. The hallmark in these cases is centrally increased pulmonary vasculature and peripherally diminished pulmonary vasculature

*From Meschan (1966), Klatte and Burko (1968), and Spitz (1968).

heart failure. Liver enlargement and ascites occasionally accompany the signs of heart failure, as may pericardial effusion (von Sandersleben, 1953; Pallaske, 1959).

CARDIAC CATHETERIZATION AND ANGIOCARDIOGRAPHY

Cardiac catheterization reveals increased pressure in the right ventricle and pulmonary artery and normal pressure in the left side of the heart. The pulmonary arterial pressure should always be greater than right ventricular pressure in this condition (Fig. 18-10). If pulmonary hypertension develops, the pulmonary arterial pressure may approximate or even surpass the aortic pressure (Fig. 18-11). This results in reversal of the shunt of blood. In asymptomatic dogs, the pulmonary arterial pressures may be normal (Schmidt, Hohaus, and Röder, 1967).

Determination of oxygen saturation of the blood in the various chambers also assists in the diagnosis of patent ductus arteriosus. The oxygen saturation is greater than 95 per cent in the aorta, and when oxygenated blood is shunted into the pulmonary artery, pulmonary arterial oxygen concentrations are higher than

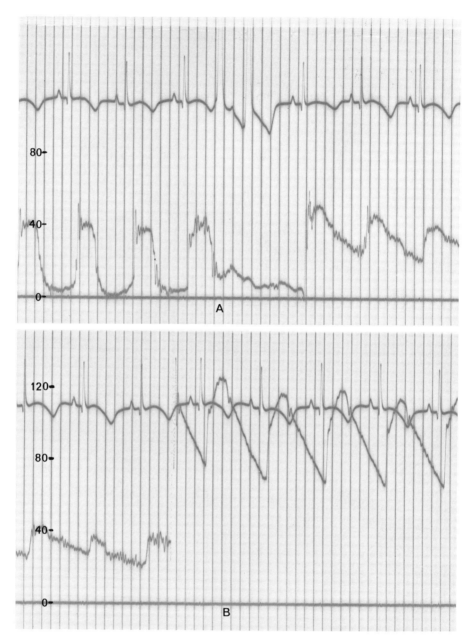

FIGURE 18-10 Patent ductus arteriosus. Pressure recordings made as catheter is withdrawn from the right ventricle into the pulmonary artery, ductus arteriosus, and finally the aorta. In *A*, the systolic pressures are slightly elevated, and the diastolic pressures are normal in the right ventricle (40/5 mm. Hg) and pulmonary artery (40/20 mm. Hg). Two ventricular premature contractions occurred as the catheter was advanced across the pulmonic valve, resulting in a temporary loss of pulse pressure. As the catheter is drawn through the patent ductus arteriosus (*B*), the pressure recording suddenly changes form, and an aortic pressure curve is recorded. The wide pulse pressure in the aortic tracing (120/65 mm. Hg) is characteristic of a patent ductus arteriosus and is responsible for the water-hammer or B-B shot arterial pulse. Withdrawal of the catheter through the patent ductus arteriosus provides positive proof of the diagnosis. Paper speed = 50 mm./sec.; time lines = 0.1 sec.

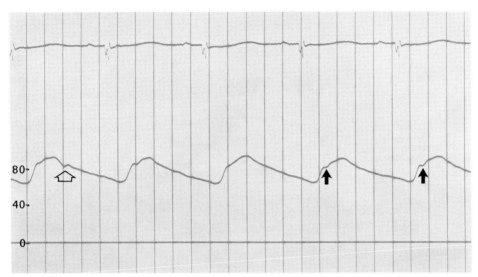

FIGURE 18-11 Hypertensive patent ductus arteriosus. Withdrawal pressure tracing made as the catheter was withdrawn from the pulmonary artery (open arrow) through the patent ductus arteriosus into the aorta (black arrows). Although there is a slight variation of the contour of the pulmonary arterial and systemic pulse curves, the pressures are the same in both. No murmur was heard in this dog because, with equal pressures in the pulmonary artery and aorta, there was no blood flow through the ductus. Pulmonary hypertension was proved by this pressure tracing and was responsible for splitting of the second heart sound.

normal. In uncomplicated cases, the oxygen saturation should be normal in the venae cavae and right atrium; it is increased in the right ventricle and is greatest in the main pulmonary artery. In one case (Brodey and Prier, 1962), the oxygen saturation in the abdominal aorta was 68 to 70 per cent, and it was 68 per cent in the main pulmonary artery. In a 6 year old, asymptomatic dog, the difference in oxygen saturation between the pulmonary artery and right ventricle or right atrium was 1.5 vol. per cent (Pierau et al., 1964). Dye-dilution or thermodilution methods can also be used to demonstrate the presence of a shunt between the right and left heart. Pierau et al. (1964) used ascorbic acid as an indicator to obtain a characteristic dye dilution curve in a dog with asymptomatic patent ductus arteriosus.

When the catheter is passed retrograde through the aorta, it may pass directly from the aorta through the patent ductus arteriosus into the pulmonary artery and right ventricle, providing positive proof of the presence of a patent ductus arteriosus. Figure 18-11 demonstrates a pressure recording made as the catheter is withdrawn from the right ventricle into the pulmonary artery, the patent ductus arteriosus, and finally the aorta.

Angiocardiography is not necessary for the routine diagnosis of patent ductus arteriosus but can be of great value in dogs without typical clinical signs such as the machinery-like murmur. It is also helpful if associated congenital cardiac lesions are suspected or if secondary signs of heart failure are present and thus mask the usually diagnostic features. Angiocardiography has been used by Buchanan (1968) to follow the condition postoperatively. Angiocardiography in patent ductus arteriosus has been discussed by Hamlin (1959), Buchanan and Patterson (1965), and Patterson (1968).

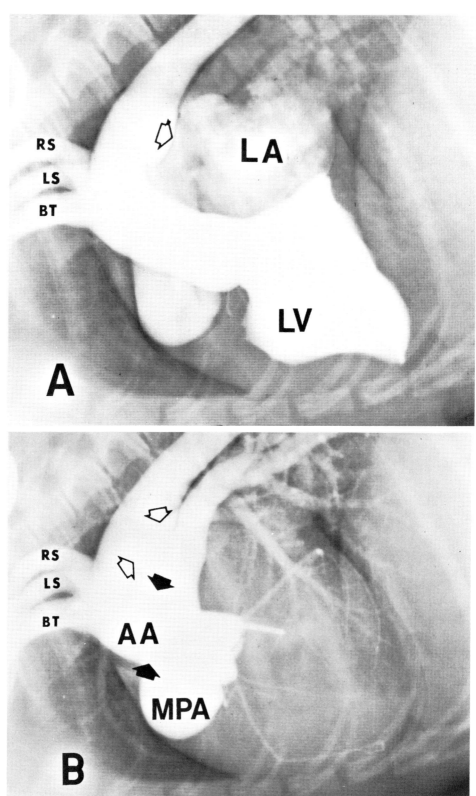

FIGURE 18-12 A & B   See legend on opposite page.

To demonstrate an uncomplicated patent ductus arteriosus with left-to-right shunt, selective injection of contrast medium at the aortic root is preferable. Because a ventricular septal defect produces radiographic signs similar to those of patent ductus arteriosus when contrast medium is injected into the left ventricle, a selective left ventricular injection is not as desirable as the aortic root injection. Ventricular injections (Fig. 18-12), however, have the advantage of indicating the presence of mitral insufficiency. When a ventricular septal defect is suspected, an additional left ventricular injection is essential. Nonselective procedures are usually not diagnostic for reasons mentioned earlier (see pp. 193-196).

The simultaneous outlining of the aorta and the main pulmonary artery after selective aortic root injection is usually diagnostic of patent ductus arteriosus. The ductus itself is not regularly outlined because of partial superimposition of the aorta and the pulmonary artery (Fig. 18-12). There is always an aneurysmal widening of the descending portion of the aortic arch at the site where the ductus originates which is considered to occur consistently and to be pathognomonic for patent ductus arteriosus (Buchanan and Patterson, 1965). An aorticopulmonary window or a rupture of the sinus of Valsalva (Kleine, Bisgard, and Lewis, 1966) and subsequent communication with the pulmonary artery or right ventricle may cause signs similar to those seen with patent ductus arteriosus. These are extremely rare conditions in the dog, however. Abnormal branching of the aortic arch is occasionally recognized as an associated anomaly. In the rare case in which a reversed shunt (right-to-left) is suspected, the injection of contrast medium into the main pulmonary artery resulting in the dye immediately entering the aorta and systemic circulation is diagnostic.

FIGURE 18-12 Selective left ventricular angiocardiograms, lateral view, 8 month old female Poodle. A continuous, machinery-like murmur with maximal intensity over the pulmonic and aortic valve regions was heard on auscultation.

A, Radiograph exposed early in the series. The left ventricle (LV) looks dilated, and contrast medium has regurgitated into the left atrium (LA). The unusual shape of the ventricle and the regurgitation suggest the possibility of a ventricular premature contraction due to the injection of contrast medium. The aortic arch is filled with contrast medium, and a small bulge (clear arrow) represents the aortic dilatation at the origin of the patent ductus arteriosus. Some contrast medium has already flowed retrograde into the main pulmonary artery, which can be differentiated from the aorta by its lesser density owing to mixing of contrast medium with blood. The branching at the aortic arch is abnormal. From top to bottom, the following arteries are seen: right subclavian artery (RS), left subclavian artery (LS), and bicarotid trunk (BT).

Radiograph *B* was exposed late in the series. The contrast medium has left the left ventricle, and the aortic valve is closed. There is simultaneous filling of the aorta and the main pulmonary artery (MPA). The patent ductus arteriosus is located between the clear arrows. The aorta or the pulmonary artery is usually partially superimposed on it. The ductus connects the dilatation of the aorta seen in *A* with the left pulmonary artery, where it branches from the main pulmonary artery. The widening of the aorta at the location of the ductus is a characteristic sign. The ascending aorta (AA), which is of the same density as the main pulmonary artery, is indicated (two black arrows). The abnormal branching at the aortic arch is the same as in radiograph (*A*). Supravalvular aortic injection of contrast medium would produce a similar angiographic appearance.

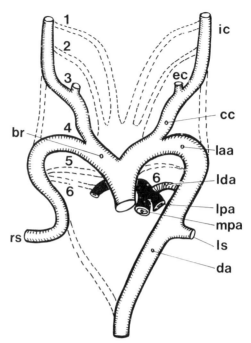

FIGURE 18-13   Schematic drawing of the normal embryologic development of the aortic arch system, ventrodorsal view. The uninterrupted lines represent the portions of the embryologic arch system that normally persist after birth, and the broken lines indicate the rudimentary or transient aortic arches. The first and second arches have involuted and do not contribute significantly to the permanent arterial system. The common carotid (cc), internal carotid (ic), and external carotid (ec) arteries originate from the third pair of arches and the aortic sac. The left aortic arch (laa) is derived from the left fourth arch and portions of the left dorsal aorta. The brachiocephalic artery (br) and the right subclavian artery (rs) originate from the right fourth aortic arch and portions of the right dorsal aorta. The fifth pair of aortic arches disappears in embryonic life, as does the dorsal right sixth aortic arch. The ventral right sixth aortic arch forms the pulmonary artery. The left ductus arteriosus (lda) originates from the left sixth or pulmonary arch and normally closes after birth to become the ligamentum arteriosum. It connects the left pulmonary artery (lpa) with the descending aorta (da). The main pulmonary artery (mpa) develops as the truncus arteriosus splits. The descending aorta (da) originates from the merged dorsal right and left aortae. The left subclavian artery (ls) normally arises from the descending aorta. (Adapted from Arey, L. B.: Developmental Anatomy. W. B. Saunders, Philadelphia, 7th ed., 1965.)

PROGNOSIS AND THERAPY

Long-term survival of dogs with patent ductus arteriosus is unusual. Although the authors have occasionally seen older dogs with the condition, most dogs that reach 6 weeks of age without developing heart failure develop congestive heart failure and die between 8 months and 3 years of age. From the studies of Patterson (1968) described previously (see page 479), it is apparent that a number of puppies with this condition die prior to 6 weeks of age and as early as a few days of age. It is therefore recommended that surgical intervention be undertaken as early as possible after the diagnosis is made (see Chapter 19). When the operation is performed, the outcome depends on the skill and experience of the surgeon and the anesthetist (Buchanan, 1968). Surgery is contraindicated if a large right-to-left shunt is proved by catheterization, since the degree of pulmonary hypertension could not be tolerated after the ductus is ligated (Buchanan, 1968). When associated congenital cardiac defects are present, the decision of whether or not to close a patent ductus arteriosus must be weighed carefully. In tetralogy of Fallot or other conditions in which there is pulmonary undercirculation, one would prefer to maintain pulmonary circulation by leaving the ductus patent.

Since most dogs are presented for surgery prior to the onset of clinical signs, no therapeutic measures, other than routine distemper-hepatitis vaccination, are necessary. Buchanan (1968) suggested that digoxin be administered orally for several days prior to surgery in those dogs with moderate or marked cardiac enlargement. In our experience, this has not been necessary unless the dog is showing clinical and/or radiographic indications of left heart failure. In those cases in which heart failure is present, the dog should be stabilized with cardiac glycosides prior to surgery. Cardiac glycosides have been shown by Linde et al. (1969) to have a beneficial effect on myocardial contractility in a dog with a patent ductus arteriosus. Diuretics may be administered if indicated, and low sodium diets and strict cage rest are recommended.

GENETIC STUDIES

The patent ductus arteriosus is more common in the female than in the male (Patterson, 1968). When Patterson (1968) bred Poodles, one or both of which had had a patent ductus arteriosus, 23 of 36 (64 per cent) offspring had congenital cardiac defects, and all 23 dogs had a patent ductus arteriosus. As a result of these breeding experiments, Patterson has concluded that patent ductus arteriosus in his series of breedings resulted from simple autosomal dominant inheritance.

PATHOLOGY

High cardiac output, increased pulmonary circulation, and increased venous return to the left heart result when the ductus arteriosus remains patent. The pulmonary arteries and veins are therefore widened, and both the right and the left ventricles become dilated and hypertrophied. Dilatation of the heart results in functional atrioventricular valvular insufficiency with consequent dilatation of the atria. Jet lesions in the pulmonary artery caused by the shunting of blood have been reported by Spörri and Scheitlin (1952). Von Sandersleben (1953) reported jet lesions in the pulmonary artery, as well as secondary changes of the pulmonic valve. A valve-like structure extending from the aortic wall partially covers the opening of the ductus arteriosus (see p. 580) (Dolowy et al., 1957; Patterson, 1965; Buchanan, 1968).

ABNORMALITIES OF THE AORTIC ARCH AND ITS BRANCHES

Abnormalities of the aortic arch were recognized and reported frequently prior to 1960. It is of historic interest to note the numerous early reports of these abnormalities (Gorton, 1925; Jex-Blake, 1926; Milks, 1929; Milks and Williams, 1935; Yamamoto and Emoto, 1935; Török, 1937-1938; Môcsy, 1939; Olafson, 1939; Brandt, 1940; Davies and Ottoway, 1943; Barry, 1951; Klotz and Brewer, 1952; van Lennep, 1952; Detweiler, 1952; Detweiler and Allam, 1955; Linton, 1956; Coward, 1957; Lawson, Penhale, and Smith, 1957). Radiographs showing esophageal dilatation probably due to vascular ring abnormalities have also been published (Fitts, 1948; Wirth, 1949; Baronti, 1950). The condition has been recognized and surgically corrected frequently in the past 10 years.

Abnormalities in the development of the aortic arch and its branches are more common than clinical reports in the veterinary literature indicate; this is so because abnormal branching that is not responsible for clinical signs is usually an incidental finding (Smollich, 1961; Vitums, 1962). Nearly 20 per cent of 136 dogs dissected in one anatomic institute had some abnormality in the branching of the aortic arch (Smollich, 1961). Only a small percentage of these abnormalities are clinically significant. These are due to the creation of a vascular ring abnormality and subsequent esophageal stricture resulting in clinical signs.

Vascular ring abnormalities of the aortic arch constrict the esophagus and/or trachea at or immediately cranial to the base of the heart. Such constrictions result from abnormal embryologic development and persistence of the fourth or sixth primitive aortic arches or portions of the dorsal and ventral aorta. In the dog, vascular ring abnormalities that have been described include persistent right aortic arch, double aortic arch, and aberrant subclavian arteries. Since the clinical signs, diagnostic procedures, and treatment are similar for all types of vascular ring anomalies reported in the dog, their clinical course will be considered as one entity following the embryologic description of the individual vascular ring anomalies. Surgical correction of vascular ring anomalies is presented in Chapter 19.

EMBRYOLOGY OF THE VASCULAR RING ANOMALIES

The branchial arches from which the aorta and some of its branches develop encircle the primitive trachea and esophagus. If the arches persist, a ring or half-ring structure referred to as a vascular ring persists that leads to esophageal constriction early in life. The normal development of the aortic system from the precursory arches has been described previously (Barry, 1951; Zietzschmann and Krölling, 1955; Arey, 1965). Abnormal development leading to the formation of vascular rings has been summarized repeatedly (Linton, 1956; Lawson, Penhale, and Smith, 1957; Frese, 1961; Vitums, 1962; Wysong, 1969).

Persistent right aortic arch. This is the most frequently encountered vascular ring abnormality in the dog, accounting for about 95 per cent of the vascular ring abnormalities that result in esophageal constriction (Buchanan, 1968). The description of the development of persistent right aortic arch has been simplified, eliminating details of little consequence to the clinical condition. In Figure 18-13, the development of the normal left aortic arch is summarized. At different times during early embryonic life, six branchial arteries connect the paired primitive ventral aortas with the paired dorsal aortas. The ventral aortas are united caudally to form the primordial heart, and the paired dorsal aortas fuse caudally early in embryonic life to form the descending aorta (Linton, 1956). The first and second pairs of aortic arches involute early and contribute only insignificantly to the permanent arterial system. The third arch and the dorsal aorta, which continues toward the head, are the precursors of the internal carotid arteries as well as the external carotid arteries and the common carotid arteries.

Each of the fourth pair of arches persists. On the left side, the fourth arch and portions of the left dorsal aorta become the permanent arch of the aorta and are referred to as the normal left aortic arch. The right fourth arch becomes the right subclavian artery and the brachiocephalic artery. The fifth pair of aortic arches is inconsistent and disappears early in embryonic life. The left side of the sixth pair of arches, also referred to as the pulmonary arches, develops into the ductus arteriosus by connecting the left or main pulmonary artery with the dorsal aorta. The right sixth arch regresses except for the ventral root, which forms the pulmonary artery.

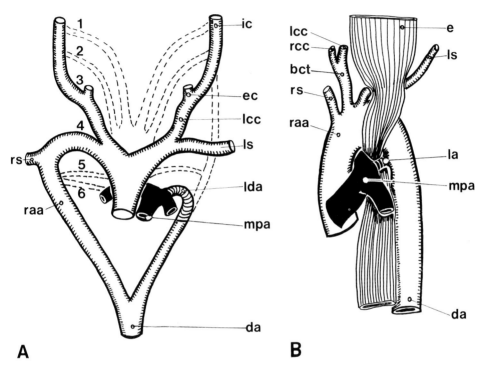

A   **B**

FIGURE 18-14   Schematic drawings of the embryologic and postnatal arrangement of the vessels in persistent right aortic arch, ventrodorsal view (compare with normal development in Fig. 18-13).

A, Embryologic development of the persistent right aortic arch. Uninterrupted lines illustrate the persistent portions of the embryologic arch system, and the broken lines indicate the transient or rudimentary portions. The transformations of arches 1, 2, 3, 5, and 6 and their respective branches, namely the internal carotid artery (ic), the external carotid artery (ec), and the common carotid artery (lcc), are the same as if development had been normal. However, the right fourth aortic arch (raa) persists instead of the left fourth arch, which in this case serves only as the origin of the left subclavian artery (ls). The left ductus arteriosus (lda) persists and remains connected to the right aortic arch and the descending aorta (da), thereby forming a closed vascular ring around the esophagus. The length of the left ductus arteriosus is schematically much longer than it is anatomically in order to show the proper relationship and development of the vessels.

B, Postnatal arrangement of the branches of the persistent right aortic arch. The esophagus (e), located to the left and ventrally of the right aortic arch (raa), is constricted by the ligamentum arteriosum (la), which completes the ring anomaly by connecting the main pulmonary artery (mpa) with the right aortic arch. Since the left subclavian artery (ls) originates from the right arch, it crosses over to the left side. As the left subclavian artery crosses retroesophageally, it often causes some indentation dorsally and on the left side of the esophagus. The branching of the aortic arch might be normal or abnormal, as it is in this case, where the brachiocephalic artery is absent. The right subclavian artery (rs) and the bicarotid trunk (bct) originate directly from the right aortic arch. The bicarotid trunk then branches into the right and left common carotid arteries (rcc, lcc).

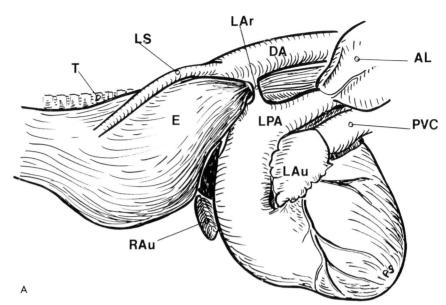

A

FIGURE 18-15 *A,* Schematic drawing from a dog with persistent right aortic arch and a vascular ring abnormality producing a stricture of the esophagus, viewed from the left side. (T) trachea; (LS) left subclavian artery; (E) esophagus with pre-cardiac saccular dilatation; (LAr) ligamentum arteriosum; (DA) descending aorta; (LPA) left pulmonary artery; (AL) left apical lobe of the lung; (PVC) caudal vena cava; (LAu) left auricle; (RAu) right auricle. *B,* Gross pathologic specimen from a puppy
Legend continues on opposite page.

When the right fourth arch persists and develops into the permanent aorta and the ductus arteriosus forms normally from the left sixth arch, a vascular ring anomaly is formed. The vascular ring connecting the right fourth and left sixth arches results in postnatal life in constriction of the esophagus and occasionally the trachea (Figs. 18-14 and 18-15). Thus, the persistent right aortic arch vascular ring abnormality in postnatal life is formed by the following structures: the ascending aorta on the right side, the ligamentum arteriosum (formerly ductus arteriosus) on the left and dorsally, the main pulmonary artery on the left and ventrally, and the heart base ventrally (Figs. 18-16, 18-17, and 18-18). The descending aorta usually remains on the left side of the spine. Shortly after birth, the ductus arteriosus closes, and the fibrous cord that remains is called the ligamentum arteriosum. It is this ligament that produces the esophageal stricture in dogs with persistent right aortic arch. Occasionally the ductus remains partially or entirely patent (see Fig. 19-16).

The development of the right aortic arch does not always lead to a vascular ring anomaly. When a mirror image transformation of the aortic arch occurs, the persistent right aortic arch is connected to the pulmonary artery by a ductus arteriosus originating from the right sixth arch. In such cases, no vascular ring forms and the esophagus remains free, as shown in Figures 18-19 and 18-20.

Double aortic arch.   In this anomaly, the vascular ring occurs because of the complete persistence of both sides of the fourth arch (Fig. 18-21). The ascending aorta divides into a right branch passing to the right and caudal of the esophagus and a left branch passing to the left and ventral to the esophagus (Klotz and

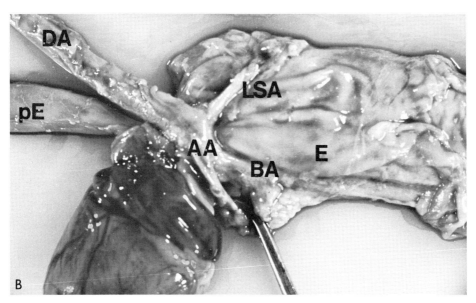

with a persistent right aortic arch. The specimen is seen from the right side. There is marked dilatation of the precardiac portion of the esophagus (E). The dilatation narrows immediately caudal to the aortic arch (AA), and the postcardiac portion of the esophagus (pE) is unremarkable. The brachiocephalic artery (BA) can be seen at the ventral border of the dilated esophagus. The left subclavian artery (LSA) produces an indentation in the esophagus as it crosses retroesophageally from the right to the left side. The stricture of the esophagus cannot be seen on this view because it is located to the left of the descending aorta (DA).

Brewer, 1952). In a case reported by Lawson, Penhale, and Smith (1957), the right aortic arch was functional, and the left aortic arch, although atretic, completed the vascular ring together with the left ligamentum arteriosum. This dog also had had respiratory distress since birth, apparently the result of an anomaly of the tracheal rings, which were composed of several parts. As a consequence, the rings could not resist pressure from the outside and collapsed. Renk and Raethel (1954) described a puppy in which abnormal tracheal cartilages were also associated with a stricture resulting in esophageal construction. Reports of a double aortic arch are extremely rare in the dog. In man, the double aortic arch is a more common vascular ring abnormality (Friedberg, 1966).

Anomalous subclavian arteries.   Anomalous branching of the aortic arch leading to clinical signs is seldom reported. In a report by Smollich (1961), nine of 136 dogs examined anatomically had an abnormality of the subclavian arteries (*arteria lusoria*). In a study by Vitums (1962), three of 275 dogs which had been examined in an anatomy laboratory had an abnormal right subclavian artery. The right subclavian artery normally arises from the brachiocephalic artery. In anomalous development of the right subclavian artery, it may arise directly from the aortic arch just distal to the left subclavian artery or together with the left subclavian artery in a short bisubclavian trunk (Fig. 18-22; see also Fig. 18-44). As the right subclavian artery crosses retroesophageally from left to right before descending to the thoracic inlet, it causes an indentation or half-ring stricture of the esophagus (Figs. 18-24 and 18-25). In these cases, the right subclavian artery, when it presses on the esophagus, results in *dysphagia lusoria*, a term

Text continues on page 505.

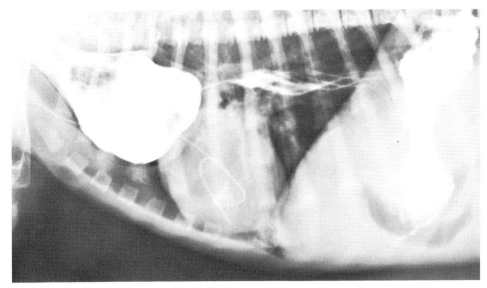

FIGURE 18-16 Left lateral esophagram made after the administration of Gastro-grafin. This 10 week old, female German Shepherd dog since it had been weaned vomited all solid food and most liquids 2 to 10 minutes after eating. The dog was dehydrated and emaciated. There is a large, contrast-filled, saccular widening of the esophagus in the area of the precardiac mediastinum. The column of contrast density suddenly narrows to barely 1 mm. in diameter and then widens again. In the postcardiac mediastinum, the normal, faint outline of the rugae is visible. The heart is unremarkable. A narrowing of the esophagus cranial to the base of the heart is a characteristic sign of constriction of the esophagus caused by a vascular ring abnormality such as a persistent right aortic arch. Aspiration of contrast medium, a complication which may occasionally occur, can cause severe secondary pulmonary changes. Utmost care in administering the contrast medium is therefore required.

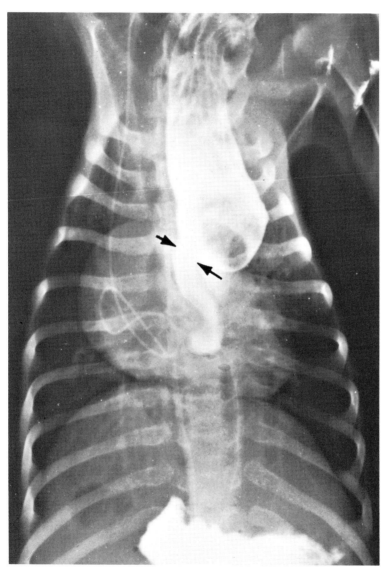

FIGURE 18-17 Dorsoventral esophagram, dog in Figure 18-16. The constriction of the esophagus begins between the two arrows and is wider in this projection than it is on the lateral view (Fig. 18-16). The saccular widening of the esophagus in the precardiac mediastinum extends to the left side. No contrast medium has been retained in the caudal portion of the esophagus.

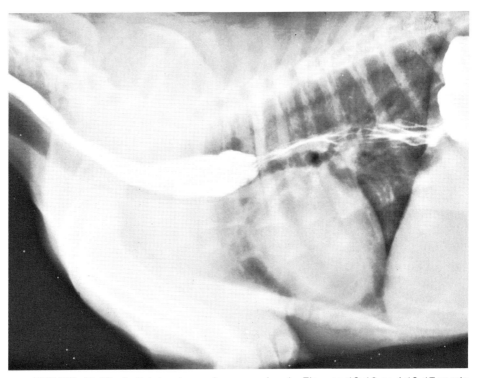

FIGURE 18-18 Left lateral esophagram, dog in Figures 18-16 and 18-17 made nearly 3 months after the constriction caused by the persistent right aortic arch on the right side, the pulmonary artery on the left side, and the ligamentum arteriosum dorsally had been relieved surgically by severing the ligamentum arteriosum. The cranial esophagus still retains contrast medium, and a widening is visible cranial to the base of the heart. There is narrowing of the esophagus over the base of the heart, but the dog had gradually improved postoperatively and seemed to swallow normally at the time when this radiograph was made.

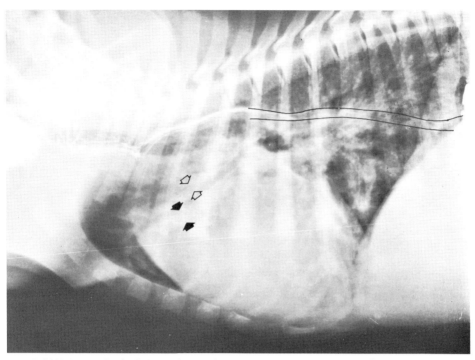

FIGURE 18-19 Left lateral esophagram, 4 month old male German Shepherd dog which had severe signs of right and left congestive heart failure. On auscultation a machinery-like murmur was heard, suggesting the diagnosis of a patent ductus arteriosus. Because of the deflection of the trachea and several unexplained densities in the precardiac mediastinum and the hilar area seen on plain radiographs, barium paste was administered orally for an esophagram. The cardiac silhouette is enlarged, and there is a remarkable cranial bulge of the cranial cardiac border, giving the impression of abnormal inclination of the apicobasilar axis. The portion of the cardiac silhouette cranial to the imaginary apicobasilar line is about five times larger than the portion caudal to it. The cranial waist has disappeared completely. Such extreme cranial bulging usually results from a greatly enlarged aortic arch or to poststenotic dilatation of the pulmonary artery. The contrast outline of the esophagus has been retouched to make it more visible. The esophagus is ventrally depressed at the thoracic inlet, then bulges dorsally over the cranial portion of the hilus and finally runs almost directly toward the hiatus in the diaphragm. Because of this dorsal deviation of the esophagus and trachea, it is likely that an abnormal aortic arch is causing the cranial bulge. The left atrium is markedly enlarged and has elevated the distal trachea and the esophagus. The trachea bends dorsally at the cranial portion of the hilus and runs parallel with the esophagus. Right atrial enlargement was therefore considered as an alternative explanation for the cardiac enlargement in the cranial direction. The left cardiac border and the caudal vena cava are unremarkable. The lung field is denser than normal, the vascular markings are blurred, and the diameters of the apical lobar arteries (clear arrows) and veins (black arrows) exceed the diameter of the proximal third of the fourth rib. The overcirculation of the lungs and the left atrial dilatation indicate a left-to-right shunting of blood. A tentative diagnosis of a patent ductus arteriosus with a greatly dilated aortic arch or a complicated ventricular septal defect was postulated.

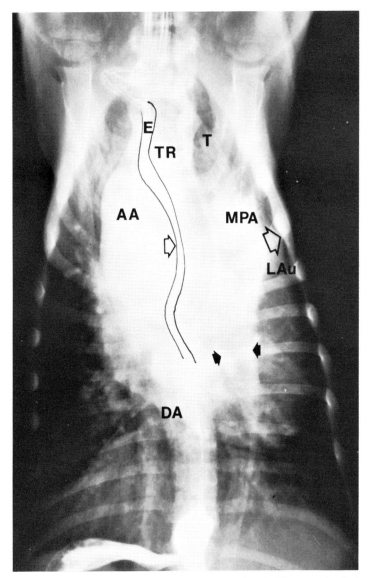

FIGURE 18-20   Dorsoventral esophagram, dog in Figure 18-19. Another barium swallow was administered, but the contrast did not adhere to the esophageal mucosa, and the outline of the mucosa remained ill-defined.

The two black lines on the radiograph follow the borders of the esophagus, in order to better delineate it. The cardiac silhouette appears markedly elongated, and the apex of the heart is wider than normal and displaced to the left side. The aortic arch (AA) is a very dense mass which obscures the right cranial quadrant of the cardiac silhouette and displaces the esophagus (E) and the trachea (TR) to the left side. The descending aorta (DA) appears to the right of the spine and the esophagus. The main pulmonary artery (MPA) is visible as a dense shadow which gradually decreases in diameter as it continues peripherally into the left pulmonary artery. A small bulge caused by dilatation of the left auricle (LAu; large, clear arrow) protrudes over the border of the enlarged left ventricle. The dilated intrapulmonary vasculature (arrows) and the blurring of the vessel outlines further support the possibility of overcirculation owing to a left-to-right shunting of blood, as was explained for the lateral radiograph (Fig. 18-19). The dense mass in the cranial right quadrant of the cardiac sil-

Legend continues on opposite page.

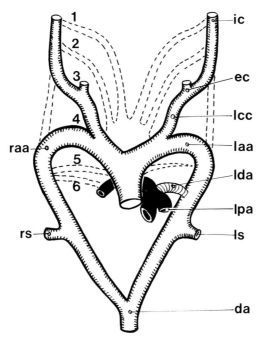

FIGURE 18-21 Schematic drawing of the embryologic development of the double aortic arch, ventrodorsal view. Uninterrupted lines illustrate the persistent portions of the embryologic arch system, and broken lines indicate the transient or rudimentary portions. The transformations of arches 1, 2, 3, 5, and 6 and their respective branches, namely internal carotid artery (ic), external carotid artery (ec), and common carotid artery (lcc), are the same as in normal development. However, the right aortic arch (raa) persists in addition to the normally developing left aortic arch (laa), creating a vascular ring anomaly which constricts the esophagus in postnatal life. The origins of the right and left subclavian arteries (rs, ls) are unchanged, as are the descending aorta (da) and the left ductus arteriosus (lda). The main pulmonary artery gives rise to the left ductus arteriosus at the origin of the left pulmonary artery (lpa).

introduced into medicine by Bayford (1789), referring to a trick or deception of nature. Brandt (1940), Detweiler and Allam (1955) and Buergelt and Wheaton (1970) encountered cases in which the left subclavian artery was responsible for constriction of the esophagus. In these cases, the right aortic arch had developed instead of the left aortic arch, and the left subclavian artery crossed retroesophageally to the left side. Henwood and Green (1964) described a case in which the subclavian arteries appeared to be reversed, ultimately resulting in esophageal constriction by the right anomalous subclavian artery.

Text continues on page 510.

houette was identified as a dilated persistent right aortic arch, displacing the esophagus and the trachea, which normally lie to the right of the aortic arch, to the left. The tentative diagnosis was confirmed angiocardiographically and at necropsy. The persistent right aortic arch and the patent ductus arteriosus were both located on the right side and had therefore caused no stricture of the esophagus. The diverticulum at the thoracic inlet could not be explained. It had not caused any signs of dysphagia. At (T), the shadow of the thymus can be identified as a sail-like density.

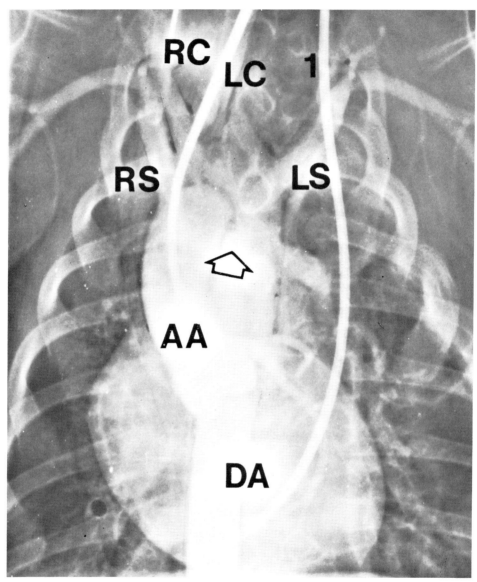

FIGURE 18-22 Selective supravalvular aortic angiogram, dorsoventral view, 3 month old male German Shepherd dog with a persistent right aortic arch, abnormal branching of the aortic arch, and persistent left cranial vena cava (see Fig. 18-23). The ascending aorta (AA), which is derived from the right aortic arch, is filled with contrast medium. The right subclavian artery arises from the aortic arch, as does a short bicarotid trunk which then further divides into the right common carotid artery (RC) and the left common carotid artery (LC). The left subclavian artery arises normally from the left side of the arch. The area where an esophageal stricture was found at the time of surgery is indicated (arrow). The descending aorta (DA) is unremarkable. A catheter (1) is in the persistent left cranial vena cava. Another catheter is seen in the left common carotid artery entering the aortic arch.

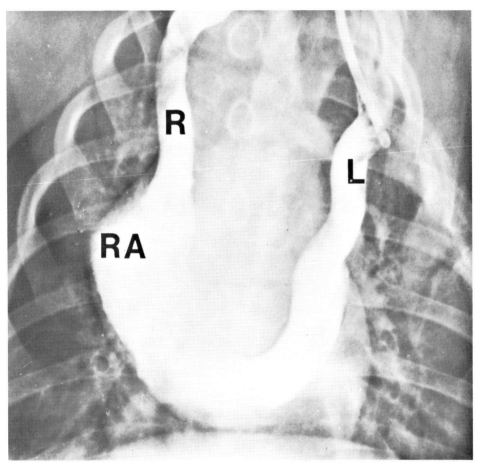

FIGURE 18-23   Dorsoventral angiocardiogram, dog in Figure 18-22. Simultaneous injection of contrast medium into the persistent left cranial vena cava and the right jugular vein results in opacification of both the normal right cranial vena cava (R), entering the right atrium (RA), and the persistent left cranial vena cava (L). The catheter in the persistent left cranial vena cava was introduced via the left jugular vein. The left cranial vena cava passes along the left border of the heart and crosses over to the right side posterior to the left atrium, where it joins the right atrium. It was not possible to determine whether the anomalous vena cava entered the right atrium directly or via the coronary sinus.

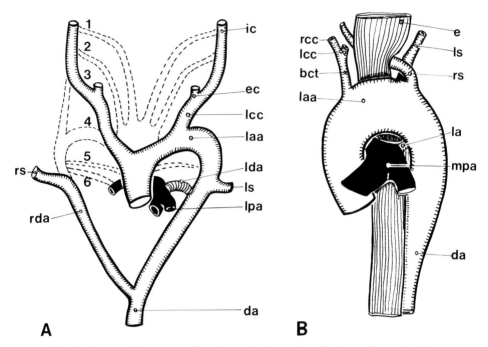

FIGURE 18-24 Schematic drawings of the embryologic and postnatal appearance of the vessels in abnormal origin of the right subclavian artery from the aortic arch, ventrodorsal view (compare to normal development in Figure 18-13). *A,* Anomalous embryologic development of the right subclavian artery. Uninterrupted lines illustrate the persistent portions of the embryologic arch system, and the broken lines indicate the transient or rudimentary portions. The transformations of arches 1, 2, 3, 5, and 6 and their respective branches, namely the internal carotid artery (ic), the external carotid artery (ec), and the common carotid artery (lcc), are the same as in normal development. The permanent left aortic arch (laa), the left ductus arteriosus (lda), and the left subclavian artery (ls) also develop normally. However, the right subclavian artery (rs) arises from portions of the normally regressing right dorsal aorta (rda), which remains connected to the descending aorta (da). The normal origin of the right subclavian artery from the right fourth arch is absent. Since the right subclavian artery originates distal to the left subclavian artery, it has to cross the esophagus retroesophageally in order to reach the right side, thereby producing esophageal stricture. (Modified from Arey, L. B.: Developmental Anatomy. W. B. Saunders Co., Philadelphia, 7th ed., 1965.) *B,* Postnatal arrangement of the branching of the aortic arch in dogs with anomalous right subclavian artery (arteria lusoria). The esophagus (e) is located to the right side of the permanent left aortic arch (laa). There is no constriction in the area of the ligamentum arteriosum (la) and main pulmonary artery (mpa). The constriction, if it occurs at all, is due to the retroesophageal crossing of the right subclavian artery (rs), originating distal to the left subclavian artery (ls) or together with the latter in a short bisubclavian trunk. The brachiocephalic artery is absent, and the right and left common carotid arteries (rcc, lcc) originate directly from the aortic arch via a bicarotid trunk (bct).

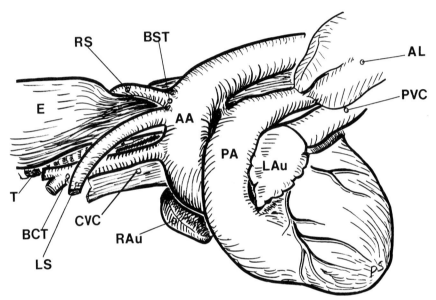

FIGURE 18-25   Schematic drawing of a retroesophageal right subclavian artery causing a stricture of the esophagus, as viewed from the left side. (RS) right subclavian artery; (E) esophagus; (BST) bisubclavian trunk (very short); (AA) aortic arch; (T) trachea; (BCT) bicarotid trunk bifurcating into the right and left common carotid arteries; (LS) left subclavian artery; (CVC) cranial vena cava; (RAu) right auricle; (PA) pulmonary artery; (LAu) left auricle; (AL) left apical lobe of the lung; (PVC) caudal vena cava.

CLINICAL SIGNS AND PHYSICAL EXAMINATION

Vascular ring anomalies may be found incidentally at necropsy in dogs which had had no clinical signs of esophageal constriction (Lawson, Penhale, and Smith, 1957). This is an unusual finding when persistent right aortic arch occurs, however.

Dogs with signs resulting from vascular ring anomalies are usually presented between 3 and 8 weeks of age because of persistent vomiting (Detweiler, 1952). However, there are reports in which the condition was diagnosed in adult dogs. Brandt (1940) described the condition in a 2½ year old dog which had been put to death because of meningoencephalitis in which clinical signs resulting from esophageal constriction had not occurred. Frese (1961) described it in a 4½ year old German Shepherd and referred to eight other cases reported in the literature in which the dog had been over 1 year old when the diagnosis was made. Some of these dogs, however, had shown pertinent signs since early life. Imhoff and Foster (1963) reported persistent right aortic arch in a 10 year old dog and referred to a previous case in which the dog had survived for 3½ years. Adkins, Farrall, and Mohart (1970) reported successful correction of this condition in a 4 year old dog.

The clinical signs typically associated with vascular ring anomalies are vomiting, a good to ravenous appetite but loss of body weight, insufficient growth, and often emaciation. Vomiting most frequently occurs shortly after eating, although it may be delayed for several hours. Some dogs will attempt to eat the vomited food immediately after regurgitating it.

The vomitus does not show signs of having been digested and is covered by mucus. It has neither the acid smell of vomitus from the stomach nor an acid pH. In dogs with large esophageal dilatations, the regurgitated food may have a bad odor, since portions of the food may have remained in the esophagus for long periods during which fermentation occurred. Pharyngitis and esophagitis often accompany advanced cases due to the irritation resulting from fermentation by-products. Esophagitis leads to further dysphagia even when fluids alone are taken.

Vomiting usually begins shortly after the puppy has been weaned—i.e., when solid foods which are unable to pass the constricted area are first fed. Since fluids do pass with ease through the constriction, clinical signs do not develop as long as the pup is fed milk or other liquid or semiliquid food.

Respiratory distress due to encroachment on the tracheal lumen, which may be more apparent after feeding, is not a common problem. Wheezy respiration and inspiratory stridor have been reported in a few cases. However, many dogs develop secondary respiratory problems due to aspiration pneumonia.

Linton (1956) and Lawson, Penhale, and Smith (1957) reported that occasionally the affected dogs take a characteristic posture, particularly during feeding, with the head held low and forward in an attempt to straighten the esophagus and the trachea. However, this is not a common sign in our experience. When the cervical portion of the esophagus has become sufficiently dilated, a bulge cranial to the thoracic inlet may become readily palpable after the dog has swallowed some food; in the short-haired breeds, the bulge can also be seen. Bulging of the cervical esophagus can be produced by holding the mouth and nares of the dog closed and simultaneously squeezing gently on the stomach, thereby increasing the pressure in the esophagus (Buchanan, 1968).

Auscultation of the heart and lungs usually does not reveal abnormal heart sounds. Lung sounds may be normal, or râles may be present, suggesting aspiration pneumonia. Occasionally, gurgling sounds are heard which are produced by the liquid retained in the dilated esophagus. The electrocardiogram, pulse, and abdomen are unremarkable in uncomplicated cases.

Persistent right aortic arch is occasionally complicated by other congenital lesions such as patent ductus arteriosus or an abnormal left subclavian artery. Coexistence of a persistent right aortic arch and a patent ductus arteriosus has been seen by the authors (see Figs. 18-19 and 18-20) and has been reported by Frese (1961) and by Buchanan (1968). Occasionally, the ligamentum arteriosum remains partially or completely patent, so that it could be argued that a patent ductus arteriosus is also present (see Fig. 19-16). Persistent left cranial vena cava and persistent right aortic arch are frequently associated (see page 572) (Buchanan, 1963; Patterson, 1968; Buergelt and Wheaton, 1970).

RADIOGRAPHIC EXAMINATION

Routine radiographs and a barium contrast study of the esophagus are essential in establishing the presence of a vascular ring anomaly. Fluoroscopy is not essential but can be useful. In some plain radiographs, the diagnosis can be made even without esophageal contrast studies. In these cases, the dog has swallowed a moderate amount of air which causes ballooning of the esophagus cranial to the heart, and a negative contrast study is effected. In other cases, the esophagus may be filled with fluid, and a large, dense, saccular opacity can be seen cranial to the heart. The size of the heart is usually unremarkable, but sometimes it is displaced ventrally and slightly caudally.

The presence of the right aortic arch can occasionally be recognized on the dorsoventral radiograph if it is made with enough penetration (Fig. 18-20). The trachea and the esophagus are displaced to the left side by a dense structure representing the right aortic arch. In most cases, the descending aorta is located to the left of the spine. However, there are cases in which the right arch is connected to a right descending aorta (Fig. 18-20). The right aortic arch and the trachea also cause the saccular widening of the esophagus to be located usually to the left of the mediastinum.

The changes suspected on the plain radiographs are substantiated by the esophagram (Figs. 18-16, 18-17, and 18-18). It is important to administer the contrast medium carefully, because dogs with a persistent right aortic arch may regurgitate and aspirate the barium. This is more common if the head of the dog is bent dorsally while the contrast is being administered. The barium suspension should be given in small doses, or, preferably, the suspension should be flavored and the dog encouraged to take it voluntarily.

The esophagram provides the differential diagnosis for persistent right aortic arch and other esophageal conditions such as congenital or acquired achalasia, esophageal diverticulum, or a foreign body. In cases of persistent right aortic arch or double aortic arch, the saccular widening is usually confined to the cranial portion of the esophagus. The dilatation stops abruptly at the base of the heart at about the fourth rib (Fig. 18-16). The cervical esophagus may or may not be affected. In long-standing conditions, the esophagus can become very large, the dilatation extending from the distal portion of the pharynx to the heart base. The distal thoracic esophagus from the base of the heart to the diaphragmatic hiatus is rarely dilated. It is often difficult to outline the distal esophagus satisfactorily, but barium in the stomach indicates that some contrast has passed the constricted region. It is not always possible to outline the area of the esophageal constriction. The dog may then be elevated cranially to force the contrast past the constriction with the help of gravity. Attempts should be made to outline the distal esophagus to obtain a reliable differential diagnosis. The stricture itself cannot be outlined in many cases.

DIFFERENTIAL DIAGNOSIS

The differential diagnosis is usually made from the esophagram. In achalasia (also referred to as cardiospasm), the esophagus is usually widened throughout its entire length. Occasionally, some degree of constriction over the base of the heart is due to the azygos vein crossing the dilated esophagus to the right side. Also, there is less room for dilatation dorsal to the heart. Segmental achalasia is uncommon and does not lead to localized, excessive constriction at the base of the heart. Foreign bodies can often be seen on the plain radiograph or are recognized by their obstructive nature after contrast has been administered. Strictures caused by formation of scar tissue that also cause marked widening of the cranial esophagus must be differentiated from persistent aortic arch, according to their different location. Diverticula are uncommon and are recognized by their localized nature. They are usually found at or near the thoracic inlet (Fig. 18-20).

The history and/or clinical examination often reveals information on the time and form of the vomiting. The specific predisposition of German Shepherds and Irish Setters to persistent right aortic arch should also be considered in the differential diagnosis (Patterson, 1968).

Although an angiogram is usually not necessary to make the clinical diagnosis, it may be of value when a complicated congenital malformation is suspected. Contrast injections into the aortic arch specifically define the branching abnormalities involved in the formation of the vascular ring. Results of angiocardiographic studies have been published by Walker and Littlewort (1964) and Buchanan and Patterson (1965). A supravalvular aortic injection is the method of choice in these cases (see Fig. 18-22). The esophagus should be filled with dilute barium suspension or air in order to demonstrate the relative positions of the vascular structures to it. If undiluted barium suspension is used, the details of the vascular structures will be obscured by the superimposed esophageal density. Radiographs should be made in both the lateral and dorsoventral projections for proper visualization of the vascular abnormalities.

PROGNOSIS

With the exception of the few cases reported and reviewed by Frese (1961) and by Imhoff and Foster (1963), the prognosis for a dog with a vascular ring abnormality in which clinical signs due to esophageal constriction are present is poor unless corrective surgery is performed early. Continued cachexia caused by malnutrition, hypoproteinemia, and the stress of aspiration pneumonia is likely to be fatal within a short period of time. Except in those cases where the dog's condition temporarily contraindicates surgical intervention, surgery should be undertaken as early as possible. The prognosis is usually good after surgical correction; however, in most cases, a certain degree of dilatation of the esophagus will remain (Fig. 18-18). Buchanan (1968) reported that some dilatation persists for several years after successful surgery. However, esophageal function is not significantly impaired after successful surgical correction unless the dog swallows large boluses of solid food. In such circumstances, occasional vomiting may occur, and the owner of the dog should be advised accordingly.

GENETIC STUDIES

Persistent right aortic arch occurs more frequently in German Shepherds and Irish Setters than in the general canine population (Frese, 1961; Patterson, 1968). Of 30 puppies resulting from experimental breeding of two dogs with persistent right aortic arches, only one had the same condition, and two others had different congenital anomalies. When the three puppies with the congenital anomalies were mated with one of their parents, none of the 16 offspring had a persistent right aortic arch, but two were found to have a persistent left cranial vena cava. Some degree of genetic control of persistent right aortic arch and persistent left cranial vena cava is suggested by Patterson (1968). In the same study, persistent left cranial vena cava (see p. 572) was found in 13 dogs, and 10 of the 13 also had a persistent right aortic arch. Persistent left cranial vena cava developed more frequently when dogs with persistent right aortic arch were bred together than when normal control dogs were mated. The two conditions are often found as coexisting vascular abnormalities.

TREATMENT

Surgical correction is recommended for all cases of persistent right aortic arch and other vascular ring abnormalities (see Chapter 19).

PULMONIC STENOSIS

Pulmonic stenosis is an obstruction which prevents the normal flow of blood from the right ventricle to the pulmonary artery. The stenosis may occur at one of three levels—at the infundibulum (or conus arteriosus), at the pulmonic valve, or above the pulmonic valve, in the pulmonary artery—and is described accordingly.

Although in the earliest reports of pulmonic stenosis the lesion was considered to be unusual in dogs (Marek and Môcsy, 1951), pulmonic stenosis is now recognized as one of the most frequently diagnosed congenital cardiac lesions in dogs in North America and Europe. In one survey, the condition was diagnosed in a higher proportion of English Bulldogs, Fox Terriers, and Chihuahuas than would have been expected to occur at random in the general clinic population (Patterson, 1968).

Valvular pulmonic stenosis is the most common form of the condition in dogs. The valve cusps are moderately to markedly thickened; when thickening is marked the commissures are lacking, and the valve appears as a dome-shaped diaphragm without distinct cusps (Patterson, 1968).

Infundibular pulmonic stenosis as a primary lesion, caused by a ring of fibrous connective tissue surrounding the right ventricular outflow tract immediately below the valve, is less common than valvular pulmonic stenosis; however, fibromuscular infundibular pulmonic stenosis (see Fig. 18-33) frequently occurs secondarily to primary pulmonic valvular stenosis due to muscular hypertrophy of the right ventricular outflow tract (Detweiler, 1962). Severin (1967) reported four dogs with subvalvular fibrous rings and one with an infundibular muscular ring.

Supravalvular pulmonic stenosis is a very unusual lesion in the dog.

Pulmonic stenosis occurs with other congenital cardiac defects such as patent foramen ovale and pericardial diaphragmatic hernia (Brodey and Prier, 1961), atrial septal defect (Ott et al., 1964; Buchanan and Patterson, 1965; Patterson, 1965; Popovic and Fleming, 1970), ventricular septal defect (Buchanan and Pyle, 1966), and aortic stenosis (Patterson, 1965). It is also one of the four primary components of tetralogy of Fallot (see pp. 554-563).

HISTORY AND PHYSICAL EXAMINATION

Dogs with pulmonic stenosis are usually asymptomatic, the condition first being recognized on cardiac auscultation during routine physical examination. As the condition progresses, cardiac signs such as dyspnea, fatigability, and right-sided decompensation may occur. Retarded development has been reported (Ripps and Henderson, 1953; Tashjian et al., 1959). Cyanosis may occur in complicated cases in which there is a right-to-left shunt of blood. Periodic episodes of cyanosis occurred in an uncomplicated case of pulmonic stenosis reported by Ripps and Henderson (1953). Patterson (1963) reported that insidious venous congestion with right heart failure develops between 6 months and 3 years

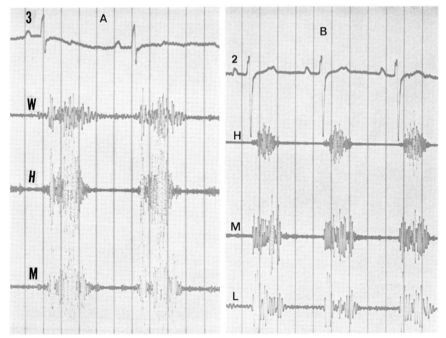

FIGURE 18-26 Phonocardiograms from two dogs with isolated valvular pulmonic stenosis. A systolic crescendo-decrescendo murmur with high-frequency accentuation is best demonstrated on the high-frequency (H) and medium-frequency (M) band phonocardiograms. It is not as clearly seen on the wide-band (W) or low-band (L) recordings. A negative lead II electrocardiogram (as in B) is consistent with severe right axis deviation.

of age, although some dogs with mild pulmonic stenosis have occasionally lived longer than five years. The authors have also observed a number of dogs with isolated pulmonic stenosis which have remained asymptomatic beyond 5 years of age. Ripps and Henderson (1953), Custer et al. (1961), and Ott et al. (1964) each reported a case of pulmonic stenosis in which syncope was the presenting sign. Polycythemia may have aggravated the clinical signs of the pulmonic stenosis in the former case, and a small atrial septal defect was present in the case of Ott et al (1964).

On auscultation, a high-frequency ejection murmur is heard between the first and second heart sounds. The murmur is of greatest intensity over the pulmonic valve region, usually near the left cranial sternal border. Occasionally, it may be loudest just to the right of the sternal border at the cranial right thoracic wall. In general, the more severe the degree of stenosis, the later is the peak of the intensity of the murmur, and very severe pulmonic stenosis can be associated with only a minimal systolic murmur. The murmur that is usually auscultated is a crescendo-decrescendo or "diamond-shaped" murmur (Fig. 18-26). This term is used to describe the increasing intensity of the murmur until middle or late systole, after which the intensity of the murmur declines rapidly. A palpable thrill over the cranioventral left thoracic wall is evident when the intensity of the murmur is severe. The second heart sound may be split (Hamlin et al. 1963a), although it is frequently difficult to isolate the second heart sound on auscultation when the intensity of the murmur is great.

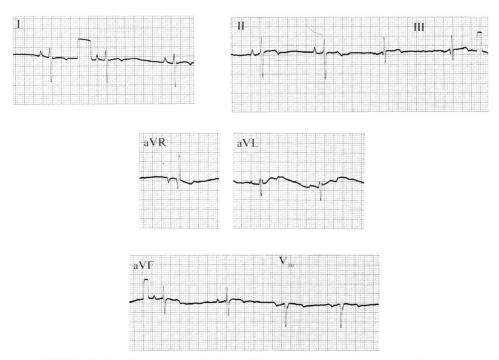

FIGURE 18-27   Right axis deviation with congenital valvular pulmonic stenosis. The mean electrical axis in the frontal plane is ± 180°. Right axis deviation of such severity is associated with marked right ventricular hypertrophy, usually resulting from a congenital cardiac abnormality.

ELECTROCARDIOGRAPHY

The electrocardiogram may be normal, but right axis deviation in the frontal plane with a mean electrical axis greater than 120° is usually encountered in moderate and advanced cases (Fig. 18-27). In severe pulmonic stenosis, the T wave in lead V_{10} is positive (i.e., T vector dorsally directed), a definitive indication of right ventricular hypertrophy (see page 143). The cardiac rhythm is normal, although atrial fibrillation has been reported to occur with the condition (Detweiler, 1957; Wallace and Hamilton, 1962). Hamlin (1963a) described a case of pulmonic stenosis in which the terminal forces were directed dextrad and craniad. In dogs with pulmonic stenosis, electrocardiography and vectorcardiography usually demonstrate that the initial forces are directed to the right in less severe cases and to the left in more advanced cases. The intermediate forces are directed rightward and craniad or caudad in moderate to advanced right ventricular hypertrophy due to pulmonic stenosis. In advanced cases, the terminal QRS forces are directed rightward, craniad, and dorsad (Fig. 18-28A) or ventrad (Fig. 18-28B).

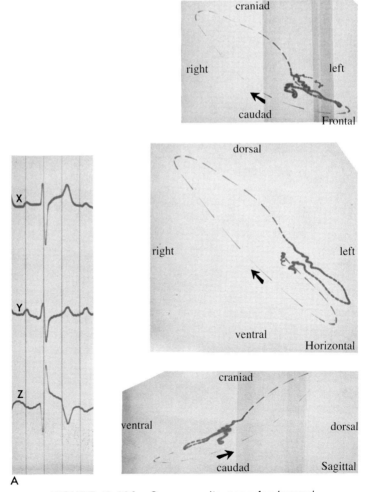

FIGURE 18-28A   *See opposite page for legend.*

RADIOGRAPHIC EXAMINATION

The characteristic radiographic signs of uncomplicated pulmonic stenosis have been well described (Ripps and Henderson, 1953; Hamlin, 1960, 1968; Detweiler, 1962; Rhodes, Patterson, and Detweiler, 1963; Ott et al., 1964). Typically, right ventricular enlargement, dilatation of the pulmonary artery segment, and normal vascularization of the lung field are seen (Figs. 18-29 and 18-30). (See Tables 18-1 and 18-2.)

On the *lateral radiograph*, the right heart is rounder than normal, which at times makes it appear semicircular. Despite the enlargement, the ventral portion of the right ventricular wall does not follow the sternum for an increased distance, as is often the case with right ventricular dilatation. In hypertrophy, the apex is frequently displaced caudodorsally. The protrusion of the dorsal portion of the cranial cardiac border varies with the degree of poststenotic dilatation present. The cranial waist is usually obliterated by the dilated pulmonary artery. When poststenotic dilatation of the pulmonary artery is great, an opaque mass is recognized in the precordial mediastinum which at times bulges dorsally, overlying the lucent band of the tracheal lumen. The left and right pulmonary arteries and the peripheral branches are usually normal in size. The trachea is slightly

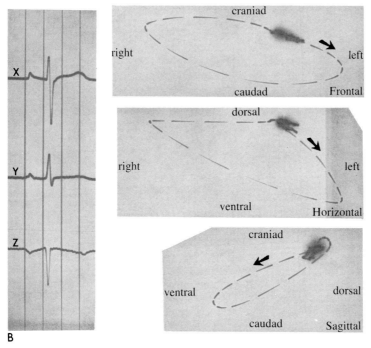

B

FIGURE 18-28 Pulmonic stenosis. *A,* Vectorcardiogram demonstrating severe right ventricular hypertrophy from a dog with valvular pulmonic stenosis. The initial forces are directed leftward, caudad, and ventrad. The major forces, which include both the intermediate and terminal forces, are directed rightward, craniad, and dorsad owing to the massive right ventricular hypertrophy. *B,* In another dog with severe right ventricular hypertrophy due to valvular pulmonic stenosis, the vectorcardiogram is similar to that in Figure 18-28*A,* except that the intermediate or major electrical activity is not directed dorsad. In both cases, direction of the horizontal loop is clockwise, which is abnormal.

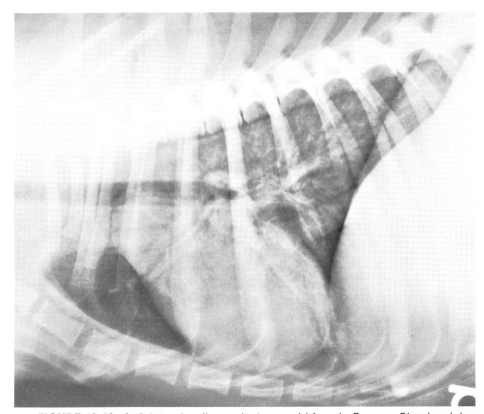

FIGURE 18-29 Left lateral radiograph, 1 year old female German Shepherd dog with valvular pulmonic stenosis. Although there were no clinical signs referable to heart failure, a high-frequency, ejection-type murmur with maximal intensity over the pulmonic valve area was auscultated. The cardiac silhouette is larger than normal because of rounding of the right ventricular border. The cranial waist has disappeared. The continuation of an ill-defined line which crosses the ventral border of the cranial vena cava outlines an indistinct mass within the precardiac mediastinum. The protrusion of the dorsal portion of the cranial cardiac border and the density in the precardiac mediastinum are both manifestations of the post-stenotic dilatation of the pulmonary artery. The apex appears to be elevated, and the apicobasilar axis is slightly more inclined than normal. This might account in part for the disappearance of the ventral bend at the distal extremity of the trachea. The caudal waist is slightly shallower than normal. However, the left heart is normal, as was also shown angiocardiographically. The accentuation of the pulmonary arteries is unusual in dogs with pulmonic stenosis.

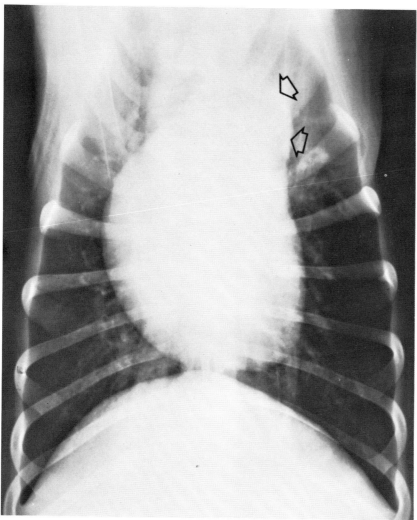

FIGURE 18-30 Dorsoventral radiograph, dog in Figure 18-29. The right heart is slightly enlarged, as indicated by the increased rounding of the right border. The large, bulging density between 12 and 2 o'clock (clear arrows) is due to marked enlargement of the main pulmonary artery. The large pulmonary artery segment represents a poststenotic dilatation of the main pulmonary artery. The increased density of the pulmonary arteries, also seen in Figure 18-29, is unusual in dogs with pulmonic stenosis.

elevated over the right ventricle, but the ventral bend of its distal extremity is always preserved. If an imaginary line is drawn from the carina at the base of the heart to the cardiac apex, it is easily demonstrated that the right ventricular surface is much larger than the left ventricular surface.

On the *dorsoventral radiograph,* the right border of the cardiac silhouette is markedly rounded and is closer to the right thoracic wall than normal. In a significant number of dogs with great right ventricular enlargement, the cardiac apex shifts to the left side and may give the false impression of left ventricular hypertrophy. The apex is rounded, and a small notch is sometimes seen at the interventricular septum. The left cardiac border remains straight. The pulmonary artery segment of the heart, although practically always dilated, varies considerably from case to case. Its size varies not only with the severity of the dilatation but also with systole, diastole, and slightly oblique positioning.

CARDIAC CATHETERIZATION AND ANGIOCARDIOGRAPHY

Sometimes great difficulty is encountered in attempting to pass a catheter through the stenotic pulmonic valve. Passing the catheter across the stenotic region is essential, since the confirmation of the diagnosis of pulmonic stenosis during cardiac catheterization relies on demonstrating a pressure gradient across the stenotic area. Elevation of right ventricular pressure and normal pulmonary arterial pressure are the expected findings on cardiac catheterization. The right atrial pressure may also be elevated, but this is not a consistent finding. Ott et al. (1964) referred to a case of pulmonic stenosis in which the preoperative pulmonary artery pressure was 45/5 mm. Hg, with a right ventricular pressure of 120/5 mm. Hg. Postoperatively, pressures recorded were 22/3 mm. Hg in the pulmonary artery and 60/3 mm. Hg in the right ventricle. In 2 other cases reported, preoperative right ventricular pressures were 100/0 mm. Hg (Hamlin, 1963a) and 132/0 mm. Hg (Tashjian et al., 1959). The pulmonary arterial pressure curve tracing in pulmonic stenosis is slow and late-rising and is similar to the aortic pressure tracing recorded from dogs with aortic stenosis (Fig. 18-32).

Angiocardiography is of value for demonstrating the location of the stenosis, the severity of narrowing at the stenotic area, the degree of narrowing of the right ventricular outflow tract, and the degree of right ventricular hypertrophy and/or right ventricular dilatation. The poststenotic dilatation of the pulmonary artery and the degree of secondary tricuspid insufficiency can also be evaluated. A number of reports concerning angiocardiography of dogs with pulmonic stenosis have been published (Ripps and Henderson, 1953; Hamlin, 1959; Tashjian et al., 1959; Rhodes, Patterson, and Detweiler, 1960, 1963; Ott et al., 1964).

The contrast medium should be injected selectively into the right ventricular outflow tract. When nonselective injection of contrast medium into the cranial vena cava or the right atrium is employed, the pulmonic valve area is often obscured by contrast remaining in the right atrium and cranial vena cava. This difficulty can be partially overcome by injecting the contrast medium into the caudal vena cava.

The lateral position is preferred to demonstrate pulmonic stenosis angiocardiographically (Fig. 18-31). In valvular stenosis, the narrowing of the contrast column between the cusps, often in the form of a cone, can be seen in adequately timed exposures. Infundibular narrowing is usually associated with valvular

Text continues on page 526.

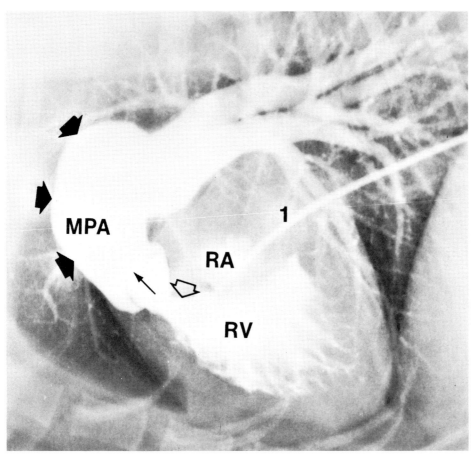

FIGURE 18-31 Selective right ventricular angiocardiogram, dog in Figures 18-29 and 18-30, exposed 1.5 seconds after the beginning of the injection of Hypaque-M 75% (1 ml./kg. body weight). Most of the contrast medium has already left the right ventricle (RV). A small jet of contrast medium indicates regurgitation into the right atrium (RA) around the catheter (1), which had been introduced antegrade via the femoral vein into the right ventricle. This regurgitation has no pathologic significance. The main pulmonary artery (MPA) is much larger than normal owing to a severe poststenotic dilatation extending from the caudal portion of the right cardiac border to approximately the level of the trachea (large black arrows). Tumors in the precardiac mediastinum are sometimes seen as masses protruding into the lucent tracheal lumen and must be differentiated from poststenotic dilatation of the pulmonary artery by examination in the dorsoventral view. The pointed, small arrow indicates the area of the valvular stenosis. There is marked narrowing of the column of contrast medium in the subvalvular area (clear arrow); this is often due to secondary muscular hypertrophy. A subvalvular fibrous ring may also be responsible for such subvalvular narrowing. The marked increase in thickness of the muscular wall between the right ventricular contrast outline and the cranial free wall indicates ventricular hypertrophy.

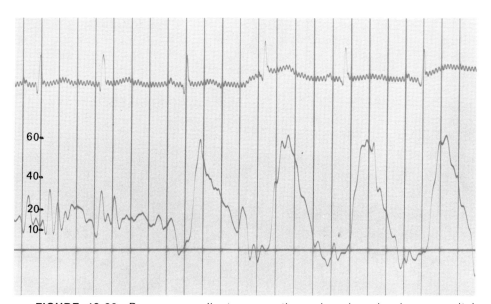

FIGURE 18-32 Pressure gradient across the pulmonic valve in congenital valvular pulmonic stenosis. The pressure in the main pulmonary artery is normal (30/10 mm. Hg), and a pressure gradient across the pulmonic valve is clearly demonstrated by the right ventricular systolic pressure (approximately 60 mm. Hg). The presence of such a gradient confirms the diagnosis of pulmonic stenosis. A gradient of this magnitude is usually not significant and is unlikely to result in clinical manifestations of heart disease.

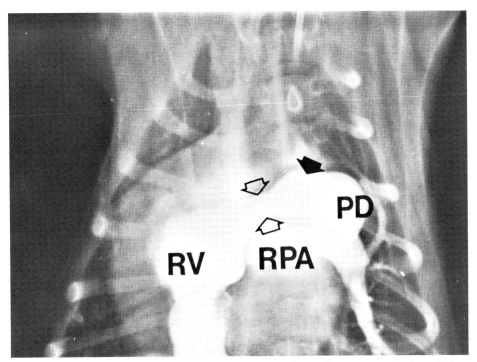

FIGURE 18-33 Selective right ventricular angiocardiogram, ventrodorsal view, 8 month old male Miniature Schnauzer with valvular pulmonic stenosis and secondary subvalvular hypertrophy. The tentative diagnosis was made on routine examination. The dog was asymptomatic and has remained asymptomatic for the last three years. Selective injection of contrast medium into the right ventricle (RV) outlined a very narrow outflow tract (clear arrows). The valvular stenosis itself (black arrow) cannot be seen clearly. The poststenotic dilatation (PD) causes the pulmonary artery segment of the cardiac silhouette to bulge. The left pulmonary artery is of normal size. The right pulmonary artery (RPA), which crosses from left to right immediately caudal to the stenosis, is also unremarkable. There is distinct right ventricular hypertrophy.

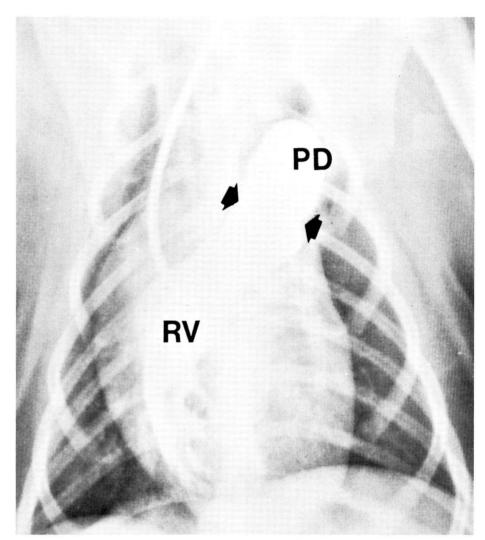

FIGURE 18-34 Selective right ventricular angiocardiogram, ventrodorsal view, 11 month old female Wirehaired Fox Terrier. A loud systolic ejection murmur with maximal intensity over the pulmonic valve area was heard on routine examination. The dog had no signs of heart disease. The valvular pulmonic stenosis was mild in this case. The heart is more oblong than the heart in Figure 18-33. The right ventricular enlargement and hypertrophy are far less obvious than in Figure 18-33. There is no infundibular narrowing. The stenosis itself is not outlined, but the location of the valve is indicated (black arrows). The poststenotic dilatation (PD) of the main pulmonary artery is thus the only characteristic sign in this case. The right and left pulmonary arteries have not yet filled with contrast medium at the time of this exposure (0.4 seconds after the beginning of the injection). Therefore, the view of the right ventricle is unobstructed.

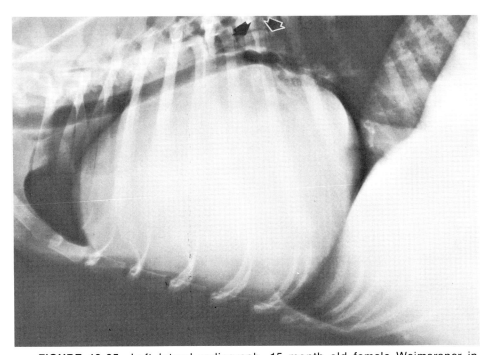

FIGURE 18-35 Left lateral radiograph, 15 month old female Weimaraner in right heart failure caused by pulmonic stenosis and tricuspid valvular insufficiency. The history indicated an enlarging abdomen and progressive weakness. A grade V/VI systolic murmur was auscultated over the right and left sternal borders. The abdominal enlargement was due to ascites. The extremely large cardiac silhouette fills most of the thoracic cavity and presses the trachea against the spine. The ventral bend at the distal extremity of the trachea has been preserved. An indistinct bulge dorsal to the tracheal bifurcation (arrows) indicates dilatation of the left pulmonary artery. Both cranial and caudal cardiac borders are globular. The caudal vena cava is distended and runs slightly craniodorsally instead of cranioventrally. The lung field is clear, and the vascular markings are barely visible. The massive cardiac enlargement in both the lateral and dorsoventral views (see Fig. 18-36) is similar to that seen with pericardial effusion. However, it is distinguished from pericardial effusion by the asymmetric enlargement, which involves primarily the right side of the heart, and by the absence of flattening of the cardiac silhouette as it touches the thoracic wall and diaphragm (see also Fig. 15-7). During cardiac catheterization, it was noticed that the enlarged cranial portion of the cardiac silhouette was due primarily to extreme enlargement of the right atrium. Right ventricular failure is indicated both by the dilated caudal vena cava and by ascites. The absence of left heart failure can be assumed from the normal-looking left atrium and the clear lung field. At necropsy, it was found that the extreme right atrial enlargement was due to severe tricuspid insufficiency caused by valvular fibrosis. There was eccentric hypertrophy of the right ventricle, which was also greatly enlarged. The commissures of the stenotic pulmonic valve leaflets adhered to each other.

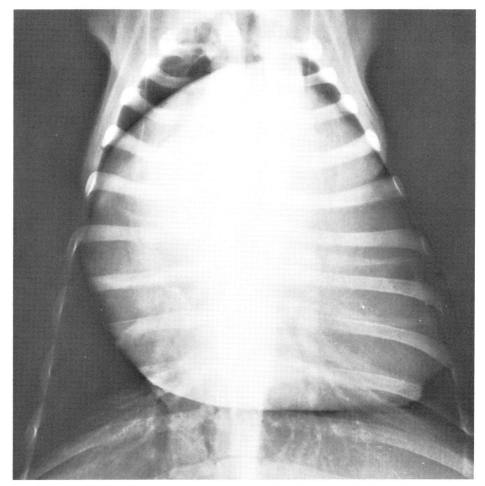

FIGURE 18-36 Dorsoventral radiograph, dog in Figure 18-35. Because of its enormous enlargement, the cardiac silhouette fills most of the thoracic cavity. However, the cardiac silhouette is not globular; a rounder right border and apical area can be differentiated. The caudal vena cava is dilated. The cardiac silhouette is not flattened where it touches the thoracic wall or the diaphragm, from which it is separated by a distinct line.

stenosis. It occurs secondarily to the valvular stenosis and results from secondary muscular hypertrophy of the right ventricular outflow tract.

The dorsoventral view is often not as characteristic as is the lateral view, and the narrowing in the valvular area might not be well visualized because of partial superimposition of the right ventricle and right pulmonary artery. The prominent pulmonary artery segment is diagnostic if no other defects can be seen and if the peripheral intrapulmonary vasculature is normal. The results of the dorsoventral view may be helpful in some cases (Figs. 18-33 and 18-34).

Tricuspid insufficiency complicating pulmonic stenosis is recognized on the angiocardiogram by regurgitation of contrast material into the right atrium, which at times is greatly enlarged (see Figs. 18-35 and 18-36). Associated congenital defects such as atrial or ventricular septal defect are best visualized when cineangiocardiography is used in preference to conventional film angiocardiography because the dye is visualized throughout its entire course in the heart. In complicated cases, the injection should be made as near to the complicating defect as possible, considering the presumed direction of the shunt as first determined by test hand injections of contrast medium.

DIAGNOSIS

The diagnosis of pulmonic stenosis is usually made on the basis of the systolic murmur heard over the pulmonic valve region, the pattern of severe right ventricular hypertrophy seen on the electrocardiogram, and the typical radiographic findings, including right ventricular hypertrophy and poststenotic dilatation of the main pulmonary artery. Other common congenital cardiac abnormalities are usually differentiated on the basis of hypervascularity of the lung field as occurs with patent ductus arteriosus, atrial septal defect, or ventricular septal defect; cyanosis and stunted growth as well as extreme hyperlucency of the lung field in tetralogy of Fallot; and left ventricular hypertrophy with poststenotic dilatation of the aortic arch in valvular and subvalvular aortic stenosis. In addition, the breed distribution of the condition, which occurs most often in the English Bulldog, Fox Terrier, and Chihuahua, is a clue for the diagnosis of congenital pulmonic stenosis.

PROGNOSIS

Although Patterson (1963) reported that most dogs with pulmonic stenosis die prior to 3 years of age, it has been the experience of the authors that death due to pulmonic stenosis may not be encountered before the dog reaches middle to old age. These observations are based on a limited number of dogs followed for more than three years which have shown no signs of heart failure.

TREATMENT

If congestive heart failure occurs, or if other signs that are related to cardiac disease develop, such as fatigability or syncope, temporary remission of signs is likely following cardiac therapy. In such cases, surgical correction probably should be considered after signs of heart failure have been relieved and the exact type of stenosis has been determined by cardiac catheterization and angiocardiography. Ripps and Henderson (1953) reported a successful valvulotomy procedure for pulmonic stenosis. Custer et al. (1961) and Ott et al. (1964) reported a successful pulmonic valve commissurotomy when surgery was performed under moderate hypothermia. Detailed descriptions of surgical approaches for pulmonic stenosis may be found in cardiovascular surgical textbooks (Cooley and Hallman, 1966).

GENETIC STUDIES

From seven matings between two dogs with valvular pulmonic stenosis, or one normal dog and one with pulmonic stenosis, eight of 41 offspring developed isolated pulmonic stenosis, proving a specific (although not a simple) hereditary transmission of the condition for this family (Patterson, 1968).

PATHOLOGY

Right ventricular hypertrophy and poststenotic dilatation of the main pulmonary artery are the prominent findings at necropsy. Microscopically, neither myocardial fibrosis nor intramural arterial lesions were found in 10 of 15 dogs with pulmonic stenosis and an intact ventriular septum. In four of the other five cases, intimal arterial thickening was recognized occasionally in the small arteries of the right ventricle, and in one case, microscopic areas of myocardial fibrosis were seen (Flickinger and Patterson, 1967).

AORTIC STENOSIS

Aortic stenosis results in obstruction of blood flow in the region of the aortic valve or proximal to it. It is classified anatomically as valvular when the obstruction is caused by a valvular anomaly; as supravalvular when the obstruction is in the ascending aorta; and as subvalvular (subaortic) when it is located in the left ventricular outflow tract. Spontaneous subvalvular aortic stenosis has been reported in dogs only as a congenital heart defect. Idiopathic hypertrophic subaortic stenosis (IHSS) has not been reported as a spontaneous disease in dogs. After toxic doses of 10 mg./kg. of amphetamine sulfate were administered once intravenously over 1 minute to each of 15 dogs, Zalis et al. (1966) reported hemodynamic, angiocardiographic, and postmortem findings that resembled the acquired clinical syndrome of idiopathic hypertrophic subaortic stenosis that occurs in man.

In purebred dogs, the incidence of aortic stenosis is higher in German Shepherds, Boxers, and Newfoundlands than would be expected according to the clinic population of these breeds (Patterson and Detweiler, 1963; Patterson, 1968). Of nine dogs with aortic stenosis in one study (Kersten, 1968), seven were Boxers, and two of the Boxers were littermates. In four litters of Newfoundlands of which at least one of the mates had subvalvular aortic stenosis, 14 of 37, or 38 per cent, of the offspring had congenital subaortic stenosis (Patterson, 1968). The condition has also been reported in a Fox Terrier, a Springer Spaniel, and an English Bulldog (Flickinger and Patterson, 1967).

In the dog, subvalvular (subaortic) stenosis usually occurs as a fibrous or fibromuscular ring (Detweiler, 1955, 1962; Patterson, 1963, 1965, 1968; Patterson and Flickinger, 1964; Flickinger and Patterson, 1967). Subvalvular aortic stenosis occurs less frequently as a membranous structure (Severin, 1967; Rowan et al., 1970). Congenital valvular aortic stenosis is unusual and appears as a dome-shaped or megaphone-type diaphragm in which the commissures are incompletely fused. Valvular aortic stenosis has been reported by Steinberg (1959) and by Patterson and Flickinger (1964). The frequency ratio of subaortic stenosis to valvular aortic stenosis in 25 cases was 24:1 (Patterson and Flickinger, 1964). In supravalvular stenosis, a ring or membrane develops above the valve. Supravalvular aortic stenosis is considered rare but has been seen in two dogs catheterized by us. Aortic stenosis has been reported to coexist with pulmonic stenosis (Patterson, 1965), a tetracuspid aortic valve (Flickinger and Patterson, 1967), tracheal stenosis and anomalous coronary ostia (Zook and Hathaway, 1966), and an anomalous right subclavian artery (Carmichael et al., 1968).

HISTORY AND PHYSICAL EXAMINATION

The dog is usually asymptomatic, and the condition is first recognized by auscultation during the first complete routine physical examination prior to vaccination. If the dog is symptomatic, syncope, panting, coughing, and pulmonary congestion or edema may occur. Patterson and Flickinger (1964) reported that one-third of all dogs with aortic stenosis examined at the University of Pennsylvania had had a history of syncopal episodes and/or sudden death. As left heart failure progresses, secondary right heart failure may also develop (Patterson, 1963). In 22 Newfoundland dogs with congenital subaortic stenosis, five developed clinical signs of heart disease, and three of the five died suddenly (Patterson, 1968).

Physically, the asymptomatic dog is in good general health. A caudally displaced apical impulse with a prominent left ventricular heave suggesting left ventricular hypertrophy may be present. A precordial thrill located at the cranial heart base may radiate to the cervical region, producing a carotid thrill (Flickinger and Patterson, 1967); occasionally, the precordial thrill is more intense on the cranioventral right thoracic wall. Palpation of the femoral pulse suggests a late-rising, small pulse. The abdomen appears normal unless secondary right heart failure has developed.

AUSCULTATION

A harsh, ejection-type, crescendo-decrescendo systolic murmur is heard over the aortic valve and usually extends to the thoracic inlet and cervical vessels. In some cases, the murmur is loudest over the cranial right thorax since the aortic arch courses to the right. On phonocardiography, the murmur appears diamond-shaped, with a midsystolic peak (Fig. 18-37). The murmur usually ends before or with the onset of the second heart sound. A systolic ejection click and paradoxical splitting of the second heart sound have been demonstrated using phonocardiography (Carmichael et al., 1968). A low-intensity diastolic murmur can develop owing to the minimal aortic insufficiency which usually accompanies congenital subaortic stenosis. When arrhythmias are present, the normal sinus rhythm is disrupted.

ELECTROCARDIOGRAPHY

The electrocardiogram of dogs with aortic stenosis may be normal or may show signs suggestive of left ventricular hypertrophy (Fig. 18-38). Ten of 19 cases reported by Flickinger and Patterson (1967) had arrhythmias. Ventricular ectopic beats were present in eight of the 10 dogs, one of which was in atrial fibrillation; another had paroxysmal atrial tachycardia, and in another atrial fibrillation developed in a dog that had previously had atrial premature contractions. It is likely that the ventricular arrhythmias result from microscopic infarctions and subsequent myocarditis in the left ventricular wall.

RADIOGRAPHIC EXAMINATION

The radiographic signs of aortic stenosis are often minimal and atypical, often incorrectly suggesting a ventricular septal defect, mitral insufficiency, atrial

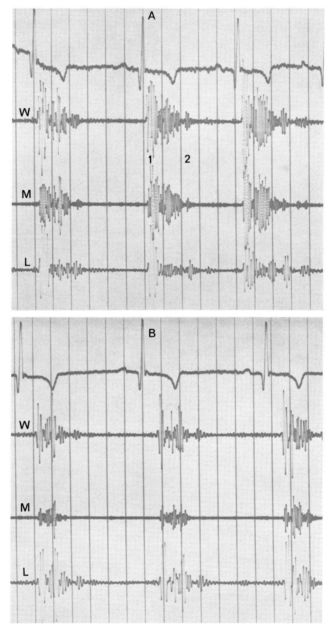

FIGURE 18-37 Subaortic stenosis. Lead II of the electrocardiogram recorded simultaneously with wide-frequency (W), medium-frequency (M), and low-frequency (L) band phonocardiograms. In A, recorded over the aortic valve region, the murmur is predominantly a medium-frequency sound occurring as a diamond-shaped crescendo-decrescendo systolic murmur. The first (1) and second (2) heart sounds are not obscured by the murmur. In B, the systolic murmur is clearly transmitted to the mid-cervical carotid artery.

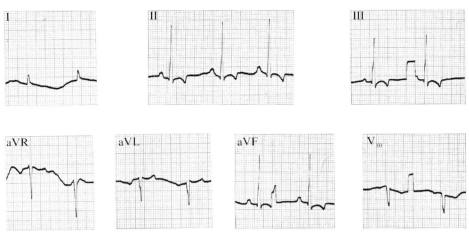

FIGURE 18-38 Subvalvular aortic stenosis. Although congenital subvalvular aortic stenosis was present in this dog, the electrocardiogram remained quite normal. The P mitrale and tall R waves would suggest left ventricular hypertrophy; however, the diagnosis of subvalvular aortic stenosis could not be made with certainty only from the electrocardiogram. In addition, slurring of the upstroke of the R wave in several of the leads is also suggestive of left ventricular hypertrophy.

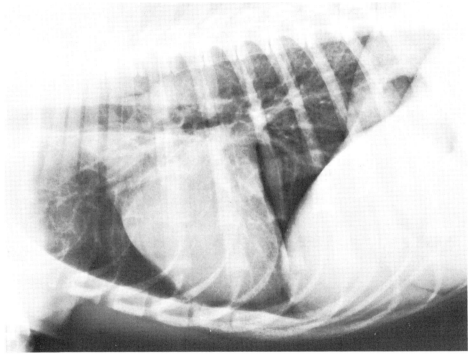

FIGURE 18-39 Left lateral radiograph, 7 month old male German Shepherd dog with a harsh systolic murmur over the cranial right ventral thorax and left cranial thorax which extended to the cervical vessels. The dog was otherwise healthy. The cranial waist has disappeared owing to slight dilatation of the aortic arch. The cranial cardiac border is slightly scalloped. The caudal cardiac border is straighter than normal. The caudal waist has disappeared, and slight left atrial enlargement has elevated the distal extremity of the trachea. The slightly narrowed angle of the trachea with the thoracic spine further supports the assumption of left heart enlargement. The radiographic signs are compatible with but not diagnostic of mild aortic stenosis (see Fig. 18-41).

531

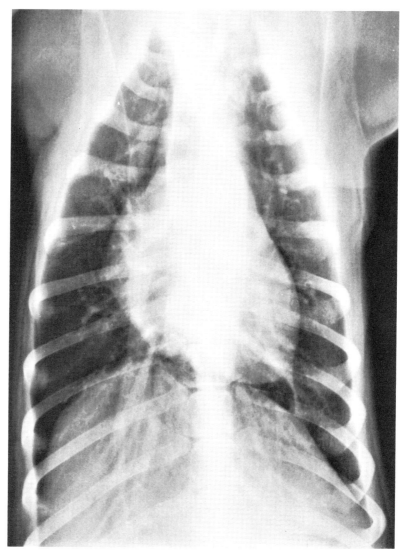

FIGURE 18-40 Dorsoventral radiograph, dog in Figure 18-39. Increased rounding in the apical and caudal left cardiac border areas indicates slight left ventricular enlargement.

septal defect, or changes secondary to anemia. In severe cases with clinical signs of heart failure, the radiographic appearance is more typical. The radiographic findings have been reported by Detweiler (1962) and by Patterson and Flickinger (1964). (See Tables 18-1 and 18-2, pp. 488-489).

In the *lateral radiograph*, the trachea is elevated, and the caudal left ventricular border may be straighter than normal (Fig. 18-39). Slight left atrial enlargement is usually seen in those cases where mitral insufficiency develops secondarily to aortic stenosis, and the pulmonary veins may become prominent because of the developing congestion. In typical cases, the aortic arch appears prominent and enlarged. The cranial waist of the cardiac silhouette may disappear, being obscured by the prominent bulge of the poststenotic dilatation of the ascending aorta. Often the poststenotic dilatation of the aorta is not large enough or is located too far caudally to be seen clearly on the plain radiograph.

In the *dorsoventral radiograph* (Fig. 18-40), the cardiac silhouette is elongated because of a prominent aortic arch, and it is rounded owing to left ventricular enlargement. The left ventricular border protrudes, and the distance between the right border and the thoracic wall is diminished. The cardiac apex may be rounder than normal. Patterson and Flickinger (1964) mentioned that in Boxers with subaortic stenosis, the apex of the heart can be in the right hemithorax. Although shifting of the apex to the opposite side is seen in left ventricular enlargement, it is not uncommon in normal brachycephalic dogs, and is probably caused by a loose cardiophrenic ligament.

CARDIAC CATHETERIZATION AND ANGIOCARDIOGRAPHY

Subaortic stenosis is characterized by subvalvular narrowing of the left ventricular outflow tract. There is a systolic pressure gradient between the left ventricular cavity and the left ventricular outflow tract (Fig. 18-42). The gradient exists across the stenotic lesion because of increased ventricular pressures with normal or near normal pressures in the aorta. The gradient ranged from 30 to 200 mm. Hg in five dogs reported by Flickinger and Patterson (1967). The pressure gradient may be increased in some cases by the infusion of dilute isoproterenol solution, which increases left ventricular pressures and has a vasodilating effect, thereby reducing aortic pressures. The small and late pulse characteristic of aortic stenosis may be recognized on arterial and left ventricular pressure tracings. The presence of an anacrotic notch on the ascending limb of the arterial tracings is highly suggestive of aortic stenosis.

When the gradient across the aortic valve is absent or small, angiocardiography often yields definitive proof of the presence of aortic stenosis. The contrast medium must be injected selectively into the left ventricle, since residual contrast in the right heart and pulmonary artery in nonselective procedures may obscure the details (see pp. 193-196).

Angiocardiography in dogs with aortic stenosis has been described by Rhodes, Patterson, and Detweiler (1963), Patterson and Flickinger (1964), Buchanan and Patterson (1965), and Carmichael et al. (1968). Left ventricular hypertrophy or dilatation and subvalvular aortic narrowing or both are seen in all cases. The degree of the stenosis varies in diameter from case to case but is usually unaltered during systole and diastole (Fig. 18-41). In some cases the stenosis is symmetric in relationship to the aortic valve cusps, but in most cases it appears asymmetric (Fig. 18-43). The degree of poststenotic dilatation of the aorta, and

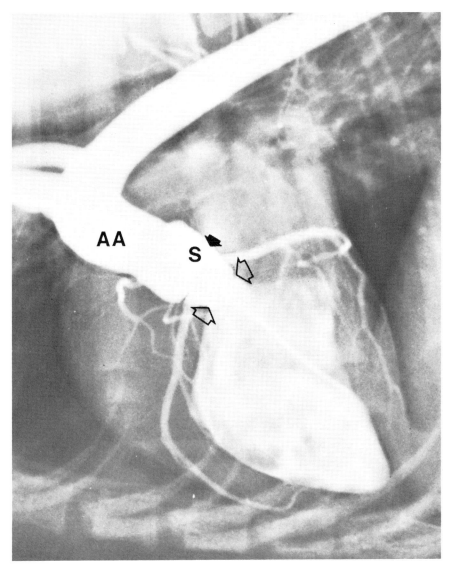

FIGURE 18-41   Selective left ventricular angiocardiogram, dog in Figures 18-39 and 18-40, made 0.3 seconds after the beginning of the injection of Hypaque-M 75% (1 ml./kg. body weight). Mild subvalvular aortic stenosis is present. The contrast medium in the ventricle has already been diluted with blood flowing into the left ventricle from the atrium. The width of the slightly constricted area of the left ventricular outflow tract (clear arrows) remained unchanged throughout systole and diastole. The valvular area is indicated (black arrow). The sinus of Valsalva of the aorta (S) from which the left coronary artery arises is usually not impaired by this defect. Notice the slight asymmetry of the stenotic subvalvular area as compared with the symmetrical valvular area. In this case there is no significant poststenotic dilatation of the ascending aorta (AA).

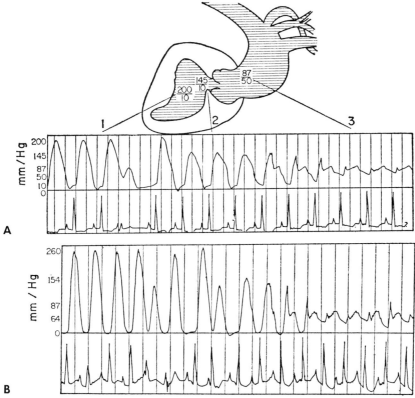

FIGURE 18-42   Subaortic stenosis. *A,* Diagram of the left ventricle, aorta, and pressure tracing indicating pressures at three stages during the withdrawal of the catheter across the subvalvular stenosis: in the left ventricle (1), in the subvalvular area (2), and in the ascending aortic arch (3). *B,* A pressure tracing obtained, indicating the gradient across the subaortic stenosis following the administration of 0.002 mg. of isoproterenol. Note the increase in gradient, the peak configuration of the left ventricular tracing, the prominent anacrotic notch, and the diminished dicrotic notch in the aortic tracing (paper speed 50 mm./sec.; time lines = 0.2 sec.). *From* Carmichael, *et al.:* 1968, p. 217 & p. 218.)

sometimes the brachiocephalic artery, is variable and in some cases barely visible; it is much less pronounced than is the poststenotic dilatation of the thin-walled main pulmonary artery in pulmonic stenosis. Aortic and mitral valvular insufficiency may be seen in some cases. Another complication is abnormal branching of the aortic arch (Fig. 18-44*A* and 18-44*B*).

The evaluation of the poststenotic aortic dilatation has been discussed in detail by Buchanan and Patterson (1965). They attribute the variation in dilatation to differences in the duration of the condition, to the degree, shape, or location of the stenosis, and to the extent that aortic pathologic changes have occurred, as well as to other undetermined factors.

The ratio between the diameter of the ascending aorta and the diameter of the aorta at the sinus of Valsalva has been referred to as the "A/S ratio." According to Buchanan and Patterson (1965), A/S is always less than 1 in normal dogs, but in dogs with subaortic stenosis it is greater than 1. The A/S ratio is useful in those cases in which the poststenotic dilatation is not obvious.

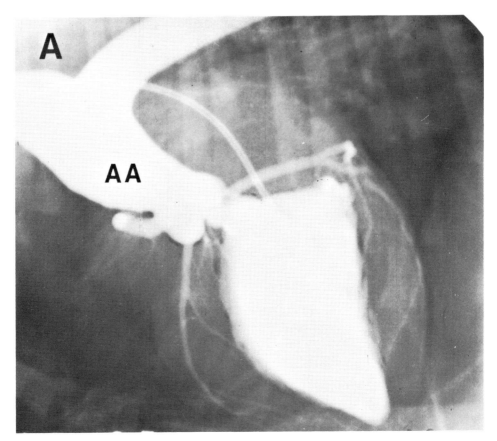

FIGURE 18-43 Selective left ventricular angiocardiograms, 9 month old male Boxer. *A,* Right lateral angiocardiogram. The left ventricle is filled with contrast medium. The narrowing of the outflow tract, which is again asymmetric in relation to the sinuses of Valsalva of the ascending aorta (AA) (see also Fig. 18-42), represents the subaortic stenotic ring. The sinuses of Valsalva of the aorta and the valve cusps look normal. A mild poststenotic dilatation is present in the distal portion of the ascending aorta and the beginning of the brachiocephalic artery. A dilated, truncated-appearing, aberrant coronary artery is seen which runs parallel with the ascending aorta. The visible catheter is located in the nonopacified right heart; the catheter in the left ventricle is obscured by the injected contrast medium.

Legend continues on opposite page.

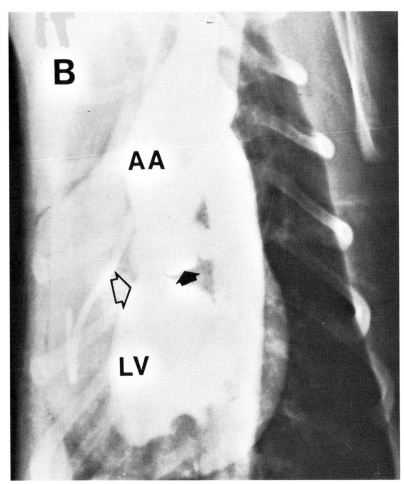

FIGURE 18-43 *B,* Ventrodorsal angiocardiogram. The stenotic subvalvular region is indicated by a clear arrow distal to the left ventricle (LV). The black arrow
points at the aortic valve. There is a mild poststenotic dilatation of the ascending
aorta (AA). Part of the descending aorta is superimposed on the left ventricle.

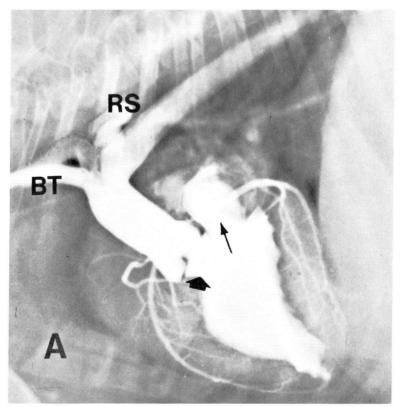

FIGURE 18-44 Selective left ventricular angiocardiograms, 10 year old male Boston Terrier with subaortic stenosis. *A*, Radiograph exposed during systole. There is a small jet of contrast medium (small, pointed arrow) regurgitating into the left atrium. Since this regurgitation was present only for a short time, it was probably a functional insufficiency due to a ventricular arrhythmia and therefore does not indicate a mitral valvular lesion. Narrowing of the subvalvular area (large arrow) indicates subaortic stenosis. It lies asymmetrically relative to the well-delineated aortic valve. The diameter of the ascending aorta is normal. However, the branching at the aortic arch is abnormal, since three separate vessels originate there, rather than the normal two. The right and left carotid arteries have a common origin, forming a bicarotid trunk (BT). The remaining two arteries are distorted and represent the left subclavian artery in the middle and the right subclavian artery (RS) dorsally. The right subclavian artery therefore originates proximally to the left subclavian artery. Its origin is obscured by the contrast density of the aortic arch. The distortion of the right subclavian artery is due to its abnormal course around the esophagus, which was also seen on a dorsoventral angiocardiogram. This abnormal branching of the aortic arch is also referred to as a retroesophageal right subclavian artery, or arteria lusoria; it sometimes causes narrowing of the esophagus and dysphagia. It was an incidental finding in the present case.

Legend continues on opposite page.

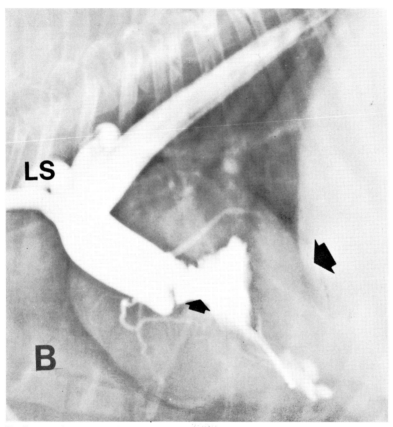

B, Radiograph exposed at the end of systole. The left ventricular chamber has narrowed to a small linear density, indicating that hypertrophy of the left ventricular musculature has caused an extreme reduction of the end systolic ventricular volume; this is typical with concentric hypertrophy. Notice the thick ventricular wall between the large, black arrow and the opacified left ventricle. Further narrowing of the stenosis than is seen in *A* can be explained by muscular hypertrophy around the outflow tract. The abnormal branching at the aortic arch into the bicarotid trunk, the left subclavian artery (LS), and the right subclavian artery is well visualized.

DIFFERENTIAL DIAGNOSIS

In advanced cases of congenital aortic stenosis, the diagnosis is usually not difficult. The high frequency of occurrence of this condition in the German Shepherd and the Boxer is an important consideration in diagnosing this condition. The clinical signs are those of syncope, sudden death, or heart failure. Radiographically, there is left ventricular hypertrophy and dilatation of the aortic arch, in contrast to the right ventricular hypertrophy and overcirculation associated with patent ductus arteriosus, atrial septal defect, and ventricular septal defect, and the right ventricular hypertrophy and undercirculation associated with pulmonic stenosis and tetralogy of Fallot.

PROGNOSIS

Detweiler (1962) mentions that dogs with aortic stenosis often die suddenly because of ventricular fibrillation. Of the 19 cases of subaortic stenosis reported by Flickinger and Patterson (1967), six dogs died in congestive heart failure, four others died suddenly, and three died during attempts at surgical correction. Five dogs were put to death, and one died of a brain neoplasm apparently unrelated to the congenital cardiac lesion. Eight of the 19 dogs with congenital subaortic stenosis examined clinically and at necropsy by Flickinger and Patterson (1967) were under 1 year of age, eight others were between 1 and 4 years of age, and three were 5, 6, and 9 years old, respectively. Approximately one-third of all dogs with aortic valvular stenosis have a history of syncopal episodes and sudden death, according to Patterson and Flickinger (1964).

TREATMENT

Digitalization, cage rest, low sodium diets, and diuretics are indicated to treat congestive heart failure. If ectopic beats are present, antiarrhythmic agents are indicated. Since the prognosis for long-term survival of dogs with symptomatic aortic stenosis with medical therapy is poor, surgical correction should be recommended in such cases. When surgical correction is considered, a complete cardiac evaluation, including cardiac catheterization and angiocardiography, is necessary to confirm the clinical diagnosis. The surgical procedure requires the use of extracorporeal circulation. For a discussion of open-heart surgical techniques and extracorporeal circulation, the reader is referred to texts on human cardiovascular surgery (Cooley and Hallman, 1966).

PATHOLOGY

Concentric hypertrophy of the left ventricle develops in aortic stenosis, and dilatation of the left atrium and ventricle occurs in about half the cases (Flickinger and Patterson, 1967) (Fig. 18-45). Fibrous endocardial thickening, encircling all or part of the left ventricular outflow tract and extending across the interventricular septum to the aortic leaflet of the mitral valve, is seen below the aortic valve (Flickinger and Patterson, 1967; Patterson, 1968). The diameter of the orifice of the subvalvular ring is narrow, and there are varying degrees of poststenotic dilatation of the ascending aorta. The edges of the valve cusps are thickened by small, firm nodules which do not noticeably impair valve closure

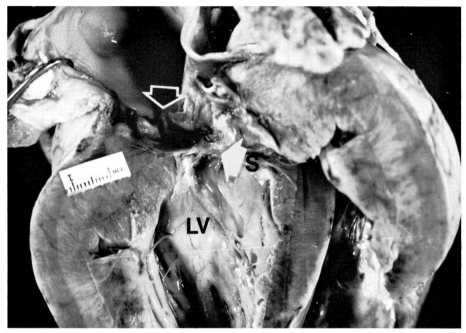

FIGURE 18-45 Gross pathologic specimen, heart of dog with subvalvular aortic stenosis. The left ventricle (LV) has been opened to demonstrate the subvalvular stenotic area (white arrow, S) formed by a fibrous band. The normal aortic valve can be seen distal to the stenosis (clear arrow). Notice the hypertrophied left ventricular wall.

(Flickinger and Patterson, 1967). Aortic insufficiency may develop secondarily to congenital subaortic stenosis because of damage to one of the aortic valve leaflets (Zook and Hathaway, 1966; Carmichael et al., 1968). At necropsy, small, irregular yellow patches probably related to recent infarctions were seen in the subendocardium of the anterior papillary muscle on the cut surface of the left ventricle in dogs with this condition (Flickinger and Patterson, 1967).

Microscopically, intramural coronary artery changes consisting of fibrous intimal thickening are confined to the left ventricle. Focal necrosis, fibrosis, and calcification of the left ventricular myocardium are recognized (Patterson and Detweiler, 1963; Flickinger and Patterson, 1967; Carmichael et al., 1968). Flickinger and Patterson (1967) suggested that the vascular lesions result from systolic occlusion of the intramyocardial arteries occurring when increased left ventricular wall tensions develop without a comparable increase in intra-arterial pressures. Similar but less obvious arterial lesions were found in 5 of 15 dogs with pulmonic stenosis that were examined by Flickinger and Patterson (1967).

ATRIAL SEPTAL DEFECT

Defects in the atrial septum may be of three types: the ostium primum defect, ostium secundum defect, and patent foramen ovale. The first two are true interatrial defects, whereas patency of the foramen ovale results from persistence of the opening existing as a circulatory pathway between the left and right atria during fetal life. Patency of the foramen ovale is usually inconsequential, and a valve-like structure normally prevents interatrial shunting of blood after birth. Defects which occur in the lower or ventral portion of the atrial septum are referred to as septum primum (ostium primum) atrial septal defects; these are uncommon in the dog. Septum secundum (ostium secundum) defects occur in the dorsal and middle portions of the interatrial septum.

Since left atrial pressure normally exceeds right atrial pressure, atrial septal defects result in a shunting of blood from the left atrium to the right atrium. Reversal of blood flow has been reported to occur in dogs secondarily to pulmonic stenosis (Buchanan and Patterson, 1965), and to tricuspid atresia, tricuspid stenosis, and tricuspid insufficiency (Ljunggren et al., 1966). In the presence of a left-to-right atrial shunt, an increased blood volume entering the right ventricle results in increased blood flow through the pulmonary vasculature, leading to an increased work load on the right ventricle. Eccentric hypertrophy of the right ventricle develops consequently.

Patterson (1968) reported 12 cases of septum secundum type of atrial septal defect. Nine of these were associated with other congenital cardiac defects. Atrial septal defects are uncommon as an isolated condition. Brodey and Prier (1961) reported that one dog had a patent foramen ovale, pulmonic stenosis, and a peritoneopericardial diaphragmatic hernia. Shive, Hare, and Patterson (1965) described chromosomal abnormalities in a dog with a tetralogy of Fallot and a patent foramen ovale. Popovic and Fleming (1970) recorded a case of an atrial septal defect and pulmonic stenosis.

CLINICAL SIGNS AND PHYSICAL EXAMINATION

Exertional dyspnea, fatigue, and weakness may occur with atrial septal defects. If heart failure occurs, it is right-sided in form, as suggested by venous engorgement and ascites. If there is reverse shunting of blood from right atrium to left atrium, cyanosis will result (Ottaway, 1949; Buchanan and Patterson, 1965).

An ejection-type systolic murmur due to relative pulmonic stenosis is auscultated over the pulmonic valve region. Splitting of the second heart sound may result from delayed closure of the pulmonic valve, and an early diastolic murmur may be detected on the phonocardiogram as increased quantities of blood pass from right atrium to right ventricle, resulting in a relative pulmonic stenosis (Hamlin, Smith, and Smetzer, 1963b). Jugular "a" waves may occur as the increased flow of blood from the left to the right atrium increases jugular venous pressure.

ELECTROCARDIOGRAPHY

Right axis deviation and right ventricular hypertrophy are associated with atrial septal defect. P pulmonale and an increased P-R interval may result from atrial dilatation. In one of the two dogs reported by Hamlin, Smith, and Smetzer (1963b), the QRS complex was directed cephalad.

RADIOGRAPHIC EXAMINATION

The radiographic findings have been described by Hamlin, Smith, and Smetzer (1963b) and Hamlin (1968). Right ventricular and right atrial enlargement, a small aortic knob, and occasionally increased intrapulmonary vascular markings with distended pulmonary arterial branches are expected on thoracic radiographs. The pulmonary artery segment may or may not be enlarged, depending on the quantity of blood shunted from left to right. Hamlin, Smith, and Smetzer (1963b) reported bulging of the main pulmonary artery in one of two dogs, and right ventricular enlargement in two dogs, with atrial septal defect. In complicated cases with a combined atrial septal defect and pulmonic stenosis, the pulmonary artery segment is usually enlarged. The pulmonary blood flow is often reduced because of the right-to-left shunting at the atrial level. (See Tables 18-1 and 18-2, pp. 488-489.)

CARDIAC CATHETERIZATION AND ANGIOCARDIOGRAPHY

Oximetry performed during cardiac catheterization reveals that the blood-oxygen content in the right atrium is increased in comparison to that in the cranial vena cava, suggesting a shunting of blood from left to right at the level of the atrium. On indicator dilution studies, the decay slope of the dilution curve is decreased if the point of sampling is distal to the point of injection of the substance (Hamlin, Smith, and Smetzer, 1963b).

It is difficult to demonstrate an atrial septal defect angiocardiographically. Selective left atrial injection may be attempted. If this is not possible, a pulmonary arterial injection should be made. With either method, simultaneous opacification of the right and left atria occurs if an atrial septal defect shunting from left to right is present. In some cases, the catheter may cross the septal defect spontaneously.

In a dog with a patent foramen ovale and pulmonic stenosis resulting in a right-to-left shunt, it was shown by Detweiler (in Brodey and Prier, 1961) that a selective caudal vena caval injection was superior to a cranial vena caval injection for outlining this defect.

DIFFERENTIAL DIAGNOSIS

Atrial septal defects produce a hypervascular lung field when the shunt is directed from left to right. Under these circumstances, the condition would need to be differentiated from a patent ductus arteriosus and a ventricular septal defect. Patent ductus arteriosus is differentiated on the basis of the pathognomonic, continuous machinery murmur, the abnormally tall electrocardiographic QRS complexes, and the typical dilated appearance of the aortic arch. Ventricular septal defects produce a loud, harsh murmur over the right thoracic wall. Complicated atrial septal defect, where the flow of blood is from right to left, results in cyanosis, and the specific diagnosis can be properly made only after cardiac catheterization and angiocardiography.

VENTRICULAR SEPTAL DEFECT

The ventricular septum separates the right and the left ventricles. Its growth is completed during the first quarter of embryonic development (Zietzschmann and Krölling, 1955). The septum is a thick, muscular wall (Septum musculare) in the apical portion of the ventricle and a membranous wall (Septum membranaceum) in the basilar region of the ventricle.

Although ventricular septal defects may occur at different levels of the interventricular septum, most occur high in the membranous or basilar portion of the septum (Buchanan and Patterson, 1965). When such defects are small and uncomplicated, and when the shunt of blood is from left to right with no significant degree of pulmonary hypertension, they are referred to as Roger's disease, in man as well as in dogs (Hamlin, Smetzer, and Smith, 1964). When viewed from the right ventricle, the membranous ventricular septal defect is located under the septal leaflet of the tricuspid valve. When viewed from the left ventricle, it is located in the left ventricular outflow tract ventral to the right coronary and noncoronary aortic cusps (Buchanan and Patterson, 1965). It is important to determine the location of the defect because the morphology and function of the aortic or pulmonic valve may be impaired. As reported by others and as seen by the authors, ventricular septal defect may be complicated by atrial septal defect (Lucam et al., 1956), patent ductus arteriosus (Hare and Orr, 1931), subaortic valvular stenosis, pulmonic stenosis, persistent left cranial vena cava, double outlet right ventricle, Eisenmenger complex, or aortic insufficiency (Buchanan and Patterson, 1965; Patterson, 1965, 1968; Shive, Hare, and Patterson, 1965).

Eyster (1969) reported 18 cases of ventricular septal defects in dogs over a three-year period. This represented 16 per cent of all canine congenital cardiac diseases recognized during that period. Patterson (1968) reported 20 cases (7 per cent) of ventricular septal defect in 290 dogs in which congenital cardiac anomalies had been diagnosed during a 12-year period.

Clark, Anderson, and Patterson (1970) reported the presence of an imperforate septal defect which passed rightward to end beneath the right atrial endocardium.

HISTORY AND PHYSICAL EXAMINATION

The ventricular septal defect is usually detected in an otherwise asymptomatic dog (Lev, Neuwelt, and Necheles, 1941) when auscultation is performed as part of the physical examination made when the dog is presented for vaccination. Occasionally the dog is presented with signs of congestive heart failure — these are usually mature dogs or puppies which cannot tolerate the hemodynamic burden initiated by the shunting of blood (Hare, 1943).

The pulse associated with a ventricular septal defect is rapid and jerky and is similar to that recognized with chronic mitral valvular fibrosis.

Pulmonary hypertension may develop if pulmonary artery pressures increase because of the increased blood flow resulting from the shunting of blood from left to right (hyperkinetic hypertension), or if hypertrophy of the walls of intrapulmonary arteries results in increased pulmonary arteriolar resistance. As the pressure in the right ventricle rises, it may equal or surpass the pressure in the left ventricle. When secondary pulmonary hypertension occurs along with right ventricular hypertrophy, and a right-to-left shunt occurs, the condition is included in the term *Eisenmenger complex* (Friedberg, 1966). This is in addition to the generally accepted anatomic definition of the Eisenmenger complex, in which an overriding aorta is present in addition to the ventricular septal defect and right ventricular hypertrophy. Ventricular septal defects with pulmonary hypertension have been reported (Buchanan and Patterson, 1965; Eyster, 1969).

When a reversed or a right-to-left shunt occurs, the dog may become cyanotic as unoxygenated blood passes from the right ventricle to the left ventricle or aorta and out to the peripheral circulation. Buchanan and Patterson (1965) reported the findings in one dog that remained acyanotic even though right ventricular pressure increased sufficiently to produce a bi-directional shunt. Pulmonic stenosis was probably responsible for elevation of the right ventricular pressure and right-to-left shunting through a ventricular septal defect in this case.

AUSCULTATION

On auscultation, a loud, harsh, holosystolic murmur is best heard slightly dorsal to or at the right sternal border over the third to fourth intercostal spaces (Fig. 18-46). The murmur is usually accompanied by a precordial thrill at the point of maximal intensity. Along the left caudal sternal border, a systolic murmur is auscultated with an intensity equal to or slightly less than that heard at the point of maximal intensity on the right. The murmur may be transmitted cranially and dorsally along the left thoracic wall, but it is of considerably lower intensity at the aortic and pulmonic valve regions. The murmur heard at the right and left points of maximal intensity is similar to that auscultated with chronic mitral valvular fibrosis (see pp. 327-330). Although only a small quantity of blood may pass through the defect, the murmur may be very loud. Splitting of the second heart sound has been reported in dogs with ventricular septal defect (Hamlin, Smetzer, and Smith, 1964). Should pulmonary hypertension be severe enough to raise right ventricular pressures and interfere with the flow of blood from the left to the right ventricle, the duration of the systolic murmur will decrease or, in the most severe cases, be obliterated.

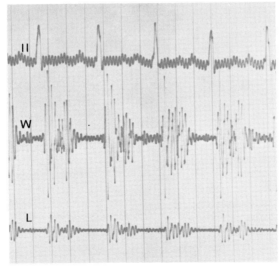

FIGURE 18-46 Ventricular septal defect. Lead II of the electrocardiogram recorded simultaneously with wide-frequency (W) and low-frequency (L) band phonocardiograms. A holosystolic murmur following the loud first heart sound was recorded over the right midthorax at the point of maximal intensity. The murmur is clinically similar to that auscultated and recorded with chronic mitral and tricuspid valvular fibrosis. With ventricular septal defects, the loudest murmur is heard over the right thorax and is composed of mixed-frequency components, so that it is best recorded on the wide band of the phonocardiogram.

ELECTROCARDIOGRAPHY

In a series of eight dogs with ventricular septal defect, Hamlin, Smetzer, and Smith (1964) reported that there was no deviation of the mean frontal plane electrical axis, and that a normal sinus rhythm was maintained in all eight dogs. It was suggested that an increase in the terminal cranial forces may have been due to early right ventricular hypertrophy or delayed activation of a portion of the right ventricle. In most cases observed by the authors, the electrocardiogram has been unremarkable. Atrial fibrillation developed in one dog with a ventricular septal defect and ultimately led to congestive heart failure.

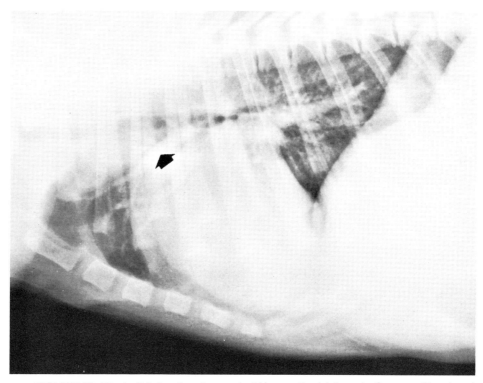

FIGURE 18-47   Left lateral radiograph, 3½ month old, female German Shepherd dog. The right ventricle is moderately enlarged and extends farther cranially than normal. The trachea is displaced dorsally, and the bend in the distal trachea has disappeared due to left atrial and left ventricular enlargement. However, the left ventricular enlargement is not as pronounced as is the right ventricular enlargement. The lung field is denser than it should be in a dog of this age. The pulmonary veins (arrow) are prominent, and the outlines of the vascular structures are blurred, indicating pulmonary congestion. Such prominent vascular markings in a young dog are suggestive of overcirculation due to a left-to-right shunt. The age of this dog, the right ventricular and left atrial enlargement, and signs compatible with overcirculation indicate a ventricular septal defect. However, the diagnosis of ventricular septal defect cannot be made from the lateral radiograph alone. The dorsoventral radiograph (Fig. 18-48) provides further characteristic signs. Angiocardiograms of this dog are shown in Figure 18-49.

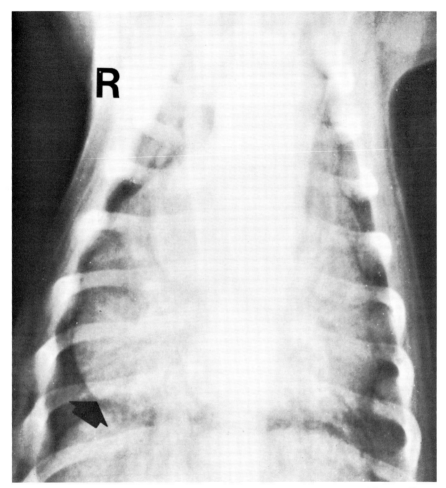

FIGURE 18-48   Dorsoventral radiograph, dog in Figure 18-47. This radiograph was made when the dog was first examined, at 2 months of age. Cardiomegaly is more obvious in this view than it is on the lateral view (Fig. 18-47). The right ventricle extends almost to the right thoracic wall and has a saccular widening in the right caudal portion (arrow). The apex has shifted slightly to the left side, which makes the left ventricular enlargement look more severe than it appeared on the lateral radiograph. The main portion of the left atrium has forced the main stem bronchi apart. The arteries and veins are more prominent than normal. Angiocardiograms of this dog are shown in Figure 18-49.

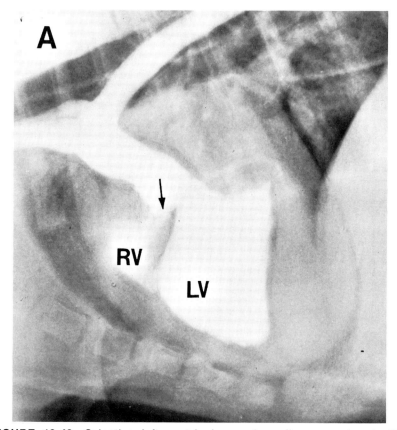

FIGURE 18-49 Selective left ventricular angiocardiograms, dog in Figures 18-47 and 18-48, made when the dog was 3 months old. Radiograph A was made 1 second after the beginning of the injection of contrast medium, and radiograph B was exposed 2 seconds after the beginning of the injection.

A, The left ventricle (LV) is at the beginning of the systolic phase, and the mitral valve is closed. There is a small jet of contrast medium just ventral to the aortic valve (black arrow). This indicates a high ventricular septal defect which, because of its location immediately ventral to the aortic valve or the pulmonic valve, may also cause abnormalities of the valve leaflets. In addition, subvalvular aortic stenosis is present, thus making this defect a complicated one. The contrast medium becomes diluted as it reaches the right ventricle (RV).

Figure continues on opposite page.

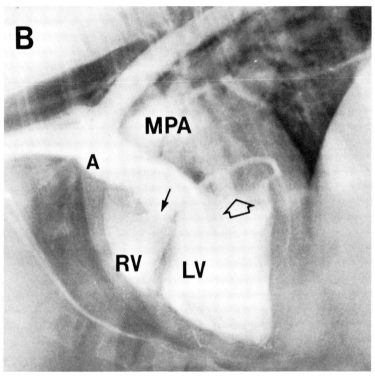

B, A small amount of contrast medium has regurgitated retrograde through the mitral valve (clear arrow); however, this is not pathologic. More contrast medium has meanwhile flowed into the right ventricle (RV) and is now opacifying the main pulmonary artery (MPA). Simultaneous filling of the main pulmonary artery and the aorta (A) after selective left ventricular injection proves that a left-to-right shunt is present. The direction of flow in a ventricular septal defect is not necessarily constant. It may be from left to right at the beginning of systole and from right to left at the end of systole.

RADIOGRAPHIC EXAMINATION

The radiographic signs produced by a ventricular septal defect depend on the size of the defect and the direction and severity of the shunt (Figs. 18-47 through 18-51). Secondary hemodynamic changes such as pulmonary hypertension result in modification of the radiographic appearance of the cardiac silhouette and the lung field. Radiographic signs of interventricular septal defect have been reported by Hamlin, Smetzer, and Smith (1964) and Buchanan and Patterson (1965). The findings on plain radiographs are usually unclear, and angiocardiography is often required for a definitive diagnosis to be made. (See Tables 18-1 and 18-2.)

Small defects in the membranous portion of the ventricular septum produce only slight changes, if any, although minimal enlargement of the right ventricle

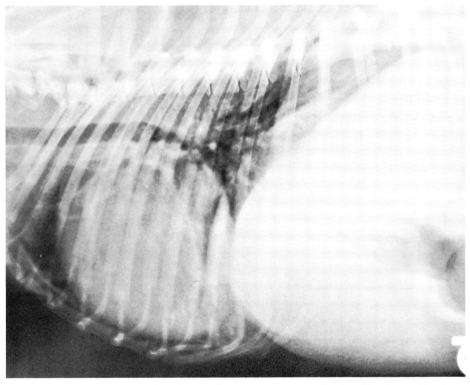

FIGURE 18-50 Lateral radiograph, 7 year old male Fox Terrier with signs referable to right and left heart failure. The dog died unexpectedly several hours after the radiographs had been made. The extreme enlargement of the cardiac silhouette is entirely due to the greatly increased size of the right ventricle. The trachea is elevated, but the ventral bend at the distal extremity has been retained. The elevation cranial to the carina may be due in part to right atrial enlargement. Despite the absence of left atrial enlargement and subsequent pulmonary congestion, the lung field is denser than normal because of fibrotic changes. The liver is very dense and greatly enlarged. Notice also the slight, localized, dorsal deviation of the thoracic spine over the base of the heart. A high interventricular septal defect and tricuspid insufficiency with signs of pulmonary hypertension and fibrosis were found at necropsy.

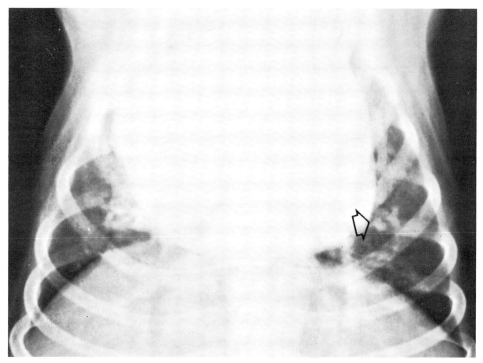

FIGURE 18-51 Dorsoventral radiograph, dog in Figure 18-50. The cardiac silhouette is greatly enlarged and appears as a transverse rather than a longitudinal oval. The right ventricle and the right atrium, which is visible as a bulge in the cranial portion of the right ventricle, have both enlarged greatly. The right ventricle has displaced the apex to the left side. The apex is difficult to recognize owing to the marked rounding. Notice the distorted appearance of the pulmonary arteries (arrow) which can result from pulmonary hypertension.

and left atrium may be seen. Enlargement of the pulmonary artery was the most consistent sign described by Hamlin, Smetzer, and Smith (1964). In some dogs, the long axis of the heart in the dorsoventral view appears elongated.

If the defect is large and if large quantities of blood are shunted from the left to the right side of the heart, right ventricular enlargement is noticeable (Fig. 18-47). The circulation in the lung field increases, and mild signs of pulmonary hypervascularity can be recognized. The hypervascularity in the cases seen by the authors has always been less pronounced than that occurring with most cases of patent ductus arteriosus. The pulmonary artery segment can be enlarged considerably. If overcirculation occurs, the left atrium gradually enlarges to accommodate the increased flow of blood to it.

CARDIAC CATHETERIZATION AND ANGIOCARDIOGRAPHY

If the defect in the ventricular septum is small and is located in the basilar portion of the ventricle, pressures in the right ventricular cavity are usually normal. However, the direction of the shunt of blood is from the left ventricle, where pressure is higher, to the right ventricular outflow tract and the pulmonary artery, where pressure is lower. Buchanan and Patterson (1965) reported that right ventricular pressures are normal when small defects are present, but that increased right ventricular pressure may be expected with large septal defects. Of eight dogs with ventricular septal defect, Hamlin, Smetzer, and Smith (1964) found right ventricular cavity pressures to be normal in six and minimally elevated in two. The authors' findings have been similar (Fig. 18-52). Right ventricular pressures should be recorded from various portions of the right ventricle, including the right ventricular outflow tract in the area just below the pulmonic valve, in an effort to detect elevations of the pressure resulting from a left-to-right shunt of blood. The increase in pulmonary arterial pressures varies with the severity of pulmonary hypertension. In uncomplicated cases, pressures from the left side of the heart are normal. Occasionally, the catheter may pass from the left ventricle through the defect and into the right ventricle.

Hamlin, Smetzer, and Smith (1964) demonstrated by blood gas analysis that the oxygen tension of blood in the main pulmonary artery is increased in dogs with ventricular septal defect. If serial samples are obtained from various portions of the right ventricle, blood oxygen tension may also be increased in the pulmonary outflow tract as compared with the right ventricular cavity.

Angiocardiography is necessary to establish the definitive diagnosis and to determine the exact location and size of the defect. Associated cardiac anomalies may also be confirmed. The contrast medium must be selectively injected into the left ventricle (Fig. 18-49*A* and 18-49*B*) unless a reversed blood flow, indicating severe pulmonary hypertension, has been suggested by elevated right ventricular pressures. When right-to-left or bi-directional shunting of blood is present, two injections should be made, one into the right ventricle and another into the left ventricle, preferably utilizing cineangiocardiography. The radiographs must always be exposed immediately following injection of the contrast medium. If

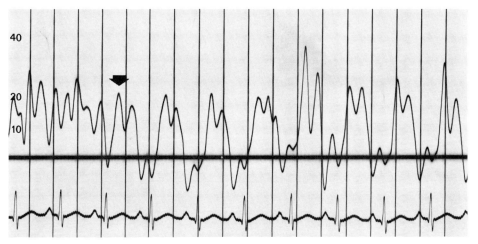

FIGURE 18-52 Ventricular septal defect. Pressures recorded during withdrawal of the catheter from the main pulmonary artery to the right ventricle. The main pulmonary arterial and right ventricular pressures are normal, and there is no pressure gradient across the pulmonic valve. This dog had a confirmed ventricular septal defect that was shunting from left to right. The arrow indicates the first right ventricular pressure curve as the catheter crosses the pulmonic valve. The tall pressure tracing (fourth from right end) is an artifact probably resulting from catheter whip.

a left ventricular injection is not possible, a pulmonary artery injection may be utilized.

Simultaneous filling of the aorta and the pulmonary artery occurs and the ventricular septal defect can be visualized subjacent to the aortic valve. Rotation of the heart frequently distorts the image, so that the defect may be projected distally into the aorta, thereby falsely suggesting an aorticopulmonary window (Fig. 18-49). Nonselective angiocardiography is inadequate for the demonstration of a ventricular septal defect for reasons already discussed (see pp. 193-196).

DIFFERENTIAL DIAGNOSIS

Uncomplicated ventricular septal defects result in a left-to-right shunting of blood. Except in unusual circumstances, large ventricular septal defects would require differentiation only from patent ductus arteriosus or atrial septal defect. The continuous murmur, the prominent aortic arch, and the excessive height of the QRS complexes on the electrocardiogram are usually sufficient to differentiate patent ductus arteriosus from ventricular septal defect. Atrial septal defects result in a systolic murmur of moderate intensity which is loudest over the pulmonic valve and would be less likely to result in marked right ventricular hypertrophy on the electrocardiogram.

PROGNOSIS

Neither death nor signs of cardiac disease was recorded in eight dogs with ventricular septal defect ranging from 1 to 8 years of age (Hamlin, Smetzer, and Smith, 1964). Eyster (1969) observed this anomaly in 18 dogs over $2\frac{1}{2}$ years of age, of which nine were in heart failure. Approximately half of those dogs with signs of heart failure had complicated congenital defects. We have occasionally seen dogs over 1 year of age with ventricular septal defect in congestive heart failure. From this meager information, it is apparent that the likely clinical course for most dogs with a ventricular septal defect is not known. It can be generally assumed that small defects do not create a serious hazard. Spontaneous closure of the septal defects is known to occur in man, but it is not known whether this occurs in dogs.

TREATMENT

No treatment is indicated when dogs with a ventricular septal defect remain asymptomatic. Surgical correction of this anomaly requires the use of cardiopulmonary bypass. Eyster (1969) has utilized the technique of pulmonary artery banding to reduce pulmonary blood flow and prevent the development of pulmonary hypertension. The same technique is used in children with heart failure resulting from a ventricular septal defect in whom open heart surgery cannot be performed. Eyster (1969) reported that some dogs with signs of congestive heart failure caused by ventricular septal defect have benefited from this procedure. When signs of congestive heart failure develop and surgical correction cannot be attempted, digitalization, restriction of exercise, and restriction of sodium intake are indicated.

TETRALOGY OF FALLOT

In tetralogy of Fallot, pulmonic stenosis is associated with right ventricular hypertrophy and a high ventricular septal defect with an overriding, dextro-positioned aorta that receives blood from both the right ventricle and left ventricle. Severe right ventricular hypertrophy is really a secondary lesion, and the dextropositioned aorta is variable in the degree of right ventricular overriding. The pulmonic stenosis, valvular, infundibular, or both, is often aggravated by narrowing of the right ventricular outflow tract as a result of myocardial hypertrophy (Dolowy et al., 1957; Clark et al., 1968). The aorta arises from either the right ventricle or both ventricles, and is usually widened. Pulmonary artery hypoplasia, a common characteristic of this syndrome in the dog according to Hamlin et al. (1962), has been recognized in most dogs with tetralogy of Fallot seen by the authors, and was reported as early as 1954 by Willis and Alai. The bronchoesophageal artery is enlarged to supply all or the majority of blood to the lungs when the pulmonary artery is hypoplastic.

HISTORY AND PHYSICAL EXAMINATION

Signs of the disease develop in the first few months of life, usually before the dog is 1 year of age. However, there have been cases of tetralogy of Fallot in which no clinical signs were present (Dolowy et al., 1957). Dyspnea and fatigability on exercise and paroxysmal anoxic spells with syncope occur. Growth is usually retarded, and most dogs are small for their age (Willis and Alai, 1954; Meredith and Clarkson, 1959; Hamlin et al., 1962; Clark et al., 1968). Cyanosis of the mucous membranes may be persistent or may be precipitated by slight exercise. The presence of cyanosis in a puppy should draw attention to the possibility of a tetralogy of Fallot. Polycythemia can be an outstanding feature; it is recognized clinically by the black or dark color of the tongue and mucous membranes.

THE CARDIAC EXAMINATION

An ejection-type systolic murmur auscultated over the pulmonic valve probably results from pulmonic stenosis. In dogs with a loud murmur, a precordial thrill is palpable (Patterson et al., 1966; Clark et al., 1968). In some cases, no murmurs can be heard because of the equal pressures in the right and left ventricles. In our experience, murmurs are not a constant finding. When they do occur, the intensity and location also vary. Whereas some dogs are presented with only a systolic ejection murmur over the aortic and pulmonic valves, others have a harsh holosystolic murmur at the right cranial midthorax (Fig. 18-53). Phonocardiography demonstrates a crescendo-decrescendo systolic murmur ending before the second heart sound. The murmur is occasionally interrupted by a midsystolic click (Clark et al., 1968).

Right axis deviation and right ventricular hypertrophy are recognized on the electrocardiogram and vectorcardiogram. The orientation of the QRS electrical axis, as reported by Hamlin et al. (1962) and Clark et al. (1968) is directed dextrad, craniad, and ventrad or dorsad (Fig. 18-54A and 18-54B). We have also seen caudally directed vectors in a dog with a tetralogy of Fallot.

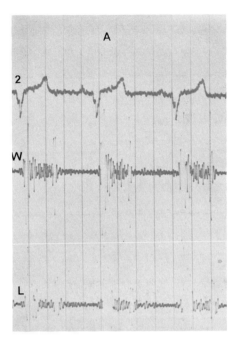

FIGURE 18-53   Tetralogy of Fallot. *A,* Wide-band (W) and low-band (L) phono-cardiograms and lead II of the electrocardiogram recorded simultaneously. A holo-systolic murmur was auscultated over the mitral and tricuspid valves of a dog with signs of exertional syncope and cyanosis. In this recording made over the right mid thorax, the holosystolic, mixed-frequency murmur is best recognized on the wide-band phonocardiogram. The negative lead II electrocardiogram is consistent with marked right ventricular hypertrophy. *B,* In some dogs with tetralogy of Fallot, no murmur or only an early systolic murmur is recorded on both the wide-frequency (W) and low-frequency (L) band phonocardiograms.

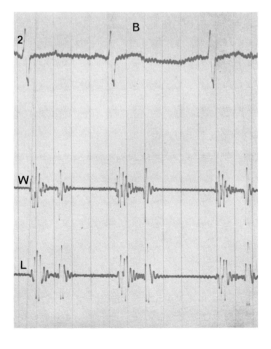

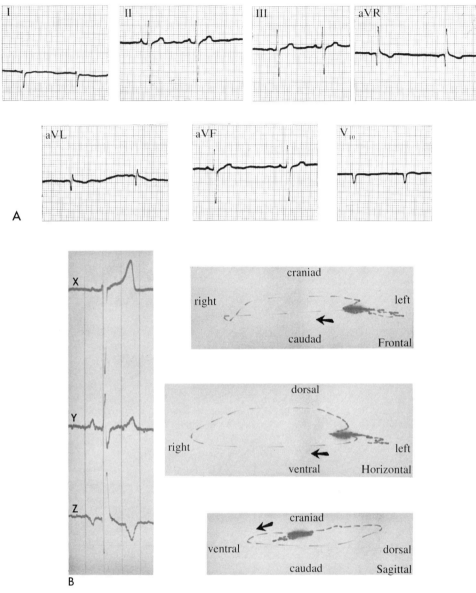

FIGURE 18-54 Tetralogy of Fallot. *A,* The electrocardiogram associated with tetralogy of Fallot usually reflects marked right ventricular hypertrophy, indicated by a shift of the mean electrical axis in the frontal plane to the right (−135°). The complexes are abnormal, since Q waves, which are usually present, are absent in leads I, II, and III, and deep S waves are abnormally present in all of these leads. This is consistent with initial leftward forces followed by a shift in the electrical forces to the right (see *B*). The negativity of leads aVF and V_{10} indicates that the electrical vectors are directed cranially and ventrally.

B, Tetralogy of Fallot. The X, Y, and Z leads are grossly abnormal and are responsible for long, narrow, constricted vector loops. The loops are oriented predominantly to the right, which indicates right heart enlargement. In addition, the horizontal loop is abnormally directed in a clockwise manner. The scalar leads were recorded at the standard amplitude and the vector loops at one-half standard amplitude.

RADIOGRAPHIC EXAMINATION

Radiographic signs referable to tetralogy of Fallot have been described by Detweiler (1962), Hamlin et al. (1962), Rhodes, Patterson, and Detweiler (1963), Patterson et al. (1966), and Clark et al. (1968).

The cardiac silhouette is usually not markedly enlarged (Figs. 18-55 and 18-56). There is often a globular appearance of the enlarged right ventricle in both the lateral and dorsoventral projections. In contrast, the left ventricle appears normal or reduced in size. In the lateral radiograph, the cranial waist is sometimes absent because of distention or displacement of the ascending aorta. Right ventricular enlargement or poststenotic dilatation of the pulmonary artery can have the same effect. The caudal waist remains essentially normal, as does the left atrium. In the dorsoventral radiograph, bulging of the right cranial border can be seen. Protrusion at the area of the pulmonary artery segment has been reported by Clark et al. (1968). However, this is often absent, or the pulmonary artery segment is reduced in size, because the main pulmonary artery is hypoplastic, and the poststenotic dilatation is therefore often not large enough to be visible.

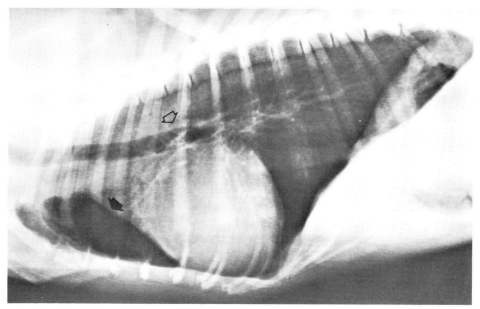

FIGURE 18-55 Lateral radiograph, 8 month old male dog of mixed breed which had severe dyspnea. The mucous membranes were cyanotic even when the dog was at rest. A loud, pansystolic murmur was auscultated. Blood analysis revealed severe polycythemia (hematocrit, 80 per cent). In spite of treatment, the dog died within a few hours after the initial examination. The right heart is rounded, and the cranial waist has disappeared owing to protrusion of the aortic arch (black arrow). The craniocaudal diameter appears enlarged, but the apicobasilar distance is unaltered, as is further indicated by the normal angle of the trachea with the thoracic spine. The left heart is normal. The lung field is lucent, giving the impression of overinflation or alveolar emphysema. The intrapulmonary vasculature is barely visible. The left pulmonary artery (clear arrow) is smaller than normal. Notice the extreme flattening of the diaphragm caused by the maximal inspiratory effort. In a young dog, right ventricular enlargement, widening of the ascending aorta, undercirculation of the lungs, and cyanosis are characteristic for tetralogy of Fallot. In a ventricular septal defect complicated by pulmonic stenosis, the radiographic appearance may be similar to that seen with tetralogy of Fallot.

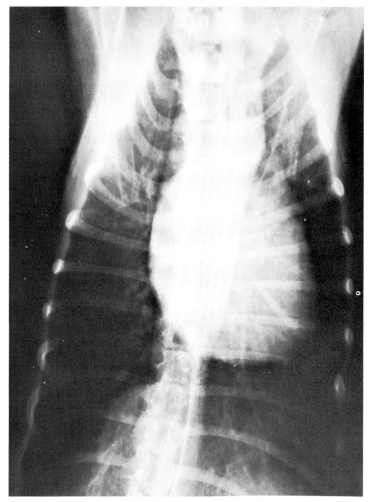

FIGURE 18-56 Dorsoventral radiograph, dog in Figure 18-55. The severe dyspnea made it difficult to obtain proper positioning; therefore, the sternum is not exactly superimposed on the thoracic spine. This results in displacement of the cardiac silhouette to the left side. However, the rounded, enlarged right ventricle can still be seen. The left cardiac border looks essentially normal. The lung field is extremely lucent, and the intrapulmonary vascular markings are barely outlined.

The lung field often exhibits a characteristic striking reduction in vascularity, making it more lucent than normal (Figs. 18-55 and 18-56) (Meredith and Clarkson, 1959). The lucency may be accentuated by overinflation of the lungs because of respiratory distress, suggesting emphysema. The vascular markings appear as thin lines in comparison to the normally visible tapering bands. (See Tables 18-1 and 18-2, pp. 488-489).

CARDIAC CATHETERIZATION AND ANGIOCARDIOGRAPHY

Right ventricular pressures are increased, and if pulmonary artery pressures can be obtained a gradient is found between the pulmonary artery and the right ventricle. It may be difficult or impossible to advance a catheter through the stenotic pulmonic valve and hypoplastic pulmonary artery. At times, the catheter is advanced through the aortic root, across the aortic valve, and then through the ventricular septal defect into the right ventricle, thus enabling pressure recordings to be obtained from both the left and the right sides. Simultaneous right ventricular and left ventricular pressure tracings indicate the direction of the shunting of blood—i.e., right to left or left to right (Fig. 18-57). Oximetry reveals that the oxygen content of the blood in the right ventricle is greater than that in the right atrium. Systemic arterial blood samples have lower oxygen concentrations than does the left ventricular sample. The dog in Figure 18-58 had the following oxygen saturations: left ventricle, 95 per cent; right ventricle, 79 per cent; and aortic arch, 90 per cent. These findings prove the existence of a right-to-left shunt at the level of the aorta or subaortic valvular ventricular septum. When injection is made into the right ventricle, indicator dilution tests reveal early arrival of the dye in a distal artery such as the aorta (Hamlin et al., 1962; Clark et al., 1968).

Angiocardiography usually demonstrates the abnormalities found in tetralogy of Fallot (Fig. 18-58). Positioning the catheter for injection of contrast medium will at times be difficult because the right ventricle resembles the left ventricle owing to the marked muscular hypertrophy and cardiac rotation, and one is often

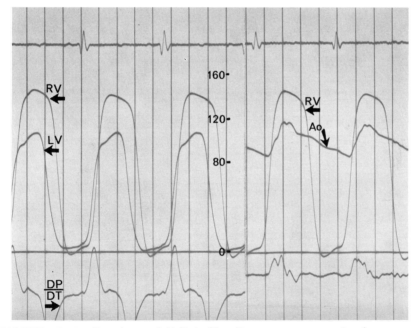

FIGURE 18-57 Tetralogy of Fallot. Simultaneous pressure tracings recorded from the left ventricle (LV) and right ventricle (RV), and from the right ventricle (RV) and aorta (Ao). The electrocardiogram is also recorded, as is the first derivative (DP/DT) of the left ventricular and aortic pressure curve. The right ventricular pressure (140/5 mm. Hg) exceeds that in the left ventricle (110/5 mm. Hg), resulting in a shunting of blood from the right ventricle to the left ventricle and aorta. Disparity between aortic and left ventricular pressure curves is due to the fact that they were not simultaneously recorded, permitting the hemodynamic state to change slightly between pressure recordings. Blood oxygen saturation was 95 per cent in the left ventricle, 79 per cent in the right ventricle, and 90 per cent in the ascending aorta. These findings indicate a right-to-left shunting of blood just above or below the aortic valve.

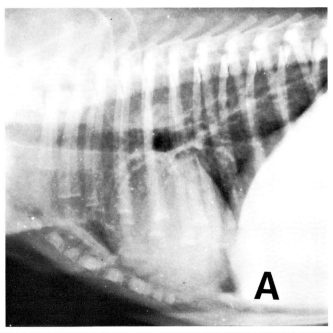

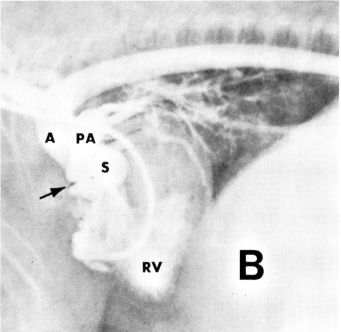

FIGURE 18-58   Plain radiographs and angiocardiograms, 3 month old female Wirehaired Fox Terrier. The dog tired easily and became cyanotic with exercise but was otherwise very alert and playful. An ejection-type holosystolic murmur was auscultated over the pulmonic valve. Polycythemia was present on hematologic examination. *A*, Lateral plain radiograph. The heart looks unremarkable in this projection. The vascular markings in the lung field are small but well delineated. *B*, Lateral selective angiocardiogram exposed 1.3 seconds after the injection of Hypaque 50% (1 ml./kg. body weight) into the right ventricle. The pulmonary artery (PA) and the aorta (A) are outlined simultaneously. The main pulmonary artery has a

Figure 18-58 and legend continues on following page.

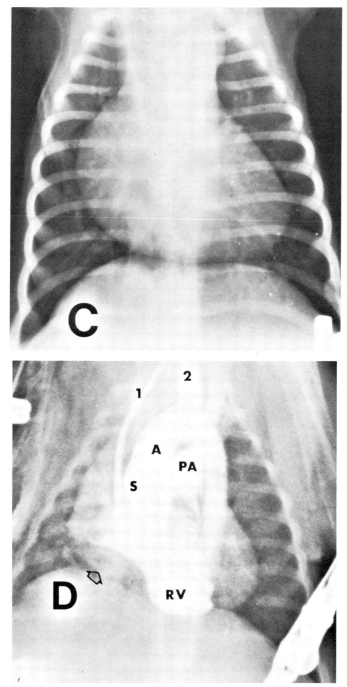

scalloped outline; its branches are much smaller than normal, indicating undercirculation. The narrowing of the pulmonic valve (arrow) appears less severe than it
was at necropsy, when the valvular opening measured approximately 1 mm. in diameter. The main pulmonary artery appears large because of a poststenotic dilatation.
The majority of contrast medium which has left the right ventricle (RV) has been
shunted into the aorta. The sinuses of Valsalva of the aorta are wide. Notice the patch
of contrast medium at the tip of the catheter. This density is due to the unintentional
intramural injection of a small amount of contrast medium.

Legend continues on following page.

not sure whether the catheter has accidentally passed through the ventricular septal defect into the left ventricle. The injection is made selectively into the right ventricle, and the aorta and the pulmonary artery are opacified simultaneously. Left ventricular injection will usually indicate some left-to-right shunting of blood and will outline the left ventricle, right ventricle, aorta, and pulmonary artery simultaneously. The ascending aorta is often dilated, as is the pulmonary artery distal to the stenotic area. In many cases, the pulmonary artery is hypoplastic, and the poststenotic dilatation is minimal. The intrapulmonary vessels are always markedly smaller then normal. The passage of contrast medium from the right ventricle into the left ventricle depends on the degree of pulmonic stenosis and hypertension in the right ventricle in contrast to the left ventricular pressures (Patterson et al., 1966). The defect in the interventricular septum may not be outlined owing to rotation of the heart. It is located high in the septum and may be obscured by the aortic sinus of Valsalva. If a selective aortic arch injection is made, the enlarged bronchoesophageal artery supplying the lungs with blood can be outlined. Occasionally, aortic insufficiency may be present.

DIFFERENTIAL DIAGNOSIS

In most cases, the presence of cyanosis in a puppy should suggest the possibility of a tetralogy of Fallot. However, pulmonic stenosis with atrial septal defect or ventricular septal defect and complete transposition of the great vessels should be considered in the differential diagnosis.

In uncomplicated pulmonic stenosis, there is no ventricular septal defect. Clinically, constant cyanosis is absent, and syncope and anoxia are infrequent. If pulmonic stenosis and an atrial septal defect occur concurrently, unoxygenated blood may pass from the right atrium, in which the pressure is higher, to the left atrium (Buchanan and Patterson, 1965). In another report (Ljunggren et al., 1966), cyanosis developed in a dog with tricuspid stenosis and insufficiency, right ventricular hypoplasia, and an atrial septal defect. Complete transposition of the great vessels would also result in cyanosis. In this anomaly, there would be an increase in pulmonary vascularity and definite cardiac enlargement.

PROGNOSIS

The prognosis for most dogs to reach adult life is poor in the authors' experience. The disease progresses with the increasing severity of the pulmonic

---

C, Dorsoventral plain radiograph. The heart is markedly enlarged, and the right ventricular border is rounded and extends farther to the right side than normal. The displacement of the apex to the left side makes the right ventricular enlargement seem less severe than it is. The left cardiac border is unremarkable.

D, Ventrodorsal selective angiocardiogram made during the same series as the angiocardiogram (*B*) using a biplane roll-film changer. This exposure was made 0.3 seconds after the beginning of the injection. The right ventricle (RV) is filled with contrast medium which, instead of flowing exclusively into the pulmonary (PA), mainly opacifies the aorta. Only a small amount of contrast medium is seen in the small main pulmonary artery. The septal defect is not outlined because it is superimposed on the density of the sinuses of Valsalva (S) of the aorta. Because of hypertrophy of the right ventricular wall (clear arrow), the right ventricle could be mistaken for the left ventricle. Notice the contrast-filled catheter (1) in the cranial vena cava which curves medially into the density of the right ventricle. The second catheter (2), placed in the aorta, is obscured by the outflowing contrast medium.

stenosis. Severin (1967) stated that dogs with tetralogy of Fallot and transposition of the great vessels usually die before weaning, and Patterson (1968) noted that large ventricular septal defects were found only in dogs with this defect that died within a few days after birth. In a review of four dogs with tetralogy of Fallot, one was put to death, two died at 10 and 20 weeks of age, respectively, and one was lost to follow-up (Clark et al., 1968). In a case reported by Hamlin et al. (1962), the dog died at 1 year of age. An exception to early death was reported by Dolowy et al. (1957), when they found tetralogy of Fallot in a clinically normal dog during experimental cardiac surgery.

GENETIC STUDIES

When two normal dogs from a family of Keeshonden in which tetralogy of Fallot was known to occur were bred, 22 per cent of their offspring had tetralogy of Fallot. When a bitch with tetralogy of Fallot was bred to a normal dog, 77 per cent of the offspring had cardiovascular abnormalities. In one instance, an affected dog was bred to a normal bitch, and the one puppy born had tetralogy of Fallot. When both the male and the female had congenital heart disease, 59 per cent of the puppies had cardiac anomalies (Patterson, 1968). In breeding Keeshonden with a history of tetralogy of Fallot, other defects involving the development of the truncoconal septal system (such as patent ductus arteriosus, ventricular septal defect, aneurysm of the membranous ventricular septum, persistent left cranial vena cava, pulmonic stenosis, fusion of pulmonic valve cusps, anomalous right subclavian artery, atrial septal defect of the ostium secundum type, persistent diverticulum of the ductus arteriosus, and tricupsid atresia) were found by Patterson (1968). In the Keeshonden family tetralogy of Fallot is not inherited as a simple Mendelian trait, but may result from a "... major autosomal gene mutation with variable penetrance and expressivity," according to Patterson (1968). Cytogenetic studies in one male mixed terrier with tetralogy of Fallot and a septum secundum atrial septal defect as well as a midline cleft of the upper lip, gingiva and maxilla demonstrated presumed autosomal translocation (Patterson et al., 1966).

TREATMENT

Medical therapy is not possible for tetralogy of Fallot. However, acute episodes of dyspnea and cyanosis may be offset with morphine and propranolol. Sodium bicarbonate is indicated for the correction of acidosis when severe shunting has developed (Cumming, 1970).

Reports of complete surgical correction are unavailable at this time. Temporary relief may be provided by anastomosing a systemic artery to a pulmonary artery, thereby increasing pulmonary blood flow and improving oxygenation of the blood (Blalock-Taussig procedure).

CONGENITAL PERITONEOPERICARDIAL DIAPHRAGMATIC HERNIA

Congenital peritoneopericardial diaphragmatic hernia is an unusual form of diaphragmatic hernia in the dog (Pommer, 1951; Clinton, 1967). In this congenital lesion, a defect is present in the ventral diaphragm, predominantly in the region which arises embryologically from the septum transversum (Arey, 1965).

In addition, the pleuropericardial membranes caudal to the heart fail to fuse, resulting in concurrent defects of the pericardium and diaphragm which result in a direct communication between the abdominal cavity and the pericardial sac. The thoracic cavity is usually separated completely from the contiguous abdominal cavity and pericardial sac. A ventral midline defect of the abdominal wall cranial to the umbilicus is often present as well.

HISTORY AND PHYSICAL EXAMINATION

The dog may be asymptomatic or may be brought to the veterinarian because of cachexia, anorexia, abdominal discomfort, dyspnea, cyanosis, or vomiting and diarrhea (Pommer, 1951; Detweiler, Brodey, and Flickinger, 1960; Cato, 1962; Baker and Williams, 1966; Clinton, 1967; Bolton, Ettinger, and Roush, 1969; Finn and Martin, 1969). Clinical signs are likely to develop in the first year of life, although they sometimes first become apparent later in life (Pommer, 1955). On physical examination, the dog is found to be in some degree of cardiac decompensation and respiratory distress. Although the dog may be asymptomatic, auscultation of the thorax reveals muffling or complete absence of heart sounds. The respiratory sounds vary with the degree of cardiac involvement and respiratory distress. Intestinal sounds or borborygmi normally heard in the abdomen may also be heard over the thoracic cavity. The cardiac apical impulse is often absent when the thorax is palpated. The abdomen may appear empty and tucked up owing to displacement of its contents into the thoracic cavity. If right heart failure has developed, ascites is present. The pulse varies from normal in asymptomatic dogs to small and rapid in dogs which have developed heart failure and cardiac tamponade.

ELECTROCARDIOGRAPHY

Decreased electrical potentials due to an increased mass in the thoracic cavity are demonstrated on the electrocardiogram by QRS complexes of low amplitude (Fig. 18-59). The heart rate and rhythm are normal, and ectopic beats are not expected. The mean electrical axis in the frontal plane is normal.

RADIOGRAPHIC EXAMINATION

The radiographic signs of peritoneopericardial hernia have been well described by Pommer (1951, 1955), Detweiler, Brodey, and Flickinger (1960), Morgan (1964), Clinton (1967), and Bolton, Ettinger, and Roush (1969). The signs are typical, and in most cases the diagnosis can be made from the plain radiographs (Figs. 18-60 and 18-61).

The cardiac silhouette is greatly enlarged, smooth, and globular in both the lateral and the dorsoventral views. The space occupied by the lungs is markedly reduced. In the lateral radiograph, the trachea is displaced dorsally and may even be slightly compressed dorsoventrally. Left atrial enlargement cannot be seen, and the lung field remains clear. The caudal cardiac border merges ventrally with the cupola of the diaphragm, and in some cases the communication between the abdomen and the pericardial sac can be seen as a defect in the ventral contour of the diaphragm.

On scrutiny of the cardiac silhouette, small, lucent, loculated areas of gas can be seen within the cardiac density, giving it a mottled appearance. Occasionally, larger pieces of bowel can be recognized readily by gas or granular fecal material retained in the lumen.

In the dorsoventral view, the defect in the diaphragm often is not outlined because it is located ventral to the cupola. The semicircular density of the cupola

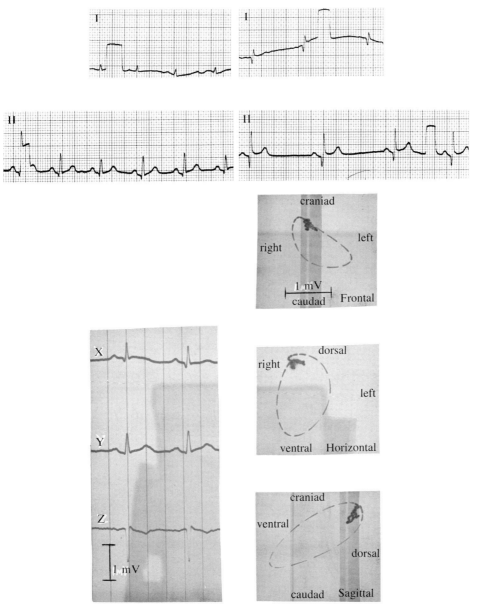

FIGURE 18-59   Peritoneopericardial hernia. *A,* Diminished amplitudes in leads I and II of the electrocardiogram are due to increased amounts of tissue (intestine) within the pericardial sac (tracings on the left). One week following removal of the intestinal mass from the pericardium, the QRS complexes were taller (tracings on the right). *B,* Vectorcardiogram of the same dog recorded prior to surgery. The amplitudes of the scalar X, Y, and Z leads, as well as of the vector loops, are diminished. The initial forces in the frontal and horizontal planes are prolonged to the right for 0.014 sec. (Tracings from Bolton, Ettinger, and Roush [1969]).

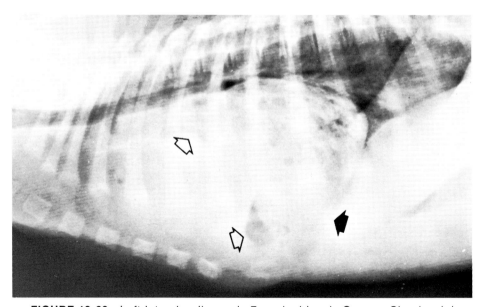

FIGURE 18-60   Left lateral radiograph, 7 week old male German Shepherd dog. Routine examination revealed absence of heart sounds. The dog had no clinical signs of disease. The cardiac silhouette fills a large part of the thoracic cavity. The trachea is compressed between the spine and the cardiac silhouette, and the main stem bronchi appear narrowed. The cranial border of the cardiac silhouette is ill-defined, and only the dorsal half of the caudal border, which extends far caudally, is well-outlined. The ventral portion of the cardiac shadow blends with the density of the diaphragm (black arrow). There are several irregular, lucent areas within the cardiac silhouette (clear arrows). There is some mottling in the caudal portion. This type of cardiac enlargement is characteristic of a pericardial lesion. The lucent areas, representing loculated gas in small bowel loops, and the mottling, caused by fecal densities, are diagnostic for a peritoneopericardial diaphragmatic hernia with prolapse of intestinal loops into the pericardial sac. The discontinuity of the diaphragmatic outline is further evidence for this diagnosis.

may thus obscure the communication with the pericardium. The dorsoventral view is often helpful in substantiating the diagnosis in that the location of the gas bubble in the stomach and the position of the liver and the spleen can be evaluated. The liver shadow may appear smaller than normal because of prolapse of one or several lobes through the diaphragm, and the gas bubble in the fundus of the stomach can be displaced toward the right side.

Abdominal radiographs should always be made when a peritoneopericardial hernia is suspected. Owing to the displacement of portions of the abdominal contents into the thorax, the abdomen appears emptied and tucked up (Finn and Martin, 1969).

When barium sulfate suspension is fed to outline the gastrointestinal tract, displacement of bowel loops or portions of the stomach into the pericardial sac is indicated by their filling with contrast material (Figs. 18-62 and 18-63) and the diagnosis is proved. It is important to continue the radiographic series until the contrast-filled loops can be seen within the cardiac silhouette, or until the contrast material has reached the colon in a negative case. The barium study is especially important for the differential diagnosis of this condition.

A similar marked enlargement of the cardiac silhouette can be seen in massive pericardial effusions caused by pericarditis or cardiac tamponade, as for example after tearing of the left atrium (see pp. 363-365). A greatly enlarged car-

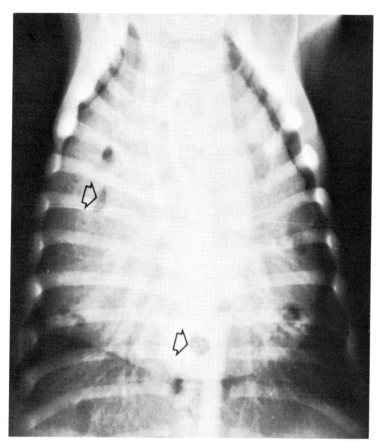

FIGURE 18-61 Dorsoventral radiograph, dog in Figure 18-60. The rather even rounding of the greatly enlarged cardiac silhouette, the flattening at the areas where the silhouette touches the thoracic wall, and the fact that the silhouette is globular in both lateral and dorsoventral projections indicate that a pericardial lesion is present. The loculated gas (arrows) within the dense silhouette is the characteristic sign which helps to make the diagnosis. There is a continuous separation between the diaphragm and the pericardium. The area of the hernia ring, which lies in the cupola of the diaphragm, is superimposed upon the pericardial density.

diac silhouette is also found in severe heart failure (see pp. 331-344). However, the presence of loculated gas and mottling within the pericardial sac, or the incomplete outline of the diaphragm in the lateral or the dorsoventral view, is diagnostic in most cases of peritoneopericardial hernia. Contrast studies secure the diagnosis in questionable cases.

A diaphragmatic hernia with prolapse of the abdominal organs into the pleural space can easily be differentiated radiographically from peritoneopericardial hernia by the absence of the enlarged cardiac silhouette and by the different location of the prolapsed organs.

Prolapse of abdominal organs into the caudal mediastinal cavity (specifically, the cavum mediastini serosum or Sussdorf's space) has been reported (Pommer, 1955) and may appear similar to a peritoneopericardial hernia.

Fluoroscopy has been advocated for diagnosis and differential diagnosis of peritoneopericardial hernia by Pommer (1951, 1955). In this condition, a zone of decreased density can be distinguished between the heart shadow and the pericardial sac containing the moderately gas-filled intestinal loops. The motility of the

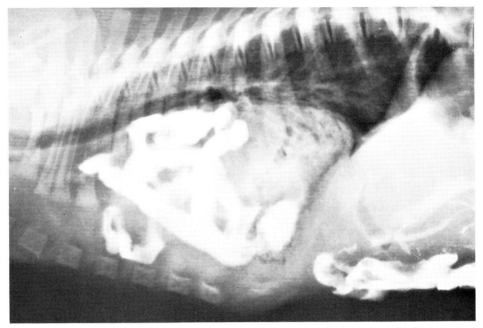

FIGURE 18-62 Lateral radiograph, dog in Figures 18-60 and 18-61. This radiograph was made one hour after a barium meal was administered to outline the intestines, which have been displaced into the pericardial sac. There are several barium-filled small intestinal loops within the cardiac silhouette. A contrast study is not needed for the diagnosis of a peritoneopericardial diaphragmatic hernia if loculated gas has been seen within the cardiac silhouette on previous radiographs. However, it can be helpful in outlining the exact location of the diaphragmatic defect, which is important for planning the surgical approach. In doubtful cases it is important to continue making radiographs until the contrast-filled intestinal loops are seen within the pericardial density or until the barium reaches the descending colon.

diaphragm is reduced, as are the cardiac contractions. Changing of the gas patterns owning to peristalsis of the intestines may occur. After changing the position of the dog, the location of the intestines within the cardiac silhouette may also change.

DIFFERENTIAL DIAGNOSIS

Thoracic diaphragmatic hernia, pericardial effusion, and congenital heart disease must be considered in the differential diagnosis. Radiographic examination before and after the barium study is likely to provide definitive differentiation of thoracic diaphragmatic hernia from peritoneopericardial diaphragmatic hernia. Congenial heart defects are eliminated on the basis of a normal electrocardiogram, possibly with diminished amplitudes, absence of typical cardiac murmurs, and the presence of diminished intensity or muffling of the heart sounds. Plain film radiographs distinguish pericardial effusion from peritoneopericardial hernia, since gas bubbles appear within the pericardial sac in the latter condition.

PROGNOSIS

Most dogs with congenital peritoneopericardial diaphragmatic hernia develop clinical signs and right heart failure within one year. Since the lesion is

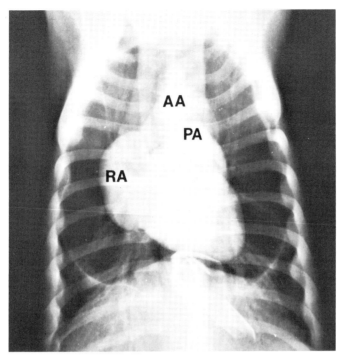

FIGURE 18-63 Pneumopericardium, dorsoventral projection, dog in Figures 18-60, 18-61, and 18-62, made one day after the hernia was repaired surgically via an abdominal approach. The pericardium is seen as a fine white line, at times touching the thoracic wall, marking the previous circumference of the pericardial sac. A drain is seen at the cupola of the diaphragm. The cardiac silhouette has a very unusual appearance. Since the pericardium has been separated from the epicardium, the details of the heart can be seen very clearly. The outlines of the notches and grooves are usually softened by the overlying pericardium. The abnormal position of the heart also contributes to its unusual appearance. The aortic arch (AA) is very prominent. The bulging density on the right side is the right atrium (RA). The left atrium is obscured by the density of the aorta. The main pulmonary artery (PA) is well delineated, as are the right and left ventricular borders.

surgically correctable, all attempts should be made to correct the defect prior to the onset of clinical signs.

TREATMENT

Surgical correction is indicated for a peritoneopericardial hernia. Successful correction of this condition has been reported by Detweiler, Brodey, and Flickinger (1960), Baker and Williams (1966), Clinton (1967), and Bolton, Ettinger, and Roush (1969). The surgical technique usually involves a midline laparotomy along the cranial abdominal wall, removal of the abdominal organs from the pericardial sac, and closure of the pericardial sac, diaphragm, and ventral abdominal wall.

CONGENITAL MITRAL INSUFFICIENCY

Normal function of the mitral valve requires the anatomic and mechanical integrity of the mitral valve anulus, the mitral valve leaflets, the chordae tendineae, and the papillary muscles. Mitral insufficiency occurs when an abnormality of one or more of these structures results in incomplete closure of the left atrioventricular valve and regurgitation of left ventricular blood into the left atrium. The term mitral incompetence is occasionally used to differentiate mitral insufficiency due to valvular defects from mitral insufficiency due to mitral anulus dilatation. The terms are used synonymously in this text because normal mitral valve function requires the integrity of all parts of the mitral valve apparatus. It may also not be possible to determine whether the valvular deformity or the anulus dilatation occurred first.

Congenital mitral insufficiency occurs both as a primary disease and as a secondary complication to some congenital cardiac defects in which function of the mitral valve apparatus is impaired. Examples of the latter are endocardial cushion defect and atrial septal defect of the ostium primum type. Mitral insufficiency also develops when congenital cardiac lesions result in volume overload or secondary left ventricular dilatation with subsequent dilatation of the mitral anulus. Examples of the latter are patent ductus arteriosus and aortic stenosis. After surgical correction of a patent ductus arteriosus, the murmur of mitral insufficiency is likely to persist for an indefinite period of time and will either diminish or disappear completely within one to two years.

Buchanan and Patterson (1965) mentioned that after successful medical treatment and a decrease in heart size as seen radiographically, a systolic murmur in three dogs with congenital mitral insufficiency had disappeared. This supports the assumption that mitral regurgitation can result from dilatation of the mitral anulus. Buchanan and Patterson (1965) further mention that acquired myocardial abnormalities may result in dilatation of the mitral valve anulus, and they therefore suggest that the term congenital mitral insufficiency might be incorrect. Of the 290 dogs with congenital cardiovascular disease described by Patterson (1968) (see Table 12-2, p. 319), nine had mitral insufficiency.

Hamlin, Smetzer, and Smith (1965) reported shortening of both leaflets of the mitral valve and reduction of their surface area to one-fourth to one-half of normal as a primary condition in eight young dogs. The size of the mitral orifice remained unchanged during diastole in these cases. Three of the seven dogs in their report died in congestive heart failure due to congenital mitral valvular insufficiency. However, the possibility that mitral regurgitation may have resulted from a functional lesion following idiopathic ventricular dilatation in the other dogs was raised. Hamlin and Harris (1969) described six Great Dane puppies with mitral insufficiency caused by dilatation of the mitral anulus. They felt that the incidence of this abnormality in the one breed constitutes more than an incidental finding.

CLINICAL SIGNS AND PHYSICAL EXAMINATION

The clinical signs in addition to retarded growth are the same as those of acquired chronic mitral valvular fibrosis—that is, fatigue, respiratory distress with dyspnea, tachypnea, and coughing, and left-sided or combined left-sided and right-sided congestive heart failure. In the two published reports describing this condition, the dogs affected were all under 1 year of age (Hamlin, Smetzer, and Smith, 1965; Hamlin and Harris, 1969). Hamlin, Smetzer, and Smith (1965) reported that a systolic murmur of variable intensity, a gallop rhythm, and occasionally a split first heart sound are present in dogs with congenital mitral insufficiency. Left ventricular hypertrophy and left atrial dilatation are indicated on the electrocardiogram. Hamlin and Harris (1969) and the authors have recognized arrhythmias such as atrial fibrillation and ventricular premature contractions in association with congestive heart failure due to apparent congenital mitral insufficiency.

Cardiac catheterization may be used to distinguish primary congenital mitral valvular insufficiency from other congenital cardiac lesions in which mitral insufficiency occurs secondarily. Hamlin, Smetzer, and Smith (1965) reported normal blood oxygen saturation in all dogs, elevated right ventricular systolic pressure in four dogs, and a decreased decay slope without a recirculation peak when indicator (dye) dilution studies were performed.

RADIOGRAPHIC AND ANGIOCARDIOGRAPHIC EXAMINATIONS

The radiographic signs of congenital mitral insufficiency are similar to those described for acquired chronic mitral valvular fibrosis (see pp. 331-344). Hamlin, Smetzer, and Smith (1965) reported ventricular enlargement in six of eight dogs; the intrapulmonary vasculature was accentuated in two dogs which were moribund. Left atrial enlargement was prominent in all cases. Left ventricular dilatation and mitral valvular insufficiency, caused by dilatation of the mitral anulus, were seen on angiocardiograms. Hamlin and Harris (1969) reported that a markedly pulsating left atrium which dilated during ventricular systole could be seen fluoroscopically. (See Table 18-1, p. 488).

PROGNOSIS

Three of the eight dogs with signs of heart disease due to congenital mitral insufficiency reported by Hamlin, Smetzer, and Smith (1965) succumbed to congestive heart failure. Of the six dogs with congenital mitral insufficiency described by Hamlin and Harris (1969), five had no clinical signs two years after being studied and did not require therapy. The sixth dog died during cardiac catheterization. When dogs with congenital mitral insufficiency considered to be of primary origin have been seen by the authors, they have usually died from congestive heart failure.

Because of the limited number of reports of congenital mitral insufficiency, definitive statements cannot be made regarding the course of the disease. A poor prognosis for long-term therapy is indicated in dogs with advanced clinical, radiographic, and electrocardiographic signs of cardiac enlargement. Those dogs with moderate cardiac enlargement, a minimal to moderate murmur, and no clinical signs or only minimal clinical signs are likely to outgrow the disease. In the latter cases, left ventricular dilatation recedes, and the functional mitral insufficiency then regresses.

TREATMENT

Medical therapy in the form of cardiac glycosides, diuretics, antiarrhythmic agents, a low sodium diet, and restriction of exercise is indicated for treatment of symptomatic congenital mitral insufficiency. In those dogs with advanced valvular lesions or those in which mitral insufficiency results from dilatation of the mitral anulus, surgical intervention should be considered after the dog has been stabilized and the congestive heart failure has been relieved medically. The surgical procedure in these cases might require valvuloplasty or total valve replacement.

PERSISTENT LEFT CRANIAL VENA CAVA

Persistence of all or part of the left cranial vena cava was reviewed by Schaller (1955) and Buchanan (1963). This condition does not produce clinical disease but is often associated with other congenital cardiac defects. Its recognition is important in the thoracic surgical patient because it may result in confusion of anatomic structures during thoracic exploration. In a review of congenital cardiac lesions in the dog, Patterson (1968) noted that 13 of 290 dogs had a persistent left cranial vena cava. Persistent right aortic arch was also present in 10 of the 13 dogs, and other congenital cardiac anomalies were present in the remaining three. Congenital cardiac defects other than persistent right aortic arch that occur with persistent left cranial vena cava include tetralogy of Fallot and retroesophageal right subclavian artery (Buchanan, 1963; Clark et al., 1968). Schaller (1955) has observed that persistent left cranial vena cava frequently occurs as an isolated anomaly. He investigated the embryonic development of the cranial vena cava and explains the condition as being due to obstruction of the opening of the coronary sinus in the right atrium during embryonic life.

The abnormally persistent left cranial vena cava, as reported in a dog by Buchanan (1963), passes through the pericardium at its left dorsocranial reflection toward the heart until its adventitia becomes continuous with the epicardium. The vessel then follows the coronary groove and receives the coronary veins. At this anatomic point it becomes the coronary sinus, entering the right atrium caudomedially near the opening of the caudal vena cava. Buchanan (1963) further refers to the occurrence of complete and incomplete forms of the anomaly. In the complete form, the anomalous vein drains venous blood from the regions cranial to the heart. The incomplete form consists of only the proximal portion of the left cranial vena cava, into which a hemiazygous vein drains. In three of 30 dogs with persistent left cranial vena cava examined or reviewed by Buchanan (1963), the right cranial vena cava was entirely absent. The persistent left cranial vena cava should not be surgically ligated unless there is sufficient proof of adequate drainage by a right cranial vena cava and branches from the left side.

This anomaly, recognized by the authors in association with a persistent right aortic arch, is illustrated in Figure 18-23.

ABSENCE OF THE CAUDAL (POSTERIOR) VENA CAVA

Absence of the caudal vena cava has been reported by Hickman, Edwards, and Mann (1949) and by Wallace (1960). There were no clinical signs in either case. Veins caudal to the heart entered the greatly distended azygos vein, which then drained into the cranial vena cava. In those cases in which the portal veins by-passed the liver, the hepatic artery was the only route of blood supply to the liver. In both reported cases, a single hepatic vein drained directly into the heart. This anomaly may be responsible for unsuccessful retrograde venous catheterization of the right heart. It also warrants consideration when a pneumonectomy is to be performed.

CONGENITAL FIBROELASTOSIS OF THE ENDOCARDIUM

In this condition, the endocardium is thickened with layers of elastic tissue and collagen, and it has a fibrous rather than a thin or nearly translucent appearance at necropsy. The condition has been reported in a puppy with congenital aortic stenosis, left ventricular hypertrophy, and generalized cardiac enlargement, by Elliot et al. (1958). The thickening and opaque appearance of the endocardium was determined microscopically to be due to increased amounts of endocardial collagen tissue.

CONGENITAL DEAFNESS AND CARDIAC ARRHYTHMIAS

James (1967) has reported that congenital deafness and cardiac arrhythmias can be associated with abnormal spotting or pigmentary abnormalities in Dalmatian dogs. Because of these defects, the dogs are usually destroyed by the experienced breeder. Four Dalmatians with the undesired confluent black spots (patches) were examined, and two of the four had electrocardiographic intermittent sinus arrest. Of nine other deaf Dalmatian dogs with various degrees of abnormal pigmentation studied in James' laboratory, three had frequent sinus pauses and periodic rhythms on the electrocardiogram. In comparison, 29 of 32 normal Dalmatians had normal electrocardiograms, and three of 32 had intermittent sinus pauses. According to James (1967), the intermittent sinus pauses may result from defective function of the sinoatrial node, and the disease is similar to a condition recognized in deaf children in which there is an abnormality of the sinus node.

CONGENITAL TRICUSPID STENOSIS AND TRICUSPID INSUFFICIENCY WITH PATENT FORAMEN OVALE

Four of 11 puppies from a litter of closely inbred Old English Sheepdogs were born with congenital cardiac anomalies (Ljunggren et al., 1966). Three puppies had congenital tricuspid stenosis and tricuspid insufficiency with a right-to-left shunt at the level of the patent foramen ovale. The diagnosis was verified at necropsy. The right-to-left shunt was apparently minimal in two dogs but was considerable in the third, resulting in cyanosis. In the latter dog, the major blood supply to the lungs came from the bronchial artery, and flow through the pulmonary artery and its branches was minimal. A loud systolic murmur was auscultated in all three dogs, and in a fourth the murmur persisted throughout systole and diastole. A precordial thrill was present in the latter dog, which had a patent ductus arteriosus. Electrocardiography suggested left atrial dilatation in two of the three puppies with tricuspid stenosis, tricuspid insufficiency, and patent foramen ovale. It is uncertain whether these abnormalities had a genetic background or not. Buchanan and Patterson (1965) reported finding an insufficient and stenotic anomalous tricuspid valve in a 2 year old German Shepherd. In a similar case seen by us, tricuspid insufficiency was due to markedly shortened chordae tendineae of the septal valve leaflet.

PSEUDOPULMONARY TRUNCUS

Wallace (1965) reported a pseudopulmonary truncus in which the pulmonary artery arose from the left common carotid artery in the middle of the neck. An overriding aorta was present at the base of the left and right ventricles, and a ventricular septal defect was also present.

SINGLE CORONARY ARTERY

A single coronary artery was reported by Day (1959). The artery arose above the right cranial aortic sinus of Valsalva. The vessel originating from the single aortic ostium then branched into two coronary arteries. One branch followed the normal course of the right coronary artery in the right atrioventricular sulcus. The anomalous branch passed in front of the conus and pulmonary artery until it assumed the normal position of the circumflex branch of the left coronary artery. Buchanan and Patterson (1965) reported a similar anomaly in a young dog with congenital subvalvular pulmonic stenosis.

References

Adkins, T. O., Farrall, J., and Mohart, C.: Persistent Right Aortic Arch in a Sentry Dog. J.A.V.M.A., 157 (1970):471.
Arey, L. B.: Developmental Anatomy. W. B. Saunders Co., Philadelphia, 7th ed., 1965.
Baker, G. J., and Williams, C. S. F.: Diaphragmatic Pericardial Hernia in the Dog. Vet. Rec., 78 (1966):578.
Baronti, A. C.: Congenital Esophageal Dilatation in a Cocker Puppy. North Amer. Vet., 31 (1950):666.
Barry, A.: Aortic Arch Derivations in the Human Adult. Anat. Rec., 111 (1951):221.
Bayford, D.: An Account of a Singular Case of Obstructed Deglutition. Mem. Med. Soc. (London), 2 (1789):271.
Bolton, G. R., Ettinger, S., and Roush, J. C.: Congenital Peritoneopericardial Diaphragmatic Hernia in a Dog. J. A. V. M. A., 155 (1969):723.
Brandt, A.: Rechtsseitiger Aortabogen mit abnormem Verlauf der A. Subclavia sinistra als Ursache von Oesophagusstenose beim. Hund. Skand. Vet.-tidskr., 30 (1940):993.
Brodey, R. S., and Prier, J. E.: Clinico-Pathologic Conference (Pulmonic Stenosis, Patent Foramen Ovale, and Diaphragmatic Pericardial Hernia). J. A. V. M. A., 139 (1961): 701.
Brodey, R. S., and Prier, J. E.: Clinico-Pathologic Conference (Patent Ductus Arteriosus and Pulmonary Hypertension). J. A. V. M. A., 140 (1962):379.
Brooks, C.: Persistent patency of the ductus arteriosus in the dog. Arch. Int. Med., 9 (1912): 44.
Buchanan, J. W.: Persistent Left Cranial Vena Cava in Dogs: Angiocardiography, Significance, and Coexisting Anomalies. J. Amer. Vet. Radiol. Soc., 4 (1963):1.

Buchanan, J. W.: Symposium: Thoracic Surgery on the Dog and Cat—III. Patent Ductus Arteriosus and Persistent Right Aortic Arch Surgery in Dogs. J. Small Anim. Pract., 9 (1968):409.

Buchanan, J. W., and Patterson, D. F.: Selective Angiography and Angiocardiography in Dogs with Congenital Cardiovascular Disease. J. Amer. Vet. Radiol. Soc., 6 (1965):21.

Buchanan, J. W., and Pyle, R. L.: Cardiac Tamponade during Catheterization of a Dog with Congenital Heart Disease. J. A. V. M. A., 149 (1966):1056.

Buchanan, J. W., Soma, L. R., and Patterson, D. F.: Patent Ductus Arteriosus Surgery in Small Dogs. J. A. V. M. A., 151 (1967):701.

Buergelt, C. D., and Wheaton, L. G.: Dextroaorta, Atopic Left Subclavian Artery, and Persistent Left Cephalic Vena Cava in a Dog. J. A. V. M. A., 156 (1970):1026.

Carmichael, J. A., Liu, S.-K., Tashjian, R. J., Radford, G., and Lord, P.: A Case of Canine Subaortic Stenosis and Aortic Valvular Insufficiency, with Particular Reference to Diagnostic Technique. J. Small Anim. Pract., 9 (1968):213.

Cato, W. R.: Diverticulum in the Diaphragm of a Dog. Vet. Med., 57 (1962):706.

Clark, D. R., Anderson, J. G., and Patterson, C.: Imperforate Cardiac Septal Defect in a Dog, J. A. V. M. A., 156 (1970):1020.

Clark, D. R., Ross, J. N., Hamlin, R. L., and Smith, C. R.: Tetralogy of Fallot in the Dog. J. A. V. M. A., 152 (1968):462.

Clinton, J. M.: A Case of Congenital Pericardio-Peritoneal Communication in a Dog. J. Amer. Vet. Radiol. Soc., 8 (1967):57.

Cordy, D. R., and Ribelin, W. E.: Six Congenital Cardiac Anomalies in Animals. Cornell Vet., 40 (1950):249.

Coward, T. C.: Persistence of the Right Primitive Aorta in a Dog with Incarceration of the Oesophagus. A Case Treated Surgically. Vet. Rec., 69 (1957):327.

Cooley, D. A., and Hallman, G. L.: Surgical Treatment of Congenital Heart Disease. Lea and Febiger, Philadelphia, 1966.

Cumming, G. F.: Propranolol in Tetralogy of Fallot (Editorial). Circulation, 41 (1970):13.

Custer, M. A., Kantor, A. F., Gilman, R. A., and DeRiemer, R. H.: Correction of Pulmonic Stenosis. J. A. V. M. A., 139 (1961):565.

Davies, J. J., and Ottoway, C. W.: A Peculiar Case of Oesophageal Obstruction in the Dog: Congenital Abnormality of the Aortic Arch. Vet. Rec., 55 (1943):102.

Day, S. B.: A Left Coronary Artery Originating from a Single Coronary Stem in a Dog. Anat. Rec., 134 (1959):55.

Detweiler, D. K.: Heart Disease in Dogs. Univ. Penn. Vet. Ext. Quart., 125 (1952):21.

Detweiler, D. K.: Clinical Aspects of Heart Disease in Dogs. Vet. Scope, 1 (1955):3.

Detweiler, D. K.: Electrocardiographic and Clinical Features of Spontaneous Auricular Fibrillation and Flutter (Tachycardia) in Dogs. Zbl. Veterinärmed., 4 (1957):509.

Detweiler, D. K.: Wesen und Häufigkeit von Herzkrankheiten bei Hunden. Zbl. Veterinärmed., 9 (1962):317.

Detweiler, D. K., and Allam, M. W.: Persistent Right Aortic Arch in Dogs. Cornell Vet., 45 (1955):209.

Detweiler, D. K., Brodey, R. S., and Flickinger, G. L.: Diagnosis and Surgical Correction of Peritoneopericardial Diaphragmatic Hernia in a Dog. J. A. V. M. A., 137 (1960): 177.

Detweiler, D. K., and Patterson, D. F.: A Phonograph Record of Heart Sounds and Murmurs of the Dog. Ann. N. Y. Acad. Sci., 127 (1965):322.

Dolowy, W. C., Lopez-Belio, M., Julian, O. C., and Grove, W. J.: Congenital Malformations of the Heart and Great Vessels in Dogs—A Report of Three Cases. J. A. V. M. A., 130 (1957):521.

Eliot, T. S., Jr., Eliot, F. P., Lushbaugh, C. C., and Slager, U. T.: First Report of the Occurrence of Neonatal Endocardial Fibroelastosis in Cats and Dogs. J. A. V. M. A., 133 (1958):271.

Eyster, G.: Incidence of Ventricular Septal Defect at Michigan State University (Abst). Acad. of Vet. Cardiol., Sci. Sessions, Spring 1969, Philadelphia, Pennsylvania.

Finn, J. P., and Martin, C. L.: Diaphragmatic Pericardial Hernia. J. Small Anim. Pract., 10 (1969):295.

Fitts, R. H.: Dilatation of the Esophagus in a Cocker Spaniel. J. A. V. M. A., 112 (1948): 343.

Flickinger, G. L., and Patterson, D. F.: Coronary Lesions Associated with Congenital Subaortic Stenosis in the Dog. J. Path. Bact., 93 (1967):133.

Frese, K.: Ueber Anomalien des Aortenbogens beim Hund. Zbl. Veterinärmed., 9 (1961): 787.

Friedberg, C. K.: Diseases of the Heart. W. B. Saunders Co., Philadelphia, 3rd ed., 1966.

Gorton, B.: Right Aortic Arch in a Dog. Vet. Rec., 5 (1925):483.

Hamlin, R. L.: Angiocardiography for the Clinical Diagnosis of Congenital Heart Disease in Small Animals. J. A. V. M. A., 135 (1959):112.

Hamlin, R. L.: Radiographic Diagnosis of Heart Disease in Dogs. J. A. V. M. A., 137 (1960):458.

Hamlin, R. L.: Analysis of the Cardiac Silhouette in Dorsoventral Radiographs from Dogs with Heart Disease. J. A. V. M. A., 153 (1968):1446.

Hamlin, R. L., and Harris, S. G.: Mitral Incompetence in Great Dane Pups. J. A. V. M. A., 154 (1969):790.

Hamlin, R. L., Marsland, W. P., Rudy, R. L., and Drenan, D. M.: Atypical Clinical Findings in a Dog with Pulmonic Stenosis. J. A. V. M. A., 142 (1963a):520.

Hamlin, R. L., Smetzer, D. L., and Smith, C. R.: Interventricular Septal Defect (Roger's Disease) in the Dog. J. A. V. M. A., 145 (1964):331.

Hamlin, R. L., Smetzer, D. L., and Smith, C. R.: Congenital Mitral Insufficiency in the Dog. J. A. V. M. A., 146 (1965):1088.

Hamlin, R. L., Smith, C. R., Rudy, R. L., and Nash, R. A.: Antemortem Diagnosis of Tetralogy of Fallot in a Dog. J. A. V. M. A., 140 (1962):948.

Hamlin, R. L., Smith, C. R., and Smetzer, D. L.: Ostium Secundum Type Interatrial Septal Defects in the Dog. J. A. V. M. A., 143 (1963b):149.

Hare, T.: Patent Interventricular Septum of a Dog's Heart. Vet. Rec., 55 (1943):103.

Hare, T., and Orr, A. B.: Patent Ductus Arteriosus with Patent Interventricular Foramen of a Dog's Heart. J. Path. Bact., 34 (1931):799.

Henwood, J. K., and Green, R. A.: Section of the Right Subclavian Artery to Relieve Associated Regurgitation of Food in the Dog. Vet. Rec., 76 (1964):1155.

Hickman, J., Edwards, J. E., and Mann, F. C.: Venous Anomalies in a Dog. Anat. Rec., 104 (1949):137.

Imhoff, R. K., and Foster, W. J.: Persistent Right Aortic Arch in a 10-year-Old Dog. J. A. V. M. A., 143 (1963):599.

James, T. N.: Congenital Deafness and Cardiac Arrhythmias. Amer. J. Cardiol., 19 (1967): 627.

Jex-Blake, A. J.: Obstruction of the Esophagus Caused by Persistent Ductus Arteriosus. Lancet, 2 (1926):542.

Kersten, U.: Klinische Untersuchungen am herzkranken Hund. Thesis. Hanover, Germany, 1968.

Klatte, E. C., and Burko, H.: The Differential Diagnosis of Cyanotic Congenital Heart Disease. Seminars Roentgenol., 3 (1968):358.

Kleine, L. J., Bisgard, G. E., and Lewis, R. E.: Rupture of the Aortic Sinus and Aortic Insufficiency in a Dog. J. A. V. M. A., 149 (1966):1050.

Klotz, A. P., and Brewer, N. R.: Double Aortic Arch in a Dog. North Amer. Vet., 33 (1952):867.

Lawson, D., Penhale, B., and Smith, G.: Persistent Right Aortic Arch in the Dog Causing Oesophageal Obstruction. Vet. Rec., 69 (1957):326.

Lev., M., Neuwelt, F., and Necheles, H.: Congenital Defect of the Interventricular Septum, Aortic Regurgitation and Probable Heart Block in a Dog. Amer. J. Vet. Res., 2 (1941): 91.

Linde, L. M., Takahashi, M., Goldberg, S. J., and Momma, K.: Effect of Acetyl Strophanthidin on Pulmonary Circulation of a Dog with Patent Ductus Arteriosus. Amer. J. Vet. Res., 30 (1969):1057.

Linton, G. A.: Anomalies of the Aortic Arches Causing Strangulation of the Esophagus and Trachea. J. A. V. M. A., 129 (1956):1.

Ljunggren, G., Nilsson, O., Olsson, S.-E., Pennock, P., Personn, S., and Sateri, H.: Four Cases of Congenital Malformation of the Heart in a Litter of Eleven Dogs. J. Small Anim. Pract., 7 (1966):611.

Lucam, F., Barone, R., Flachat, Ch., Cottereau, Ph., and Valentin, F.: Malformations cardiaques congénitales chez un Chien et chez un Chat. Rev. Méd. Vét., 107 (1956): 674.

Marek, J., and Môcsy, J.: Klinische Diagnostik der Inneren Krankheiten der Haustiere. Gustav Fischer, Jena, Germany, 4th ed., 1951.

Meredith, J. H., and Clarkson, T. B.: Tetralogy of Fallot in the Dog. J. A. V. M. A., 135 (1959):326.

Meschan, I.: Roentgen Signs in Clinical Practice. Vol. II. W. B. Saunders Co., Philadelphia, 1966.

Milks, H. J.: Diverticulum of the Esophagus Due to Congenital Malformation. Vet. Med., 24 (1929):227.

Milks, H. J., and Williams, W. L.: Persistence of the Right instead of the Left Primitive Aorta in the Dog Incarcerating the Esophagus and Causing Its Dilatation. Cornell Vet., 25 (1935):365.

Môcsy, J. von: Zwei Fälle von Schlundröhren-Abschnürung beim Hunde. Jahresber. Vet. Med., 65 (1939):335.

Morgan, J. P.: What Is Your Diagnosis? (Pericardial Diaphragmatic Hernia). J. A. V. M. A., 144 (1964):533.

Olafson, P.: Congenital Cardiac Anomalies in Animals. J. Tech. Methods, 19 (1939):129.

Ott, B. S., Raymond, B. A., North, R. L., and Pickens, G. E.: Diagnosis and Surgical Repair of Congenital Pulmonic Stenosis in the Dog. J. A. V. M. A., 144 (1964):851.

Ottaway, C. W.: Patent Foramen-Ovale in a Puppy. Vet. Rec., 61 (1949):503.

Pallaske, G.: Tödliche Kreislaufstörungen beim Hund durch Persistenz des Ductus arteriosus. Deutsch. Tierärztl. Wschr., 66 (1959):203.

Patterson, D. F.: Clinical and Epidemiologic Studies of Congenital Heart Disease in the Dog. Sci. Proc. Amer. Vet. Med. Ass., (1963):128.

Patterson, D. F.: Congenital Heart Disease in the Dog. Ann. N. Y. Acad. Sci., 127 (1965):541.

Patterson, D. F.: Epidemiologic and Genetic Studies of Congenital Heart Disease in the Dog. Circ. Res., 23 (1968):171.

Patterson, D. F., and Detweiler, D. K.: Predominance of German Shepherd and Boxer Breeds among Dogs with Congenital Subaortic Stenosis. Amer. Heart J., 65 (1963): 429.

Patterson, D. F., and Detweiler, D. K.: Hereditary Transmission of Patent Ductus Arteriosus in the Dog. Amer. Heart J., 74 (1967):289.

Patterson, D. F., and Flickinger, G. L.: Clinico-Pathological Conference (Subaortic Stenosis). J. A. V. M. A., 145 (1964):363.

Patterson, D. F., Hare, W. C. D., Shive, R. J., and Luginbühl, H. R.: Congenital Malformations of the Cardiovascular System Associated with Chromosomal Abnormalities (A Report of the Clinical, Pathologic, and Cytogenetic Findings in 2 Dogs). Zbl. Veterinärmed., 13 (1966):669.

Pierau, F. K., Olesch, K., Klussmann, F. W., and Frese, K.: Cardiologische Diagnostik mit Indikator-Verdünnungsmethoden beim Haustier. Ductus arteriosus apertus beim Hund. Berlin. Münch. Tierärztl. Wschr., 77 (1964):221.

Pommer, A.: Hernia Diaphragmatica Pericardialis bei Hunden. Wien. Tierärztl. Mschr., 38 (1951):497.

Pommer, A.: Röntgenbefund bei Zwerchfellhernien und Rupturen der Hunde. Zbl. Veterinärmed., 2 (1955):173.

Popovic, N., and Fleming, W.: Pulmonic Stenosis with Atrial Septal Defect and Heartworms. J. A. V. M. A., 157 (1970):485.

Renk, W., and Raethel, S.: Trachea- und Oesophagusstenose durch abnormen Verlauf der Aorta beim Hund. Berlin. München. Tierärztl. Wschr., 67 (1954):174.

Rhodes, W. H., Patterson, D. F., and Detweiler, D. K.: Radiographic Anatomy of the Canine Heart, Part I. J. A. V. M. A., 137 (1960):283

Rhodes, W. H., Patterson, D. F., and Detweiler, D. K.: Radiographic Anatomy of the Canine Heart, Part II. J. A. V. M. A., 143 (1963):137.

Ripps, J. H., and Henderson, A. R.: Congenital Pulmonic Valvular Stenosis in a Dog. J. A. V. M. A., 123 (1953):292.

Rowan, P., Lukban, S., Ettinger, S., and Carmichael, J. A.: Surgical Correction of Congenital Subaortic Stenosis in the Dog. 1970 Unpublished data.

Saunders, E. C.: Surgical Closure of Patent Ductus Arteriosus in the Dog. North Amer. Vet., 38 (1957):185.

Schaller, O.: Die Vena cava cranialis sinistra persistens bei unseren Haussäugetieren, insbesondere den Fleischfressern. Z. Anat. Entwicklungsgesch., 119 (1955):131.

Schmidt, D., Hohaus, B., and Röder, F.: Offener Ductus arteriosus (Botalli) beim Hund. Berlin. Münch. Tierärztl. Wschr., 80 (1967):168.

Schmutzer, K., Marable, S. A., and Maloney, J. V.: Successful Closure of a Patent Ductus Arteriosus in the Dog. Report of a Case. Cornell Vet., 48 (1958):404.

Shive, R. J., Hare, W. C. D., and Patterson, D. F.: Chromosomal Studies in Dogs with Congenital Cardiac Defects. Cytogenetics, 4 (1965):340.

Severin, G. A.: Congenital and Acquired Heart Disease. J. A. V. M. A., 151 (1967):1733.

Smollich, A.: Abweichungen im Bereich der Äste des Aortenbogens und ihre Bedeutung. Arch. Exp. Veterinärmed., 15 (1961):986.

Spitz, H. B.: Eisenmenger's Syndrome. Seminars Roentgenol., 3 (1968):373.

Spörri, H., and Scheitlin, M.: Klinisch physiologische und pathologische-anatomische Untersuchungen in zwei Fällen von persistierendem Ductus arteriosus (Botalli). Schweiz. Arch. Tierheilk., 94 (1952):387.

Steinberg, I.: Angiocardiography in Congenital Heart Disease. In *Cardiology, An Encyclopedia of the Cardiovascular System.* Edited by A. A. Luisada, Vol. 3. McGraw-Hill Book Company, New York, (1959).

Tashjian, R. J., Hofstra, P. C., Reid, C. F., and Newman, M. M.: Isolated Pulmonic Valvular Stenosis in a Dog. J. A. V. M. A., 135 (1959):94.

Török, J.: Zwei seltene klinische Fälle. Jahresber. Veterinärmed., 62 (1937-1938):24.

Van Lennep, E. W.: Een geval van Rechter arcus Aortae bij de Hond. T. Diergeneesk., 77 (1952):381.

Vitums, A.: Anomalous Origin of the Right Subclavian and Common Carotid Arteries in the Dog. Cornell Vet., 52 (1962):5.

Von Sandersleben, J.: Aszites beim Hund infolge Persistenz des Ductus arteriosus. Deutsch. Tierärztl. Wschr., 60 (1953):476.

Walker, R. G., and Littlewort, M. C. G.: Angiography in the Pre-Operative Assessment of Vascular Ring Obstruction of the Oesophagus in the Dog. Vet. Rec., 76 (1964):215.

Wallace, C. R.: Absence of Posterior Vena Cava in a Dog. J. A. V. M. A., 136 (1960):27.

Wallace, C. R.: Spontaneous Congestive Heart Failure in the Dog. Ann. N. Y. Acad. Sci., 127 (1965):570.

Wallace, C. R., and Hamilton, W. F.: Study of Spontaneous Congestive Heart Failure in the Dog. Circ. Res., 11 (1962):301.

Walters, B., and Bramer, C. N.: Patent Ductus Arteriosus. North Amer. Vet., 33 (1952): 252.

Willis, T. E., and Alai, J.: Congenital Cardiac Defect: Diagnosis and Treatment (A Case Report). North Amer. Vet., 35 (1954):838.

Wirth, D.: Einführung in die klinische Diagnostik der inneren Erkrankungen und Hautkrankheiten der Haustiere. Urban und Schwarzenberg, Vienna, 3rd ed., 1949.

Wysong, R. L.: Embryology of Persistent Right Aortic Arch. Vet. Med., 64 (1969):203.

Yamamoto, S., and Emoto, O.: Ein Fall von Speiseröhrenverengerung eines junges Hundes auf Grund kongenitalen abnormalen Sitzes derselben. J. Jap. Soc. Vet. Sci., 14 (1935): 20.

Zalis, E. G., Inmon, T. W., Lundberg, G. D., and Knutson, R. A.: Dynamic Left Ventricular Outflow Obstruction Experimentally Induced. Amer. Heart J., 71 (1966):488.

Ziezschmann, O., and Krölling, O.: Lehrbuch der Entwicklungsgeschichte der Haustiere. Paul Parey, Berlin, 1955.

Zook, B. C., and Hathaway, J. E.: Tracheal Stenosis and Congenital Cardiac Anomalies in a Dog. J. A. V. M. A., 149 (1966):298.

CHAPTER

19

SURGICAL CORRECTION OF PATENT DUCTUS ARTERIOSUS AND VASCULAR RING ANOMALIES

William D. DeHoff, D.V.M., M.S.
Head, Department of Surgery
The Animal Medical Center
New York, New York

The surgical techniques and considerations for closure of patent ductus arteriosus and correction of vascular ring anomalies are presented because proper treatment of these common congenital and developmental cardiovascular lesions is feasible and safe in veterinary practice.

Cardiovascular surgery requires a thorough knowledge of the anatomy and physiology of the thorax and its structures; an understanding of the pathophysiology of the disease conditions involved; the ability to reach as specific a diagnosis as possible; the technical training and equipment necessary to perform the required surgery; and the facilities and trained personnel for postoperative care and treatment of the animal.

The success of cardiovascular surgery is dependent upon complete attention to every detail from the time the anesthetic is administered until the animal awakens in the recovery area. This is best accomplished by a thorough review of the surgical plan prior to the procedure with all staff involved so that they know what is expected and are able to act efficiently should a crisis arise. After surgery has been completed, the staff should review the procedure and record changes that could be beneficial in preparation for future cases.

DEVELOPMENT AND CLINICAL SIGNS
OF THE ANOMALIES

PATENT DUCTUS ARTERIOSUS

The ductus arteriosus is located at the level of the fourth rib and lies between the bifurcation of the pulmonary artery near the origin of the left pulmonary artery and the left ventrolateral wall of the aorta. In the normal fetal circulation, blood flow is from right to left; blood is shunted from the pulmonary artery to the descending aorta via the ductus arteriosus, thereby by-passing the nonfunctional lung tissue. At birth or shortly thereafter the ductus constricts, and as the vascular system develops it is obliterated, enabling the blood to flow from the pulmonary artery into the lung. In the dog, proliferation of the vessel wall and fibrosis of the tissue completes anatomic closure of the vessel by approximately 1 month of age (Buchanan, 1968). Normally, the ligamentum arteriosum is the remnant of the ductus arteriosus (see p. 478).

With failure of the ductus arteriosus to close, the reasons for which are unknown, blood begins to flow from the aorta to the pulmonary artery as the aortic pressure increases and pulmonary artery pressure decreases after birth. This left-to-right shunting, opposite from the normal right-to-left fetal shunt, usually causes a continuous murmur as a result of the turbulence from blood "jetting" into the pulmonary artery. As the aortic blood pressure continues to rise after birth and pulmonary artery pressure decreases, the abnormal flow of blood becomes even greater because of the increased pressure gradient. The murmur is continuous because the aortic pressures are higher than the pulmonary artery pressures throughout both systole and diastole (Figs. 18-2 through 18-5).

Clinical signs of the anomaly (see p. 479) may be apparent any time from birth (Patterson, 1968) to 10 years of age; however, in the majority of cases, clinical signs are evident between 8 months and 3 years of age. It is generally agreed that heart failure will develop in all dogs with a patent ductus arteriosus, and the longer the abnormality is present, the more severe will be the secondary pathologic changes. Consequently, surgery should be performed at the earliest possible date (see pp. 494–495).

In time, the aorta and the pulmonary arteries become dilated and thin-walled, and the aorta often dilates to such an extent that a postductal aneurysmal bulge develops owing to the turbulent blood flow in the region of the ductus. A valve-like flap forms on the inner ventrolateral surface of the aorta, cranial to the opening into the ductus (Detweiler et al., 1962). This flap may interfere with the view of the ductus both angiographically and at the time of surgery; the ductus appears to enter the aorta more ventrally than it actually does. The openings of the ductus into the aorta and pulmonary artery often widen as the vessels dilate (Buchanan, Soma, and Patterson, 1967), sometimes causing the ductus to become twice as wide as it is long. These secondary changes occur in children with this condition, and it has recently been shown that the prognosis is better when surgery is performed as early as possible, and before clinical signs of cardiac disease are present (Kilman et al., 1970).

If patent ductus arteriosus is diagnosed early and if the need for early correction is realized, the surgical procedure is generally technically easier; there are fewer postoperative complications, and the morbidity and mortality rates are lower. An uncomplicated procedure on a young dog can easily be accomplished in a minimum of surgical time, and is well tolerated.

The presurgical confirmation of the specific diagnosis of patent ductus arteriosus and indications, contraindications, and medical preparation of the dog with a patent ductus arteriosus for surgery have been discussed in Chapter 18.

VASCULAR RING ANOMALIES

Vascular ring anomalies are congenital cardiovascular malformations of the great vessels, and they do not interfere with cardiac function or cause heart disease. These anomalies have been found in most species of domestic animals and in man. The dog is the domestic animal most often affected by anomalies such as double aortic arch, anomalous subclavian arteries, and, most commonly, persistent right aortic arch (see p. 496). This section is concerned only with those vascular ring anomalies that constrict the trachea or, more commonly, the esophagus at the base of the heart, which results in regurgitation of food.

Approximately 95 per cent of all reported vascular ring anomalies in dogs have been due to persistent right aortic arch (Buchanan, 1968). In this situation, the right fourth aortic arch develops embryologically in place of the normal left fourth arch; therefore, the aorta is abnormally located to the right of the trachea and esophagus instead of to the left, as it is normally. The aorta does function normally, but the problem arises from the ligamentum arteriosum or patent ductus arteriosus, which runs from the bifurcation of the pulmonary artery near the origin of the left pulmonary artery to the aorta. The ductus arteriosus has been shown to remain patent in dogs with persistent right aortic arch, but in most cases the constricting structure is a solid fibrous structure, the ligamentum arteriosum, and it will be referred to as such throughout the discussion.

The ligamentum arteriosum now crosses over the dorsal and left lateral surfaces of the esophagus (retroesophageal), squeezing the esophagus between the pulmonary artery, the trachea, and the aorta. The resulting constriction prevents passage of solid food and rapid swallowing of fluid (see p. 510 and Figs. 18-16 and 18-17) (Lawson, Penhale, and Smith, 1957; Buchanan, 1968). As the dog continues to eat, the portion of the esophagus cranial to the constriction becomes mechanically dilated. Without surgical correction, the esophagus continues to dilate and stretches beyond its capacity to return to normal. Ventral pouches develop in the stretched cranial esophagus, and there is loss of some if not all ability to contract (Fig. 19-1). If the vomiting is recognized early and occurs only after ingestion of solid food, and if the dog is maintained on oral fluids, the secondary signs and pathologic changes normally associated with the disease can be delayed and the dog strengthened prior to surgical correction of the malformation.

The diagnosis is made based on the history and clinical signs and on specialized radiographic examination (see pp. 510-512). The disease must be differentiated from dilatation of the esophagus due to other pathologic conditions (see p. 512). The definitive diagnosis is made radiographically (Figs. 18-16 through 18-18).

The onset of clinical signs is rapid, and because of their increasing severity and the progressive pathologic complications, *immediate surgical intervention is recommended*. Regardless of the cause, the esophageal stricture must be corrected to prevent further esophageal dilatation and foreign body pneumonia in those dogs not advanced in the course of the disease. In those presented in a

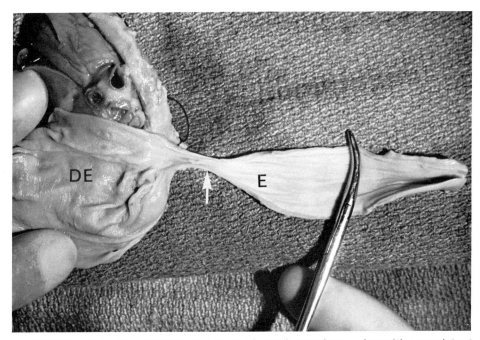

FIGURE 19-1 Postmortem specimen of esophagus from a dog with a persistent right aortic arch. The esophagus is from a 12 week old German Shepherd puppy which had signs of persistent right aortic arch for four weeks. The dilated thoracic esophagus (DE) cranial to the area of constriction is seen to be thin and pouchy and to lack the normal longitudinal rugae seen in the normal esophagus (E) caudal to the area of the constriction. The narrowest part of the esophageal specimen (arrow) is the area of the esophagus that was constricted by the ligamentum arteriosum. This area could be dilated and does dilate in the intact animal postoperatively as food is ingested.

debilitated condition, attempts to improve their condition prior to surgery, other than restoring their immediate fluid imbalance, have been of little value. It is well recognized that it is difficult to maintain a puppy's nutritional requirements by intravenous feeding without elaborate clinical laboratory facilities, and major surgical esophageal by-pass procedures such as gastrotomies or enterostomies are as traumatic to the dog as correction of the aortic arch anomalies.

GENERAL SURGICAL CONSIDERATIONS FOR PATENT DUCTUS ARTERIOSUS AND VALVULAR RING ANOMALIES

The same surgical approach is required for correction of both patent ductus arteriosus and vascular ring anomalies, and the immediate postoperative management is similar as well.

ANESTHESIA

Most vascular ring anomalies require surgical correction when the dog is very young. Surgery for correction of patent ductus arteriosus is encouraged if not essential at a young age. Anesthesia during correction of vascular ring anomalies is made more difficult because clinical problems such as emaciation, dehydration, and inhalation pneumonia due to chronic vomiting are present. In addition, if the cranial esophageal pouches are very large, expansion of the apical and cardiac lobes of the lung will be reduced. Dogs with a patent ductus arteriosus have an extremely high but possibly inadequate cardiac output owing to the presence of a significant left-to-right shunting of blood. In the presence of pulmonary congestion resulting from left heart failure, there will be an alteration in the alveolar ventilation perfusion ratio due to the reduction in diffusion of oxygen across the alveolar membrane. These factors contribute to the increased risk of anesthesia when surgery is contemplated. For these reasons, the anesthetist plays a vital role in the outcome of either procedure. Without absolute control of anesthesia and adequate oxygenation of the dog, the operations in question should not be undertaken.

For maximum control of anesthesia, a suitable pre-anesthetic agent should be employed to reduce apprehension and excitement when it exists. Atropine is routinely administered in all cases. Induction for endotracheal intubation is usually safe using a short-acting intravenous barbiturate. However, in the bad risk case in which there is no upper respiratory obstruction, mask induction with nitrous oxide and fluothane in the presence of 50 per cent oxygen is advised.

Controlled ventilation should begin immediately after induction of anesthesia to ensure adequate pulmonary oxygen and carbon dioxide levels. Maintenance of inhalation anesthesia is accomplished with agents such as fluothane or methoxyflurane, with or without nitrous oxide. Adequate intermittent positive pressure ventilation must be maintained via either a circle system for the larger dogs or an Ayres T-piece for smaller dogs. A muscle relaxant such as succinyl choline may be used to advantage, especially in larger dogs. A muscle relaxant permits greater control of ventilation and a greater degree of muscle relaxation at lighter levels of anesthesia.

Cardiac monitoring of the anesthetized dog is essential. Rate, rhythm, and appearance of the electrocardiogram should be followed on an oscilloscope. A patent jugular catheter enables the administration of drugs and infusion of fluids directly into the right heart. Central venous pressure can also be measured when necessary.

Adequate drugs for the treatment of cardiac emergencies, as well as fluids, blood, or plasma expanders to alleviate hemorrhage or shock, should be available.

Following surgery, respiration must be supported until the dog can ventilate itself adequately. Only after self-ventilation is possible should the endotracheal tube be removed. The postoperative condition of the dog can be improved considerably by the alleviation of pain resulting from the thoracotomy wound. Low dosages of meperidine (Demerol) or other narcotic agents are recommended for this purpose.

SURGICAL APPROACHES

The surgical approach to the thorax for patent ductus arteriosus and vascular ring anomalies is best accomplished through the fourth intercostal space (Weipers and Lawson, 1965) or the fifth intercostal space, or by resection of the fifth rib. Since the corrective procedures are most often performed on dogs when they are small, it is important to gain as large a thoracic opening as possible to afford good visualization and to enable manipulation of the structures involved. These procedures cannot be done with maximum control through small incisions.

The ductus arteriosus lies directly under the fourth rib and is easily reached through the fourth intercostal space. However, if the dog has a wide, barrel chest, is very small, or has an enlarged heart, or if division and suturing of the ductus is anticipated, then resection of the fifth rib or exposure through the fifth intercostal space will provide a wider thoracic opening and easier use of instruments without impairing direct vision of the ductal area throughout the procedure.

The dog is placed in right lateral recumbency. An insulating blanket or towel is placed under small, thin, or young dogs to control unnecessary heat loss. The left forelimb is held in moderate extension, keeping the elbow away from the surgical field but not to the extent that it inhibits expansion of the thorax (Fig. 19-2). The left lateral thorax is clipped and prepared aseptically from the dorsum of the back to the right sternal border and over the scapula to the caudal extent of the rib cage. The primary incision is made through the skin, subcutaneous tissues, and cutaneous trunci muscles over the area of the fifth rib, extending from just lateral to the dorsal spinous processes to half the distance between the costochondral junction and the sternum. As an aid in maintaining sterile technique, lap pads or towels can be attached to the skin edges at this time.

The thoracic incision is continued with curved dissecting scissors, cutting the latissimus dorsi and dorsal portion of the serratus ventralis muscles which cover the ribs (Miller, Christensen, and Evans, 1964). The ribs can now be counted

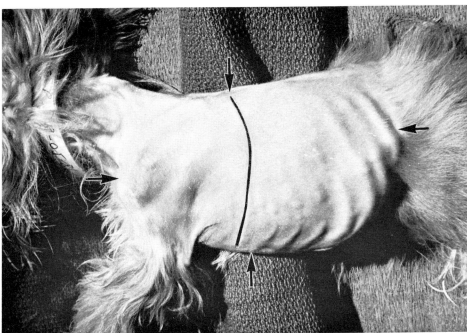

FIGURE 19-2 Surgical preparation of dog for left lateral thoracotomy for thoracic exposure at the fourth intercostal space or by resection of the fifth rib. The dog's hair is clipped from the point of the shoulder (arrow) cranially to the caudal extent of the rib cage (arrow) and from across the dorsum of the back (arrow) to across the sternum (arrow). The left forelimb is extended away from the operative field. The skin incision (black line) should extend from just lateral to the dorsal spinous processes to halfway between the costochondral junction and the midline of the sternum. The dog's thorax can be stabilized and supported with sand bags or with a folded towel, as was used for this dog.

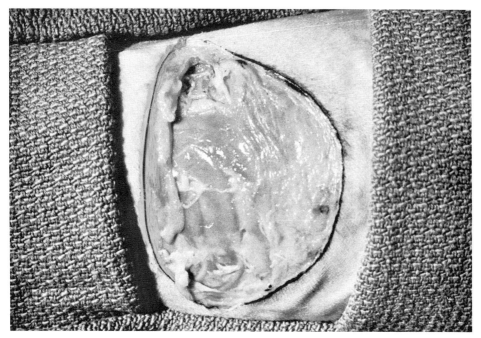

FIGURE 19-3 Thoracic exposure through the skin and sling muscles of the forelimb. The skin and subcutaneous muscles have been incised. The sling muscles of the forelimb, the latissimus dorsi, and the serratus ventralis have also been severed. The ribs can be counted accurately after the major sling muscles of the forelimb have been divided. Lap pads moistened with warm saline solution are normally applied when the skin and subcutaneous tissues are incised.

accurately to ensure proper placement of the thoracic opening (Fig. 19-3). The incision is continued in the fourth intercostal space, over the fifth rib, or in the fifth intercostal space, depending on the surgical approach selected.

Approach through the fourth or fifth intercostal space. The ventral fibers of the serratus dorsalis cranialis muscle are separated, and the dorsal portion covering the intercostal space is transected. The dorsal end of the thoracic incision is then extended to above the angle of the rib, requiring the iliocostalis thoracis muscle and the ventral portion of the longissimus muscle to be severed to the body of the spinalis and semispinalis muscles. This dorsal extension of the thoracic incision into the deeper muscles in the area of the dorsal spine permits greater rib retraction, which enlarges the thoracic exposure over the area of the aorta and pulmonary artery. The scalenus muscle is cut, and the aponeurosis of the rectus abdominus muscle should be incised distally to the level of the skin incision (Miller, Christensen, and Evans, 1964).

The intercostal space is now exposed, and the external and internal intercostal muscles are cut with scissors from the angle of the rib dorsally, to below the costochondral junction. The incision should be parallel to the contour of the ribs and midway between them, with care being taken not to incise along the caudal aspect of the rib where the intercostal artery and vein are located. The pleura is punctured, with care being taken not to damage the lung lobe beneath, and the lungs are allowed to fall away from the pleural surface. Blunt-tipped scissors are then used to incise the pleura for the entire length of the incision. As soon as the pleura is opened, respiratory functions for the dog *must* be assumed by the anesthetist.

Approach via resection of the fifth rib. After the ribs have been counted accurately, the serratus dorsalis muscle is elevated from the fifth rib. The periosteum on the lateral surface of the rib is incised with a scalpel from the angle of the rib to midway between the costochrondral junction of the rib and the sternebrae. A small periosteal elevator is used to elevate the edges of the periosteum off the lateral surface of the rib, being particularly careful not to puncture the pleura and penetrate the thoracic cavity. The periosteum is now stripped off the medial side of the rib for the entire length that is to be resected. When the periosteum has been elevated from the angle of the rib dorsally and to the ventral extent of the thoracic opening, bone cutters are used to cut the rib away. A small incision is made through the periosteum, the lungs are permitted to fall away, and the incision is extended the entire length of the elevated periosteum, staying in the middle of the periosteum parallel to the adjacent ribs.

These two techniques of lateral thoracic incision are complicated somewhat by the fact that surgery for patent ductus arteriosus and vascular ring anomalies is often performed on small dogs and very young dogs; therefore, gentle dissection and as atraumatic a technique as possible are required, since the landmarks used are often small and sometimes indistinct, and the tissues are delicate.

After the thorax has been opened, the lungs are evaluated for proper inflattion and the presence of atelectatic areas or other pathologic changes. Attempts to correct these changes are made before the thorax is closed and are noted for evaluation and postoperative treatment. Lap pads moistened with warm saline solution are placed along the rib borders, and a self-retaining rib retractor is inserted after a final examination of the thoracic wall tissues is made. The moistened pads should cover all exposed tissues of the thoracic wall completely, and the retractor should be light and compact, permitting maximum expansion of the thoracic opening without interfering with the surgical field or putting pressure on the heart and major vessels.

The apical and cardiac lobes of the lung are collapsed manually and packed off gently with lap pads moistened with warm saline solution in a caudal direction, exposing the operative area, the base of the heart, the aorta, the main pulmonary artery, the left pulmonary artery, and the esophagus for correction of patent ductus arteriosus or a vascular ring anomaly. The time should be noted so that the lung lobes can be unpacked and reinflated for a few minutes every 20 minutes. The heart, the best monitoring device for the surgeon, should be observed as to rate, color, and strength of movement throughout the procedure. All monitoring devices and administration of fluids should be checked for proper function before continuing with the major part of the surgical procedure.

CLOSURE OF THE THORAX

After the procedure has been completed, the thoracic cavity is thoroughly flushed with warm saline solution to remove all blood clots and other debris, and an opening is made through the mediastinum so that any fluid or air trapped on the opposite side of the thoracic cavity can be removed.

The left lung lobes are gently reinflated, ensuring that no atelectatic areas remain. A small stab incision is made in the skin three to four ribs caudal to the thoracic incision in the upper half of the thorax. A fine, curved hemostat is used to tunnel under the skin a short distance cranially, and the thoracic cavity is punctured one to two ribs caudal to the operative site. A thoracic drainage tube is drawn retrograde from the thoracic cavity and out through the stab wound in the skin. The drainage tube is positioned forward in the thoracic cavity, without kinks, so that the last side hole is safely within the thoracic cavity. A purse-string suture is placed around the wound and is tied; it is then secured to the drainage tubing to prevent the tube from being pulled out accidentally. Many commercial thoracic drains are available, but we have found Brunswick feeding tubes, French sizes 14 to 18, depending on the size of the dog, to be effective; four to five additional small, smooth side holes, similar to the ones already present, are cut near the tip of the tube (Fig. 19-4). The thoracic drainage tube is left open to the outside while positive pressure ventilation is maintained and the thorax is being closed.

If the fourth or fifth intercostal space exposure was used, the thoracic wall is closed by preplacing six or more size 2-0 to 1 chromic catgut sutures, depending on the size of the dog, around the ribs and then approximating the ribs with a rib approximator or large Bachaus towel clamp, taking care that the ribs do not overlap. The sutures are then tied. If the fifth rib was resected, then the fourth and sixth ribs are drawn closer together with a rib approximator, eliminating tension on the periosteum of the fifth rib, while a continuous suture pattern of size 2-0 to 0 chromic catgut is placed in the periosteum.

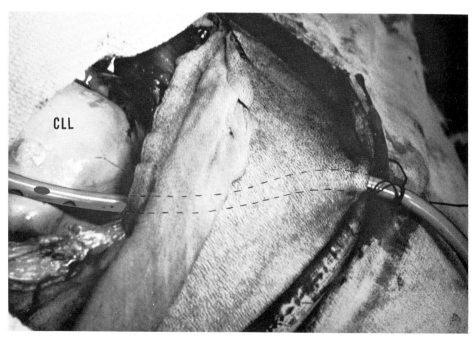

FIGURE 19-4 Thoracic drain implanted in thorax. The cardiac lobe of the left lung (CLL) has been re-expanded after having been packed off. The lap pads sewn to the skin have been pulled cranially to expose the point of exit of the thoracic drain from the thoracic cavity. The skin and subcutaneous tissues are sealed around the tube with a purse-string suture. This suture is then secured to the drainage tube to prevent the tube from being pulled out of the thorax.

The remaining muscle layers are usually closed with 2-0 chromic catgut, using two layers of continuous suture. In very young or small dogs, however, a single-layer continuous suture pattern may help to develop a more air-tight seal because of the small muscle masses and delicate subcutaneous tissues. Closure of the subcutaneous tissues and skin is routine. A light gauze compression dressing is applied to the wound to prevent formation of dead spaces in the area of closure in which blood or air might accumulate. However, the dressing should not be applied so tightly that expansion of the thorax is restricted (Fig. 19-5). After closure of the thoracic wall, the lungs are fully expanded, expelling the remaining air and fluid in the thorax, and the drainage tube is clamped off with a hemostatic forceps.

A radiograph is taken immediately after the procedure to evaluate the position of the thoracic drainage tube and the inflation of the lungs, and to determine whether air or fluid is present in the thoracic cavity. The thoracic drain is connected to an underwater seal or other device such as a Heimlich valve (Sauer, 1969), enabling air and fluid to be expelled from the thorax while preventing backflow into the thorax. Intermittent manual or automatic suction devices can be used if the dog requires a respiratory support system to aid respiration and remove larger quantities of air or fluids accumulating in the thorax. Suction is usually not needed after the first few hours if the surgery was uncomplicated. The drain is left in place, and a second radiograph is taken 12 to 24 hours after the last air or

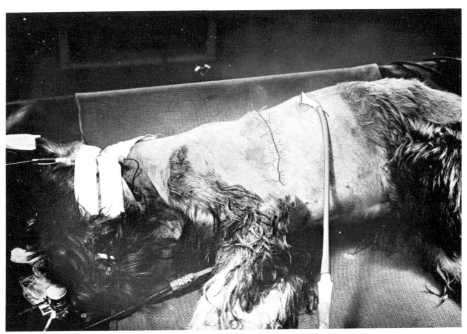

FIGURE 19-5 Thorax after completion of procedure. This picture of a 7 month old Standard Schnauzer immediately postoperatively demonstrates the jugular catheter used for administration of fluids and monitoring of central venous pressure. The electrocardiographic leads are in place, and the thoracic drainage tube has been attached to an underwater seal. A light, sterile gauze dressing will now be applied over the skin incision, and a postoperative radiograph will be taken.

fluid was removed from the thoracic cavity. If the thorax is free of air and fluid at this time, the drain is removed. A petrolatum-coated gauze sponge is held around the tube, and it is rapidly withdrawn from the thoracic cavity to prevent formation of a pneumothorax.

The skin opening for the drainage tube may be sutured closed, or it may be covered with the petrolatum-coated gauze sponge until the wound has sealed.

SURGICAL TECHNIQUE

PATENT DUCTUS ARTERIOSUS

The thorax is opened and the lungs are packed off as described above. The left phrenic and left vagus nerves are identified, and the main pulmonary artery is palpated to locate the area of greatest thrill. The thrill is then followed dorsally to the aorta to locate the ductus, which lies under the vagus nerve. The rate and size of the heart and the size of abnormal bulges of the aorta and left pulmonary artery should be noted (Fig. 19-6).

The mediastinal pleura is incised parallel to the aorta and dorsal to the left vagus nerve with blunt, fine, thumb forceps and small, fine, blunt-tipped dissecting scissors. Enough tissue is freed to permit the vagus nerve to be retracted and held ventrally by an encircling heavy silk suture and then tagged with a hemostatic forceps. The left recurrent laryngeal nerve, which branches medially from the vagus nerve and circles back around the caudal aspect of the ductus arteriosus, is now exposed. *This is the landmark for locating the caudal aspect of the ductus arteriosus* (Figs. 19-7 and 19-8).

When the ductus has been located, the mediastinal pleura and adventitial tissues are dissected away from the aorta, ductus, and pulmonary artery, beginning with the aorta and working ventrally. In most cases, all dissection is carried out extrapericardially; however, when the ductus is very short, the pericardium must be entered to expose the junction of the ductus with the pulmonary artery (Fig. 19-9).

When the ductus and its attachments to the aorta and pulmonary artery are clearly visualized, the medial blind dissection of the ductus and its junctions with the aorta and pulmonary artery is begun. A fine, blunt-tipped, right-angle forceps with its tip always directed toward the aorta is used for this dissection, which is started at the caudal aspect of the ductus. The blind dissection of this area is a difficult part of the procedure, since the craniomedial area of the ductus is shortest, thin-walled, and in close apposition with the right pulmonary artery (Fig. 19-10). Hemorrhage at this point is not uncommon and is usually due to puncture of the right pulmonary artery; this hemorrhage is controlled by digital pressure for 3 to 5 minutes.

After the ductus has been dissected free, two oiled or moistened size 0 to 2 silk ligatures are passed around the ductus, ensuring that the strands have not overlapped medially. The large diameter silk is used to prevent cutting of the ductal tissue, as well as to prevent recanalization of the ductus. Keeping very gentle traction on the pulmonary artery side of the ductus with one strand, the other is tied *gently* to the aortic side of the ductus as close to the aortic wall as

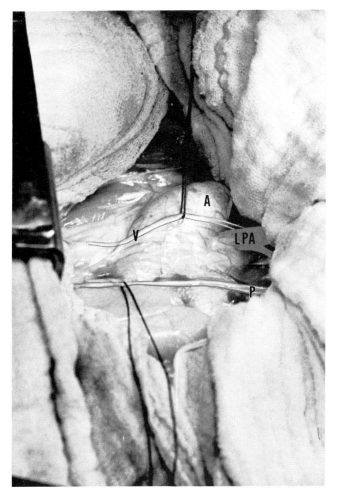

FIGURE 19-6 Exposure of the operative site for a patent ductus arteriosus prior to dissection. The ribs are retracted, and the lungs have been collapsed and packed off in a caudoventral direction with lap pads moistened with warm saline solution. This is the view the surgeon has standing at the dog's sternal border. The vagus (V) and phrenic (P) nerves have been tagged with silk ligatures. The aorta (A) is seen to bulge dorsal to the vagus nerve. The left pulmonary artery (LPA) is located ventral to the vagus nerve. The important anatomic structures in the following photographs have been highlighted to enable clearer visualization.

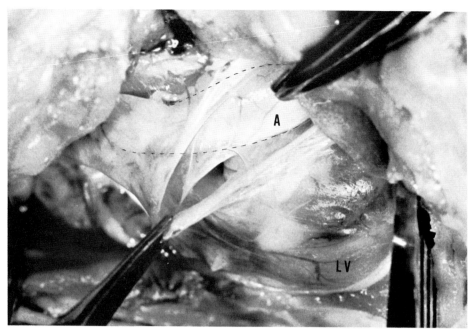

FIGURE 19-7 Dissection of the mediastinal pleura for surgery for patent ductus arteriosus. The mediastinal pleura and adventitia are dissected away from the aorta (A), the patent ductus arteriosus, and the main pulmonary artery. This dissection begins at the aorta and is gently worked through the different tissue planes ventrally. This connective tissue is very thin and delicate. The left ventricle (LV) is seen ventrally.

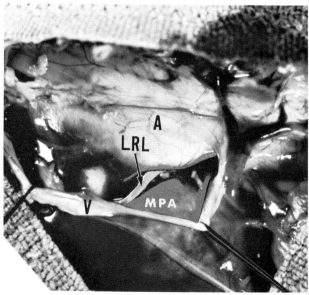

FIGURE 19-8 Location of the patent ductus arteriosus. The pleural and adventitial tissues have been dissected away, permitting the vagus nerve (V) to be freed and retracted ventrally. The left recurrent laryngeal nerve (LRL) is seen coursing around the caudal extent of the patent ductus arteriosus. The main pulmonary artery (MPA) can be seen bulging ventral to the aorta (A). The main pulmonary artery should be palpated for the area of thrill from the ductus, and the thrill is followed dorsally to the aorta to locate the ductus.

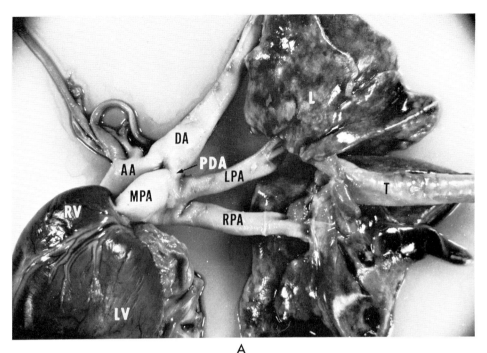

A

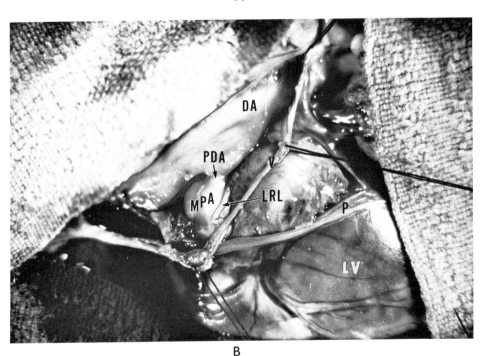

B

FIGURE 19-9 *A,* Postmortem specimen of patent ductus arteriosus. The adventitia has been stripped from the aortic arch (AA), descending aorta (DA), main pulmonary artery (MPA), left pulmonary artery (LPA), right pulmonary artery (RPA), and patent ductus arteriosus (PDA). The pericardium has been removed so that the left ventricle (LV) and the right ventricle (RV) can be seen. The lungs (L) and trachea (T) have been retracted to expose the major vessels involved with patent ductus

Legend continued on following page.

possible by laying the knot upon the junction of the ductus and the aorta and slowly tightening it. In older dogs, in which the ductus is not as pliable, the ductus is partially tied off. At this time, the electrocardiogram should be closely watched for changes in the cardiac rate or rhythm. After a few minutes, the turbulent blood flow in the aorta at the area of the ductus adjusts, and pulmonary artery pressures decrease, lessening the tension on the ductus. Then the suture can more safely be secured. The decrease in pressure on the pulmonary artery side of the ductus also permits the second suture to be easily tied at the junction of the ductus and the pulmonary artery. A third suture, size 4-0 or 5-0 silk, with a small cardiovascular needle attached, should be used as a transfixing ligature between the first two sutures (Figs. 19-10 through 19-12).

If the ductus is wider than it is long, a technique of dividing the ductus and suturing, rather than simple ligation, is recommended, especially in older dogs in which the ductal tissues are not as pliable. Two vascular forceps are used to divide the ductus arteriosus after it has been dissected free; we prefer a small Satinsky type clamp for the aortic side and a straight Potts ductal clamp for the pulmonary artery side (Tsuji, Redington, and Kay, 1968), although other vascular type clamps may be used. The Satinsky clamp is placed around the ductus and against the aortic wall at right angles to where the ductus leaves the aorta, and it is gently and slowly closed. After the turbulent blood flow in the aorta is reduced, the grip of the forceps is tightened to ensure a good grasp of the tissues without crushing them. The Potts clamp is applied to the ductus on the pulmonary artery side, placing it as close as possible to the main pulmonary artery and its left branch without grasping the right pulmonary artery. The ductus is transected with a scalpel midway between the clamps. If insufficient tissue to suture either side of the ductus is available at this time, another clamp is placed behind the first clamp, which is then released.

The ductal stump on the pulmonary artery side is closed first so that all unnecessary instruments are removed from the surgical site. This permits an unobstructed view of the aortic ductal stump, which is potentially more difficult to close because of the higher blood pressure in the aorta and because of the degenerative changes that have developed in the arterial wall. Therefore, as little manip-

---

arteriosus. The aorta (A) is seen to bulge around the junction with the ductus. The main pulmonary artery is also widely dilated. The junction of the ductus with the main pulmonary artery is seen to be at the origin of the left pulmonary artery just cranial to the bifurcation of the pulmonary artery. In this particular case, the pulmonary arteries appear as thick as the other arteries because severe pulmonary hypertension was present.

B, Thorough dissection of the operative site for patent ductus arteriosus. This dog was dissected at necropsy for clearer demonstration of the important structures involved in closure of a patent ductus arteriosus. The descending aorta (DA) is seen to be dilated from the area of the patent ductus arteriosus (PDA) distally. The bulging main pulmonary artery (MPA) has been exposed by removing the pericardium. The patent ductus arteriosus can be seen between the aorta and the main pulmonary artery. The left recurrent laryngeal nerve (LRL) is seen at the caudal aspect of the patent ductus arteriosus and branches medially from the vagus nerve (V). The phrenic nerve (P) and the left ventricle (LV) are seen in the ventral half of the picture. The phrenic nerve is used only as an identifying landmark, but the left ventricle is exposed so that the heart's action can be observed during surgery.

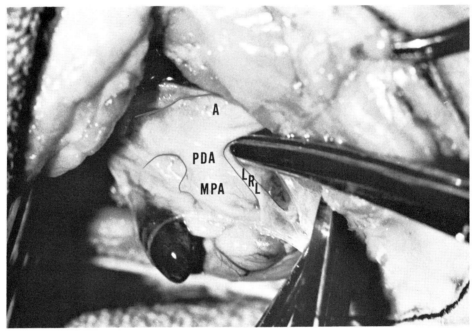

FIGURE 19-10 Medial dissection of a patent ductus arteriosus. The aorta (A), main pulmonary artery (MPA), and patent ductus arteriosus (PDA) have been dissected laterally, yielding good visualization of the structures. Medial dissection of the patent ductus arteriosus is started at the caudal aspect of the ductus where the left recurrent laryngeal nerve (LRL) courses.

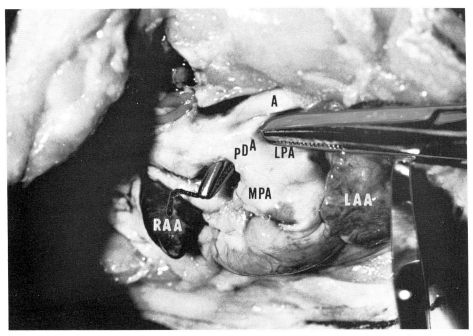

FIGURE 19-11 Thorough dissection of a patent ductus arteriosus, demonstrating placement of the first suture. A dog at postmortem with a patent ductus arteriosus. The pericardium has been removed to demonstrate the anatomic relationships and placement of the first suture. This can be a troublesome part of the surgical procedure. The dissection must be gentle to avoid tearing the right pulmonary artery. The aorta (A), patent ductus arteriosus (PDA), main pulmonary artery (MPA), and left pulmonary artery (LPA) are shown. The right and left auricular appendages (RAA and LAA) are seen cranially and caudally.

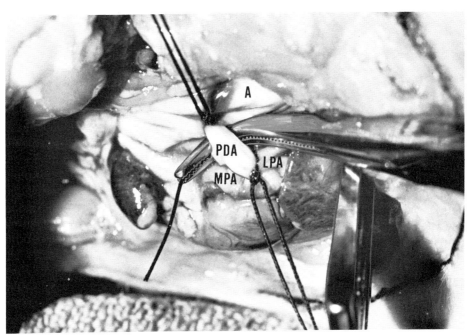

FIGURE 19-12 Ligation of the patent ductus arteriosus. This view, demonstrating the ligation technique for a patent ductus arteriosus, shows a collapsed aorta (A), main pulmonary artery (MPA), and left pulmonary artery (LPA) because it is a postmortem specimen. Large silk ligatures, size 0 to 1, are used to prevent the suture from cutting the ductal tissue. The sutures are placed at the junctions of the ductus (PDA) with the aorta and main pulmonary artery.

ulation of the vascular clamp as possible is recommended. The ductal stumps are then closed using moistened or oiled 5-0 silk or other nonabsorbable cardiovascular suture. Using a simple continuous pattern, a row of sutures is placed in the tissue in front of the clamps, and the ends of the sutures are tied and then tagged with small hemostatic forceps. The suture pattern is then repeated over the first layer of continuous suture, starting at the opposite end of the ductal stump and oversewing in a similar pattern so that a criss-cross pattern over the end of the stump results.

The vascular forceps is gently released, and if hemorrhage occurs the forceps is replaced for 3 to 5 minutes to allow formation of a clot, after which the vascular forceps is again released. The tagged suture ends are used to guide replacement of the vascular forceps should bleeding occur. If no bleeding occurs, the vascular forceps is removed, and the suture tags are cut (Fig. 19-13). If slight seepage persists, digital pressure is applied to the area for several minutes. If all conservative efforts to control seepage fail, the vascular clamp is again secured to the stump, and a simple interrupted suture is placed through the area of hemorrhage.

If severe hemorrhage occurs during surgery, first try to control all bleeding with digital pressure, at least until a plan to control more serious hemorrhage is developed. Have sufficient quantities of fluid and whole blood available for rapid transfusion. If massive bleeding should occur, be prepared to place clamps around the aorta cranial and caudal to the ductus to enable rapid localization and clamping of the troublesome area.

Upon closure of the ductus, the heart rate immediately slows, and the rhythm

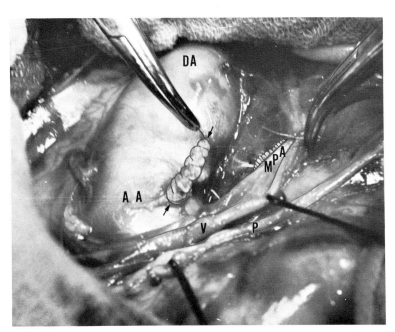

FIGURE 19-13 Appearance of the aorta and pulmonary artery after closure of a patent ductus arteriosus by division and suturing. In this 5 year old dog with patent ductus arteriosus, the ductus was closed by division and suturing with size 4-0 silk. The aortic arch (AA) and descending aorta (DA) are seen to be widely dilated. The sutured ductal stump on the aortic side (→ ←) is very wide and could not have been ligated successfully. The edge of the main pulmonary artery (MPA) and its sutured stump can be seen. The vagus (V) and phrenic (P) nerves are being retracted with silk sutures.

is regular. Digital palpation of the pulmonary artery suggests that the pressure is reduced, that the vessel is less distended, and that the thrill is absent.

Postoperatively, the dog's activity is restricted. No excitement is permitted, and cage rest with limited exercise is enforced for 5 to 10 days, depending upon the type of closure and the surgical difficulties encountered. Penicillin and streptomycin are administered prophylactically for approximately 5 days after surgery. The dog is re-examined at 1 month, 6 months, and 1 year after surgery by auscultation, electrocardiography, and radiography to determine whether the ductus has recanalized and to evaluate cardiovascular and pulmonary function. These follow-up evaluations are of greatest importance in those dogs which had signs of cardiac disease prior to surgery and in those in which serious secondary changes of the major vessels were seen at the time of surgery. These examinations also enable the surgeon to observe the thoracic and cardiovascular changes taking place and indicate what should be expected postoperatively in future cases.

VASCULAR RING ANOMALIES

The surgical approach to the thorax has already been described. When the anomaly is a persistent right aortic arch, the constriction is caused by the same structure that is approached in the operation for patent ductus arteriosus, but the structure is now longer, narrower, less friable, and more accessible, and it is easily identified. The structure in dogs with persistent right aortic arch is sometimes a patent ductus arteriosus, and it is therefore divided using the same precautions taken when closing a major artery.

After the appearance and function of the lungs have been evaluated, the lungs are collapsed and packed off in a caudoventral position using lap pads moistened with warm saline solution. The left vagus and phrenic nerves are identified, and the esophagus is located cranially and caudally from the base of the heart (Fig. 19-14). It is not unusual to find that a persistent left cranial vena cava coexists with a vascular ring anomaly. If it is present, this vessel should be gently freed and retracted ventrally with umbilical tape before major dissection is begun. The mediastinal pleura over the base of the heart is dissected free, starting at the bulging cranial esophagus and working caudally to the normal esophagus. This maneuver is repeated through the fine tissue planes until the area of esophageal constriction is completely visualized (Fig. 19-15).

Using fine, blunt-tipped right-angle forceps, the dissection is continued under the middle of the constricting structure over the esophagus dissecting toward the aorta and then toward the pulmonary artery. Two vascular clamps are placed on the middle third of the structure after it has been dissected free, and the structure is transected between them. Both ends are ligated with size 2-0 silk

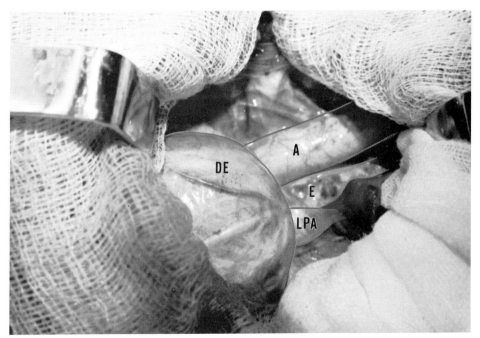

FIGURE 19-14 View of the operative site prior to dissection for correction of a persistent right aortic arch. The thorax has been opened through the fourth intercostal space. The lungs have been collapsed and packed off with lap pads moistened with warm saline solution in a caudoventral direction. This exposure enables clear visualization of the large, dilated esophagus (DE) cranial to the constricted area. The normal esophagus (E) is clearly visualized ventral to the aorta (A). A small portion of the left pulmonary artery (LPA) is seen at the cranioventral border of the normal esophagus. Note the extreme difference in size between the dilated portion of the esophagus and the normal esophagus.

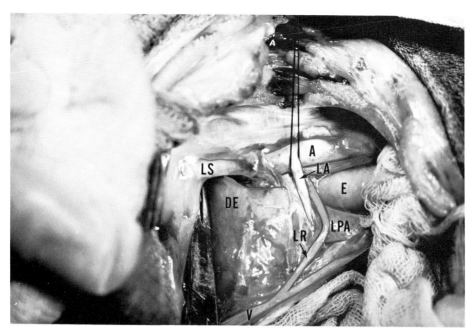

FIGURE 19-15 View of the operative site after dissection and before ligation of the ligamentum arteriosum. The mediastinal pleura and adventitia have been dissected away starting cranially over the dilated portion of the esophagus (DE) and working caudally, exposing the normal esophagus (E). The dilated esophagus (DE) is being retracted cranioventrally with a hemostatic forceps to demonstrate the structures clearly visualized after dissection is completed. The left subclavian artery (LS) and the aorta (A) with the ligamentum arteriosum (LA), the remnant of the ductus arteriosus, come into full view, as does the left pulmonary artery (LPA), to which the ligamentum arteriosum connects. The left vagus nerve (V) with its branching left recurrent laryngeal nerve (LR) is seen to course immediately caudal to the ligamentum arteriosum. Around the ligamentum arteriosum and close to the aorta, the first suture of size 0 silk is ready to be tied. This view also demonstrates the excellent exposure of the dorsal thoracic structures when the thoracic cavity is opened to the angle of the rib by dividing the ventral fibers of the longissimus muscle.

near the junctions with the major vessels, and both ends are transfixed with size 4-0 or 5-0 silk. The major band constricting the esophagus has not been removed, but the surrounding adventitia and mediastinal pleura that remains often prevents the esophagus from dilating fully (Fig. 19-16). These tissues must be dissected away for approximately 2 cm. on either side of the original stricture.

When the dissection has been completed, a small stomach tube is passed into the cervical esophagus, and the esophagus is distended with air. The entire esophagus should now bulge along its entire length, without any areas of restriction by surrounding tissues. The surgical technique is complete at this point except for closure of the thorax. None of the tissues dissected away from the esophagus should be closed, since the esophagus must not be inhibited from maximal dilation in this area (Fig. 19-17).

If other anomalous vessels such as a double aortic arch or a persistent subclavian artery are found to cause the esophageal stricture, the vessel constricting the esophagus must be divided and the esophagus freed in the same way as the persistent right aortic arch. These vessels are patent and should be ligated and

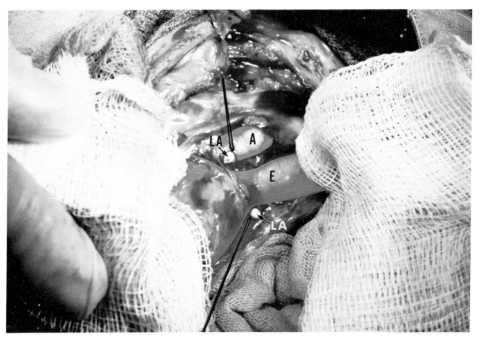

FIGURE 19-16 View of the operative site after the ligamentum arteriosum has been divided. The ligamentum arteriosum (LA) has been ligated with size 0 silk and severed near its junction with the aorta (A) and the pulmonary artery. The ligamentum arteriosum is seen to be patent on the aortic side but not on the pulmonary artery side of the stump. Because this is not an uncommon finding, the ligamentum arteriosum (LA) should be treated as a patent vessel. The stump end was transfixed on the pulmonary artery side and oversewn on the aortic side (A) with a continuous suture pattern using size 5-0 silk. The esophagus has been freed of the major restricting structure, the ligamentum arteriosum, but is not able to dilate fully because of the remaining adventitia at the site of the stricture.

transfixed or oversewn with a continuous suture pattern close to where they branch from their main vessel.

Postoperative care is very important after surgical correction of vascular ring anomalies. The basic goals of postoperative care of dogs with vascular ring anomalies are to stop the vomiting as quickly as possible and to feed a high-protein diet which will enable the dog to regain its strength. The amount and type of care required postoperatively, as well as the length of time that the dog must remain on a special feeding and watering program, is dependent upon both the degree of esophageal dilatation cranial to the constriction and the individual response to different types of feeding programs.

Generally, if the esophageal constriction is corrected early, or if clinical signs are mild and the dog is in good health, the dog should be able to eat and drink normally. Small amounts of food of normal consistency should be fed frequently throughout the day after surgical correction. However, if there is severe pouching of the cranial esophagus and if signs of esophagitis are present, then a regimen of small amounts of a high-protein diet in the form of a gruel fed five or more times daily is recommended. This watery mixture is fed while the dog is held up on its hindlimbs. The position is maintained for 5 to 10 minutes after feeding as well. To ensure that food and fluids do not collect in the cranial esophageal pouches following each feeding, the dog should be rotated back and forth, with his back being

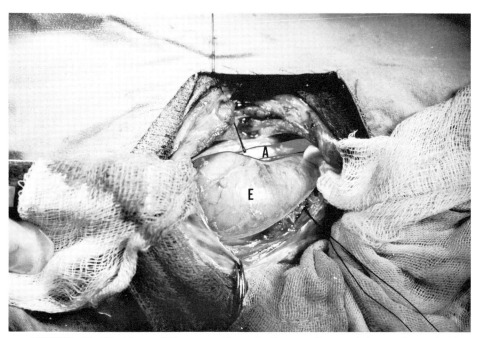

FIGURE 19-17 View of the operative site for persistent right aortic arch after completed dissection of the esophageal constriction. The esophagus (E) has been freed of all tissue restricting full dilation. The connective tissue remaining at the constricted portion of the esophagus has been dissected away. If this step of the surgical procedure is not followed, the clinical signs associated with the disease will persist. The aorta (A) is seen dorsally, coming from behind the esophagus; this demonstrates the developmental malformation of a persistent right aortic arch, in which the aorta forms from the right fourth aortic arch rather than from the normal left fourth aortic arch. The two ligatures on the ligamentum arteriosum are seen to be widely separated. None of the tissues dissected away to expose the esophagus and the ligamentum arteriosum are closed. This area is left open to permit full esophageal dilation and to reduce the chance of any restricting scar tissue developing around the esophagus. The thoracic cavity is now ready for closure.

held at an angle of at least 90° to the floor. If food and fluids are permitted to stagnate in the esophageal pouches, the mixture will ferment and further irritate the already inflamed esophagus. This more demanding postoperative care is gradually decreased as the dog begins to regain its strength and can tolerate eating and drinking without vomiting.

Depending on the dog's response, this type of feeding program must usually be maintained for 3 to 10 days. Dogs with more severe esophageal dilatation must be fed with the forelimbs raised off the floor for a month or more, but this is not common.

To evaluate the progress of the patient postoperatively and to have some indication of the condition of the esophagus, a barium swallow 3 months after surgery is of prognostic value. The cranial esophageal pouches often remain, to some degree, for the remainder of the dog's life (see Fig. 18-18). If the esophagus is severely dilated, the situation may be corrected at the time of surgery by left dorsolateral longitudinal resection or by dorsal wall imbrication of the dilated portion of the esophagus. However, we have found that this is usually unnecessary if the malformation is corrected shortly after clinical signs have become evident and if the postoperative feeding regimen outlined above is adhered to strictly. If the results of surgery are inadequate, the above technique permits the animal to be strengthened prior to the elective second stage operation of esophageal imbrication, resection, or both.

References

Buchanan, J. W.: Symposium: Thoracic surgery in the dog and cat—III. Patent ductus arteriosus and persistent right aortic arch surgery in dogs. J. Small Anim. Pract., 9 (1968):409.

Buchanan, J. W., Soma, L. R., and Patterson, D. F.: Patent ductus arteriosus surgery in small dogs. J. A. V. M. A., 151 (1967):701.

Detweiler, D. K., Botts, R. P., Patterson, D. F., Hubben, K., and Cushmore, J. B.: Heart disease in dogs: Prevalence and diagnosis. Small Anim. Clin., 2 (1962):79.

Kilman, J. W., Sirak, H. D., Clatworthy, H. W., Jr., Cralnen, J., and Hosier, D. M.: The case for early closure of a patent ductus arteriosus. Surgery, 67 (1970):197.

Lawson, D., Penhale, B., and Smith, G.: Persistent right aortic arch in the dog causing oesophageal obstruction. Vet. Rec., 69 (1957):326.

Miller, M. E., Christensen, G. C., and Evans, H. E.: Anatomy of the Dog. W. B. Saunders Co., Philadelphia, 1964.

Patterson, D. F.: Epidemiologic and Genetic Studies of Congenital Heart Disease in the Dog. Circ. Res., 23(1968):171.

Sauer, B. W.: Valve drainage of the pleural cavity of the dog. J. A. V. M. A., 155 (1969): 1997.

Tsuji, H. D., Redington, J. V., and Kay, J. H.: A technique for division of the patent ductus arteriosus. Arch. Surg., 96 (1968):85.

Weipers, W. L., and Lawson, D. D.: Heart and Great Vessels. In Canine Surgery. Edited by J. Archibald. 1st Archibald ed. American Veterinary Publications, Inc., Santa Barbara, California, 1965:421.

INDEX

Note: Page numbers in *italics* refer to illustrations; (t) refers to tables.

Abdomen, palpation of, 9
Abdominal breathing, 7, 447
Abdominal fluid, detection of, 9
Abdominal infection, ascitic fluid analysis in, 10
Abdominal lesions, vs. tricuspid insufficiency, 375
Abdominal organs, in right heart failure, 218
 infarction of, embolism and, 461
 passive congestion of, signs of, 9
Abdominal pain, in right heart failure, 219
Abdominal paracentesis, 263
Aberrant conduction, 290
Accrochage, 290, *291*
Acetazolamide, 255
Addison's disease, heart disease and, 469
 radiographic appearance of, 71
Addisonian crisis, *470*
Adrenal cortical dysfunction, heart disease and, 469
Adrenergic blocking agents, 264, 266
Adrenergic receptor sites, drugs affecting, 263
Air alveologram, 90
Air bronchogram, 90
Aldactazide (spironolactone), 255
Aldactone (spironolactone), 255
Aldosterone-inhibiting agents, 255
Allergic disorders, 266
Alligator clips, *110*
Alpha-adrenergic blocking agents, 266
Aminophylline, 250, 359(t)
Amphetamine, 265
Amplitude, 109
 measurement of, 126
Anatomy, normal cardiac, 47
Anemia, and right heart failure, 218
 heart disease and, 8, 465
 heart sounds in, 10, 15
Anemic heart murmur, 38, 353, *464*
Anesthesia, arrhythmias during, 308
Aneurysm, 458
 aortic, angiocardiographic technique in, 172(t)
Angiocardiogram, normal, 194, *200-202, 204, 205*

Angiocardiography, 189-206
 complications of, 203-206
 contrast media for, 193
  hemodynamic changes due to, 203
 equipment for, *173, 174,* 190-192
 injection sites for, 172(t)
 intravenous, 193-196
 methods of, 190
 non-selective, 190, 193
 opacification time in, 172(t)
 selective, 196-203
  injection sites for, 172(t), 198
 techniques in various disorders, 172(t)
Angiography, 203
Anomalous pulmonary venous drainage, heart sounds in, 19, 37
Antiarrhythmic therapy, 239-248
Antibiotic therapy, in heart failure, 262
Aorta, aneurysm of, 458, *459*
 angiocardiographic techniques in, 172(t)
 ascending, position of, *52*
 atresia of, radiographic findings in, 489(t)
 descending, position of, *50, 55, 59*
 embolism of, 458
 hypoplasia of, radiographic findings in, 489(t)
 pressure in, *188*
Aortic arch, abnormalities of, 82, 495
 branching of, *508*
 double, 498
  development of, *505*
  surgical correction of, 599
 persistent right, 496
  development of, *497*
  dilated, *503-505*
  esophagus in, 582
  radiographic findings in, 488(t)
  surgical correction of, 598-600
 position of, *50, 52,* 53
Aortic arch system, development of, *494*
Aortic body tumor, 417(t), 472
Aortic insufficiency, angiocardiography in, 172(t), 203
 digitalis therapy in, 228

603

Aortic insufficiency (*Continued*)
 heart sounds in, 32, *33*
 left heart failure with, 216
 mitral insufficiency with, heart sounds in, 32
 pulse in, 10
 radiographic signs of, 79(t)
Aortic stenosis, 528-541
 angiocardiography in, 172(t), 199
 congenital, pulse in, 10
  vectorcardiographic findings, *162*
  vs. mitral insufficiency, 356
 heart sounds in, 15, 32, *34*
 left heart failure with, 216
 radiographic findings in, 488(t)
 subvalvular, *534-539*
Aortic thrombosis, 458
 angiocardiographic techniques in, 172(t)
Aortic valve, heart sounds related to, auscultation of, 14
Aortic valvular insufficiency, 376-378
 decrescendo murmur in, *377*
Aorticopulmonary window, radiographic findings in, 489(t)
Apicobasilar line, *52*
Aramine (metaraminol), 265
Arrhythmia(s), 269-309
 classification of, 276
 conduction disturbances in, 272(t)
 congenital, deafness and, 573
 digitalis in, 225-238
 digitalis-induced, 232, 238
  adrenergic blocking agents in, 266
  treatment of, 243
 due to cardiac catheterization, 182
 incidence in dogs, 271(t)
 isoproterenol in, 265
 myocardial irritability and, 386
 pulse in, 10
 rhythmic, 25
 sinus, 273, *274*
 supraventricular, *346*
 therapy for, 239-248. See also *Antiarrhythmic therapy.*
 ventricular, lidocaine in, 244
Arterial hypertension, 457
Arteriosclerosis, mitral valvular fibrosis and, 359
Arteriotomy, pulmonary, 435
Arteriovenous fistula, 456. See also *Patent ductus arteriosus.*
 and right heart failure, 218
Artery(ies), pruning of, in heartworm disease, 426, 433
Artifacts, in electrocardiography, 153
A/S ratio, 535
Ascites, 9
 evaluation of, 219
 fluid analysis, 9
 in congestive heart failure, 219
 in heartworm disease, 423
 in right heart failure, 218, 219
 low sodium diets in, 260
 radiographic appearance of, 93
Asthma, bronchial, vs. cor pulmonale, 450, 451(t)

Asthma (*Continued*)
 cardiac, 217
  xanthines for, 250
Atrial activation, 126
Atrial beat, 276
Atrial fibrillation, 292-299, *330, 389*
 beta-adrenergic blocking agents in, 267
 conversion by drug therapy, *298*
 digitalis therapy in, 228
 electrocardiographic signs in, *349*
 electroshock in, 246
 heart rate in, 25, *26*
 heart sounds in, 15
 in idiopathic cardiomyopathy, 392, *393*
 paroxysmal, *297*
 patent ductus arteriosus and, *481*
 pulse deficit with, 10
 quinidine for, 240
 with ventricular premature contractions, *294*
Atrial flutter, 299
 artifactual, *158*
 cardioversion in, 247
 digitalis in, 229
Atrial junctional tachycardia, paroxysmal, digitalis in, 229
Atrial premature contraction, 276-279
 associated disease states, 282
Atrial septal defect, 541-543
 angiocardiography in, 172(t), 198, 199
 heart sounds in, 19, 37
 radiographic findings in, 76(t), 79(t), 488(t), 542
Atrial tachycardia, 265, 283, *285*
 paroxysmal, *346*
  methoxamine in, 265
Atrioventricular block, 301, 303-308
 accrochage and synchrony with, 290
 atrial tachycardia and, 284
 atropine for, 263
 in digitalis intoxication, 232
 vs. atrioventricular dissociation, 289
Atrioventricular dissociation, 287, *290, 391*
 in digitalis intoxication, 232
 incomplete, beats in, 288
Atrioventricular groove, *52*
Atrioventricular junctional rhythm, due to adrenal cortical hypofunction, *470*
 in digitalis intoxication, 232
Atrioventricular junctional tachycardia, paroxysmal, digitalis in, 229
Atrioventricular nodal beat, 276. See *Junctional beat.*
Atrioventricular node, 124, *125*
Atrium, enlargement of, atrial fibrillation and, 294
 bilateral, 135, *136-137*
  electrocardiographic findings in, 134
 splitting of, 361-366
 tear of, *362*
 tumors of, 471
  angiocardiography in, 198
Augmented limb leads, 117
Auscultation, of heart sounds, 12-14
Atropine, in cardiac disease, 263
A-V node. See *Atrioventricular node.*
Axis, electrocardiographic, 107
Azygos vein, *60*

Backward heart failure, 216
Bacterial endocarditis, 378
  embolism and, 461
Bailey six-axis reference system, *119*
B-B shot pulse, 327, 480
  in patent ductus arteriosus, 10
  pulse pressure and, *490*
Belladonna alkaloids, 263
Benzhydroflumethiazide (Benuron), 253
Benzothiadiazide diuretics, 252
Beta-adrenergic blocking agents, 266
Bicarotid trunk, 508, 509
Bigeminy, 282
Biplane x-ray unit, *191*
Bipolar leads, 115
Biventricular failure, vs. tricuspid insufficiency,
  375
Biventricular hypertrophy, electrocardiographic
    findings in, 143, *148*
  vectorcardiographic findings in, *166*
Blocking agents, adrenergic, 264, 266
Blood, clotting, in cardiac catheterization, 182
  density and viscosity of, and heart murmurs, 27
  oxygen content of, determination of, 172(t)
    in patent ductus arteriosus, 491
  pH determinations, 207
Blood gas analysis, 207
Blood pressure, adrenergics and, 266
  amphetamines and, 265
  central venous, with pericardial effusion, 406
  intracardiac, measurements of, 172(t), 183
    in congestive heart failure, 216
    normal values for, 184-188, 186(t)
  methoxamine and, 265
  normal values for, 186(t)
Body planes, *121*
Body-section technique, 99
Body surface area, determination of, 210
Body temperature. See *Temperature.*
Brachial veins, position of, *55*
Brachiocephalic artery, position of, *50, 52, 59*
Bradycardia, 126, 306
  syncope and, atropine in, 263
Branham test, 456
Breathing, abdominal, 7, 447
Bronchial asthma, vs. cor pulmonale, 450, 451(t)
Bronchial bifurcation, *52*
Bronchitis, chronic, vs. tracheal collapse, 446
  cor pulmonale and, *448*
Bronchodilators, 359
Bronchogram, 90
Bronchopneumonia, cough in, 7
Bronchoscopy, in tracheal collapse, 445
Bronchography, 442-445
Bundle branch block, electrocardiographic
    findings in, 149, *151*
  heart sounds in, 15, *17*
Bundle of His, 124
  blocking of, 149

Cachexia, cardiac, 220
Cannon "a" waves, 219, 291
Caparsolate (thiacetarsamide sodium), 436, 437

Capture beat, 288, 347
Carbon dioxide, as contrast medium, 193
Carbonic anhydrase inhibitors, 255
Cardiac apex. See *Heart, apex of.*
Cardiac arrest, adrenergics in, 265
Cardiac arrhythmias, 269-309. See also *Arrhythmias.*
Cardiac asthma, 217, 250
Cardiac border, 53
Cardiac catheterization, 170-188
  anesthesia for, 178
  blood oxygen and pH determinations in, 207
  catheters for, *177*, 181(t)
  complications of, 182
  entry sites for, *179*
  instruments for, *176*
  laboratory equipment for, 171, *173*
  left heart, 182
  methods of, 178
  monitoring and recording devices for, *173, 174*
  retrograde, and angiocardiography, 197
  uses of, 171, 172. See also under specific
    anomalies.
Cardiac conduction, aberrant, 290
  disturbances in, 272(t), 301-308
Cardiac conduction system, 124, *125*
Cardiac contraction(s), auscultation of, 10
  premature, *27*. See also *Premature cardiac
    contractions.*
  synchronous with diaphragm contractions, 461,
    462
Cardiac cough, 7. See *Cough, cardiac.*
Cardiac decompensation, acute, aggravating and
  precipitating factors, 220
Cardiac dilatation, *84*
  biventricular, 392
Cardiac disease. See *Heart disease.*
Cardiac glycosides, 225-238
  dosage rates, 231
  metabolism of, 230
  sources of, 226
Cardiac hypertrophy, 83
Cardiac index, 209
Cardiac mensuration, 63
Cardiac murmur, 27-39. See also *Heart mur-
  mur(s).*
Cardiac muscle fiber, electrical stimulation of,
  104
Cardiac output, decreased. See also *Congestive
    heart failure.*
  sodium and water retention in, 250
  determination of, 209
    Fick method, 170
    special equipment for, 174
  diminished, and cyanosis, 8
  epinephrine and, 265
  inadequate, 215
  increased, in heart failure, 227
    pulmonary overcirculation in, 88
Cardiac pacemaker, 272, *274*
Cardiac puncture, direct, in cardiac catheterization, 178
Cardiac ratio, 63
Cardiac reflex pressor effects, 266
Cardiac resuscitation, norepinephrine in, 264

Cardiac silhouette, dorsoventral view, 54-58
 in congenital heart disease, 488(t)
 in left ventricular hypertrophy, 77
 lateral view, 49-54
 measurement of, 65, 68
 normal, 46-61
 size of, 84
 with pericardial effusion, 405
Cardiac tamponade, and right heart failure, 218
 in pericardial effusion, 450
Cardiac tomography, 99
Cardiac vector, 107, 108
Cardiogenic shock, 216
Cardiohemic system, 15
Cardioinhibition, 227
Cardiomegaly. See Heart, enlargement of.
Cardiomyopathy(ies), 383, 385-391. See also
 Myocardial disease.
 idiopathic, 392-400
 left heart failure with, 216
 mitral insufficiency due to, 353
 vs. cor pulmonale, 451(t)
Cardiophrenic ligament, 55, 55
Cardiothoracic ratio, 65
Cardiovascular clinic examination report, 4, 5
Cardiovascular disease, clinical approach to, 314
Cardiovascular surgery, 579
Cardiovascular system, radiographic examina-
 tion of, 40-101
 turbulence in, 27
Cardioversion, 246, 298-299, 349
 in ventricular tachycardia, 292
Caricide (diethylcarbamazine), 437
Carotid body tumor, 473
Carotid sinus reflex, hyperactive, atropine in, 263
Catecholamines, 264
Catheter(s), for cardiac catheterization, 177,
 181(t)
Caudal waist, in left ventricular hypertrophy, 77
Central venous pressure, with pericardial effusion, 406
Chemodectoma, 472
Chlorthiazide (Diuril), 253
Chordae tendineae, rupture of, 353, 366-371,
 367, 369
Chronic mitral valvular fibrosis, 141, 322-361
 atrial fibrillation in, 297
 atrial premature contractions in, 278, 282
 clinical course of, 326
 clinical signs of, 322
 electrocardiographic findings in, 135, 344-350,
  345, 350, 354, 391
 etiology of, 360
 heart failure and, 304
 heart sounds in, 10, 327
 incidence of, 322
 laboratory findings in, 351
 mucous membranes in, 8
 pathologic findings in, 358
 phases of, clinical and radiographic description, 324-325(t)
 physical signs of, 326
 radiographic findings in, 331, 356
 treatment of, 357
 vectorcardiographic findings in, 351, 352

Cinchonism, 242
Cineangiographic unit, 173
Circulation time, 210
Circulatory system, transfusion overloading of,
 220
Click, systolic, 15, 17
Clinical examination, in cardiac disease, 1-11
 report of, 4, 5
Clotting, in cardiac catheterization, 182
CMVF (chronic mitral valvular fibrosis), 322-361
Codeine, for acute congestive heart failure, 261
Collapsed trachea, 439-447. See Tracheal
 collapse.
Compensatory pause, 276, 277
 ventricular premature contractions and, 280
Complications, of angiocardiography, 203
 of cardiac catheterization, 182
Concentric hypertrophy, 84
Conduction, cardiac, aberrant, 290
 disturbances in, 272(t), 301-308
Conduction system, cardiac, 124, 125
Congenital aortic stenosis, pulse in, 10
 vectorcardiographic findings in, 162
 vs. mitral insufficiency, 356
Congenital heart defects, and right heart failure,
 218. See also specific defects.
Congenital heart disease, 477-578
 classification of, 313
 cyanosis in, 8
 incidence of, 318, 319(t)
 roentgen analysis of, 488(t), 489(t)
Congenital subaortic stenosis, 142
Congestive heart disease, digitalis in, 225-238
 pulmonary sounds in, 11
Congestive heart failure, 215
 ascites with, 9
 bilateral, 503
 chronic, malnutrition in, 220
 digitalis therapy in, 228
 digitalization in, 235
 due to mitral insufficiency, vs. heartworm
  disease, 434(t)
 low sodium diets in, 260
 mitral valvular fibrosis and, 304, 391
 mitral valvular insufficiency and, 322
 narcotics in, 261
 ophthalmologic signs in, 11
 oxygen therapy in, 262
 phlebotomy in, 262
 precipitating and aggravating factors in, 220
 pulmonary edema and, digitalization in, 235
 pulse in, 10
 radiographic findings in, 82, 83(t), 342
 sodium as precipitating factor in, 6
 sodium retention in, 258
 supraventricular tachycardia and, 287
 ventricular tachycardia in, 291
 with pulmonary edema, differentiation of, 353
  radiography in, 88
 xanthines in, 25
Contractility, cardiac, digitalis and, 227
Contraction, cardiac. See Cardiac contraction
 and Premature cardiac contractions.
Contrast media, angiocardiographic, 193
Conus arteriosus, position of, 50, 51, 59

Convallotoxin, 226
Cor pulmonale, 421-455
    and right heart failure, 218
    differential diagnosis of, radiographic, 451(t)
    due to bronchitis, *448*
    due to heartworm disease, differential diagnosis of, 434(t)
    due to primary lung disease, 447-452
    due to tracheal collapse, 439-447. See also *Tracheal collapse.*
    etiology of, 421
    radiographic signs in, 76(t)
Coronary arteriosclerosis, mitral valvular fibrosis and, 359
Coronary artery, anomalies, radiographic findings in, 489(t)
    disease, left heart failure with, 216
    single, 574
Coronary embolism, 400
Cough, cardiac, 7
        xanthines for, 250
    causes of, differentiation of, 7
    in heartworm disease, 423
    in left heart failure, 216
    in mitral valvular fibrosis, 323
    in tracheal collapse, 439
    narcotics for, 261
    nocturnal, 7, 323
    noncardiac, 6
    paroxysmal, 217
Cournand catheter, *177,* 181(t)
Coving, 102
Cranial waist, 53
    in enlarged right atrium, 76
Crescendo-decrescendo murmur, *514*
    in aortic stenosis, 32
    in pulmonic stenosis, 32
Cushing's syndrome, heart disease and, 468
Cyanosis, 218
    in congenital heart disease, 8
        and radiographic differentiation, 488(t), 489(t)

Deafness, congenital, arrhythmias and, 573
Death, sudden, in Doberman Pinschers, 457
Decrescendo murmur, *377*
Defibrillation, 300
Dehydration, in heartworm disease, 423
Deslanoside, 230
Diamond-shaped heart murmur, 32, *34, 35, 328*
    in subaortic stenosis, *530*
Diamox (acetazolamide), 255
Diaphragm, contractions of, simultaneous with cardiac contractions, 461, *462*
Diaphragmatic hernia, heart sounds with, 10
    peritoneopericardial, 563-569
Diarrhea, due to quinidine intoxication, 242
    in digitalis intoxication, 232, 237
Dibenzyline (phenoxybenzamine), 266
Dicrotic notch, *185*
Diet, and cardiac disease, 6
    therapy, 259-261
Diethylcarbamazine (Caricide), 437

Digilanids, 226
Digitalis, 225-238
    contraindications to, 229
    in atrial fibrillation, 295
    indications for, 228
    intoxication, 229
        atrioventricular block in, 306
        junctional beats in, 282
        lidocaine for, 245
        treatment of, 237
    metabolism of, 230
    pharmacologic activity of, 227
    preparations of, 230
    therapeutic effects of, 231
Digitalization, 231
    electrocardiographic changes in, 232
    in ventricular premature contractions, 282
    rapid parenteral, dosage for, 236(t)
    slow oral, 233
        recommended dosage for, 234(t)
    toxic effects of, 232
Digitoxin, 226, 230
Digoxin, 230
    dosage, 233
    metabolism of, 230
Dihydrocodeinone (Hycodan), 261
Dilantin (diphenylhydantoin), 246
Dilatation, cardiac, *84,* 392
Dipetalonema reconditum, 422
    vs. Dirofilaria immitis, 429
Diphenylhydantoin, 246
Dirofilaria immitis, life cycle of, 438
    vs. Dipetalonema reconditum, 429
Dirofilariasis, 422-439. See also *Heartworm disease.*
Dithiazanine iodide (Dizan), 437
Diuretics, 249-256
Diuril (chlorthiazide), 253(t)
Dizan (dithiazanine iodide), 437
Doberman Pinschers, sudden death in, 457
Double aortic arch, 498
    development of, *505*
    surgical correction of, 499, 599
Dysphagia lusoria, 499
Dyspnea, 7, 323
    abdominal paracentesis in, 263
    cardiac, vs. cor pulmonale, 450
    exertional, 217
    neurogenic, vs. cor pulmonale, 450
    paroxysmal, 217

Eccentric hypertrophy of heart, *84*
Ectopic beats, classification of, 276
    ventricular, second heart sound in, 19
Edecrin (ethacrynic acid), 254
Edema, cardiac, thiazides in, 252
    subcutaneous peripheral, origins of, 8
Einthoven's law, 117
Einthoven three-lead system, 115
Einthoven triangle, 115, *116*
Eisenmenger complex, 489(t), 544
Ejection sounds, 15
Electric shock, precordial, 246

Electrocardiogram, 13
  normal, *16, 128, 129*
    criteria for, 102
Electrocardiography, 102-169
  abnormalities on, 135-148
  artifacts due to errors in recording, 153-158
  baseline in, irregular, 153, *154, 155*
  electrode placement, reversed, 153
  in evaluation of digitalis therapy, 231
  leads in, 115-122
  normal values, 132-133(t)
  panting and shivering and, 153, *154*
  paper for, 113
  positioning in, 109, *111-113*
  60-cycle interference in, 110, *154*
  standardization pulse in, 111
  technical errors in, 153
  techniques of, 109-113
  theories of, 105
  time intervals in, 113
Electrode(s), attachment of, 111-113
  reversed placement of, 153, *157*
Electrophysiology, 103
Embolism, 458
  and infarction of abdominal organs, 461
  coronary, 400
Emphysema, heart sounds in, 15
Endocarditis, 378
  aortic embolism and, 461
  bacterial, 378, 461
Endocardium, congenital fibroelastosis of, 572
  disease of, 321
  rupture of, 361-366, *363*
Environment and cardiac disease, 6, 8
Ephedrine, 265
Epinephrine, 264
Equivalent generator theory, 105
Esidrex (hydrochlorthiazide), 253
Esophageal lead, 120
Esophagram, 98
Esophagus, displacement of, 98
  stricture of, *581, 582*
    vascular ring anomalies and, *498, 500-502*
Ethacrynic acid (Edecrin), 254
Ethylpapaverine hydrochloride, 359(t)
Exertional dyspnea, 217
Expiratory grunt, 447
Exposure factors, radiographic, 41, 47
Exposure time, radiographic, 41
Exudate, pericardial, 403. See also *Pericardial effusion.*

Fainting. See *Syncope.*
Fallot, tetralogy of. See *Tetralogy of Fallot.*
Femoral arteries, palpation of, 10
Femoral pulse, 10
  absence of, 461
  in mitral insufficiency, 327
Fever, heart sounds in, 10
  recurrent, in bacterial endocarditis, 379
Fibrillation. See *Atrial fibrillation* and *Ventricular fibrillation.*
Fibroelastosis, of endocardium, 572
  radiographic findings in, 489(t)

Fick method, 170
Fick principle, 210
First heart sound, 15, *17*
Fistula, arteriovenous, 218, 456
Fluoroscopy, 96
Flutter, atrial, 299. See *Atrial flutter.*
Foramen ovale, patent, 541, 573
  position of, *51*
Forward heart failure, 216
Fourth heart sound, 21, *23, 28, 329*
Functional heart murmur, 38
Functional syncytium of heart muscle, 104
Furosemide (Lasix), 253
Fusion beat, 288, *347*

G-strophanthin, 226
Gallop rhythm, 21-24, *329*
  presystolic, 21
  protodiastolic, 21
    in mitral insufficiency, 29, *31*
  summation, 21, *24*
Galvanometer, 107
Gastrointestinal tract, edema of, and right heart failure, 218
Gitalin, 226
Gitoxin, 226
Globular heart, 489(t)
Glycosides, cardiac, 225-238
Goodale-Lubin catheter, *177,* 181(t)
Great vessels, aneurysm of, 458
  anomalies of, *506-509*
  dilatation of, ejection sounds in, 15
  relative position of, 58-61
Grunt, expiratory, 447

Head, edema of, right heart failure and, 218
  examination of, 9
Heart, aneurysm of, 458
  apex of, 53, 55
    displacement of, 9
    in right ventricular hypertrophy, 73
    on radiographic examination, 48
  auscultation of, 12-14
  axis, length, in left vs. right ventricular hypertrophy, 77
  border of, 53
  catheterization of. See *Cardiac catheterization.*
  chambers of, 58-61
  clinical examination of, 1-11
  conduction disturbances, 272(t), 301-308
  contractility of, digitalis and, 227
  contractions of. See *Cardiac contractions.*
  cranial waist of, 53
  decompensation, 220
  defects, congenital. See *Congenital heart defects.*
  decreased size, 69
  dilatation of, *84,* 392
  electrophysiology of, 103
  enlargement of, 69
    dilatation vs. hypertrophy in, *84*

Heart (*Continued*)
  electrocardiographic findings in, 134-148
    empirical evaluation of, 66
    radiographic evaluation of, 62-69
  globular, 489(t)
  horizontal positioning of, 131
  hypertrophy of, *84*
  innervation of, 125
  left, radiographic anatomy of, *52, 58*
  muscle, electrophysiology of, 103
    functional syncytium of, 104
  normal radiographic anatomy of, 47
  right, *51, 52*
    enlargement of, quantitative evaluation of, 77
  shape of. See *Cardiac silhouette.*
  size of, decrease in, 69, *71*
    increased, in hemorrhagic shock, *466*
  topography of, *50, 58-61*
  tumors of, 471
    and right heart failure, 218
  valvular disease of, 321. See *Valvular heart disease* and specific types.
Heart attack, 400
Heart base tumor, 473
Heart beat, premature, 276. See *Cardiac contractions, premature.*
Heart block, 303
  adrenergics in, 265
  complete, accrochage and synchrony with, 290
    first heart sound in, 15
  diagnosis of, 25
  digitalization and, 232
  due to digitalis intoxication, 229
  first degree, 127
  jugular venous pulsations in, 219
  medical therapy for, 307
Heart disease, acquired, 317
    classification of, 313
  adrenal cortical dysfunction and, 468
  anemia and, 8, 218, 465
  clinical examination in, 1-11
  clinical signs of, 214
  congenital, 477-578. See also *Congenital heart disease.*
  congestive. See *Congestive heart failure.*
  cough in, 7. See also *Cough, cardiac.*
  diagnosis of, radiographic, 40-101
  endocardial, 321
  environmental factors in, 6, 8
  extracardiac signs of, 85-96
  hyperthyroidism and, 464
  incidence in dogs, 313-320
  jaundice in, 8
  low sodium diets in, 257-261
  pharmacologic therapy in, 223-256
  phases of, 215(t)
  polycythemia vera and, 468
  prevalence ratios by age, *315, 316*
  pulmonary circulation in, 85, *86*
  pulse deficit in, 10
  recognition of, 1, 214-223
  renal function and, 249
  symptoms of, 6
  syncope in, 6
  uremia and, 463

Heart failure, body fluid protein concentrations in, 220(t)
  chronic. See *Congestive heart failure.*
  congestive. See *Congestive heart failure.*
  due to mitral insufficiency, heart sounds in, 29
  due to patent ductus arteriosus, 488
  gallop rhythm in, 21, *22*
    summation, *24*
  hemodynamic changes in, 83
  left, 216. See *Left heart failure.*
  radiographic signs of, 82-85, 83(t)
  renal function in, 249
  right. See *Right heart failure.*
  right vs. left, *94, 95*
  sodium retention in, 257
  thoracic fluid accumulation in, clinical signs of, 7
Heart murmur(s), 27-39
  anemic, 38, 353, *464*
  as diagnostic feature, 10
  classification of, 27
  crescendo-decrescendo, *514*
  decrescendo, *377*
  diamond-shaped, 32, *34, 35, 328*
  differentiation of, 353
  due to noncardiac causes, 39
  frequencies of, 12, *13*
  functional, 38
  innocent, 38
  intensity of, 28
  machinery-like, *480*
  pitch of, 29
  systolic vs. diastolic, 29
  timing of, 27
Heart rate, 10, 126
  and congestive heart failure, 220
  and P-R interval, 127
  as diagnostic sign, 8
  decreased, digitalization and, 232
  digitalis and, 227
  disturbances in, 269-309. See *Arrhythmias.*
  electrocardiographic determination of, 113
  in atrial fibrillation, 293
  normal, 102
  vagal tone and, 273, 275
  variability in, 25
Heart sounds, 14-21
  as diagnostic feature, 10
  auscultation of, 10, 12-14
  decreased, 406
  differentiation of, 15
  first, 15
    splitting of, 15, *17*
  fourth, 21, *23, 28.* See also *Gallop rhythms.*
  frequencies of, 12, *13*
  intensity of, variation in, 25, 282
  irregularity of, 10, 25
  muffled, 405
  normal, electrocardiogram of, *16*
  origin of, 14
  second, 19
    splitting of, 19, *20*
  third, 21. See also *Gallop rhythms.*
Heartworm disease, 422-439
  and right heart failure, 218
  angiocardiography in, 172(t), 199, 431, *432*

Heartworm disease (*Continued*)
blood findings in, 430
cardiac catheterization in, 430
cardiac dyspnea in, vs. cor pulmonale, 450, 451(t)
cardiac examination in, 423
clinical signs of, 7
complications of, 436
differential diagnosis of, 434(t)
electrocardiographic findings in, 145, 424
$S_1S_2S_3$ pattern in, 148
heart sounds in, 15, 19, 20, 424
hypertension due to, radiographic appearance of, 86
incidence of, 6, 422
junctional tachycardia in, 286
pathologic changes in, 429, 438
physical findings in, 423
prevention of, 437
pulmonary vascular changes due to, 427
pulmonic insufficiency and, 378
radiographic findings in, 76(t), 425
right ventricular hypertrophy due to, vector-cardiographic findings in, 165
therapy for, 434-437
vascular changes in, 432
vectorcardiography in, 165, 425
vs. cor pulmonale, 451(t)
Heat prostration, 8
vs. cor pulmonale, 450, 451(t)
Hemodynamic studies, cardiac catheterization in, 172(t), 203
Hemopericardium, causes of, 403
endocardial splitting and, 363
Hemorrhage, intra-abdominal, ascitic fluid in, 9
Hemorrhagic shock, 466
Hepatojugular reflex, 372
Hepatomegaly, in right heart failure, 219
radiographic assessment of, 92
Hernia, diaphragmatic, heart sounds with, 10
peritoneopericardial, 366, 563-569
History, in diagnosis of cardiac disease, 3-6
Humidity, and cardiac disease, 221
Hycodan (dihydrocodeinone), 261
Hydrochlorthiazide, 253
Hydrothorax, in diagnosis of heart failure, 92
Hypaque, in angiocardiography, 193
Hyperkalemia, 463
in Addison's disease, 469
Hyperkinetic state, 465
Hypertension, arterial, 457
pulmonary. See *Pulmonary hypertension.*
systemic arterial, left heart failure with, 216
Hyperthyroidism, heart disease and, 464
Hypokalemia, and digitalis intoxication, 229, 237
electrocardiographic changes in, 468, 469
methoxamine in, 265

Idiopathic cardiomyopathy, 387, 392-400
Image intensifier, 173
Infarction, myocardial, 400
Infection, abdominal, ascitic fluid analysis in, 10
and congestive heart failure, 220
Innocent heart murmur, 38

Interfered P wave, 287
Interpolated beat, 276, 277
Intervenous crest, 51
Intracardiac pressure, determination of, 172(t), 183, 355
normal values for, 186(t), 184-188
Ischemic myocardial disease, 383, 400
Isoproterenol, 264
for heart block, 307
Isorhythmic dissociation, 290
Isuprel (isoproterenol), 264, 307

Jaundice, heart disease and, 8
Jet lesions, 359, 360
Jugular venous pulse, 219
prominent, 404
Junctional beat(s), 276, 279
associated disease states, 282
Junctional premature contractions, 279
Junctional tachycardia, 284
digitalis in, 229

Kennel cough, 7
Kidney function, in heart disease, 249
Knott technique, 429
Kyphoscoliosis, 421

Laminagraphy, 99
Lanatosides, 226, 230
Lasix (furosemide), 253
Lead(s), electrocardiographic, 107, 109, 115-122
Left atrial pressure, 187
Left atrial rupture, 362
Left atrium, angiography of, 199
enlargement of, 79
on vectorcardiogram, 162
Left axis deviation, 142
on electrocardiogram, 345
Left bundle branch block, electrocardiographic findings in, 149, 151
Left heart, catheterization of, 182
enlarged, quantitative evaluation of, 82
Left heart failure, 216
causes of, 216
clinical findings in, 217
extracardiac signs of, 83(t)
pathologic findings in, 216
pulmonary edema due to, 91
pulmonary venous pressure in, 216
radiographic signs of, 88, 342
Left ventricular hypertrophy (LVH), 77
associated cardiac conditions, 79(t)
differentiation of, 72
electrocardiographic findings in, 135, 141, 151, 349
QRS complex in, 138
slight, radiographic findings in, 532
T wave in, 143
vectorcardiographic findings in, 160, 162
Left ventricular pressure, 187

Lehman ventriculography catheter, *177*, 181(t)
Levophed (norepinephrine), 264
Lidocaine, as antiarrhythmic agent, 244-246
Liver, cirrhotic, right heart failure and, 218
    function, in right heart failure, 219
    "nutmeg," 218
    palpation of, 9
Liver failure syndrome, 422
Loading principle, 233
Local effect theory, 105
Longus colli muscle, *59*
Low sodium diets, 257-261
Lung(s), overcirculation, *503*
    primary disease of, cor pulmonale due to, 447-452
    vasculature of, 61, 86
    zones of, 62
Lung fields, radiographic examination of, 61
LVH. See *Left ventricular hypertrophy*, 135

McFee orthogonal lead system, *121*
    corrected, 160
Machinery murmur, 480
Malnutrition, in chronic congestive heart failure, 220
Mean electrical axis (MEA), determination of, 122-124, *128*
    deviation of, in right ventricular hypertrophy, 143, *144-147*
Mediastinal pleura, dissection of, *591*
Mephentermine (Wyamine), 265
Meralluride (Mercuhydrin), 252
Mercurial diuretics, 251
Mesothelioma, *413*
Metaraminol (Aramine), 265
Methamphetamine, 265
Methoxamine (Vasoxyl), 265
Microfilariae, chemotherapy for, 436
    identification in blood, 429
Microscopic intramural ventricular myocardial infarction (MIMI), 359
Minute cardiac volume, 209
Mitral incompetence, 569
Mitral insufficiency, *78*, 321
    angiocardiography in, 172(t), 199, 343, 353
    aortic insufficiency with, heart sounds in, 32
    atrial fibrillation in, 295
    cardiac catheterization in, 351
    cardiac dyspnea in, vs. cor pulmonale, 450, 451(t)
    congenital, 569
    congestive heart failure and, vs. heartworm disease, 434(t)
    differential diagnosis of, 353-356
    digitalis therapy in, 228
    due to chronic mitral valvular fibrosis. See *Chronic mitral valvular fibrosis*.
    electrocardiographic findings in, *135*
    etiology of, 321
    functional, in angiocardiography, 203
    heart failure due to, heart sounds in, 29
    heart sounds in, 15, 21, *22*, 29, *30*, *31*
    left heart failure with, 216
    phases of, *332-339*

Mitral insufficiency (*Continued*)
    pulmonary congestion with, *89*
    pulse in, 10
    radiographic findings in, 79(t), 488(t)
    systolic click in, 19
    vectorcardiographic findings in, *162*
    vs. congenital aortic stenosis, 162
    vs. tricuspid insufficiency, 375
Mitral regurgitation, fourth heart sound in, *23*
Mitral stenosis, 378
    heart sounds in, 29
    left heart failure with, 216
Mitral valve, disease of, atrial fibrillation and, 295
    fibrosis of, chronic. See *Chronic mitral valvular fibrosis*.
    heart sounds related to, auscultation of, 14
    location of, *52*
Monitors, for cardiac catheterization, *175*
Monophasic action potential, 104
Morphine, for acute congestive heart failure, 261
Multifocal premature contractions, 281
Multiple premature contractions, 281, *282*
Murmur. See *Heart murmur*.
Myocardial contraction, digitalis and, 227
Myocardial degeneration, 383, 385-391
Myocardial disease, acquired, 283. See also *Cardiomyopathy*.
    atrial fibrillation and, 295
    gallop rhythm in, 21
    heart sounds in, 15
    incidence of, 384
    ischemic, 383, 400
    left heart failure with, 216
    primary, radiographic signs of, 79(t)
Myocardial infarction, 400
    microscopic intramural ventricular, 359
Myocarditis, 383, 385-391
    and right heart failure, 218
    idiopathic, *387*
    left heart failure with, 216
    ventricular tachycardia in, 291, *390*

Narcotics, in acute congestive heart failure, 261
Neck, examination of, 9
Neoplasms, abdominal, vs. tricuspid insufficiency, 375. See also *Tumor*.
    cardiac, 471
        right heart failure and, 218
        vs. cor pulmonale, 451(t)
Neo-Synephrine (Phenylephrine), 265
Nerves, cardiac, 125
Nervous system, and cardiac conduction system, 124
Nodal premature contractions, 279
Nodal tachycardia. See *Junctional tachycardia*.
Norepinephrine, 264
Normal sinus rhythm, 273, *277*
Nutmeg liver, 218

Obesity, heart sounds in, 10, 15, 421
    radiography in, 46, 48

Odman-Ledin catheter, *177*, 181(t)
Opacification time, 172(t)
Ophthalmologic signs, in congestive heart failure, 11
Optical cardiac output system, *174*
Oretic (hydrochlorthiazide), 253
Orthogonal lead systems, 120
Orthopnea, 217, 323
  cardiac cough and, 7
Ostium primum defect, 541
Ostium secundum defect, 541
Ouabain, 226, 230
  dosage, 237
Oxygen, as contrast medium, 193
  blood, determination of, 172(t)
    in patent ductus arteriosus, 491
  dissociation curve, *208*
  therapy, 262

P loop, 160
P mitrale, 135, *135*, *151*, 344, *346*, *349*
  atrial premature contractions in, 278
P pulmonale, 134, *134*, *152*
  in cor pulmonale, 448
  in mitral valvular fibrosis, *345*
P wave, 124, 126
  absence of, 293
  in atrial premature contractions, 276, *278*
  interfered, 287
  negative, *330*
  normal, 102
  notching of, 127, *135*
  prolongation of, 134, *135*
Pacemaker, 272
  electrical, accrochage and synchrony with, 290
  wandering, *274*
Pair of ectopic beats, 282
Pancreas, congestion of, right heart failure and, 218
Panting, during electrocardiography, 153, *154*
Paracentesis, abdominal and thoracic, 263
Parietal block, 138
Paroxysmal atrial tachycardia (PAT), 283, *285*, *346*
Paroxysmal dyspnea, 217
Paroxysmal supraventricular tachycardia, 241
PAT (Paroxysmal atrial tachycardia), 283, *285*
Patent ductus arteriosus, 477-495
  anatomic findings in, *478*
  and right heart failure, 218
  aneurysmal widening of aorta in, 580
  angiocardiography in, 172(t), 199
  aortic arch in, 82
  atrial fibrillation and, 295
    murmur in, *480*, *481*
  blood oxygen saturation in, 491
  cardiac catheterization in, 489-493
  clinical signs of, 480
  development and clinical signs of, 580
  dissection of, *594*, *595*
  electrocardiographic findings in, 483
  heart failure due to, 488
  heart sounds in, 34, *36*, 480
  postmortem specimen, *592*
  pulmonary arteries in, *592*

Patent ductus arteriosus (*Continued*)
  pulmonary hypertension and, *482*, *491*
  pulmonary signs in, *87*
  pulmonic insufficiency and, 378
  pulse in, 10
  radiographic signs in, 76(t), 79(t), 485, *486*, *487*, *492*
  surgical correction of, 583-602
  surgical location of, *591*
  vectorcardiographic findings in, *483*, *485*
  vs. cor pulmonale, 451(t)
Patent foramen ovale, 541, 573
pCO$_2$, determination of, 207
Pentaerythritol tetranitrate, 359(t)
Pentalogy of Fallot, 489(t)
Pericardial effusion, 92, 404-419
  and right heart failure, 218
  aspiration of fluid in, 418
  differential diagnosis of, 404
  electrocardiographic signs in, *473*
  heart sounds in, 10
  radiographic findings in, 97, *407*
  types of, 403
Pericarditis, 403-419
Pericardium, diseases of, 403-420
Peritoneopericardial hernia, 366, 563-569
Persistent left cranial vena cava, 571
Persistent right aortic arch. See under *Aortic arch.*
Persistent subclavian artery, surgical correction of, 599
Pharmacologic therapy, 223-256
Phenoxybenzamine (Dibenzyline), 266
Phentolamine hydrochloride (Regitine), 266
Phenylephrine (Neo-Synephrine), 265
Pheochromocytoma, arterial hypertension due to, 457
Phlebotomy, in acute congestive heart failure, 262
Phonocardiogram, 13
  logarithmic, 13, *18*
Phonocardiography, 12-39
Phrenic nerve, hyperirritability of, 462
Physical examination, 7-11
Pickwickian syndrome, 421
Planigraphy, 99
Pleura, mediastinal, dissection of, in PDA, *591*
Pleural effusion, heart sounds in, 10
  radiographic signs of, 92, *407*
PMI. See *Point of maximum intensity.*
pO$_2$, determination of, 207
Point of maximal intensity (PMI), palpation of, 9, 14
Polycythemia, in tetralogy of Fallot, 554
  mucous membranes in, 8
Pneumonia, vs. cor pulmonale, 451(t)
  vs. heart disease, 353
Pneumopericardium, *409*, *410*
  after hernia repair, *569*
Pneumoperitoneum, *93*
Polycythemia vera, heart disease and, 468
Positioning for radiographic examination, 41-46
Potassium supplementation by food, 252(t)
Potter-Bucky diaphragm, 41
P-R interval, 124, 127
  duration of, 127

P-R interval (*Continued*)
  normal canine, 102
  prolonged, 127, *349*
    first heart sound in, 15
P-R segment, 124, 127
Precordial electric shock, 246
Precordial leads, unipolar, 118
Precordial thrill, 29
  in mitral valvular fibrosis, 326
  in pulmonic stenosis, 32
Premature beats, classification of, 276
  differentiation of, 25
Premature cardiac contractions, atrial, 276-279,
    282, *346*
  ectopic, 25
  first heart sound in, 15
  in mitral valvular fibrosis, *330, 346*
  pulse deficit with, 10
  supraventricular, 276
  ventricular, *346, 387, 389*
Pressure measurements, intracardiac, 183
Pressure overload, 73, 138
Procainamide, as antiarrhythmic agent, 242-243
Proscillaridin A, 226
Pruning of arteries, in heartworm disease, 426,
    433
Pseudopulmonary truncus arteriosus, 573
Pulmonary arterial hypertension, radiographic
    appearance of, *86*
Pulmonary arterial wedge pressure, *186*
Pulmonary arteriotomy, 435
Pulmonary artery(ies), enlargement of, 74
  in patent ductus arteriosus, *592*
  position of, *50, 51, 55, 57, 59, 60*
  radiographic identification of, 53
Pulmonary artery pressure, normal, *185*
Pulmonary artery segment, 74, 75
Pulmonary circulation, and cardiac disease,
    85, *86*, 489(t)
  decreased, 85
  fetal, 478
Pulmonary congestion, in mitral insufficiency, *89*
  radiographic appearance of, *86, 89*
Pulmonary disease, chronic, electrocardiographic
    findings in, *134*
  clinical signs of, 11
Pulmonary edema, 217
  congestive heart failure and, digitalization in,
    235
  due to left heart failure, *91*
  furosemide in, 253
  in rupture of chordae tendineae, 368
  interstitial, 89
  paroxysmal, in mitral valvular fibrosis, 323
  phlebotomy in, 262
  radiographic signs of, 90
Pulmonary hypertension, 88
  in patent ductus arteriosus, 479, 483, 489
    electrocardiogram in, *482, 491*
  radiographic findings in, *86*, 450
  right heart failure and, 218
  second heart sound in, 19
  ventricular septal defect and, 544
Pulmonary overcirculation, 87, 489(t)
  with left-to-right shunt, *503*

Pulmonary undercirculation, 85
Pulmonary vascular obstruction, due to heart-
    worm disease, 422
  radiographic findings in, 489(t)
Pulmonary vasculature, anatomy of, 61
  in heartworm disease, *427*
  radiographic appearance of, *86*
    arterial and venous densities in, 62
Pulmonary vein(s), position of, *52*
  anomalous, radiographic findings in, 489(t)
Pulmonary venous drainage, anomalous, heart
    sounds in, 19, 37
    radiographic findings in, 489(t)
Pulmonary venous pressure, in left heart failure,
    216
Pulmonic insufficiency, heart sounds in, 32
Pulmonic stenosis, 513-528
  and right heart failure, 218
  angiocardiography in, 172(t), 199, 520
  atrial fibrillation and, 295
  cardiac catheterization in, 520
  congenital, electrocardiographic findings in,
    146
    right axis deviation in, *515*
    vectorcardiographic findings in, *163, 164*
  diamond-shaped murmur in, *35*
  electrocardiographic findings in, 516
  heart sounds in, 32, 515
    ejection, 15
    second, 19
  phonocardiogram in, *514*
  pressure gradient in, *522*
  radiographic findings in, 76(t), 488(t), 489(t),
    517, *518-529*
  right ventricular hypertrophy in, *74*
  subvalvular hypertrophy and, *523*
  vectorcardiogram in, *517*
  vs. cor pulmonale, 451(t)
  vs. heartworm disease, 434(t)
  vs. mitral insufficiency, 356
Pulmonic valve, heart sounds related to, auscul-
    tation of, 14
Pulmonic valvular insufficiency, 378
Pulse, B-B shot, 10, 327, 480
  femoral, 10
    absence of, 461
    in mitral insufficiency, 327
  irregular, 10
  "jerky," 10
  normal, 10
  standardization, 111
  thready, 327
  waterhammer, 480
Pulse deficit, 10
  in mitral insufficiency, 327
Pulsus alternans, 10
Purkinje fibers, 124

QRS complex, 124, 127-131
  normal, 102
  prolonged, 138, *151, 152*
QRS loop, 160
Quinidine, in antiarrhythmic therapy, 239-242

R wave, amplitude of, *139*
Radiographic examination, body-section technique, 99
  dorsoventral view, 42, *44, 45,* 54-58
  exposure factors in, 47
  exposure times in, 41
  positoning for, 41-46
  techniques of, 40-46
    special, 96
Radiographs, evaluating standard of, 47
  serial, in angiocardiography, 189
Râles, 90, 217
Regitine (phentolamine hydrochloride), 266
Renal function, in cardiac disease, 249
Resetting of cardiac rhythm, 276, *277*
Respiration, disturbances in, clinical signs of, 7
  effect on vagal tone, 273
Respiratory distress, in left heart failure, 217
  tracheal collapse and, 439
Respiratory sinus arythmia, *274*
  and cardiac rate, 25
Resting transmembrane potential (ERP), 104
Resuscitation, cardiac, norepinephrine in, 264
Retinal venous congestion, in right heart failure, 219
Reynolds' number, 27
Rhythm, cardiac, 10, 102
  disturbances, 269-309. See also *Arrhythmias.*
  gallop, 21-24. See also *Gallop rhythms.*
  epinephrine and, 265
  resetting of, 276, *277*
  trigeminal, *280*
  variations in, 25
Rib cage, angulation of, in heartworm disease, 7
Right atrial pressure, *184*
Right atrium, enlargement of, 75
  angiocardiography in, 198
Right axis deviation, *145*
  in heartworm disease, *425*
  in valvular pulmonic stenosis, *514, 515*
  on electrocardiogram, *345*
Right bundle branch block, electrocardiographic findings in, 149, *152*
  second heart sound in, 19, *20*
  vectorcardiographic findings in, 167
Right heart failure, 218
  abdominal pain in, 218
  causes of, 218
  clinical signs of, 219
  due to mitral valvular insufficiency, 323
  due to pulmonic stenosis and tricuspid insufficiency, *525*
  extracardiac signs of, 83(t)
  hepatic function in, 219
  intractable, abdominal paracentesis in, 263
  pathologic findings in, 218
  radiographic signs of, 90, *93,* 373
Right heart pressure, in heartworm disease, 431(t)
Right ventricular enlargement, tricuspid insufficiency and, 374
Right ventricular hypertrophy (RVH), acquired, vectorcardiographic findings in, *165*
  associated cardiac conditions, 76(t)
  cardiac silhouette in, 73
  differentiation of, 72, 73
  eccentric, *525*

Right ventricular hypertrophy (RVH) (*Continued*)
  electrocardiographic findings in, 143, *145*
  in heartworm disease, *425*
  in pulmonic stenosis, *74,* 517
  radiographic findings in, 73
  right heart failure and, 218
  vectorcardiographic findings in, 160, *163*
Right ventricular outflow tract, position of, *50, 51, 59*
Right ventricular pressure, *184*
Right ventriculotomy, for heartworm disease, 435
RP. See *Resting transmembrane potential.*
Run of ectopic beats, 282, *346*
RVH. See *Right ventricular hypertrophy.*

S waves, 143
S-A node. See *Sinoatrial node.*
Saddle thrombus, *459*
Second heart sound, 19-21
  splitting of, in heartworm disease, 424
Seldinger needle, *177*
Septal defects. See *Atrial septal defect* and *Ventricular septal defect.*
  interventricular, *550-551*
  vs. cor pulmonale, 451(t)
Shivering, during electrocardiography, 153, 154
Shock, alpha-adrenergic blocking agents in, 266
  cardiogenic, 216
  first heart sound in, 15
  hemorrhagic radiographic appearance, 69, *466*
  norepinephrine in, 264
Shunting, 478, 488(t), 489(t)
  causing pulmonary overcirculation, 86, 87
  causing pulmonary undercirculation, 85
  in atrial septal defects, 542
  in ventricular septal defects, 553
Silhouette, cardiac, 46-61. See *Cardiac silhouette.*
Single dipole theory, 105
Sinoatrial arrest, 301, *302*
  atropine for, 263
  due to adrenal cortical hypofunction, *470*
Sinoatrial block, 301
Sinoatrial (S-A) node, 124, *125*
  discharge cycle, of, 272
Sinus arrhythmia, 273
Sinus rhythm, normal, 273
Sinus tachycardia, 283, *285*
  beta-adrenergic blocking agents in, 267
Sinus of Valsalva, position of, *52, 58*
Sodium loading, and congestive heart failure, 6, 220
Sodium retention, in heart failure, 257
Spironolactones, 255
Spleen, rupture of, hemorrhagic shock due to, *466*
Splenomegaly, detection of, 9
  in right heart failure, 219
Splitting, endocardial, *363*
  of first heart sound, 15, *17*
  of second heart sound, 19, *20*
$S_1S_2S_3$ pattern, 143, *148*
S-T segment, 125, 131
  normal, 102

Standardization pulse, 111
Statham pressure transducer, *173*
Stethoscope, types of, 12
Stokes-Adams seizures, adrenergics in, 265
    ventricular tachycardia and, 291
Stroke volume, 210
Subaortic stenosis, congenital, *142*, 528-541
    electrocardiogram in, *530*
    radiographic findings in, *534-539*
Subclavian artery, anomalous, 499
    persistent, surgical correction of, 599
    position of, *50, 52, 59*
    right, abnormal origin of, *508*
Sudden death in Doberman Pinschers, 457
Summation gallops, 21, *24*
Supraventricular arrhythmia, *346*
Supraventricular beat, 276
Supraventricular premature contraction, 276
Supraventricular tachycardia, 283-287
    cardioversion in, 246
    diagnosis of, beta-adrenergic blocking agents
        in, 267
    digitalization for, 235
    due to digitalis intoxication, 229
    paroxysmal, quinidine in, 241
Surgery, arrhythmias during, 308
    cardiovascular, 579
Sympathomimetic drugs, 264
Synchrony, 290, *290*
Syncope, and cardiac disease, 6
    causes of, differentiation of, 6
    in mitral valvular fibrosis, 323
    paroxysmal atrial tachycardia and, 287
Systemic venous pressure, increased, in right
    heart failure, 219
Systolic whoop, *328*

T loop, 160
T wave, 125, 131
    normal canine, 102
T$_a$ wave, 134
Tachycardia(s), 25, 126, 283-301
    atrial, 283. See also *Atrial tachycardia.*
    classification of, 283
    digitalis therapy in, 229
    heart sounds in, 10, 15
    incidence of, 272(t)
    irregular, in idiopathic cardiomyopathy, 393
    junctional, digitalis in, 229
    supraventricular 283-287. See also *Supraven-
        tricular tachycardia.*
    ventricular, 287, *288*. See also *Ventricular
        tachycardia.*
Tachypnea, 323
Tamponade, cardiac, and right heart failure, 218
    and pericardial effusion, 450
Temperature, and cardiac disease, 221
    changes in, 8
Tetralogy of Fallot, 554-563
    and right heart failure, 218
    angiocardiography in, 172(t), 199
    ejection sounds in, 15
    electrocardiographic findings in, *556*
    radiographic findings in, 76(t), 488(t), *557-562*

Tetralogy of Fallot (*Continued*)
    vectorcardiogram in, *556*
    vs. cor pulmonale, 451(t)
Theophylline, 250, 359(t)
Thiacetarsamide sodium (Caparsolate), 436, 437
Thiazides, 252
Third heart sound, 21, *22*
Thoracocentesis, 263
Thoracotomy, incision for, *584*
Thorax, auscultation of, 11
    cross section of, *59, 60*
    deformity of, *48*
    draining, postsurgical, *587*
    examination of, percussion in, 10
    fluid accumulation in, clinical signs of, 7
    measurement of, *65*
    palpation of, 9
    radiographs of, 40
    wall of pulsations of, *462*
Threshold potential (TP), 104
Thrill, 9
Thrombosis, aortic, angiocardiographic tech-
    niques in, 172(t)
    in cardiac catheterization, 182
Thrombus, saddle, *459*
Time, on electrocardiogram, measurement of,
    126
Timing, of heart murmurs, 27
Tomography, cardiac, 99
Tourniquets, in acute congestive heart failure,
    262
Total peripheral resistance, 210
TP (Threshold potential), 104
Trachea, displacement of, 76
Tracheal bifurcation, *52*
Tracheal collapse, 439-447
    cough in, 7
    differential diagnosis of, 446
    radiographic findings in, 440-445
    therapy for, 446
Tracheogram, 445
Tracheal rings, calcification of, *448*
Tracheitis, vs. tracheal collapse, 446
Tracheobronchitis, cough in, 7
Transfusion, and congestive heart failure, 220
Transthoracic puncture, in angiocardiography,
    197
Transudate, pericardial, 404
Tricuspid insufficiency, and right heart failure,
    218
    angiocardiography in, 172(t), 199
    atrial fibrillation in, 295
    differential diagnosis of, 353
    due to tricuspid valvular fibrosis, 371-376
    electrocardiographic findings in, *145*
    heart sounds in, *30*
    murmur of, 353
    radiographic signs in, 76(t)
    vectorcardiographic findings in, *162*
Tricuspid stenosis, angiocardiography in, 198
    atrial septal defect and, radiographic findings
        in, 488(t)
Tricuspid valve, heart sounds related to, auscul-
    tation of, 14
Tricuspid valvular fibrosis, *141*, 371-376
    electrocardiographic findings in, *345*

Tricuspid valvular insufficiency, mitral valvular insufficiency and, 323
Trigeminy, *280, 282*
Trilogy of Fallot, 489(t)
Truncus arteriosus, pseudopulmonary, 573
roentgen findings in, 489(t)
Tumor, atrial, 198
aortic body, 472
cardiac, *413-416,* 471. See also under *Neoplasm.*
vs. cor pulmonale, 451(t)

Underexposure, radiographic, 89
Unifocal premature contractions, 281
Unipolar limb leads, augmented, 117
Uremia, cardiac disease and, 463, *464*

Vagal activity, 273
Vagal tone, heart rate and, 273-275
Valsalva, sinus of. See *Sinus of Valsalva.*
Valvular fibrosis, chronic, myocarditis and, 385
Valvular heart disease, acquired, 321
Valvular insufficiency, acquired causes of, 321
atrioventricular, mucous membranes in, 8
Van Slyke manometric technique, 207
Vascular pressures, normal values, 186(t)
Vascular ring anomalies, 496-513
development and clinical signs, 580
embryology of, 496
esophageal stricture with, *498, 506*
radiographic findings in, 488(t)
surgical correction of, 579-602
Vasoxyl (Methoxamine), 265
VCG. See *Vectorcardiogram.*
Vector, cardiac, 107, *108*
Vectorcardiogram, normal, 160, *161*
Vectorcardiography, 158-169
leads in, 115
Vena cava, caudal, absence of, 572
persistent left cranial, 571
radiographic findings in, 488(t)
position of, *50, 51, 59*
Vena caval syndrome, acute, due to heartworm disease, 423, 430
cranial, angiocardiography in, 198
Venous congestion, in right heart failure, 219
Venous cut-down, in cardiac catheterization, 180
Venous pressure overload, and right heart failure, 218

Ventricular activation, 127, 130
Ventricular beat, 276
Ventricular depolarization, 127, 130
Ventricular fibrillation, 300, *301*
electroshock in, 246
Ventricular premature contractions, 280
first heart sound in, 15
in digitalis intoxication, 232
procainamide in, 243
quinidine for, 240
Ventricular repolarization, 131
Ventricular septal defect, 543-553
and right heart failure, 218
angiocardiography in, 172(t), 199
electrocardiogram in, *545*
heart sounds in, 37
pressure tracings in, *552*
pulse in, 10
radiographic findings in, 76(t), 79(t), 488(t), 489(t), *546-549*
vs. mitral insufficiency, 356
Ventricular tachycardia, 287, *288*
accrochage and synchrony with, 290
beats in, 288
cardioversion in, 246
drug-induced, 291
due to myocarditis, *390*
in digitalis intoxication, 232
jugular venous pulsations in, 219
procainamide in, 243, 244
quinidine for, 240
vs. supraventricular, 290
with capture and fusion, *347*
Ventriculotomy, 435
Volume overload, 73, 83, 138
Vomiting, due to quinidine intoxication, 242
due to vascular ring anomalies, 510
in digitalis intoxication, 232, 237

Wandering pacemaker, *274*
Waterhammer pulse, 10, 327, 480
in patent ductus arteriosus, *490*
Wenckebach phenomenon, 303, *305*
Wheatstone bridge, 183
Whoop, systolic, *328*
Wyamine (mephentermine), 265

Xanthines, 250
X-ray machine, minimal requirements for, 40
X-ray unit, biplane, *191*